ATION

Attention-Deficit Hyperactivity Disorder in Adults and Children

Attention-Deficit Hyperactivity Disorder in Adults and Children

Edited by

Lenard A. Adler
Professor of Psychiatry and Child and Adolescent Psychiatry, Director of the Adult ADHD Program, New York University School of Medicine, NY, USA

Thomas J. Spencer
Associate Professor of Psychiatry, Harvard Medical School and Associate Chief, Clinical and Research in Pediatric Psychopharmacology, Massachusetts General Hospital, Boston, MA, USA

Timothy E. Wilens
Chief of the Division of Child and Adolescent Psychiatry and Director at the Center for Addiction Medicine, Massachusetts General Hospital, Boston, MA, USA

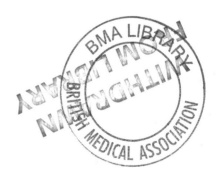

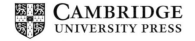

CAMBRIDGE
UNIVERSITY PRESS

CAMBRIDGE
UNIVERSITY PRESS

University Printing House, Cambridge CB2 8BS, United Kingdom

Cambridge University Press is part of the University of Cambridge.

It furthers the University's mission by disseminating knowledge in the pursuit of education, learning and research at the highest international levels of excellence.

www.cambridge.org
Information on this title: www.cambridge.org/9780521113984

© Cambridge University Press 2015

First published 2015

Printed and bound in the United Kingdom by Clays, St Ives plc

A catalog record for this publication is available from the British Library

Library of Congress Cataloging in Publication data
Attention-deficit hyperactivity disorder in adults and children /
edited by Lenard Adler, Thomas J. Spencer, Timothy Wilens.
   p. ; cm.
Includes bibliographical references and index.
ISBN 978-0-521-11398-4 (hardback)
I. Adler, Lenard, editor.   II. Spencer, Thomas J., editor.   III. Wilens,
Timothy E., editor.
[DNLM: 1. Attention Deficit Disorder with Hyperactivity. WS
350.8.A8]
RC394.A85
616.85′89 – dc23   2014012379

ISBN 978-0-521-11398-4 Hardback

....

Every effort has been made in preparing this book to provide accurate and up-to-date information which is in accord with accepted standards and practice at the time of publication. Although case histories are drawn from actual cases, every effort has been made to disguise the identities of the individuals involved. Nevertheless, the authors, editors, and publishers can make no warranties that the information contained herein is totally free from error, not least because clinical standards are constantly changing through research and regulation. The authors, editors, and publishers therefore disclaim all liability for direct or consequential damages resulting from the use of material contained in this book. Readers are strongly advised to pay careful attention to information provided by the manufacturer of any drugs or equipment that they plan to use.

Contents

Contributors

Andrew Adesman, MD
Chief, Developmental and Behavioral Pediatrics, Steven and Alexandra Cohen Children's Medical Center of New York, and Professor of Pediatrics, Hofstra North Shore-LIJ School of Medicine, Hempstead, NY, USA

Lenard A. Adler, MD
Professor of Psychiatry and Child and Adolescent Psychiatry, Director of the Adult ADHD Program, New York University School of Medicine, NY, USA

Samuel Alperin, BS
Hofstra North Shore-LIJ School of Medicine at Hofstra University, Hempstead, NY, USA

Kira E. Armstrong, PhD, ABPP-CN
Independent practice, Woburn, MA, USA

L. Eugene Arnold, MD, MEd
Nisonger Center and Department of Psychiatry, Ohio State University, Columbus, OH, USA

Amy F. T. Arnsten, PhD
Department of Neurobiology, Yale University School of Medicine, New Haven, CT, USA

Russell A. Barkley, PhD
Clinical Professor of Psychiatry, Medical University of South Carolina, Charleston, SC, USA

Craig W. Berridge, PhD
Department of Psychology, University of Wisconsin, Madison, WI, USA

Joseph Biederman, MD
Director, Clinical and Research Programs in Pediatric Psychopharmacology and Adult ADHD, Massachusetts General Hospital, and Professor of Psychiatry, Harvard Medical School, MA, USA

F. Xavier Castellanos, MD
Center for Neurodevelopmental Disorders, NYU Child Study Center, NYU Langone Medical Center, New York, and Nathan S. Kline Institute for Psychiatric Research, Orangeburg, NY USA

Barbara J. Coffey, MD, MS
Director, Tics and Tourette's Clinical and Research Program, Division of Tics, OCD and Related Problems, Icahn School of Medicine at Mount Sinai, and Professor, Department of Psychiatry, Research Psychiatrist, Nathan Kline Institute for Psychiatric Research, Mount Sinai Behavioral Science Unit, New York, NY, USA

Alison M. Cohn, BA
Ferkauf Graduate School of Psychology, Yeshiva University, Bronx, NY, USA

C. Keith Conners, PhD
Professor Emeritus, Department of Psychiatry and Behavioral Sciences, Duke University Medical Center, Durham, NC, USA

Joan M. Daughton, MD
Assistant Professor of Psychiatry, University of Nebraska Medical Center, Nebraska Medical Center, Omaha, NE, USA

Stephen V. Faraone, PhD
Departments of Psychiatry and Neuroscience & Physiology, SUNY Upstate Medical University, Syracuse, NY, USA

John Fayyad, MD
Institute for Development, Research, Advocacy and Applied Care (IDRAAC), Department of Psychiatry and Clinical Psychology, St. George Hospital University Medical Center and Faculty of Medicine, Balamand University, Beirut, Lebanon

Lisa G. Hahn, PhD, ABPP-CN
Independent practice, Neuropsychology Associates of New Jersey, Morristown, NJ, USA

Laura Hans, MD, FAAP
Research Scientist, Duke University, Durham, NC, USA

Elizabeth Hurt, PhD
Nisonger Center, Ohio State University, Columbus, OH, USA

Gagan Joshi, MD
Assistant Professor of Psychiatry, Director of Autism Spectrum Disorder Program in Pediatric Psychopharmacology, Massachusetts General Hospital, Harvard Medical School, Boston, MA, USA

Rahil Jummani, MD
Assistant Clinical Professor and Medical Director, NYU Langone Medical Center Child Study Center, Long Island Campus, Lake Success, NY, USA

Jesse M. Jun, BS
NYU Langone Medical Center School of Medicine, New York, NY, USA

Ronald C. Kessler, PhD
Department of Health Care Policy, Harvard Medical School, Boston, MA, USA

Scott Haden Kollins, PhD
Department of Psychiatry and Behavioral Science, Duke University Medical Center, Durham, NC, USA

Kimberly Kovacs, MA
Department of Psychiatry, NYU School of Medicine, NY, USA

Christopher J. Kratochvil MD
Professor of Psychiatry and Pediatrics, Assistant Vice Chancellor for Clinical Research, University of Nebraska Medical Center, Omaha, NE, USA

Beth Krone, PhD
Department of Psychiatry, Icahn School of Medicine at Mount Sinai, and Assistant Professor, Adjunct, Psychology Department, City University of New York, New York, NY, USA

Nicholas Lofthouse, PhD
Private Practice, Columbus, OH, USA

Michael J. Manos, PhD
Head, Center for Pediatric Behavioral Health, Children's Hospital, Cleveland Clinic, Cleveland, OH, USA

Francis Joseph McClernon, PhD
Department of Psychiatry and Behavioral Science, Duke University Medical Center, Durham, NC, USA

Joel E. Morgan, PhD, ABPP-CN
Independent practice, Neuropsychology Associates of New Jersey, Morristown, NJ, USA

Nicholas R. Morrison, BA
Staff in Pediatric Psychopharmacology, Child Psychiatry Service, Massachusetts General Hospital, Boston, MA, USA

Sonali Nanayakkara, MD
Assistant Professor of Clinical Psychiatry, The University of Illinois at Chicago, Chicago, IL, USA

Jeffrey H. Newcorn, MD
Associate Professor Psychiatry and Pediatrics and Director, Division of ADHD and Learning Disorders, Icahn School of Medicine at Mount Sinai, New York, NY, USA

Phillip L. Pearl, MD
William G. Lennox Chair and Professor of Neurology, Harvard Medical School, Boston, MA, USA

Juan D. Pedraza, MD
Assistant Professor Psychiatry, Icahn School of Medicine at Mount Sinai, New York, NY, USA

Guy M. L. Perry
Departments of Psychiatry and Medicine, SUNY Upstate Medical University, Syracuse, NY, USA

Steven R. Pliszka, MD
Professor and Interim Vice Chair, Chief of Division of Child and Adolescent Psychiatry, University of Texas Health Science Center, San Antonio, TX, USA

Jefferson B. Prince, MD
Director of Child Psychiatry Massachusetts General Hospital for Children at North Shore Medical Center, Staff Pediatric Psychopharmacology Clinic, Massachusetts General Hospital, and Instructor in Psychiatry, Harvard Medical School, Boston, MA, USA

J. Russell Ramsay, PhD
Perelman School of Medicine of the University of Pennsylvania, Philadelphia, PA, USA

Anthony L. Rostain, MD, MA
Perelman School of Medicine of the University of
Pennsylvania, Philadelphia, PA, USA

David M. Shaw, BA
Department of Psychiatry, NYU School of Medicine,
NY, USA

Mary V. Solanto, PhD
Adjunct Associate Professor of Psychiatry,
Mount Sinai School of Medicine, New York, NY,
USA

Mark A. Stein PhD, ABPP
Professor of Psychiatry and Behavioral Sciences and
Adjunct Professor of Pediatrics, University of
Washington, Seattle, WA, USA

Jonathan R. Stevens, MD, MPH
Staff in Pediatric Psychopharmacology Unit,
Massachusetts General Hospital; Department of
Child Psychiatry, North Shore Medical Center; and
Instructor in Psychiatry, Harvard Medical School,
Boston, MA, USA

Brigette S. Vaughan, MSN, APRN-BC, NP
University of Nebraska Medical Center, Nebraska
Medical Center, Omaha, NE, USA

Margaret Weiss, MD PhD FRCP (C)
Clinical Professor, University of British Columbia,
and Weiss Clinic for ADHD Care, West Vancouver,
BC, Canada

Roy E. Weiss, MD, PhD, FACP, FACE
Professor, Chairman of Department of Medicine, The
University of Miami Miller School of Medicine,
Miami, FL USA Metabolism, Departments of
Medicine and Pediatrics, University of Chicago,
Chicago, IL, USA

Timothy E. Wilens, MD
Chief, Division of Child and Adolescent Psychiatry,
Director, Center for Addiction Medicine,
Massachusetts General Hospital, Boston, MA, USA

Janet Wozniak, MD
Associate Professor of Psychiatry, Massachusetts
General Hospital, Harvard Medical School, Boston,
MA, USA

Foreword

Over the past two decades, extraordinary work on attention-deficit hyperactivity disorder (ADHD) has changed the way we think and treat this disorder. *Attention-Deficit Hyperactivity Disorder in Adults and Children* is an important work that will help those seeking authoritative information to understand ADHD in a contemporary manner as a serious neurobiological disorder with available, excellent and varied therapeutic options. Far from earlier thoughts that ADHD is a fleeting mild disorder affecting only a small number of boys that remits by adolescence, we now know that ADHD is among the most common neurobehavioral disorders estimated to afflict up to 10% of children and 5% of adults worldwide. We also now know that ADHD is frequently associated with a wide range of other psychiatric, addictive, and cognitive disorders across the lifespan, and carries with it a very substantial personal and societal burden including academic and occupational underachievement, delinquency, motor vehicle safety, and difficulties with personal relationships. New findings on genetic liabilities, emotional dysregulation, and cognitive deficits have also been elucidated. A convergence of findings linking neuropsychological deficits, specific brain anatomy, and specific neurocircuitry are disentangling the neural basis of ADHD and related conditions in a developmentally sensitive manner.

Although historically ADHD was thought to remit by adolescence, well-conducted, long-term controlled follow-up studies have clearly shown the persistence of the disorder and its associated impairments onto adulthood. Research has also established the syndromatic continuity between pediatric and adult ADHD. The recognition of ADHD as a valid disorder in adults has led to the increasing identification and treatment of adults with ADHD. While no textbook can cover every aspect of a complex disorder such as ADHD, *Attention-Deficit Hyperactivity Disorder in Adults and Children* provides a broad depth of coverage of key aspects of this disorder written by a group of accomplished experts in the field. Without any doubt, readers of this book will be better able to understand and appreciate the voluminous new information on ADHD, and by doing so will better the lives of those touched by this disorder.

Sincerely
Joseph Biederman, MD
Director, Clinical and Research Programs in
Pediatric Psychopharmacology and Adult ADHD,
Massachusetts General Hospital;
Professor of Psychiatry, Harvard Medical School

Chapter 1

History of attention-deficit hyperactivity disorder (ADHD)

C. Keith Conners

If we take in our hand any volume…let us ask, Does it contain any abstract reasoning concerning quantity or number? No. Does it contain any experimental reasoning, concerning matter of fact and existence? No. Commit it then to flames: for it can contain nothing but sophistry and illusion.
David Hume [1]

Introduction

Historians recognize that there are many different forms of historical investigation [2]. However, Hume's dictum reminds us that a truly *scientific history* of ADHD has yet to be written; that is, a quantitative account of how various antecedent variables contributed to ADHD as a dependent variable. Consider, for example, the number of peer-reviewed papers using the keywords, "Attention Deficit Hyperactivity Disorder" (Figure 1.1).

The exponential growth in scientific papers shows an approximate doubling in number of references with each half-decade. This beautiful law-like curve calls out for an explanation in quantitative terms. An exact scientist would be inclined to ask, to what extents do various scientific discoveries; modes of thinking; social, political, economic, or other forces act as causes for the remarkable rise in awareness of the concept of ADHD? Some weighted combination of variables might then resolve the persisting controversies of what caused the upsurge of interest in ADHD and how much each component variable contributed to the outcome. However, until such a history is written it will be necessary to opt for Aristotle's advice that, "If you would understand anything, observe its beginning and its development."

There are already several competing views of the history of ADHD. Regarding the basic symptoms

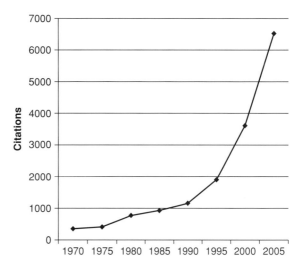

Figure 1.1. The number of citations of ADHD in titles of Ovid Medline citations database. "Attention Deficit Hyperactivity Disorder" was used as a search term for all English and foreign language citations for each 5-year period between 1970 and 2009.

of ADHD, one such recent account by Rafalovich assumes that, "The history of compiling these symptoms into formal diagnoses represents an increasing drive to medicalize unconventional childhood behavior." [3, p. 94]. He rejects both the "child control" explanations for ADHD by Schrag and Divoky [4] and Peter Breggin [5]; as well as Barkley's [6–8] and Kessler's [9] characterization of ADHD as the slow progress towards scientific validity. He finds those different approaches both too brief and "disturbingly ideological" ways of serving their own agendas. Another recent account sees ADHD's hold on scientific interest as the product of a down-and-out struggle between psychoanalysis, social psychiatry, and modern neurosciences, in which the neurological basis of the disorder was a recent outcome of the winner of the struggle [10].

Attention-Deficit Hyperactivity Disorder in Adults and Children, ed. Lenard A. Adler, Thomas J. Spencer and Timothy E. Wilens. Published by Cambridge University Press. © Cambridge University Press 2015.

While there are undoubtedly *some* truths buried in each of those accounts, I will argue that the neurological and scientific basis of ADHD began in the early eighteenth and nineteenth centuries with a particular model of mental illness, the idea that overstimulation causes disinhibited and immoral behavior due to a neurological weakness. This idea was later followed by a paradigm shift in taxonomic thinking about diagnosis which revolutionized how the illness was defined, allowing a union of the older ideas of inattention and overstimulation with recent developments in neuropharmacology and neurosciences.

Our history of ADHD will focus on the various factors leading to and enhancing the growth of the scientific awareness of ADHD in our time, though one cannot ignore the non-scientific outcries against it, since in its own way vocal resistance to the concept also contributes to the notoriety, if not true understanding, of the concept.

Pre-scientific origins of ADHD: *Zeitgeist* and famous men

I believe that the *idea* of ADHD did not begin with the commonly mentioned pioneers given credit for initiating the "medicalization" of the concept, but rather with a deep-seated model of mental illness which dominated eighteenth- and nineteenth-century thinking, and which to a large extent still pervades our own culture. This period formed the *zeitgeist* or background for a particular paradigm of scientific understanding.

"The inscrutable *Zeitgeist*" was Goethe's term that he used in 1827 for "the source of events that occur neither by agreement nor by fiat, but self-determined under the multiplicity of climates of opinion," (quoted from Edwin Boring's classic paper on the *Zeitgeist* and Psychology of Science, in which he contrasts the *Zeitgeist* with the "Great Man Theory" of scientific progress) [11, p. 13]. The history of ADHD has *both* famous men and a *Zeitgeist*, which partially accounts for the steady progress towards today's conception of ADHD. As it usually turns out, the "famous man" chosen by history as the innovator of a turning point merely represents the confluence of ideas already widely current in his or her time.

Palmer and Finger called attention to one such famous man [12], a very early neglected figure who succinctly described in 1798 what is now known as the Inattentive Subtype of ADHD. Sir Alexander Crichton was a Scottish physician widely known in his time for

his treatise on mental illness [13]. With amazing prescience he stated:

> The incapacity of attending with a necessary degree of constancy to any one object, almost always arises from an unnatural or morbid sensibility of the nerves, by which means this faculty is incessantly withdrawn from one impression to another. When born with a person it becomes evident at a very early period of life, and has a very bad effect, inasmuch as it renders him incapable of attending with constancy to any one object of education. But it seldom is in so great a degree as totally to impede all instruction; and what is very fortunate, it is generally diminished with age.... In this disease of attention, if it can with propriety be called so, every impression seems to agitate the person, and gives him or her an unnatural degree of mental restlessness. People walking up and down the room, a slight noise, in the same, the moving of a table, the shutting a door suddenly, a slight excess of heat or cold, too much light or too little light, all destroy constant attention in such patients, inasmuch as it is easily excited by every impression. [p. 272]

Note how Crichton refers to patients with this "disease" – one he obviously was familiar with from his own practice. He was aware that the condition existed in various degrees in otherwise normal individuals, had a deleterious impact on educational attainment, and that it often diminished in severity with age. The "morbid sensibility of the nerves" squarely points to a neurological basis of the disorder.

Crichton's work was in general accord with the thinking of the time, as may be seen in another widely read and respected work of the nineteenth century on mental illness, George Mann Burrows' 1828 *Commentaries on the Causes, Forms, Symptoms and Treatment, Moral and Medical, of Insanity* [14]. He published his commentaries just 30 years after Crichton's treatise, based upon his own clinical experience and a scholarly review of world literature. He was probably well aware of Crichton's treatise in the tightly knit British Royal Society.

> The moderns divide the cause of insanity into moral and physical. Every impression on the sensorium, through the external senses, and every passion in excess, may become a moral cause of insanity. Thus all, however opposite, act as exciting causes, and will produce this result: joy and grief, anger and pain, love and hatred, courage and fear, temperance and ebriety, repletion and inanition, application and indolence may have the same effect. Vices, also, which occasion

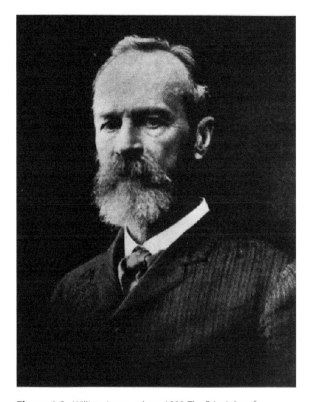

Figure 1.2. William James, whose 1890 *The Principles of Psychology* contained a chapter on attention which is still highly quoted today.

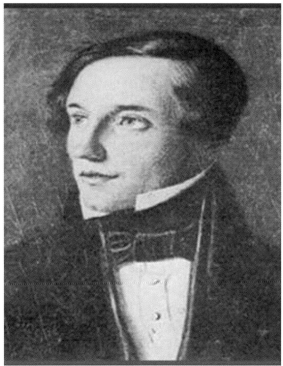

Figure 1.3. Heinrich Hoffman (1845), whose descriptions of "Fidgety Phil" or "Slovenly Peter" popularized the character of a restless, obnoxious, and careless youngster.

changes in the physical constitution, act as remote moral causes, and induce mental derangement. [p. 9]

What today appears as a quaint preoccupation with "moral" causes was in fact a specific theory in which moral behavior depended upon the regulation of stimulation to the brain. Too much stimulation acted to divert action away from correct choices towards immoral, unlawful, or antisocial behavior. *Attention* and its opposite state of *distraction* were the keys for selecting the correct or "moral" choice.

This theme of the centrality of attention in behavior was reinforced in 1890 by William James (Figure 1.2) [15], the most widely known scholarly psychologist of the day.

Every one knows what attention is. It is the taking possession by the mind, in clear and vivid form, of one out of what seem several simultaneously possible objects or trains of thought. Focalizations, concentration, of consciousness are of its essence. It implies withdrawal from some things in order to deal effectively with others, and is a condition which has a real

opposite in the confused, dazed, scatter-brained state which in French is called *distraction*. [p. 403]

Thus, a coherent picture emerged in the nineteenth century in which overstimulation of any kind could produce a picture of misbehavior, due to some fundamental weakness in the nervous system. This idea was widely known in both academic medicine and psychology, as well as among the general public.

The awareness of physicians and the lay public of the impulsive, disruptive behavior pattern was particularly influenced by a German psychiatrist, Heinrich Hoffman (Figure 1.3), whose doggerel verse and charming picture book appeared in 1845, and became very popular throughout Europe. Influences from Hoffman's observations continue even to the current day in art, music, and literature; for example in the movie of Edward Scissorhands, stage plays, commemorative stamps, and new editions in English [16]. Hoffman's book portrays several troublesome children, each teaching a particular moral lesson. "Fidgety Phil," or "Slovenly Peter" as Mark Twain called him from his own translation into English, is an impulsive, naughty

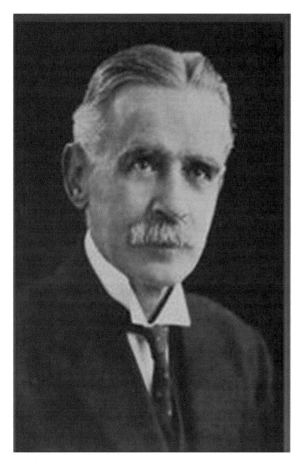

Figure 1.4. Sir George F. Still, British physician generally considered the father of pediatrics, whose Goulstonian lectures are often credited as the beginning of ADHD.

extensive commentary linking many of Still's observations to current interpretations of causes for ADHD.

In keeping with the beliefs of his time, Still argued that the children he studied suffered from a "moral" defect, which meant that their behavior, which was "against the good of all," arose from a defect in focusing of conscious attention towards correct behavioral choices. He alludes to William James' theory of attention as the basis for that force of will, which is required for channeling one's behavior along acceptable societal and educational paths. He included in his list of behavioral characteristics a "passionate" or highly emotional state, lawlessness, spitefulness, cruelty, and dishonesty. (Some might argue that Still should be considered the father of Conduct Disorder, or Oppositional Defiant Disorder, rather than ADHD.) But undeniably he put his finger on some key features of ADHD such as a failure of volitional control or inhibition, and excitable or impulsive behavior in otherwise normal children.

Rafalovich, a historian of sociology of medicine, argues that the nineteenth century's accepted wisdom regarding the nature of mental illness, rather than Still's lectures, was the driving force that is the true progenitor for the ADHD concept [3]. He gives Still credit for realizing that there was a continuum of intelligence extending from the imbecile to normal children, and that there was a deviant behavior pattern that could be observed in the otherwise normal children:

> It is more germane to study medical concepts that were *en vogue* at the time of Still's research: idiocy, and, more significant for Still, imbecility…I argue that Still was the first to link the notion of imbecility to the morality of children, even though he failed to provide an official diagnosis for this childhood behavior. [p. 98]

Rafalovich points out that the idea of moral insanity ("moral imbecility") involving reckless and shameful behavior in children antedated Still's report by several years [p. 102]. His historical analysis treats Still's work as a plea to the medical community rather than a critical medical discovery, with modern accounts by Barkley and Kessler also simply dismissed as a misrepresentation "which distorts the experimental and conceptual history that has given us the legacy of ADHD." [p. 104]. This comment should be seen as an example in which the *Great Man Theory* of history is less preferred than The *Zeitgeist* as an explanatory model for scientific progress. It is in line with the historian Boring, who says what matters is not any particular man,

youngster who typically creates chaos at the dinner table, more from his careless and impulsive acts than merely oppositional or intentional misbehavior.

He is the archetype of the hyperactive bull in the china shop (ironically, commemorative china plates depict him at the dinner table, pulling the table cloth from under the dishes as he grabs it on his way over backwards in his chair). The late psychiatrist Dennis Cantwell suggested that ADHD be called "Hoffman's Disease" after the author who first characterized the syndrome (personal communication).

Much has been written regarding the seminal contribution of George Still (Figure 1.4), whose lectures to the British Royal Society and publication in *The Lancet* of his Goulstonian lectures [1902] are often credited with the first clinical description of ADHD [17].

Key excerpts from these lectures are available in a current journal [18], where Barkley provides an but "the total body of knowledge and opinion available at any time to a person living within a given culture" [11, p. 13].

Rafalovich also argues for the importance of the behavioral picture resulting from the pandemic of *Encephalitis Lethargica* as more relevant to the origins of ADHD than Still's lectures. There can be no argument about the relevance of that great pandemic to the line of investigation which ultimately led to the discovery of the role of stimulant drugs, and the subsequent upsurge of research on ADHD. Regardless of which position one takes on the issue of Still's priority in the development of the ADHD concept, there is little doubt that events shortly *after* his presentation had a major impact on the history of ADHD. Sixteen years after Still's lectures a pandemic of influenza caused a disastrous episode of *Encephalitis Lethargica* or sleeping sickness, known as *von Economo's encephalitis* [19], in which 20 million people worldwide were estimated to have died from the illness. The disease was complex, with many sequelae and an uncertain course, often re-occurring after long periods of apparent recovery.

A key feature of *Encephalitis Lethargica* was the contrast of the normal personality preceding the illness with the subsequent deranged behavior [20]. However, the disease was complicated by as many as 27 different symptoms [9] and apart from the obvious motor signs, there were personality features that mimicked the cunning antisocial behavior and moral lapses of children without the disease [21]. Because of the complexity of the disease and cases with a long interval between onset and re-occurrence of symptoms, there were bound to be cases of behavior disorder that could be attributed to an unknown earlier episode of encephalitis. Therefore the classic logical error of *post-hoc, ergo propter hoc* ("after this, therefore because of this") was sometimes made. Thus began a period of uncertainty when it was not always clear whether a behavior problem in a child was due to "brain damage" or some other "functional" cause.

Encephalitis and early psychopharmacology

Pasteur's "fortune favors a prepared mind," was never more apt than in Charles Bradley's serendipitous discovery of the role played by stimulants in the treatment of behavior disordered children. Bradley's great uncle, George Bradley, had a daughter severely impaired by *Encephalitis Lethargica,* which caused him to found a

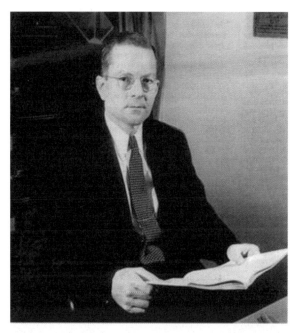

Figure 1.5. Charles Bradley, MD, first medical director of the Emma Pendleton Bradley Hospital for Children.

hospital in Providence, Rhode Island for her care, subsequently known as the Emma Pendleton Bradley Hospital for Children. George Bradley appointed his great nephew Charles as the first medical director of the hospital. Charles Bradley was a psychiatrist fresh out of his residency at New York's famous Bellevue Hospital, where he developed a strong belief in the biological origins of mental illness (Figure 1.5).

In his new role at the Bradley Hospital, Charles was confronted with the common problem of distinguishing the post-encephalitic behavior disorders from those without a known history of infection or brain injury. Using the only available brain imaging technique of the day, he routinely collected pneumo-encephalograms (sometimes known as PEG) on the new cases. This technique requires draining cerebrospinal fluid and replacing it with air in order to allow the structure of the brain to show up more clearly on X-ray. It was introduced in 1919 by the neurosurgeon Walter Dandy at the height of the pandemic of von Economo's encephalitis. Fortunately Bradley had received training in this technique during his residency. Now totally abandoned due to the superior imaging technologies of MRI and CT scans, PEG typically produced severe, painful headaches.

Bradley reasoned that if he could stimulate the choroid plexus surrounding the ventricles he

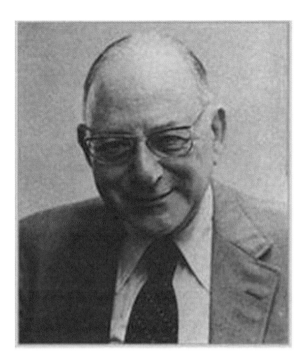

Figure 1.6. Maurice Laufer, second medical director of the Emma Pendleton Bradley Hospital for Children.

studies on children they described as having *Hyperkinetic Impulse Disorder*. What was unique was the creation of a set of formal criteria for selecting the patients for their studies [24–26]. These included:

- Hyperactivity
- Short attention span
- Poor concentration
- Variability in performance
- Impulsiveness
- Inability to delay gratification
- Irritability and explosiveness
- Poor school work.

These criteria anticipated by more than three decades a very similar symptom list in the new *Diagnostic and Statistical Manual* (DSM) in its various revisions. Laufer and colleagues thought of hyperkinesis as the "cardinal" symptom for their new appellation of a *Hyperkinetic Impulse Disorder*.

Laufer and Denhoff were careful to point out that many of these hyperkinetic children were anxious, but not in the sense of neurotic anxiety often seen in the clinic; but rather as a result of their difficulties at school and in relationships with peers. They also were careful to note the difference between poor school work as a part of the syndrome, and more specific learning disorders. Perhaps regrettably, the DSM committee later removed poor school work from their list, as well as the criteria of variability and irritability/explosiveness. (The latter is likely to be reinstated, controversially, in the form of temper dysregulation disorder in DSM-5.)

Also unique in their day was the hypothesis that defective filtering of external stimuli by the diencephalon was responsible for the behavior of the hyperkinetic impulse disorder. Thus, the venerable notion that pervaded nineteenth-century thinking, *excess stimuli flooding the brain* and causing the behavioral and attentional syndrome, reappeared with Bradley and his successors at the Bradley Hospital. They based this idea on their findings from a daring (and now impossibly controversial) experiment, measuring the threshold of photo-stimulation activation of metrazol-induced seizure patterns on the EEG. They reported that this threshold was lower for children with the hyperkinetic impulse disorder. This experiment has never been repeated, and presumably never will, given the risk/reward problem in such an experiment.

could alleviate the headaches. To accomplish this he treated 43 of the children with Benzedrine, the trade name of the racemic mixture of amphetamine (d,l-amphetamine). Bradley was promptly informed by his teachers and staff that about half of the children had suddenly become more calm, organized, and effective in their learning. The children came to view the pills as "math pills" because of their apparent effect in allowing them to do sums that heretofore had been difficult or impossible because of their unfocused and restless behavior. Bradley noted that although the children became subdued, they also remained alert and focused [22]. The results prompted him to continue the treatment and he later published a series of 100 children between ages 5 and 12 years, including 77 boys and 23 girls [23].

Bradley's ultimate influence on the progress towards ADHD went far beyond this introduction of stimulant treatment, for he established a tradition of close observation and experiment at the Bradley Hospital which continued well after he departed. Maurice Laufer, a child psychiatrist, was to become the new medical director of the Bradley Hospital (Figure 1.6).

Laufer and his child neurologist colleague, Eric Denhoff, began a series of experiments and clinical

There is little doubt that the striking clinical effect of the stimulant drugs, which began with Bradley and

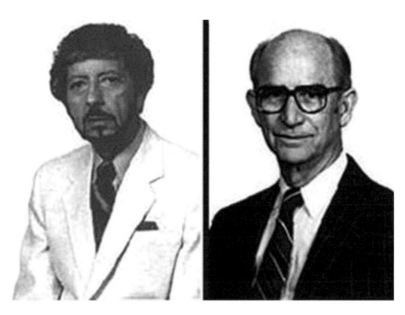

Figure 1.7. Samuel Clements and John Peters, important contributors to the concept of Minimal Brain Dysfunction (MBD).

his colleagues, propelled a movement towards a true period of psychopharmacology with children, as well as the search for a more satisfactory diagnostic framework. The next several decades would see a flourishing of efforts to characterize a specific syndrome or diagnostic entity that is both reliable and valid, and which would eventually allow a true scientific union with genetics, neuroscience, and therapeutic trials.

Minimal brain dysfunction

In 1908, soon after Still's lectures, it was hypothesized by Tredgold that children with disruptive, hyperactive behavior without demonstrable brain damage may have suffered mild injuries during birth, or *minimal brain damage* [27]. The term *"organic drivenness,"* also soon entered the literature, referring to a characteristic behavior pattern in children without verified brain damage or illness [28].

Influential educators then began recognizing the importance of special methods of education for such children [29], coming explicitly to the conclusion that "we are justified in diagnosing on the basis of functional rather than neurological signs." [30, p. 42]. The influential developmental psychologists Gesell and Amatruda (1941), who had enormous impact on child-rearing ideas, stated that "an entirely negative birth history and an uneventful neonatal period may nevertheless demand a diagnosis of minimal injury because of persisting or gradually diminishing behavior signs

[31, p. 231]. Thus, it came to be common practice to accept the behavior pattern alone as evidence of brain damage. Between the 1950s and 1970s there was a growing awareness among pediatricians and public health researchers of the impact of early birth and perinatal problems on later development and behavior [31–35]. The notion of a "continuum of reproductive casualty" gave a more substantive meaning to the idea of a behavior syndrome with brain involvement of a possible subtle or minimal level of damage.

In this atmosphere, Sam Clements and John Peters (Figure 1.7), first coined the term *Minimal Brain Dysfunction* (MBD) [36].

Clements and Peters were part of a remarkable group of physicians, psychologists, and educators at the University of Arkansas, which also included Roscoe Dykman and Peggy Ackerman. This team was responsible for many early clinical and laboratory studies on MBD as well as innovative assessment and educational interventions with learning-disabled and educationally handicapped children. Their early suggestion that *specific learning disability*, along with its associated behavioral characteristics, constituted an *attentional deficit syndrome* had a significant impact on subsequent nomenclature. Although others are often given credit for the re-introduction of attention into the diagnostic discourse of ADHD (such as the classic paper by Virginia Douglas called *Stop, look, and listen*) [37], the Arkansas group was actually the first to provide this insight [38]. In a later 1993 discussion of this point, Dykman and Ackerman point out:

This was the first paper to suggest specifically that MBD be replaced by the label attention deficit syndrome. Many people reading the 1971 paper believed that we were talking only about LD [Learning Disability] children, but in fact most of our studies at that time included children who were hyperactive alone [but typically underachieving in one area or another], LD alone, or both. Our belief was that the majority of children referred to our clinic for academic problems were both hyperactive and LD...Our research is very consistent in supporting the idea that attention problems are common to the majority of LD as well as ADD [Attention Deficit Disorder] children. [39, p. 14]

Peters *et al.* also developed a special neurological examination, a battery of psychological tests, and clear descriptions of the clinical assessment procedures for MBD [40]. Their *Physician's Handbook* [41] was an influential teaching guide for recognizing MBD, which brought the condition to the awareness of a generation of medical students, pediatricians, and psychiatrists.

Neurologists resisted the growing trend of attributing the behavior pattern to brain damage. Shortly after the 1963 Clements and Peters paper appeared, the Oxford International Study Group on Child Neurology decided to adopt Clements' and Peters' term for the behavior pattern as *Minimal Brain Dysfunction* or *MBD*. They elected to retain the notion of *brain damage* only for those cases in which a known disease preceded the pattern and in which classic focal neurological signs could be detected [42].

Responding to a growing need for a consensus on the features of MBD, a Public Health Service committee headed by Clements in 1966 arrived at an official statement:

This term as a diagnostic and descriptive category refers to children of near average, average or above average intellectual capacity with certain learning and/or behavioral disabilities ranging from mild to severe, which are associated with deviations of function of the central nervous system. These deviations may manifest themselves by various combinations of impairment in perception, conceptualization, language, memory and *control of attention, impulse or motor function* [emphasis ours]. These aberrations may arise from genetic variations, biochemical irregularities, perinatal brain insults, or other illnesses or injuries sustained during the years critical for the development of the central nervous system [43].

(Interestingly, the last set of symptoms in this list, "control of attention, impulse or motor function," was the primary concept retained in later formulations of ADHD by DSM-III and DSM-IV. The much broader concept of MBD was winnowed down to subtypes of Hyperactivity/Impulsivity, Inattention, and their combination.)

Wender's 1971 monograph on MBD further elaborated the clinical description and proposed a central mechanism to account for the clinical picture [44]. In this monograph and subsequent articles [45] he advanced the hypothesis that the disorder was genetic in origin, mediated by decreased activity in dopaminergic systems in the brain. This suggestion of a dopaminergic mechanism preceded confirmation of the hypothesis by several decades, when it became possible to image dopamine synaptic markers with positron emission tomography in ADHD adults [46].

Despite a wealth of historical, epidemiological, clinical, and laboratory studies employing the MBD diagnostic concept, it gradually lost favor for a number of reasons. Critics of the concept of a single syndrome, which includes hyperkinesis, learning disabilities, inattention, and minor motor signs, cited several problems. First, there appeared to be no single or "cardinal" symptom that invariably appeared with the syndrome. Even though Donald and Rachel Klein pointed out in 1974 that a syndrome need not be monothetic, but could instead be characterized by a list of several symptoms from which some minimal number always appeared (i.e., a polythetic taxonomic structure) [47], the long list of qualifying symptoms for MBD inevitably led to study samples of widely differing characteristics.

Second, the role of the brain was always inferential; there were at this period very few direct measures of brain structure or integrity specific enough to warrant consideration. As a result, the diagnosis was often circular, the only evidence for the role of the brain being the behavioral symptoms alone. This is tantamount to the joke about the parent who asks why their child cannot read, and is told that they have dyslexia; and then when asked what causes dyslexia, is told, "Inability to read."

Third, much of the behavioral evidence showed that hyperactive or disruptive behavior was situational. For example, that the disturbances might be evident only at school, not at home, or vice versa, resulting in a low correlation between measures taken from teachers and parents. The lack of a criterion of pervasiveness waited for a remedy in the later concept of ADHD.

Fourth, there was an obvious overlap of the proposed symptoms of MBD with other psychiatric disorders. This fatal flaw of the MBD concept was stated by Rutter:

> …the nosological status of the hyperkinetic or attentional deficit syndrome remains quite uncertain and lacking in empirical validation. Much of the difficulty stems from the very pervasiveness of the phenomena. Both epidemiological…and clinical studies…have shown that a high proportion of children with psychiatric disorders of all kinds tend to be restless, fidgety, overactive, inattentive, and lacking in concentration…The available evidence suggests that, in and of themselves, the mere presence of overactivity or poor concentration is of no diagnostic importance. Both symptoms may have many quite different causes. Thus, for example, it is well recognized that high levels of anxiety may lead to restlessness and that depression tends to be accompanied by deficits in concentration. [48, p. 581]

Perhaps the strongest *empirical* indictment of the MBD concept came from the results of the massive perinatal project of the National Institute of Neurological and Communicative Disorders and Stroke (NINCDS) [49]. This project followed over 30 000 children whose mothers were examined from the antenatal period, and whose children were examined from birth to 7 years of age. Symptoms were examined in four major categories: behavior, cognitive/perceptual-motor, academic, and neurological. Factor analyses reduced the number of variables to hyperkinetic-impulsive behavior, learning difficulties, and neurological "soft signs." (A fourth category of social immaturity was to be analyzed later.) No single "MBD factor" was identified, but the three main groups of "MBD" symptoms became the dependent measures for the predictive analyses.

From the pre- and postnatal periods, 331 variables were screened as possible predictors of symptoms of MBD. These included family history, socioeconomic data, maternal characteristics, pregnancy, labor, delivery, speech/language, and hearing tests. Only about 5% of the three main groups were considered suspicious. These were then contrasted with the completely "normal" remainder of the sample, consisting of 12 511 children. Discriminant function analyses searched for independent contributions to the variance.

The only consistent finding across the three symptom groups was maternal smoking and poor prenatal care. Learning difficulties were more related to demographic variables such as large family size, low socioeconomic status, and frequent changes in residence, than to pregnancy, labor, and delivery factors. The family factors appeared to be associated with demographic rather than genetic variables. (The hyperactive–impulsive factor measures at age 4, however, were consistently related to various impairments in learning and behavior at 7 years of age.) But there were few overlaps between this factor and the neurological indices, suggesting that the "brain" part of MBD had little support from the neurological examination.

Paradigm shift: the diagnosis of ADHD

The historian Thomas Kuhn referred to a scientific paradigm as the set of practices that define a scientific discipline at any particular period of time [50]. He included in its meaning *what* is to be observed and scrutinized, the kind of *questions* to be asked, *how* these questions are to be structured, and how the *results* of scientific investigations should be interpreted. By all of these criteria, the diagnosis of ADHD, beginning with the DSM-III, 1980, stands as a revolutionary *paradigm shift* [51, 52]. The major feature of this shift was a change from an etiological model to a descriptive behavioral model of mental illness. DSM-I had designated the hyperkinetic behavior syndrome as a *reaction* disorder in childhood, in keeping with the current psychiatric thinking attributing the behavior to parental and family environment and neurotic conflict. Although the term "reaction" was dropped in the 1968 version, DSM-II, *neurosis* was still included.

Robert Spitzer, the chair of the DSM-III committee, championed a "neo-Kraeplinian" model of descriptive categories, modified to be similar to the Washington University ("Feighner") and Research Diagnostic Criteria developed by workgroups at the Washington University of St. Louis and New York State Psychiatric Institute, respectively. These concepts included criteria regarding the age and course of the illness, response to treatment, associated features, and level of impairment.

There is little doubt that the science of ADHD was markedly enhanced by the shift from an etiological approach embodied in both the nineteenth-century *Zeitgeist* and in the MBD concept. Laufer and

Denhoff's listing of the criteria for the hyperactive–impulsive behavior disorder, and the Clements and Peters list of symptoms for MBD were important transitional influences because they laid out specific symptomatic criteria, but were framed within the classical medical tradition of an etiological model of disease processes. The rather simple hypothesis of a single brain mechanism in the diencephalon, itself a carryover from nineteenth-century ideas of over-stimulation as the source of mental disease, could now be abandoned in favor of a more refined exploration of the many directly measured brain mechanisms involved in ADHD.

However, despite many criticisms of the MBD concept, researchers looking for a brain-based cause of MBD, once new brain imaging tools became available, would eventually return to neurological explanations. This caused Judith Rapaport and Xavier Castellanos to remark:

> Since the publication of DSM-3-R in 1987…a number of anatomical MRI studies…have in fact documented minimal but significant brain anatomical deviations – ironically, minimal brain dysfunction now takes on new meaning! [53, p. 267]

But the explosive growth of the neurosciences in ADHD was only possible by virtue of stricter behavioral guidelines for selecting cases within a new diagnostic framework.

Therapeutics of ADHD: pharmacotherapy and behavior therapy

The new era of pharmacotherapy, initiated by Bradley's serendipitous discovery of the impact of stimulants, along with application of the new diagnostic framework using controlled clinical trials, led to a significant burst in the use of stimulants with ADHD. Meta-analyses of stimulant use over a period of several decades showed a consistent enhancement of behavioral improvement with effect sizes ranging from 0.6 to 0.8 [54, 55]. A recent meta-analysis showed mean effect sizes of 0.77 and 1.03 for methylphenidate and amphetamine, respectively [56]. Significant, but lesser effect sizes occurred for academic as opposed to behavioral targets.

Much had been written during the period of MBD attesting to the importance of behavioral methods of treatment, particularly relating to educational intervention, in mitigating the impact of the MBD syndrome on both academic and behavioral functioning. Safer and Allan gave perhaps the earliest and most comprehensive coverage of the concept of multimodal therapy. As Eisenberg stated in the foreword to their 1976 book,

> There is enough evidence now to support the authors' conclusion that a *combined* "multimodal" coordinated plan of management makes the most sense. Either-or formulations do violence to clinical reality. A significant feature of this book is its skillful synthesis of multiple approaches into a comprehensive plan of care for children very much in need of our help. It is clear to me that the book is a major contribution. [57]

Almost two decades later hundreds of studies attested to the validity of this prescient statement. In 1992 in response to overwhelming evidence that each treatment individually was effective, the National Institute of Mental Health (NIMH) and the US Department of Education sponsored the largest controlled trial of multimodal treatment of ADHD, known as the Multimodal Treatment of ADHD (MTA) Study. Figure 1.8 shows the members of the MTA project. Almost 600 children were treated in six university sites by investigators deemed competent in both pharmacological and behavioral management of ADHD. As Eisenberg predicted, the study was designed to test the idea that the combined treatments would be more effective than either treatment alone.

The rationale, design, subject selection, composition of treatments, and major findings for this large, complex long-term treatment of ADHD have been well described by Jensen *et al.* elsewhere [58]. Suffice it to say, the findings clearly demonstrated the superiority of multimodal therapy, as well as the superiority of the carefully scripted delivery of the drug and behavioral treatments over the usual care found in the community. Long-term follow-up of the initial findings continues to support the value of combined multimodal therapy over single treatment approaches.

Adult ADHD

One of the major factors in the recent upsurge of scientific notice of ADHD has been the rediscovery that adults have ADHD. Despite Crichton's remarkable very early 1798 identification of an ADHD subtype in adults, and Wender's early revival of the concept, the

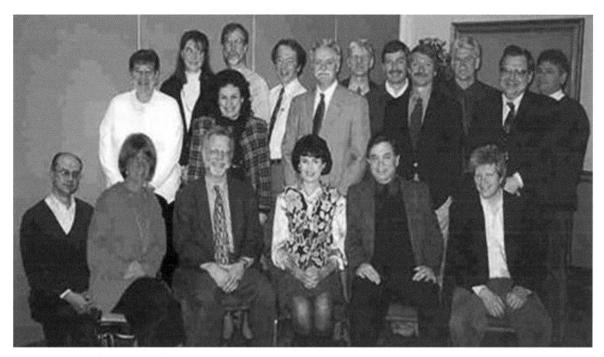

Figure 1.8. The MTA Cooperative Group. From left to right, bottom to top: Ben Vitiello Joanne Severe, Howard Abikoff, Karen Wells, Larry Greenhill, Jeffrey Newcorn, Helen Kraemer, Lily Hechtman, C. Keith Conners, Stephen Hinshaw, Glen Elliott, Betsy Hoza, William Pelham, Peter Jensen, Eugene Arnold, John March, James Swanson, Tim Wigal.

diagnosis and treatment of adults still provokes controversy [59, 60]. Possibly this simply relates to a lag in public perception due to the incorrect belief, long held in the literature, that ADHD is a childhood disorder that disappears in adulthood. That error is probably the result of a tradition in which hyperactivity was considered to be the primary symptom; and indeed, hyperactivity *does* tend to decline with age, but continues to disrupt attention and behavior in the form of *mental* restlessness. In addition, there are several technical problems in making a diagnosis in adults. These have been succinctly noted by Jensen in a book review [61, p. 97]:

(a) Problems with the accuracy of retrospective recall based on adults' reports of their childhood ADHD symptoms;

(b) Variations in severity or comorbidity thresholds leading to differing times to diagnosis;

(c) Socioeconomic and family factors that differ across patients and within patients over time;

(d) Discontinuities in who serve as key informants during the childhood versus adult years;

(e) Substantial differences in the tasks of children with ADHD versus adults with ADHD;

(f) Gradual development and accumulation of positive skills in coping with and/or negative consequence of ADHD, and

(g) Vast differences to which children versus adults with ADHD have control over their selection of environments in which ADHD symptoms may be most manifest.

Despite these barriers, research strongly supports the validity of an adult diagnostic category. This research stems primarily from both long-term follow-up of children diagnosed with ADHD, and cross-sectional studies comparing diagnosed ADHD with normal controls and with other psychiatric conditions [62–64].

Barkley and colleagues chose to bypass peer review in order to present a wealth of data from two extraordinary studies, in a manner that was both readable and cogent. While peer-reviewed detailed monographs or journal articles will undoubtedly follow, there seems little doubt that their work firmly establishes the importance of the adult diagnostic category, albeit with important changes needed to rectify shortcomings of the DSM-IV version, particularly the age of onset and number of criteria needed for diagnosis. Though more complicated by comorbidity and physical status, considerable work also demonstrated the robust effects of stimulant medications for adult ADHD [65–71].

Non-scientific causes of the rise of ADHD

Space does not permit an account of all of the *non-scientific* reasons why ADHD has thrived as a diagnosis and treatment over the past several decades, including the many controversial attacks on the concept and its treatments. However, a recent comprehensive and scholarly account by Rick Mayes and colleagues clearly shows the significant impact of several factors [72]:

1. A confluence of *trends* [clinical, economic, educational, political];
2. An alignment of *incentives* [among clinicians, educators, policy makers, health insurers, the pharmaceutical industry];
3. The growth in *knowledge* about ADHD and stimulants;
4. Decreasing stigma associated with mental disorders. [p. 2]

These factors in turn led to changes in assistance through the Supplemental Security Income Program, lobbying pressures from parents of children with ADHD, and the Individuals with Disabilities Education Act (IDEA), and finally expanded eligibility for reimbursement through Medicaid.

As an example of one of the most significant non-scientific influences, it is instructive to examine the impact of the US Food and Drug Administration (FDA) Modernization Act of 1997 on the growth of new drug treatments for ADHD. This act, which extended the patent exclusivity life for new drugs, immediately prompted investment in research on new medication formulations such as long-acting methylphenidate and amphetamine, molecular alterations of older drugs, new uses for older drugs, and promising drugs that had failed in treatment of other disorders (Figure 1.9).

Note the relatively stable lack of interest in methylphenidate and amphetamine for the 15 years prior to the 1997 Act. Cooperation between drug companies and researchers on ADHD was quite limited until it became possible for the major pharmaceutical companies to recoup the investment required to gain approval of a new drug prior to the 1997 Act and then

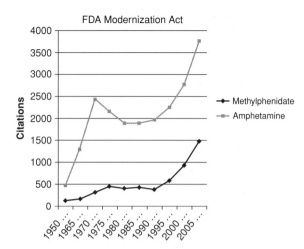

Figure 1.9. Half-decade Medline citations for *methylphenidate* and *amphetamine* as keywords in the Ovid Medline database. Interest in the drugs reached a plateau for several years, prior to the FDA Modernization Act of 1997.

a great burst of activity for the stimulant drug research took place.

Summary and conclusions

What accounts for the remarkable increase in the scientific awareness of ADHD with which we began this brief history? Over the course of several centuries a few intrepid and dedicated clinicians made careful observations on children, eventually leading to a relatively clear understanding of those we now diagnose as having ADHD. These clinicians and scientists began with a simple notion of mental disturbances arising from overstimulation, leading to a disordered behavior pattern in children that appeared incongruous given their intellect and upbringing, and immoral according to the standards of the community. From the beginning they saw a neurological basis for the susceptibility to misguided attention and distraction.

This subtle combination of inattention and disordered behavior was from its beginning assumed to be due to either an illness affecting the brain or unknown constitutional factors. But it took "thinking outside of the box," a shift to a new biomedical paradigm, away from an *etiological* paradigm to a *behavioral* paradigm, before advances could be made in casting the diagnosis specifically enough for real neuroscience to enter the discussion. For instance, at last there was a phenotype that allowed partial confirmation of strong genetic influences [73, 74].

Even so, there is still considerable concern over the heterogeneity of the phenotype provided by DSM-IV. In the future, the search for *endophenotypes* may eventually provide a more refined set of phenotypes from which more specific causal factors can be discovered [75, 76].

I have argued here that the explosion of scientific interest in ADHD is a cumulative effect of the gradual transformation from the pre-scientific era involving astute observations of clinical details in an *etiological framework* of mental disorders, to a *behavioral framework* of the DSM period. During the early period leading up to modern conceptions of ADHD, there was a universal belief that the behavior pattern of ADHD (under other names) was the result of inattention and distraction, caused by a neurologically based deficit. Overstimulation was the key proximate cause of inattention and thus the trigger which revealed the underlying weakness in the ability to inhibit socially inappropriate actions.

I have touched upon some of the non-scientific influences accounting for the explosive attention to the ADHD concept, but believe that an abundance of strong data from neuroscience and clinical trials strongly affirm the role of genuine science in the validity of this concept, and largely accounts for the wide interest in the concept of ADHD. Confirmation of this conclusion from a *quantitative* point of view awaits the next intrepid scientific historian of science. I have made a slight gesture in the direction of a quantitative account with a kind of bibliometric demonstration of possible dependent variables in some doctoral student's future opus. Until then we have to admit full disclosure and accept that our ideas are themselves subject to the overriding *zeitgeist* of our times, a belief that true credibility stems from data, not opinion.

References

1. Hume D. *Enquiries Concerning the Human Understanding and Concerning the Principles of Morals.* Reprinted from the 1748 edition and edited by Selby-Bigge L. London: Oxford University Press; 1748.

2. Anonymous. Introduction to historical method: what is history? Cliopolitical.blogspot.com/.

3. Rafalovich A. The conceptual history of attention deficit hyperactivity disorder: idiocy, imbecility, encephalitis and the child deviant, 1877–1929. *Deviant Behav.* 2001;**22**:93–115.

4. Schrag P, Divoky D. *The Myth of the Hyperactive Child and Other Means of Child Control.* New York, NY: Pantheon; 1975.

5. Breggin P. *Talking Back to Ritalin.* Monroe, ME: Common Courage Press; 1998.

6. Barkley RA. *Attention Deficit Hyperactivity Disorder: A Handbook for Diagnosis and Treatment.* New York, NY: Guilford Press; 1990.

7. Barkley RA. *Attention Deficit Hyperactivity Disorder: A Clinical Workbook.* New York, NY: Guilford Press; 1991.

8. Barkley RA. *ADHD and the Nature of Self-control.* London: Guilford Press; 1997.

9. Kessler JW. History of minimal brain dysfunctions. In: Rie H, Rie E, eds. *Handbook of Minimal Brain Dysfunction: A Critical View.* New York, NY: Wiley-Interscience. 1980; 18–42.

10. Smith M. Psychiatry limited: hyperactivity and the evolution of American psychiatry, 1957–1980. *Social Hist Med.* 2008;**21**:541–59.

11. Boring EG. Eponym as Placebo. In: Watson RI, Campbell DT, eds. *History, Psychology, and Science: Selected Papers by Edwin G Boring.* New York, NY and London: John Wiley & Sons, Inc. 1963; 5–25.

12. Palmer ED, Finger S. An early description of ADHD [Inattention Subtype]: Dr. Alexander Crichton and the "Mental Restlessness" [1798]. *Child Psychol Psychiatry Rev.* 2001;**6**:66–73.

13. Crichton A. *An Inquiry into the Nature and Origin of Mental Derangement: Comprehending a Concise System of the Physiology and Pathology of the Human Mind and a History of the Passions and their Effects.* London: T. Cassell Jr. & W. Davies; 1798.

14. Burrows GM. *Commentaries on the Causes, Forms, Symptoms, and Treatment, Moral and Medical, of Insanity.* London: Thoms and George Underwood; 1828.

15. James W. *The Principles of Psychology.* New York, NY: Henry Holt; 1890.

16. Hoffman H. Der Struwwelpeter ["Shaggy Peter"]. 1845; Available from: http://en.wikipedia.org/wiki/Struwwelpeter.

17. Still GF. Some abnormal psychical conditions in children: the Goulstonian lectures. *Lancet.* 1902;**1**:1008–12.

18. Still GF. Some abnormal psychical conditions in children: Excerpts from three lectures. *J Atten Disord.* 2006;**10**:126–36.

19. von Economo C. Die Encephalitis lethargica. *Wien Klin Wochenschr.* 1917;**30**(May 10, 1917): 581–5.

20. Ebaugh FG. Neuropsychiatric sequelae of acute epidemic encephalitis in children. *Am J Dis Child.* 1923;**25**:85–97.

21. Strecker EA. Behavior problems in encephalitis. *Arch Neurol Psychiatry.* 1929;**21**:127–44.

22. Bradley C. The behavior of children receiving benzedrine. *Am J Psychiatry.* 1937;**94**:577–85.

23. Bradley C, Bowen M. School performance of children receiving amphetamine [benzedrine] sulfate. *Am J Orthopsychiatry.* 1940;**10**:782–8.

24. Laufer M, Denhoff E. Hyperkinetic behavior syndrome in children. *Pediatrics.* 1957;**50**:463–74.

25. Laufer MW, Denhoff E, Solomons G. Hyperkinetic impulse disorder in children's behavior problems. *Psychosom Med.* 1957;**19**:38–49.

26. Laufer MW, Denhoff E, Rubin EZ. Photo-Metrazol activation in children. *Electroencephalogr Clin Neurophysiol.* 1954;**6**:1–8.

27. Tredgold AF. *Mental Deficiency [Amentia].* London: Bailliere, Tindall, & Cox; 1908.

28. Kahn E, Cohen LH. Organic drivenness: a brain-stem syndrome and an experience. *N Engl J Med.* 1934;**210**: 748–56.

29. Strauss AA, Lehtinen LE. *Psychopathology and Education of the Brain-Injured Child.* New York, NY: Grune and Stratton; 1947.

30. Strauss AA, Kephart NC. *Psychopathology and Education of the Brain-Injured Child: Vol. II: Progress in Theory and Clinic.* New York, NY: Grune and Stratton; 1955.

31. Gesell A, Amatruda CS. *Developmental Diagnosis.* New York, NY: Hoeber; 1941.

32. Pasamanick B, Rogers ME, Lilienfeld AM. Pregnancy experience and the development of behavior disorder in children. *Am J Psychiatry.* 1956;**112**:613–18.

33. Lapouse R. An epidemiologic study of behavior characteristics in children. *Am J Public Health.* 1958;**48**:1134–44.

34. Rogers ME, Lilienfeld AM, Pasamanick B. Prenatal and paranatal factors in the development of childhood behavior disorders. *Acta Psychiatr Neurol Scand Suppl.* 1955;**102**:1–157.

35. Pasamanick B, Knobloch H. Brain damage and reproductive casualty. *Am J Orthopsychiatry.* 1960;**30**: 285–305.

36. Clements SD, Peters JE. Minimal brain dysfunctions in the school-age child. *Arch Gen Psychiatry.* 1962;**6**: 185–97.

37. Douglas V. Stop, look and listen: the problem of sustained attention and impulse control in hyperactive and normal children. *Can J Behav Sci.* 1972;**4**:259–82.

38. Dykman RA. Specific learning disabilities: an attentional deficit syndrome. In: Mykelbust H, ed. *Progress in Learning Disabilities*, Vol. 2. New York, NY: Grune and Stratton. 1971; 56–93.

39. Dykman RA, Ackerman PT. Cluster versus dimensional analysis of attention deficit disorders. In: Matson JL, ed. *Handbook of Hyperactivity in Children.* Needham Heights, MA: Allyn & Bacon. 1993; 11–34.

40. Peters JE, Dykman RA, Ackerman PT, Romine JS. The special neurological examination. In: Conners CK, ed. *Clinical Use of Stimulant Drugs in Children.* Amsterdam: Excerpta Medica. 1974; 53–66.

41. Peters JE, Davis J, Goolsby C, Clements SD, Hicks T. *Screening for MBD: Physician's Handbook.* Summit, NJ: CIBA Medical Horizons; 1973.

42. Bax M, MacKeith R, eds. *Minimal Cerebral Dysfunction: Clinics in Developmental Medicine.* London: William Heinemann; 1963.

43. Clements SD. *Minimal Brain Dysfunction in Children: NINDB Monograph.* Washington, DC: US Public Health Service; 1966.

44. Wender P. *Minimal Brain Dysfunction in Children.* New York, NY: Wiley; 1971.

45. Wender P. Hypothesis for a possible biochemical basis of minimal brain dysfunction. In: Knights RM, Bakker DJ, eds. *Neuropsychology of Learning Disorders: Theoretical Approaches.* Baltimore: University Park Press; 1976.

46. Volkow N, Wang G-J, Kollins SH, *et al.* Evaluating dopamine reward pathway in ADHD: Clinical implications. *JAMA.* 2009;**302**:1084–91.

47. Klein DF, Klein RG. Diagnosis of minimal brain dysfunction and hyperkinetic syndrome. In: Conners CK, ed. *Clinical Use of Stimulant Drugs in Children.* Amsterdam: Excerpta Medica. 1974; 1–11.

48. Rutter M. Concepts of "minimal brain dysfunction": issues and prospects in developmental neuropsychiatry. In: Rutter M, ed. *Developmental Neuropsychiatry.* New York, NY: Guilford Press. 1983; 577–98.

49. Nichols PL, Chen T-C. *Minimal Brain Dysfunction: A Prospective Study.* New Jersey: Lawrence Erlbaum Associates; 1981.

50. Kuhn TS. *The Structure of Scientific Revolutions*, 3rd edn. Chicago and London: University of Chicago Press; 1996.

51. Mayes R, Horvitz AV. DSM-III and the revolution in the classification of mental illness. *J Hist Behav Sci.* 2005;**41**(3):249–67.

52. Wilson M. DSM-III and the transformation of American psychiatry: a history. *Am J Psychiatry.* 1994;**50**(3):399–410.

53. Rapoport JL, Castellanos FX. Attention deficit/hyperactivity disorder. In: Wiener JM, ed. *Diagnosis and Psychopharmacology of Childhood and Adolescent Disorders*. New York, NY: John Wiley and Sons, Inc. 1996; 265–92.

54. Conners CK. Forty years of methylphenidate treatment in Attention-Deficit/Hyperactivity Disorder. *J Atten Disord*. 2002; **6**(Suppl 1):S17–30.

55. Swanson JM, McBurnett K, Wigal TL, *et al*. Effect of stimulants: on children with attention deficit disorder: a "review of reviews." *Except Child*. 1993;**60**:154–62.

56. Faraone SV, Buitelaar J. Comparing the efficacy of stimulants for ADHD in children and adolescents using meta-analysis. *Eur Child Adolesc Psychiatry*. 2010;**19**:353–64.

57. Safer DJ, Allen RP. *Hyperactive Children: Diagnosis and Management*. Baltimore: University Park Press; 1976.

58. Jensen P, Hinshaw SP, Swanson JM, *et al*. Findings from the NIMH Multimodal Treatment Study of ADHD [MTA]: implications and applications for primary care providers. *J Dev Behav Pediatr*. 2001; **22**(1):60–73.

59. Spencer T, Biederman J, Wilens TE, Faraone SV. Adults with attention-deficit/hyperactivity disorder: a controversial diagnosis. *J Clin Psychiatry*. 1998; **59**(Suppl 7):59–68.

60. McGough JJ, Barkley RA. Diagnostic controversies in adult attention deficit hyperactivity disorder. *Am J Psychiatry*. 2004;**161**(11):1948–56.

61. Jensen P. Book Review of *ADHD in Adults: What the Science Says. J Atten Disord*. 2009;**13**(1):97–8.

62. Weiss G, Hechtman LT. *Hyperactive Children Grown Up*, 2nd edn. New York, NY: Guilford Press; 1993.

63. Manuzza S, Klein RG, Bessler A, Malloy P, LaPadula M. Adult psychiatric status of hyperactive boys grown up. *Am J Psychiatry*. 1998;**155**(4):493–8.

64. Barkley RA, Murphy KR, Fischer M. *ADHD in Adults: What the Science Says*. New York, NY: Guilford Press; 2008.

65. Biederman J, Monuteaux M, Mick E, *et al*. Young adult outcome of attention deficit hyperactivity disorder: a controlled 10 year prospective follow-up study. *Psychol Med*. 2006;**36**:167–79.

66. Biederman, J, Petty CR, Evans M, Small J, Faraone SV. How persistent is ADHD? A controlled 10-year follow-up study of boys with ADHD. *Psychiatry Res*. 2010;**177**:299–304.

67. Biederman J, Mick E, Surman C, *et al*. A randomized, placebo-controlled trial of OROS methylphenidate in adults with attention-deficit/hyperactivity disorder. *Biol Psychiatry*. 2006;**59**(9):829–35.

68. Faraone SV, Spencer T, Aleardi M, Pagano C, Biederman J. Meta-analysis of the efficacy of methylphenidate for treating adult attention-deficit/hyperactivity disorder. *J Clin Psychopharmacol*. 2004;**24**(1):24–9.

69. Spencer T, Wilens T, Biederman J, *et al*. A double-blind, crossover comparison of methylphenidate and placebo in adults with childhood-onset attention-deficit hyperactivity disorder. *Arch Gen Psychiatry*. 1995;**52**(6):434–43.

70. Spencer T, Biederman J, Wilens T. Stimulant treatment of adult attention-deficit/hyperactivity disorder. *Psychiatr Clin North Am*. 2004;**27**(2): 361–72.

71. Spencer T, Biederman J, Wilens T, *et al*. A large, double-blind, randomized clinical trial of methylphenidate in the treatment of adults with attention-deficit/hyperactivity disorder. *Biol Psychiatry*. 2005;**57**(5):456–63.

72. Mayes R, Bagwell C, Erkulwater J. *Medicating Children: ADHD and Pediatric Mental Health*. Cambridge, Massachusetts and London, England: Harvard University Press; 2009.

73. Faraone SV, Biederman J, Lehman BK, *et al*. Evidence for the independent familial transmission of attention deficit hyperactivity disorder and learning disabilities: results from a family genetic study. *Am J Psychiatry*. 1993;**150**(6):891–5.

74. Faraone S V, Mick E. Molecular genetics of attention deficit hyperactivity disorder. *Psychiatr Clin North Am* 2010;**33**;159–80.

75. Nigg JT. Attention-deficit/hyperactivity disorder: endophenotypes, structure, and etiological pathways. *Curr Dir Psychol Sci*. http://www.psychologicalscienceorg/journals/cd/19_inpress/Nigg_finalpdf [serial on the Internet]. 2009.

76. Nigg JT, Blaskey L, Stawicki J, Sachek J. Evaluating the endophenotype model of ADHD neuropsychological deficit: results for parents and siblings of children with DSM-IV ADHD combined and inattentive subtypes. *J Abnorm Psychol*. 2004;**113**:614–25.

Diagnosing ADHD in children and adults

Lenard A. Adler, David M. Shaw, Kimberly Kovacs, and Samuel Alperin

Introduction

Attention-deficit hyperactivity disorder (ADHD) is one of the most common psychiatric disorders, affecting 6–9% of children worldwide [1]. Once considered to occur only in children, ADHD has now been well documented to persist into adolescence and adulthood in approximately half of childhood cases [2–6]. Recent data suggest that the prevalence of ADHD in adults is 4.4%, indicating that approximately 8 million adults in the United States have the disorder [4]. Although recognition of ADHD in adults has grown in recent years, it remains vastly under-recognized and under-treated as only 10–25% of adults with the disorder are diagnosed and adequately treated [7]. A recent survey found that more than 40% of respondents who met the criteria for adult ADHD had not been previously diagnosed despite seeing a healthcare professional in the previous year. Furthermore, only 10% of respondents with adult ADHD had received treatment for the disorder in the previous year [4, 8]. The individual, societal, and familial costs due to untreated ADHD across the lifespan are vast and result in higher rates of academic underachievement, unemployment, underemployment, divorce, marital separation, early-onset substance abuse, cigarette smoking, and motor vehicle accidents [9–14]. All of these factors highlight the importance of making an accurate diagnosis of ADHD in children, adolescents, and adults.

History of ADHD in the *Diagnostic and Statistical Manual of Mental Disorders* (DSM)

The first clinical description of ADHD was made by Sir George F. Still in 1902 [15] but the disorder was not included in the *Diagnostic and Statistical Manual of Mental Disorders* (DSM) until 1968 when the condition "Hyperkinetic Reaction of Childhood" appeared in the second edition of DSM (DSM-II) [16]. Early definitions of ADHD classified it primarily as a type of hyperactivity disorder, emphasizing hyperactive behaviors and restless symptoms [16, 17]. The third edition of DSM (DSM-III) published in 1980 changed the name of the disorder to attention deficit disorder (ADD) and expanded its definition by acknowledging that symptoms of inattention can occur independently of hyperactive and impulsive symptoms [18]. DSM-III also presented two subtypes of the disorder, ADD with hyperactivity and ADD without hyperactivity [18]. The revised third edition of DSM (DSM-III-R) changed the name to ADHD and consolidated the symptoms into a unidimensional disorder by removing the two subtypes found in DSM-III [19].

The fourth edition of DSM (DSM-IV) published in 1994 reclassified the symptoms of ADHD into three subtypes based on a series of factor analyses published at the time and the DSM-IV field trials: predominately inattentive, predominately hyperactive, and a combined subtype that includes both inattentive and hyperactive symptoms of ADHD [20, 21]. A text revision of DSM-IV was published in 2000 (DSM-IV-TR) [22] but no substantive changes were made to ADHD.

ADHD diagnostic criteria

The DSM-IV-TR diagnostic criteria for ADHD are the same for children and adults and can be reliably used to diagnose individuals who are currently experiencing symptoms of the disorder and who, in the case of older adolescents and adults, have a history

Attention-Deficit Hyperactivity Disorder in Adults and Children, ed. Lenard A. Adler, Thomas J. Spencer and Timothy E. Wilens. Published by Cambridge University Press. © Cambridge University Press 2015.

of such symptoms since childhood. Establishing the childhood onset of symptoms in older adolescents and adults can be done by careful questioning of the individual, which is combined with parental or teacher reports for adolescents [23].

According to DSM-IV-TR, individuals must currently have at least six significant symptoms of inattention and/or six symptoms of hyperactivity/impulsivity (Criterion A) that have persisted for a minimum of 6 months and are "to a degree that is maladaptive and inconsistent with developmental level" [22]. Some of the symptoms must have been present before the age of 7 (Criterion B) and occur in at least two settings, such as at home and at school or work (Criterion C) [22]. There must also be clear evidence of impairment in "developmentally appropriate social, academic, or occupational functioning" (Criterion D) [22]. Lastly, the symptoms cannot occur exclusively during the course of a pervasive developmental disorder, schizophrenia, or other psychotic disorder and are not better accounted for by another mental health disorder (Criterion E) [22]. The symptoms of inattention and hyperactivity/impulsivity are shown in Table 2.1. A diagnosis of ADHD requires that an individual meet all criteria from A through E.

As previously mentioned, the factor analysis and the DSM-IV field trials classified ADHD into three subtypes. Individuals presenting with six or more inattentive symptoms and five or fewer hyperactive/impulsive symptoms meet the criteria for the inattentive subtype. Individuals presenting with six or more hyperactive/impulsive symptoms and five or fewer inattentive symptoms meet the criteria for the hyperactive/impulsive subtype. Individuals with at least six inattentive symptoms and six hyperactive/impulsive symptoms meet the criteria for the combined subtype.

Although research has shown hyperactive/impulsive symptoms to decline with age [17, 24, 25], the combined subtype is the most prevalent in children, adolescents, and adults [1]. Trials of atomoxetine in 536 patients with ADHD showed that 31% of the study participants were classified with the inattentive subtype, 3% were classified with hyperactive subtype, and 66% were classified with the combined subtype [26]. However, in another clinical trial, an equal number of participants were classified with the inattentive subtype as with the combined subtype [27]. Longitudinal studies of youths with ADHD have shown that symptoms of hyperactivity and impulsivity

Table 2.1. DSM-IV-TR criteria symptoms of ADHD (Criterion A)

Symptoms of inattention
(a) Often fails to give close attention to details or makes careless mistakes in schoolwork, work, or other activities
(b) Often has difficulty sustaining attention in tasks or play activities
(c) Often does not seem to listen when spoken to directly
(d) Often does not follow through on instructions and fails to finish schoolwork, chores, or duties in the workplace (not due to oppositional behavior or failure to understand instructions)
(e) Often has difficulty organizing tasks and activities
(f) Often avoids, dislikes, or is reluctant to engage in tasks that require sustained mental effort (such as schoolwork or homework)
(g) Often loses things necessary for tasks or activities (e.g., toys, school assignments, pencils, books, or tools)
(h) Is often easily distracted by extraneous stimuli
(i) Is often forgetful in daily activities

Symptoms of hyperactivity
(a) Often fidgets with hands or feet or squirms in seat
(b) Often leaves seat in classroom or in other situations in which remaining seated is expected
(c) Often runs about or climbs excessively in situations in which it is inappropriate (in adolescents or adults, may be limited to subjective feelings of restlessness)
(d) Often has difficulty playing or engaging in leisure activities quietly
(e) Is often "on the go" or acts as if "driven by a motor"
(f) Often talks excessively

Symptoms of impulsivity
(a) Often blurts out answers before questions have been completed
(b) Often has difficulty awaiting one's turn
(c) Often interrupts or intrudes on others (e.g., butts into conversations or games)

Source: American Psychiatric Association [22]. Reprinted with permission from *Diagnostic and Statistical Manual of Mental Disorders, Fourth Edition* (Copyright © 2000) and the *Diagnostic and Statistical Manual of Mental Disorders, Fifth Edition* (Copyright © 2013). American Psychiatric Association. All rights reserved.

tend to wane, whereas inattention tends to persist into adulthood [28, 29]. Other studies have found clinically significant levels of hyperactivity and impulsivity in approximately half of ADHD-diagnosed adults and prominent inattention symptoms in up to 90% [28]. Consistent with previous studies of children growing up with ADHD, in a study of 107 adults (mean age 37 years) with ADHD presenting for treatment, higher rates of inattentive symptoms were found relative to hyperactive–impulsive symptoms [30]. In fact, over 90% of adults with ADHD endorsed inattentive symptoms of the disorder (see Figure 2.1, adapted from Wilens *et al.* [30]).

In the recently published DSM-5 the age of onset criteria has been increased from 7 years of age to 12 years of age [31]. The increase in the age of onset

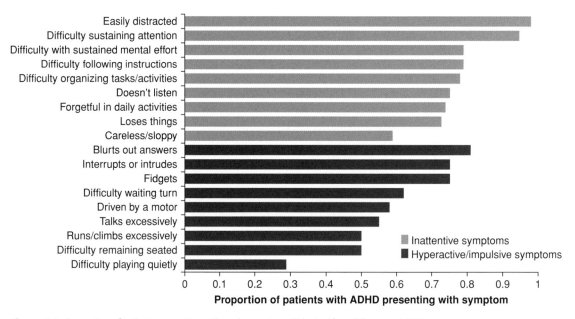

Figure 2.1. Proportion of patients presenting with each symptom. (Adapted from Wilens *et al.* [30].)

criteria is based on studies indicating: (1) that many bright individuals with ADHD will not have significant symptom onset until middle school and (2) that the subgroup of individuals identified with this later age of onset is virtually indistinguishable from individuals with an age of onset prior to the age of 7 in terms of symptoms, impairments, and comorbidity [5].

Diagnosing children with ADHD

Diagnosing ADHD in young children can be extremely tricky due to the irregularity of the developmental process during that time. Inattention and impulsivity are considered appropriate behaviors as children explore their surroundings, the impairment is determined by the child displaying symptoms that are inappropriate for their developmental stage. Diagnosing a child with ADHD begins with a detailed evaluation of the child's prenatal, birth, developmental, medical and psychiatric history; an evaluation of academic performance; and finally a review of the family and social history [32]. This evaluation should rule out other disorders or medical problems that can mimic some of the symptoms of ADHD like developmental disabilities, learning disorders, autism, depression, anxiety disorder, pediatric bipolar disorder, hyperthyroidism, or tic disorders [32, 33].

Many children with ADHD also show comorbid symptoms of other psychiatric or physical conditions,

67% according to some studies, most significantly oppositional defiant disorder (35–39.9%), conduct disorder (14.3–30%), and anxiety disorder (25–38.7%) [33, 34]. Due to the frequent coexistence of comorbid psychiatric conditions and disorders, it has been recommended by most clinicians, the American Academy of Child and Adolescent Psychiatry [35], and the American Academy of Pediatrics [36] that children also be examined for symptoms of depression, anxiety, tics, substance abuse, mania, psychosis, and learning disabilities. Furthermore, a thorough clinical evaluation will help with treatment decisions, as efficacy of treatment has been shown to be related to subtype of ADHD as well as comorbidity [32, 34, 37].

One of the key elements in diagnosing a child with ADHD is demonstrating functional impairment in two settings, usually home and school. Symptoms tend to present themselves in more structured settings requiring a child to sit and attend to a task. Assessing symptoms is done through parent reports at home and teacher observations and reports in the school. In certain situations, such as one-on-one interactions or unstructured time, symptoms of ADHD may be absent. Nonetheless, in older children and adolescents, it is important to interview the patient separately from the parents, so as to allow the child to speak freely and reveal all possible symptoms [35]. The one-on-one interview is not for purposes of diagnosis of ADHD, but rather to identify symptoms inconsistent with ADHD and possibly suggestive of comorbid problems.

A variety of rating scales can be used to help the clinician in gathering information from the parents and children and scales should be chosen carefully so that they are age appropriate. Common ADHD symptom rating scales include the Conners' Rating Scales; the ADHD Rating Scales-IV; Swanson, Nolan, and Pelham IV Questionnaire (SNAP-IV); Swanson, Koktin, Agler, M-Flynn, and Pelham Scale (SKAMP); Brown ADD Rating Scales; Child Behavior Checklist; and each has its own limitations and benefits depending on length, informant, versions, age, and normative data [35, 36, 38]. These rating scales should only be used to assist in making the diagnosis through symptom ascertainment and not to provide a diagnosis by themselves. Furthermore, it should be noted that differences in ratings may appear, as parents and teachers see the child in different settings. It has been posited that parents' reports of symptoms may have a higher diagnostic value and teachers' reports may have a greater prognostic validity [37]. While parents may observe their child doing homework, chores, and playing videogames, teachers see the child during social settings with other children and during lessons, and their ratings have some comparative validity.

As a child develops and grows, the presentation of ADHD symptoms may also evolve. During preschool, a child with ADHD may display gross motor hyperactivity such as running and climbing on furniture. Fewer than 50% of children diagnosed between 3 and 5 years of age continue to have ADHD during the rest of their childhood [33]. Children with ADHD often have more difficulty remaining quiet and adapting to more focused activities, less developed social skills, more difficulty transitioning to new activities, and are more noncompliant with adults than their non-ADHD peers [37].

By the time children with ADHD enter elementary school, they begin to display difficulties in the academic arena, usually through poor organizational skills, forgetfulness, losing important items, and difficulty focusing, leading to the child performing under their academic potential and delivering messy or sloppy work. Conflicts with peers also begin to emerge during elementary school [37]. As the child grows older, symptoms of hyperactivity and impulsivity both decrease and also seem to shift into other behavioral manifestations, such as inability to finish long-term

projects, unwillingness to do household chores, and overall sense of "being on the go" [37]. These behavioral issues can lead to underachievement in school and are related to higher rates of repetition of grades, suspension from school, dropping out of school, and disruption of family life, not only affecting the child but also leading to higher rates of depression and interpersonal relationship issues in the parents [39]. The majority of ADHD diagnosis occurs during early elementary school, and around 60–80% of children diagnosed with ADHD continue to show significant symptoms as adolescents [35, 37].

Adolescents with ADHD may appear more immature than their peers and are often in trouble with their parents and teachers, and increasing academic demands result in underperforming in school as they have difficulties with completing class assignments and homework. The adolescent with ADHD also tends to engage in more high-risk activities than adolescents without ADHD, leading to increased rates of substance abuse, motor vehicle accidents, academic and occupational impairments, unplanned pregnancy, and sexually transmitted diseases [32]. Around 60% of adolescents continue to have ADHD into adulthood [32, 33].

Diagnosing adults with ADHD

Many adults are not diagnosed with ADHD in childhood because of the structure of their environments and the minimal demands required of them and it is suggested that these individuals show greater impairment as adults [23, 28, 40].

To accurately evaluate ADHD in adults, clinicians review childhood onset, and persistence and pervasiveness of current symptoms [41]. Clinicians must assess symptoms from the previous 6 months as well as symptoms which occurred prior to the age of 7. Currently, diagnosing ADHD cannot occur without demonstrating that significant impairment was present in childhood. Although retrospective self-reports have been considered questionable, studies have shown them to be a reliable method of diagnosis [25]. Research studies on ADHD show that symptoms of hyperactivity and impulsivity often diminish with age [17, 24, 28, 29, 42]. Adults often seek help due to impairment from academic, professional, or interpersonal difficulties.

In childhood, boys outnumber girls in diagnosis on the order of up to four to five to one, primarily in response to the way in which their ADHD symptoms present themselves [43, 44]. The discrepancy in diagnosis is usually due to the fact that girls display more inattentive symptoms while boys are more hyperactive, which often leads to increased behavioral disturbances [45]. Since hyperactive symptoms tend to be less severe in adults, the difference in diagnoses between men and women is much smaller, circa two to one or even equal in gender distribution [43, 45].

Three subtypes were established from factor analyses: predominately inattentive, predominately hyperactive, and a combination of both inattentive and hyperactive symptoms, which is the most common of the subgroups [46].

Functional and educational impairment

According to data from the Milwaukee Young Adult Outcome Study, individuals with ADHD are more likely than their peers to be held back in school, be suspended, or be expelled. Individuals with ADHD drop out of school more often than their non-ADHD peers and community surveys have shown that many do not complete higher education programs [10, 13, 47, 48].

The effects of ADHD can be seen in the work place in employees who consistently have problems completing tasks or interacting with coworkers [49]. Many adults with ADHD tend to switch jobs frequently either because they lose interest rapidly or because of their inability to live up to the employer's expectations [41, 50]. By examining longitudinal studies, it is evidenced that adults with ADHD are more likely to be fired or receive low work performance ratings compared to their non-ADHD peers. These adults with ADHD often display a low frustration tolerance and behavioral disturbances in the work environment which frequently result in increased numbers of job switches [51]. By looking at the results of a community survey conducted in the United States, researchers have discovered that not only are adults with ADHD more likely to be of a lower social class but they are also three times as likely to be unemployed, more likely to frequently switch jobs, and have increased rates of divorce and police arrests. The survey compared 500 adults with ADHD to 501 non-ADHD adults and revealed that adults with ADHD are less satisfied with their family life, profession, and social interactions [13].

Related impairments

Adults who present with significant inattentive symptoms often have deficits in executive functioning [29, 52–56]. Executive functioning includes components of attention, reasoning, planning, inhibition, set shifting, interference control, and working memory [53, 57] so it is clear that deficits in any of these routinely used skills can be extremely impairing. Poor control over executive functioning is attributed to low functioning frontal regions of the brain [58].

Difficulties with regulating one's mood is commonly present among individuals with ADHD [51]. Many individuals with undiagnosed ADHD report lower self-esteem and it can be tricky to distinguish between depressive symptoms that are a result of living with ADHD and those of a primary diagnosis of major depression or dysthymia [59]. When ADHD is the primary diagnosis, depressive mood-related symptoms are usually in response to consequences of the individual's ADHD symptoms and are usually fleeting [59].

As for depressive disorders, difficulties regulating one's mood can also make it difficult to identify ADHD symptoms from pervasive mood changes in bipolar disorder.

Recognizing ADHD in adults: presenting signs and coping strategies

The symptoms of ADHD are extremely varied and, depending on the individual, may present in completely different ways. Most clinicians are aware that they should screen a patient who presents with symptoms such as difficulty concentrating and poor organization and planning, but it is also important to screen individuals who report low self-esteem and poor self-discipline. Symptoms that may go undetected that also warrant screening are: poor memory, forgetfulness, trouble thinking clearly, and mood lability [51]. Patients may report trouble in their work environment or of constantly changing jobs, as well as having difficulties maintaining meaningful relationships. In many cases, patients may get treatment for a comorbid disorder and treatment may remain unsuccessful due to the persistence of ADHD symptoms. During a clinical interview, four key objectives must be met: (1) an early childhood onset, (2) at least six of the nine significant symptoms of either inattention or hyperactivity/impulsivity, (3) significant impairment in at least two settings, and (4) symptoms that are best explained by ADHD and not another psychiatric disorder [22].

An important part of the diagnosis process is to account for the coping mechanisms that patients develop over the years. Coping strategies may make it seem that a patient has fewer symptoms or that the symptoms are less severe, but are less likely to mask more severe symptoms [40]. Individuals with ADHD may also be living well below their potential as a way to deal with their symptoms. It is important that clinicians uncover a full picture of the disorder and that they account for any misconceptions that coping mechanisms may present.

References

1. Faraone SV, Sergeant J, Billberg C, Biederman J. The worldwide prevalence of ADHD: is it an American condition? *World Psychiatry*. 2003;**2**(2):104–13.

2. Dulcan M. Practice parameters for the assessment and treatment of children, adolescents, and adults with attention-deficit/hyperactivity disorder. American Academy of Child and Adolescent Psychiatry. *J Am Acad Child Adolesc Psychiatry*. 1997;**36**(Suppl 10): 85S–121S.

3. Barkley RA, Fischer M, Smallish L, Fletcher K. The persistence of attention-deficit/hyperactivity disorder into young adulthood as a function of reporting source and definition of disorder. *J Abnorm Psychol*. 2002; **111**(2):279–89.

4. Kessler RC, Adler LA, Barkley R, *et al.* Patterns and predictors of attention-deficit/hyperactivity disorder persistence into adulthood: results from the national comorbidity survey replication. *Biol Psychiatry*. 2005; **57**(11):1442–51.

5. Faraone SV, Biederman J, Spencer T, *et al.* Diagnosing adult attention deficit hyperactivity disorder: are late onset and subthreshold diagnoses valid? *Am J Psychiatry*. 2006;**163**(10):1720–9.

6. Barkley RA, Murphy KR, Fischer M. *ADHD in Adults: What the Science Says*. New York, NY: Guilford Press; 2008.

7. Castle L, Aubert RE, Verbrugge RR, Khalid M, Epstein RS. Trends in medication treatment for ADHD. *J Atten Disord*. 2007;**10**(4):335–42.

8. Kessler RC, Adler L, Barkley R, *et al.* The prevalence and correlates of adult ADHD in the United States: results from the National Comorbidity Survey Replication. *Am J Psychiatry*. 2006;**163**(4):716–23.

9. Mannuzza S, Klein RG. Adolescent and adult outcomes in attention-deficit/hyperactivity disorder. In: Quay HC, Hogan AE, eds. *Handbook of Disruptive Behavior Disorders*. New York, NY: Kluwer Academic/Plenum Publishers 1999; 279–94.

10. Barkley RA. Major life activity and health outcomes associated with attention-deficit/hyperactivity disorder. *J Clin Psychiatry*. 2002;**63**(Suppl 12): 10–15.

11. Eakin L, Minde K, Hechtman L, *et al.* The marital and family functioning of adults with ADHD and their spouses. *J Atten Disord*. 2004;**8**(1):1–10.

12. Wilens TE, Dodson W. A clinical perspective of attention-deficit/hyperactivity disorder into adulthood. *J Clin Psychiatry*. 2004;**65**(10):1301–13.

13. Biederman J, Faraone SV, Spencer TJ, Mick E, Monuteaux MC. Functional impairments in adults with self-reports of diagnosed ADHD: A controlled study of 1001 adults in the community. *J Clin Psychiatry*. 2006;**67**(4):524–40.

14. Biederman J, Monuteaux MC, Mick E, *et al.* Young adult outcome of attention deficit hyperactivity disorder: a controlled 10-year follow-up study. *Psychol Med*. 2006b;**36**(2):167–79.

15. Still G. The Goulstonian lectures on some abnormal psychical conditions in children. *Lancet*. 1902; **159**(4102):1008–12.

16. American Psychiatric Association. *Diagnostic and Statistical Manual of Mental Disorders*, 2nd edn (DSM-II). Washington, DC: American Psychiatric Association; 1968.

17. Biederman J, Mick E, Faraone SV. Age-dependent decline of symptoms of attention deficit hyperactivity disorder: impact of remission definition and symptom type. *Am J Psychiatry*. 2000;**157**(5):816–18.

18. American Psychiatric Association. *Diagnostic and Statistical Manual of Mental Disorders*, 3rd edn (DSM-III). Washington, DC: American Psychiatric Association; 1980.

19. American Psychiatric Association. *Diagnostic and Statistical Manual of Mental Disorders*, 3rd edn, rev (DSM-III-R). Washington, DC: American Psychiatric Association; 1987.

20. American Psychiatric Association. *Diagnostic and Statistical Manual of Mental Disorders*, 4th edn (DSM-IV). Washington, DC: American Psychiatric Association; 1994.

21. Lahey BB, Applegate B, McBurnett K, *et al.* DSM-IV field trials for attention deficit hyperactivity disorder in children and adolescents. *Am J Psychiatry*. 1994; **151**(11):1673–85.

22. American Psychiatric Association. *Diagnostic and Statistical Manual of Mental Disorders,* 4th edn, text rev (DSM-IV-TR). Washington, DC: American Psychiatric Association; 2000.

23. Adler L, Cohen J. Diagnosis and evaluation of adults with attention-deficit/hyperactivity disorder. *Psychiatr Clin North Am.* 2004;**27**(2):187–201.

24. Biederman J, Faraone S, Milberger S, *et al.* Predictors of persistence and remission of ADHD into adolescence: results from a four-year prospective follow-up study. *J Am Acad Child Adolesc Psychiatry.* 1996;**35**(3);343–51.

25. Murphy P, Schachar R. Use of self-ratings in the assessment of symptoms of attention deficit hyperactivity disorder in adults. *Am J Psychiatry.* 2000;**157**(7):1156–9.

26. Michelson D, Adler L, Spencer T, *et al.* Atomoxetine in adults with ADHD: two randomized, placebo-controlled studies. *Biol Psychiatry.* 2003;**53**(2):112–20.

27. Spencer T, Biederman J, Wilens T, *et al.* Efficacy of a mixed amphetamine salts compound in adults with attention-deficit/hyperactivity disorder. *Arch Gen Psychiatry.* 2001;**58**(8):775–82.

28. Millstein RB, Wilens TE, Biederman J, Spencer TJ. Presenting ADHD symptoms and subtypes in clinically referred adults with ADHD. *J Atten Disord.* 1997;**2**(3):159–66.

29. Kessler RC, Green JG, Adler LA, *et al.* Structure and diagnosis of adult attention-deficit/hyperactivity disorder: analysis of expanded symptom criteria from the adult ADHD clinical diagnostic scale. *Arch Gen Psychiatry.* 2010;**67**(11):1168–78.

30. Wilens TE, Biederman J, Faraone SV, *et al.* Presenting ADHD symptoms, subtypes, and comorbid disorders in clinically referred adults with ADHD. *J Clin Psychiatry.* 2009;**70**(11):1557–62.

31. American Psychiatric Association. *Diagnostic and Statistical Manual of Mental Disorders,* 5th edn. Arlington, VA: American Psychiatric Publishing; 2013.

32. Kratochvil CJ, Vaughan BS, Barker A, *et al.* Review of pediatric attention deficit/hyperactivity disorder for the general psychiatrist. *Psychiatr Clin North Am.* 2009;**32**(1):39–56.

33. Floet AMW, Scheiner C, Grossman L. Attention-deficit/hyperactivity disorder. *Pediatr Rev.* 2010;**31**(2):56–69.

34. Jensen PS, Hinshaw SP, Swanson JM, *et al.* Findings from the NIMH Multimodal Treatment Study of ADHD (MTA): implications and applications for primary care providers. *J Dev Behav Pediatr.* 2001;**22**(1):60–73.

35. Pliszka SR; AACAP Work Group on Quality Issues. Practice parameter for the assessment and treatment of children and adolescents with attention-deficit/hyperactivity disorder. *J Am Acad Child Adolesc Psychiatry.* 2007;**46**(7):894–921.

36. Subcommittee on Attention-Deficit/Hyperactivity Disorder; Steering Committee on Quality Improvement and Management, Wolraich M, Brown L, *et al.* ADHD: clinical practice guideline for the diagnosis, evaluation, and treatment of attention-deficit/hyperactivity disorder in children and adolescents. *Pediatrics.* 2011;**128**(5):1007–22.

37. Greenhill LL. Diagnosing attention-deficit/hyperactivity disorder in children. *J Clin Psychiatry.* 1998;**59**(Suppl 7):31–41.

38. Kaplan G, Newcorn JH. Pharmacotherapy for child and adolescent attention-deficit hyperactivity disorder. *Pediatr Clin North Am.* 2011;**58**(1):99–120.

39. Katragadda S, Schubiner H. ADHD in children, adolescents, and adults. *Prim Care.* 2007;**34**(2):317–41.

40. Murphy KR, Adler LA. Assessing attention-deficit/hyperactivity disorder in adults: focus on rating scales. *J Clin Psychiatry.* 2004;**65**(Suppl 3):12–17.

41. Spencer TJ, Adler L. Diagnostic approaches to adult attention-deficit/hyperactivity disorder. *Prim Psychiatry.* 2004;**11**(7):49–53.

42. Kessler RC, Adler L, Ames M, *et al.* The World Health Organization Adult ADHD Self-Report Scale (ASRS): a short screening scale for use in the general population. *Psychol Med.* 2005;**35**(2):245–56.

43. Biederman J, Faraone SV, Spencer T, *et al.* Gender differences in a sample of adults with attention deficit hyperactivity disorder. *Psychiatry Res.* 1994;**53**(1):13–29.

44. Gaub M, Carlson CL. Gender differences in ADHD: a meta-analysis and critical review. *J Am Acad Child Adolesc Psychiatry.* 1997;**36**(8):1036–45.

45. Biederman J. Impact of comorbidity in adults with attention-deficit/hyperactivity disorder. *J Clin Psychiatry.* 2004;**65**(Suppl 3):3–7.

46. Kooij JJ, Buitelaar JK, van den Oord EJ, *et al.* Internal and external validity of attention-deficit hyperactivity disorder in a population-based sample of adults. *Psychol Med.* 2005;**35**(6):817–27.

47. Barkley RA, Fischer M, Smallish L, Fletcher K. Young adult follow-up of hyperactive children: antisocial activities and drug use. *J Child Psychol Psychiatry.* 2004;**45**(2):195–211.

48. Barkley RA, Fischer M, Smallish L, Fletcher K. Young adult outcome of hyperactive children: adaptive functioning in major life activities. *J Am Acad Child Adolesc Psychiatry.* 2006;**45**(2):192–202.

49. Shekim WO, Asarnow RF, Hess E, Zaucha K, Wheeler N. A clinical and demographic profile of a sample of adults with attention deficit hyperactivity disorder, residual state. *Compr Psychiatry.* 1990;**31**(5):416–25.

50. Biederman J, Wilens T, Mick E, *et al.* Psychoactive substance use disorders in adults with attention deficit hyperactivity disorder (ADHD): effects of ADHD and psychiatric comorbidity. *Am J Psychiatry.* 1995; **152**(11):1652–8.

51. Wolf LE, Wasserstein J. Adult ADHD. Concluding thoughts. *Ann N Y Acad Sci.* 2001;**931**:396–408.

52. Barkley RA. Behavioral inhibition, sustained attention, and executive functions: constructing a unifying theory of ADHD. *Psychol Bull.* 1997;**121**(1):65–94.

53. Sergeant JA, Geurts H, Oosterlaan J. How specific is a deficit of executive functioning for attention-deficit/ hyperactivity disorder? *Behav Brain Res.* 2002; **130**(1–2):3–28.

54. Biederman J, Petty C, Fried R, *et al.* Impact of psychometrically defined deficits of executive functioning in adults with attention deficit hyperactivity disorder. *Am J Psychiatry.* 2006;**163**(10): 1730–8.

55. Biederman J, Petty CR, Fried R, *et al.* Stability of executive function deficits into young adult years: a prospective longitudinal follow-up study of grown up males with ADHD. *Acta Psychiatr Scand.* 2007;**116**(2): 129–36.

56. Biederman J, Petty CR, Fried R, *et al.* Can self-reported Behavioral scales assess executive function deficits? A controlled study of adults with ADHD. *J Nerv Ment Dis.* 2007;**195**(3): 240–6.

57. Pennington BF, Ozonoff S. Executive functions and developmental psychopathology. *J Child Psychol Psychiatry.* 1996;**37**(1);51–87.

58. Barkley RA. *Attention-Deficit Hyperactivity Disorder: A Handbook for Diagnosis and Treatment.* New York, NY: Guilford Press; 2005.

59. Wender PH. *Attention-Deficit Hyperactivity Disorder in Adults.* New York, NY: Oxford University Press; 1995.

Chapter 3

The epidemiology and societal burden of ADHD

John Fayyad and Ronald C. Kessler

Introduction

This chapter presents an overview of the voluminous literature on the epidemiology and societal burden of attention-deficit hyperactivity disorder (ADHD). ADHD has long been known to be a common childhood mental disorder [1, 2], but adult ADHD has been less well studied because it was long assumed that ADHD remits in the transition to adulthood. Clinical follow-up studies have now made it clear, though, that children with ADHD often continue to have symptoms in adulthood and that adults with a history of childhood ADHD have a comparatively high prevalence of other mental disorders that develop subsequent to ADHD [3, 4]. These observations have led to a growing interest in adult ADHD [5], although controversy exists about appropriate diagnostic criteria [6]. Our review focuses separately on child–adolescent and adult ADHD.

Childhood and adolescent ADHD

Prevalence

Several comprehensive reviews exist on the prevalence of childhood and adolescent ADHD [7–9]. Prevalence estimates vary widely from over 20% to less than 1%, but with a central tendency of 4–6%. A recent quantitative analysis of worldwide studies reported a pooled estimate of 5.3% current prevalence (6.5% for children and 2.7% for adolescents) [7].

While most child–adolescent ADHD epidemiological studies have taken place in the USA, Australia, and Europe, more recent studies have been carried out in all regions of the world, both in developed and developing countries (e.g., Farah *et al.* [10]).

When comparable instruments and classification systems are used, the estimated prevalence of ADHD is similar in these other parts of the world to estimates in the USA, Australia, and Europe [11], although there is a trend for prevalence to be somewhat lower in these other populations [8].

Comparison of prevalence estimates is complicated by methodological variation across studies, including differences in the classification system used to make diagnoses (higher prevalence when *Diagnostic and Statistical Manual of Mental Disorders* [DSM] criteria are used than *International Statistical Classification of Diseases* [ICD] criteria [12], and higher using DSM-IV [13] than DSM-III-R [14] criteria), whether or not impairment is required to qualify for a diagnosis (lower prevalence when impairment is required), using the either/or rule for criteria by informant, the type of informant (higher prevalence when the informant is a parent or teacher than child), and the instrument used to measure prevalence (higher using rating scales than structured interviews).

Three subtypes of ADHD are distinguished in the DSM-IV: the primarily inattentive, primarily impulsive–hyperactive, and combined subtypes. It is difficult to estimate the relative prevalence of these three subtypes both because the cut-points for determining primacy are not well established and because the distinctions are sometimes unstable over time [15]. There is nonetheless reason to believe that the subtype distinctions are real in light of the fact that they differ in their correlates [16]. Indeed, the suggestion has been made that the primarily inattentive subtype might be a distinct disorder from ADHD involving impulsivity–hyperactivity [17], although a systematic review of the available evidence suggests that it would be

Attention-Deficit Hyperactivity Disorder in Adults and Children, ed. Lenard A. Adler, Thomas J. Spencer and Timothy E. Wilens.
Published by Cambridge University Press. © Cambridge University Press 2015.

premature to draw this conclusion [18]. A recent analysis of the National Comorbidity Survey Replication indicates that there may be an additional factor related to executive functioning (EF) that is specific to predicting persistence of ADHD into adulthood [19].

Comorbidity

Epidemiological surveys consistently find high comorbidity among mental disorders [20]. Numerous cross-sectional studies have examined the underlying structure of this comorbidity [21, 22], while a number of longitudinal studies have examined temporal progression between specific earlier and later disorders [23]. These studies typically find stronger patterns of comorbidity within, rather than between, two broadly defined clusters of disorders that are generally referred to in childhood as *internalizing* (anxiety and mood) and *externalizing* (disruptive behavior and substance) disorders. Patterns of comorbidity with ADHD are similar in childhood/adolescence to those in adulthood.

ADHD is one of the externalizing disorders and is consistently found to have especially strong comorbidity with conduct disorder (CD) and oppositional defiant disorder (ODD). Similar patterns are found in clinical samples [24, 25]. The ADHD subtypes involving impulsivity–hyperactivity are consistently found to have higher comorbidity with CD and ODD than the primarily inattentive subtype [16].

Longitudinal studies aimed at teasing apart the relative importance of ADHD, CD, and ODD on each other are few in number (e.g., Costello *et al.* [26], Fergusson *et al.* [27]), but consistently show that ADHD usually has an earlier age of onset than the other disorders [28], suggesting that ADHD is either a causal risk factor or a risk marker for subsequent comorbidity. However, recent research found evidence consistent with the possibility that common genetic influences might account for this predictive association of ADHD with subsequent CD and ODD [29]. Furthermore, despite the temporal priority of ADHD over CD and ODD, longitudinal studies show that CD and ODD both have predictive effects on subsequent outcomes that are distinct from those of ADHD [26, 27].

There is a great deal of interest in, as well as considerable controversy about [30, 31], comorbidity between childhood–adolescent ADHD and pediatric bipolar disorder (BPD). Some studies suggest that

these two disorders are highly comorbid [32], while others suggest that this kind of comorbidity is quite uncommon [33]. Although the central tendency in high-quality studies of unrestricted samples is to find relatively high comorbidity between pediatric ADHD and BPD [34], the enormous range in the estimated magnitude of ADHD–BPD comorbidity is striking and at least indirectly suggestive that methodological confounding of some sort is involved [35]. A number of bases for diagnostic confusion exist that could account for this wide variation in estimates of pediatric ADHD–BPD comorbidity, all related to the possibility that symptoms of pediatric BPD might mistakenly be interpreted as due to ADHD or vice versa [35].

The possibility of diagnostic confusion is thought to increase when CD and ODD are added to the multimorbid profile [36]. Although guidelines have been developed to improve the accuracy of differential diagnosis of such cases [37], few empirical studies have followed these guidelines in making diagnoses. There is some limited evidence for common risk factors [11, 38] that might argue for ADHD–BPD comorbidity being genuine rather than artifactual. Given that ADHD has a much earlier age of onset than BPD, there is also the possibility that ADHD is a causal risk factor for the subsequent onset of BPD. A suggestion has been made that comorbid ADHD–BPD with a pediatric onset of BPD might be a distinct subtype [39], but the fact that symptoms of ADHD do not remit along with BPD symptoms when patients with ADHD–BPD are treated for BPD but do remit with subsequent conventional ADHD treatment [40] has been taken to undercut the plausibility of this idea [35]. Carefully crafted developmental genetic epidemiological studies will almost certainly be needed to sort out all this complexity in a satisfactory fashion.

The impairments caused by childhood and adolescent ADHD

One interesting characteristic of ADHD from a research perspective is that it creates impairments in cognitive functioning that can be assessed objectively with neuropsychological tests. Such tests show clear impairments that are specific to pediatric ADHD and that vary significantly across ADHD subtypes. For example, a recent study of EF among Chinese boys with ADHD documented significant decrements in a wide range of EF tests compared to healthy boys who were matched to the patients in terms of age and IQ [41]. The patients with exclusively impulsive–hyperactive ADHD had a narrower range of EF deficits than those who also had symptoms of inattentiveness, while comorbid CD and ODD were unrelated to EF deficits. This specificity of the effects on EF of ADHD compared to CD and ODD has been replicated for other objective measures of neurocognitive impairment in other studies (e.g., Barnett et al. [42], Qian et al. [43]), although differentiation in objective neurocognitive tests across ADHD subtypes has been less well replicated [44, 45].

The costs of childhood and adolescent ADHD

The costs of illness include both direct costs of obtaining treatment and a variety of indirect costs associated with such things as lost productivity due to the illness. Costs can be considered not only in economic terms but also in psychological terms, such as the burden of the illness on caregivers and the psychological toll the illness takes on family members. A large body of research has documented significant indirect costs of childhood and adolescent ADHD [46–50]. The impact and burden of ADHD are even greater when the high rates of secondary comorbid conditions associated with ADHD (e.g., anxiety, mood, substance and behavioral disorders) are taken into consideration. We examine some of these indirect costs of childhood-adolescent ADHD by focusing on studies of educational attainment, risk behaviors, healthcare costs, and family burden.

Educational attainment

Research in clinical samples has shown consistently that youth undergoing treatment for ADHD have significant decrements in educational attainment. Mannuzza et al. [51], for example, found that subjects with ADHD had an average of 2 years less education than controls in addition to much higher rates of not finishing high school, while the Young Adult Outcome Study showed that adolescents with ADHD were more likely to be suspended, expelled, and held back from school than controls [52]. These kinds of adverse effects are also found in studies of community samples of youth with untreated ADHD. A recent comprehensive review of these epidemiological studies found that untreated ADHD was consistently associated with low grades, poor performance on standardized tests for both verbal and quantitative performance, grade retention, expulsion, failure to complete secondary

school, and failure to go on to obtain post-secondary education after completing secondary school [53]. The latter results are consistent with those in epidemiological surveys of adults, which consistently find low levels of educational attainment among adults with a retrospectively reported history of childhood–adolescent ADHD. Most of the prospectively followed samples, however, were untreated, and the potential effect of long-term treatment on mitigating these impairments remains unclear [54, 55].

Risk behaviors

Accidents and injuries are much more common among both children and adolescents with ADHD than without ADHD [56, 57]. It is not known if this elevation is due to inattentiveness, impulsivity–hyperactivity, or a combination, but there are good conceptual reasons to suggest that both inattentiveness [58] and impulsivity–hyperactivity [59] are risk factors for accidents and injuries. In addition, a recent study suggested that the combination of inattentiveness and hyperactivity was an especially powerful risk factor for accidents and injuries [60]. Impulsivity in ADHD is also known to be associated with a number of other risk behaviors, including child and adolescent violent aggression [61], adolescent substance abuse [62], and adolescent suicidality [63].

Use of healthcare services

Children with diagnosed ADHD have been found consistently to have higher use of healthcare services than matched youth without ADHD [47, 48, 50]. These elevated rates of treatment include, but are not limited to, school-based services for the treatment of ADHD [53]. A recent review of this literature, most of it from the USA, found that the total annual healthcare costs of youth diagnosed with ADHD are twice as high as those of other youth [64]. At least part of this association is to be expected by virtue of the fact that some of these studies detected cases through treatment records, thereby over-representing active help-seekers [65]. However, youth diagnosed with ADHD in these studies not only have higher healthcare utilization for the treatment of emotional problems but also higher use of services for physical health problems and emergency room visits. As noted above, accident-proneness is a correlate of ADHD [56, 57].

Studies that identified ADHD through school records rather than only through medical records also document elevated healthcare costs associated with ADHD for a wide variety of conditions, including emergency room visits, injuries, and hospital admissions, rather than only costs for the treatment of emotional problems [66]. It has generally been assumed that the hyperactive component of ADHD accounts for these healthcare costs. However, a study of 124 children with ADHD in Spain found no difference in rates of health utilization among the inattentive, hyperactive–impulsive, and combined subtypes of ADHD [67]. Based on this finding, further research is needed to investigate the causal processes that lead to high rates of healthcare utilization among youth with ADHD. The literature is very clear in showing that these costs exist, but much remains to be learned about causal pathways and plausible targets of intervention aimed at reducing these costs.

Family burden

It is to be expected that the experience of having a child with impairments as substantial as those related to ADHD will take a toll on families. Research has consistently shown this to be the case, as parent–child relationships of children with ADHD are less positive than with other children [68, 69]. In addition, family conflict, parental depression, and parental divorce are all more common in families where one or more children have ADHD [70, 71]. Pediatric ADHD is also associated with impairment in parental role functioning, as the parents of youth with ADHD have increased time demands associated with the excess healthcare needs and behavioral problems of their children. Parents of children with ADHD report more lost work time associated with caring for the needs of their child and a greater likelihood of having to change jobs to accommodate the needs of their child than other parents [72]. A recent European survey of the parents of children with ADHD and matched controls found that having a child with ADHD is associated with increased time demands throughout the day related to disruptive, impulsive, and disorganized behavior [71]. Disruption of family routines and parent interactions with other children were cited as additional problems. What probably compounds parenting difficulties are situations where mothers or fathers have ADHD themselves, resulting in their reacting more impulsively and impatiently to their children than parents without adult ADHD.

Quantifying the costs of pediatric ADHD

Although numerous studies have attempted to document impairments in functioning associated with ADHD, we are aware of only one that tried to estimate the total costs of illness of child–adolescent ADHD. That study, which was carried out by Pelham and colleagues [50], reviewed the results of 13 reports on the costs of ADHD in the domains of health care, special education, parental work loss, and juvenile justice. Results were synthesized across these published reports to estimate annual per-patient costs across these areas. These estimated costs averaged $12 005–17 458 per patient per year in the USA.

Sociodemographic correlates

Gender differences in ADHD include a higher prevalence among boys than girls and a higher relative prevalence of the predominantly inattentive subtype among girls than boys [73]. Although earlier estimates indicated a male-to-female ratio of 9:1, a recent meta-analysis of worldwide studies estimated that the ratio is 2.45:1 among non-referred community samples [8]. This finding suggests that previously reported higher ratios may have been a function of referral or treatment bias, as it is known that a higher proportion of boys than girls with ADHD receive treatment [74].

There does not seem to be a significant association of ADHD prevalence with either race-ethnicity or parent socioeconomic status. However, as noted above, ADHD prevalence is related to age, with up to half of childhood cases remitting by the end of adolescence. Inattentive symptoms tend to persist more than those of hyperactivity–impulsivity, resulting in the proportion of adolescent cases with a predominantly inattentive symptom profile being higher than among childhood cases. However, as detailed below, the available evidence suggests that remitted adolescent cases often continue to have clinically significant residual symptoms, which means that they might more accurately be characterized as in partial remission than full remission.

Adult ADHD

Prevalence

Although it has long been known from clinical follow-up studies that children with ADHD often continue to have symptoms in adulthood [75] and that adults with a history of pediatric ADHD have a comparatively high prevalence of other mental disorders that develop subsequent to ADHD and might be, to some extent, consequences of primary ADHD [76], there is much less agreement about the extent to which ADHD persists as a disorder in adulthood [77, 78]. As the traditional view was that ADHD remitted in the transition to adulthood as part of the natural process of childhood impulsivity resolving with maturation [3], adult ADHD was not included in any of the major psychiatric epidemiological surveys carried out in the 1980s and 1990s in response to the landmark Epidemiologic Catchment Area (ECA) study [79, 80]. However, prevalence estimates have been generated by more recent studies based on three different approaches: indirect assessments, screening assessments, and direct assessments.

Indirect assessments of prevalence

One way to obtain an accurate prevalence estimate of adult ADHD is to build on the firmer set of prevalence estimates of pediatric ADHD with information about persistence into adulthood. A number of early studies did this by following up clinical samples of youth treated for ADHD to determine how many of them continued to meet criteria in adulthood. A limitation in doing this, of course, is that adults whose childhood ADHD was treated might have a lower prevalence of adult ADHD than adults whose ADHD was not treated. On the other hand, the low treatment rate of ADHD at the time these studies were initiated means that the children studied might have been especially severe cases with atypically high persistence [4]. The fact that diagnostic criteria for ADHD at baseline in these studies differed from current criteria raises further questions. Another limitation is that baseline cases lost to follow-up are known to represent a healthier group than those who participate [81], presumably biasing estimates of persistence upwards.

Even in the face of all these limitations, information about the persistence of treated pediatric ADHD into adulthood could be useful. An influential meta-analysis of the first generation of these clinical follow-up studies carried out by Hill and Schoener [82] is usually cited in support of the view that adult ADHD is rare. That report, which synthesized the results of nine prospective studies of children who were diagnosed with ADHD and subsequently followed for between 4 and 16 years into early adulthood, concluded that

ADHD prevalence decreases by approximately 50% every 5 years. Based on this conclusion, adult ADHD was projected to have a prevalence of less than 1% by age 40.

Critics of Hill and Schoener's work noted a number of methodological flaws (e.g., small number of studies, non-representative studies, inappropriate statistical model, sample attrition, reporting bias) that could have introduced bias into their estimate of ADHD persistence [4, 83]. In addition, Hill and Schoener required full diagnostic criteria to qualify for a diagnosis of adult ADHD even though subsequent research showed that many adults with a history of childhood ADHD continue to have clinically significant impairment associated with remaining symptoms even when those symptoms do not meet full diagnostic criteria [84]. Based on these problems, Faraone and colleagues [85] carried out a second meta-analysis that deviated from the Hill and Schoener approach in distinguishing between syndromal and sub-syndromal persistence of adult ADHD. The analysis showed, consistent with Hill and Schoener, that while only a relatively small proportion of cases (approximately 15%) in the studies examined continued to meet full criteria for ADHD in early adulthood, a majority (approximately two-thirds) continued to have enough symptoms and impairment to qualify for a DSM-IV diagnosis of ADHD in partial remission. These results suggest, then, that the population prevalence of broadly defined ADHD in early adulthood might be as much as two-thirds as high as the prevalence in childhood. It is noteworthy, though, that the follow-up studies examined by Faraone et al. included clinical samples in which the most serious childhood cases are presumably over-represented. This is important because of evidence that severity of childhood symptoms strongly predicts adult ADHD persistence [86].

Screening assessments of prevalence

Another way to estimate the prevalence of adult ADHD is to screen for the disorder in samples of the general population. Two important studies of that sort were done by Faraone and Biederman [87] and Kooij et al. [88]. Faraone and Biederman carried out a telephone survey with 966 adults in the USA that used semi-structured research clinical interviews to assess adult ADHD using DSM-IV criteria. The authors estimated that 2.9% of respondents met full DSM-IV criteria for ADHD and that 16.4% met subthreshold criteria [87]. Kooij *et al.* carried out a self-report survey of a representative sample of 1813 adults selected from an automated primary care physician registry in the Netherlands [88]. A fully structured questionnaire was used to estimate the prevalence of adult ADHD. No clinical follow-up interviews were carried out to validate these self-reports. The authors estimated the prevalence of adult ADHD to be 1.0% when full DSM-IV criteria were required and 2.5% when the criteria were relaxed to require four rather than six current symptoms.

Direct assessments of prevalence

A more definitive way to assess prevalence is to include adult ADHD in large-scale community epidemiological surveys of mental disorders. As noted above, this was not done in the epidemiological surveys carried out in the wake of the landmark ECA study. However, the more recent World Health Organization (WHO) World Mental Health (WMH) surveys [89] did include an assessment of adult ADHD. The WMH surveys are a series of coordinated large-scale community epidemiological surveys administered in nearly two dozen countries throughout the world in an effort to obtain information for health policy planning purposes. A fully structured retrospective assessment of childhood ADHD and a comparable assessment of current adult ADHD were both included in the WMH surveys as part of the revised WHO Composite International Diagnostic Interview (CIDI) [90]. The estimated prevalence of DSM-IV adult ADHD was 4.4% in the US WMH survey [55] and 3.4% (range: 1.2–7.3%) pooled across all 10 surveys (Table 3.1) [54]. Prevalence estimates were significantly higher than this average in France (7.3%) and significantly lower in Colombia, Lebanon, Mexico, and Spain (1.2–1.9%).

Importantly, a blinded clinical reappraisal study was carried out in a probability subsample of WMH respondents using the Adult ADHD Clinical Diagnostic Scale version 1.2 (ACDS v1.2) [91, 92], a semi-structured interview that includes the ADHD Rating Scale (ADHD-RS) [93] for childhood ADHD and an adaptation of the ADHD-RS to assess current adult ADHD [55]. The ADHD-RS has been used in clinical trials of adult ADHD [94, 95]. A strong association (with an area under the receiver operating characteristic curve of 0.86) was found between the questions about ADHD in the WMH assessment and

Table 3.1. Estimated prevalence of DSM-IV adult ADHD in community surveys carried out across 10 countries in the WHO World Mental Health Survey Initiative

	%	(Standard error [se])	(n)
Belgium	4.1	(1.5)	(486)
Colombia	1.9[*]	(0.5)	(1731)
France	7.3[**]	(1.8)	(727)
Germany	3.1	(0.8)	(621)
Italy	2.8	(0.6)	(853)
Lebanon	1.8[*]	(0.7)	(595)
Mexico	1.9[*]	(0.4)	(1736)
Netherlands	5.0	(1.6)	(516)
Spain	1.2[*]	(0.6)	(960)
USA	5.2	(0.6)	(3197)
Total	3.4	(0.4)	(11 422)

[*] The upper end of the 95% confidence interval of this estimate is below the prevalence estimate for the total sample.
[**] The lower end of the 95% confidence interval of this estimate is above the prevalence estimate for the total sample.
Source: Originally appeared in: Fayyad J, de Graaf R, Kessler RC, *et al*. Cross-national prevalence and correlates of adult attention-deficit hyperactivity disorder. *Br J Psychiatry*. 2007;**190**(5):402–9. ©2007 The Royal College of Psychiatrists. Used with permission.

the clinical diagnoses, confirming the accuracy of the WMH assessment.

The appropriateness of current diagnostic criteria for adult ADHD

All the above prevalence estimates of adult ADHD can be criticized based on the claim that existing diagnostic criteria are not valid. Diagnostic criteria for ADHD were originally developed for children [96, 97]. We know that the clinical profile and manifestations of ADHD evolve with age [4, 98, 99], raising questions about the most appropriate diagnostic criteria for adults. Many studies have found that symptoms of hyperactivity and impulsivity decline with age, although they persist in some cases and sometimes are the presenting complaints of adult ADHD, while deficits in attention persist and become more varied among adult cases [84, 100–106]. These results raise the possibility that the symptoms of adult ADHD might profitably be modified in future DSM and ICD revisions. Indeed, in anticipation of planned revisions of this type in DSM-5 and ICD-11, several proposals were made in recent years to improve accuracy of assessment of adult ADHD by increasing the variety of symptoms assessed [107], reducing the severity threshold [108], or reducing the DSM-IV six-of-nine symptom requirement [88]. As it happened, DSM-5 did reduce the number of required symptoms from six to five for adults and added new examples of adult ADHD symptom profiles to assist clinicians in diagnosis, but did not adopt any of the recommendations for broadening symptoms. The reduction in number of symptoms means that the prevalence estimates in the studies reviewed here are conservative with regard to DSM-5 criteria.

Only a few of the recommendations for revising diagnostic criteria have been based on empirical studies [100, 109, 110]. Barkley and colleagues evaluated patients at an ADHD clinic, clinic controls, and a convenience sample of community controls [100]. They compared the predictive validity of DSM-IV and theoretically derived non-DSM symptoms of adult ADHD in distinguishing between cases and non-cases. Of the seven discriminating items found in that study, only one was a DSM-IV symptom, while most others described deficits in EF. Faraone and colleagues [109] compared ADHD and non-ADHD adults on the same items used by Barkley et al. and concluded that the Barkley algorithm was an efficient predictor of DSM-IV adult ADHD. Kessler et al. administered clinical interviews to subsamples of respondents in two community epidemiological surveys with enriched subsamples of those who screened positive for a history of ADHD [19]. Consistent with previous studies, they found that symptoms of inattention were more common than those of hyperactivity–impulsivity among adult cases, but factor analysis also found a factor of EF problems. Stepwise logistic regression found EF problems to be the most consistent and discriminating predictors of adult DSM-IV ADHD based on the fact that inattention-hyperactivity and impulsivity were strongly comorbid with other adult mental disorders and EF problems were more specific to adult ADHD. The authors conclude that the number of EF symptoms used to define adult ADHD should be increased in the upcoming DSM and ICD revisions.

Predictors of the persistence of pediatric ADHD into adulthood

Given the high persistence of ADHD into adulthood, estimated to be in the range 30–60% of pediatric cases

in the WMH data, predictors of persistence become of considerable interest. Although these predictors have been examined in several clinical follow-up studies, these studies focused mainly on associated features of childhood ADHD [111, 112] with number and severity of childhood symptoms found to be the strongest predictors of adult persistence. Two other prospective studies examined a broader set of predictors [101, 102], but those studies were limited to follow-ups into adolescence rather than adulthood. History of ADHD in relatives, presence of comorbid childhood disorders (especially CD), and childhood psychosocial adversities were the strongest predictors of persistence in these studies.

The same limitations of clinical follow-up samples in estimating adult prevalence (i.e., sample selection bias, attrition bias, and the fact that course of illness can be affected by early intervention) also limit analysis of predictors of adult persistence in these studies. We are aware of only one general population study that addressed these limitations [104]. That study, which was based on the WMH data, used retrospective adult reports to assess childhood predictors of adult ADHD persistence. The results could have been biased by recall error, but nonetheless provide a useful counterpoint to results based on clinical follow-up studies. These results showed that persistence was unrelated to gender after controlling for childhood ADHD symptom profile, but strongly related to that symptom profile, with the highest persistence associated with the attentional plus impulsive–hyperactive type compared to the lowest associated with the impulsive–hyperactive type.

Other significant predictors of persistence included childhood ADHD symptom severity (more severe symptoms were associated with high persistence), high comorbidity (i.e., three or more child–adolescent disorders in addition to ADHD), and parental psychopathology (anxiety-mood and antisocial personality disorders). Childhood adversities (e.g., physical abuse, sexual abuse, neglect) and traumatic life events (e.g., traumatic death of a loved one, exposure to a natural or man-made disaster), in comparison, did not predict persistence. It is noteworthy that the predictive associations involving comorbid child–adolescent disorders might indicate aspects of pediatric ADHD symptom severity that were not assessed as accurately in the retrospective WMH reports as in the prospective clinical studies. Another possibility is that high comorbidity

Table 3.2. Bivariate comorbidity between DSM-IV adult ADHD and other DSM-IV disorders in the pooled WHO World Mental Health surveys (n = 11 422)[1]

	ADHD/CO[2]		CO/ADHD[2]			
	%	(se)	%	(se)	OR	(95% CI)
I. Classes of co-occurring disorders						
Mood	11.1	(1.2)	24.8	(2.6)	3.9[*]	(3.0–5.1)
Anxiety	9.9	(1.0)	38.1	(3.1)	4.0[*]	(3.0–5.2)
Substance	12.5	(2.3)	11.1	(2.0)	4.0[*]	(2.8–5.8)
II. Number of co-occurring disorders						
Exactly one	5.4	(0.7)	20.4	(2.1)	1.6[*]	(1.3–2.1)
Exactly two	10.3	(1.5)	12.9	(1.6)	3.2[*]	(2.4–4.2)
Three or more	20.3	(2.4)	16.2	(2.4)	7.2[*]	(5.1–10.2)
Any	8.5	(0.8)	49.5	(3.6)	3.9[*]	(3.0–5.2)

[*] Significant at the 0.05 level, two-sided test.
[1] Based on bivariate logistic regression equations.
[2] The percentages in the ADHD/CO column are the conditional prevalence estimates of adult ADHD in the subsamples of respondents with the comorbid disorders. The percentages in the CO/ADHD column are the conditional prevalence estimates of the co-occurring disorders in the subsample of respondents with adult ADHD.
Source: Originally appeared in: Fayyad J, de Graaf R, Kessler RC, *et al.* Cross-national prevalence and correlates of adult attention-deficit hyperactivity disorder. *Br J Psychiatry.* 2007;**190**(5):402–9. ©2007 The Royal College of Psychiatrists. Used with permission.

somehow interferes with the processes that bring about recovery from ADHD in adolescence. Prospective studies that use information about adolescent severity and comorbidity to predict adult persistence will be needed to investigate this possibility and, if positive, to determine if successful treatment of secondary comorbid child–adolescent disorders might help reduce risk of persistence of ADHD into adulthood.

Comorbidity of adult ADHD with other mental disorders

Adult ADHD has been found to be significantly comorbid with a wide range of other DSM-IV disorders both in clinical [76, 113] and epidemiological [54, 55] samples. In one large US community epidemiological survey [55], odds ratios (ORs) for adult ADHD in association with other DSM-IV disorders were in the range 3.3–6.1 for mood disorders, 2.6–5.3 for anxiety disorders, 2.1–14.9 for substance disorders, and 3.8–9.8 for disruptive behavior disorders. Very strong ORs with 12-month drug dependence (14.9) and ODD (9.8) were especially noteworthy. ORs were generally larger for 12-month than lifetime prevalence, suggesting indirectly that adult ADHD is associated not only with the occurrence but also the persistence of comorbid disorders.

Very similar patterns were found cross-nationally in the WMH surveys (Table 3.2) [54]. A dose–response relationship was also found between ADHD and a number of other disorders, with the highest OR associated with having three or more other disorders. Within-country patterns in the WMH data were very similar to those in the combined sample, with a predominantly positive sign pattern (95% of within-country ORs greater than 1.0) and 56% of the within-country ORs significant at the 0.05 level. As one might expect with a disorder that has as early an age of onset as ADHD, comparison of age-of-onset reports in the WMH data showed that the comorbidity of adult ADHD with other adult DSM-IV disorders is due largely to temporally primary ADHD predicting subsequent first onset of later disorders (Table 3.3). The only exception is comorbid-specific phobia, which tends to have an earlier age of onset than ADHD.

The controversy noted earlier about comorbidity between pediatric ADHD and BPD extends as well to adult ADHD [114, 115]. A recent systematic literature review found few rigorous studies [116], but concluded that this type of comorbidity is quite common among adults and associated with severe-persistent course of ADHD. These studies also suggested that ADHD–BPD comorbidity in adulthood is commonly associated with *multimorbidity*, that is, with the co-occurrence of a number of different disorders, including comorbid

Table 3.3. Temporal priorities in first onset of comorbid DSM-IV adult ADHD and other DSM-IV disorders in the pooled WHO World Mental Health surveys

Co-occurring disorder	ADHD first		Other disorder first		Both same year		
	%	(se)	%	(se)	%	(se)	(n)[1]
Mood disorder	85.6	(2.5)	9.5	(2.4)	4.9	(1.3)	(310)
Anxiety disorder	49.6	(3.9)	41.2	(4.0)	9.2	(2.0)	(312)
Specific phobia	34.3	(5.3)	54.8	(5.1)	11.0	(2.8)	(185)
Any other anxiety disorder	68.5	(4.1)	19.7	(3.2)	11.8	(2.2)	(244)
Substance disorder	99.0	(0.7)	0.5	(0.5)	0.4	(0.4)	(145)

[1] Number of respondents with co-occurrence of adult ADHD and the class of disorders in the row.
Source: Originally appeared in: Fayyad J, de Graaf R, Kessler RC, *et al*. Cross-national prevalence and correlates of adult attention-deficit hyperactivity disorder. *Br J Psychiatry*. 2007;**190**(5):402–9. ©2007 The Royal College of Psychiatrists. Used with permission.

anxiety, substance, and disruptive behavior disorders. This high comorbidity creates treatment challenges and makes it difficult to sort out the relative importance of individual component disorders in naturalistic studies. Given the high persistence and severity of multimorbid ADHD–BPD, further research is needed on prevalence, correlates, and treatment response.

Impairments associated with adult ADHD

Clinical research consistently documents that adult ADHD is associated with considerable impairment in many areas of role functioning, including unemployment, underemployment, marital disruption, and social isolation [117]. A large US community survey of adults, for example, found respondents with ADHD to have significantly more unemployment, job changes, arrests, and divorces than age/sex-matched controls [118]. Another large US survey of a sample of 21 000 adult managed care subscribers screened for adult ADHD and then evaluated for numerous aspects of functional and psychosocial impairment [119]. Subscribers with undiagnosed ADHD were found to have significantly more difficulties in emotional and interpersonal functioning and higher rates of physical and mental comorbidity than controls.

Consistent with this evidence, the WMH surveys found that adult ADHD was associated with significantly elevated ORs (95% confidence intervals) of disability on the WHO Disability Assessment Schedule (http://who.int/icidh/whodas) dimensions of mobility (2.2 [1.6–2.9]), cognition (3.9 [2.8–5.4]), high days out of role (2.6 [2.0–3.5]), and social functioning (3.1 [2.1–4.5]) [54]. Within-country patterns were very similar to those in the combined sample, with only a handful of within-country ORs differing significantly from the

cross-national averages. Objective tests of neurocognitive functioning document substantial deficits among adults with ADHD that might underlie these disabilities [120].

A separate WMH report examined the work performance of employed people with and without adult ADHD [121]. Across countries, employees with ADHD were found to have decrements in work performance equivalent to an average of 22 annual days of excess lost work. More than half this lost work performance was associated with reduced quantity/quality of work performance on days at work rather than with excess days out of work. No between-occupation difference was found in the association between ADHD and work performance.

As with pediatric ADHD, adult ADHD is associated with significantly elevated rates of healthcare utilization for a wide range of conditions [122, 123]. Accidents and injuries, in particular, are much more common among adults with than without ADHD [124]. Controlled studies of simulated performance tasks suggest that this elevated accident/injury risk is linked primarily to inattentiveness when performing routine tasks that carry injury risk [125].

Sociodemographic correlates

As noted in the last section, persistence of pediatric ADHD into adulthood is not related to gender after controlling for pediatric symptom profiles. However, as noted above, these symptom profiles are associated with gender, as girls are more likely than boys to have a primarily inattentive symptom profile and less likely than boys to have a predominantly impulsive–hyperactive symptom profile. As the predominantly impulsive–hyperactive profile is least likely to persist into adulthood, we would expect that the gender difference in adult ADHD would be smaller than the gender difference in pediatric ADHD. Community epidemiological data show that this is the case, as the elevated risk of adult ADHD among men versus women is only about 50% that of the male:female risk of pediatric ADHD [54]. One plausible explanation for this difference is that females with ADHD are more likely than males to have predominantly inattentive symptoms and that these symptoms are more likely to persist into adulthood than are the impulsive–hyperactive symptoms more characteristic of males. Results from recent analyses of adult ADHD symptom subtype data in an epidemiological study of the US general population are consistent with this explanation [19].

Some controversy exists about the possibility that the prevalence of ADHD among adult women might be even higher than this relative to men due to hyperactivity–impulsivity and their adverse consequences being less prominent among female than male cases and the recognition of female cases consequently being lower than the recognition of male cases [126]. However, although future nosological analyses aimed at revising diagnostic criteria for adult ADHD might find that current criteria do, in fact, under-represent the symptoms of women relative to those of men, available evidence from epidemiological surveys using current DSM-IV criteria find no evidence for this being the case.

Because of the adverse effect of childhood–adolescent ADHD on educational attainment, adult ADHD is also associated with reduced socioeconomic status. This could be due to low educational achievement or to the impairments in work performance with adult ADHD [54]. Adults with ADHD also appear to have high rates of marital disruption, presumably associated with difficulties in interpersonal relationships associated with inattention and impulsivity [54].

Treatment of adult ADHD

The most reliable data on the treatment of adult ADHD come from the WMH surveys, where the proportion of respondents with 12-month adult ADHD who reported receiving treatment for emotional problems at some time in the past 12 months differed markedly across countries [54]. The highest proportion of cases receiving treatment was in the USA, where nearly half (49.7%) reported getting some type of care, followed by roughly half as many (19.9–23.8%)

receiving treatment in three of the European countries (Belgium, the Netherlands, and Spain), roughly half this number (9.4–12.4%) in four other countries (Colombia, France, Germany, and Mexico), and only 1.1% in Lebanon. The majority of cases in treatment were seen in the specialty mental health sector in all countries other than France and Italy, where the majority were seen in the general medical sector. Cases in treatment were generally not seen for problems with attention, concentration, impulsivity, or hyperactivity, but rather for other comorbid emotional and behavioral problems. In other words, their ADHD was overlooked even when they obtained treatment for a mental disorder. Even in the USA, where close to half the survey respondents with 12-month adult ADHD received treatment for some type of emotional problem, only 10.9% received treatment specifically for their ADHD [54].

The total cost of ADHD

Bernfort et al. proposed a model in which the total cost of ADHD to society can be calculated by taking into consideration the cost of ADHD during childhood and adolescence in addition to the cost in adulthood derived from probabilities of unwanted outcomes such as criminality, material damage, lost life years, production loss, healthcare consumption, and other indirect costs [127]. The authors concluded, though, that currently available data are too imprecise to make accurate quantitative estimates. Birnbaum and colleagues nonetheless attempted to estimate the costs of all ADHD (both childhood–adolescent and adult) in the USA for a limited set of cost domains (health care and work loss) by combining data from a number of published reports with data from a case–control sample of roughly 300 000 health plan subscribers [122]. Excess per capita healthcare and work loss costs of *treated* ADHD patients (both children and adults) and their family members were calculated using administrative claims data. The excess costs of *untreated* individuals with ADHD and their family members were estimated based on survey data regarding prevalence and extrapolation from claims data for estimates of cost. The total annual cost of ADHD was estimated in this way to be somewhat more than $30 billion.

Less than one-fourth (23%) of this total estimated cost of ADHD was attributed to children or adolescents. The other 77% was attributed to adult ADHD. On reflection this might not seem surprising in light of the fact that the number of adults is five times the number of children and adolescents in the US population, while the estimated prevalence of ADHD is 30–60% as high among adults as children–adolescents. However, this dominance of costs associated with adult ADHD is striking in that it deviates so markedly from the major focus of clinicians on ADHD among youth rather than adults. Another somewhat surprising result of the Birnbaum *et al.* analysis is that less than 5% of the total estimated costs of ADHD were due to direct costs of treating ADHD. A much higher proportion (one-third of the total) was attributed to other healthcare costs of people with ADHD, treatment of patients, and an additional roughly comparable component to excess healthcare costs of family members of people with ADHD. Close to 10% of the total estimated costs of ADHD, finally, were attributed to income loss associated with reduced work due to ADHD (either the work loss of parents of children with ADHD or of adults with ADHD).

Discussion

The data reviewed in this chapter document clearly that ADHD is a commonly occurring and seriously impairing childhood and adolescent disorder in many parts of the world; that pediatric ADHD is associated with the subsequent onset and persistence of a number of secondary comorbid mental disorders in childhood, adolescence, and adulthood; and that the persistence of ADHD into adulthood, which occurs in 30–60% of pediatric cases, is associated with substantial subsequent impairment. Although some of the impairment associated with adult ADHD is accounted for by comorbid conditions, this might be considered an indirect effect of persistent ADHD to the extent that the latter is a causal risk factor for the onset, persistence, and severity of secondary adult mental disorders.

The typically earlier age of onset of ADHD than comorbid disorders raises the question whether early successful treatment of pediatric ADHD might influence the onset and course of secondary disorders. This question has not so far been investigated in controlled studies. However, suggestive evidence can be found in a naturalistic study of boys who were referred in childhood for the treatment of ADHD and then followed for a decade into young adulthood [128]. This follow-up study showed that the boys who received stimulant treatment for their ADHD as children were

significantly less likely than other boys to go on to develop subsequent anxiety, mood, and disruptive behavior disorders.

A related question is whether treatment of adult ADHD would have an effect on the persistence or severity of comorbid adult disorders. We are aware of no research that has addressed this question. The results reviewed here highlight the importance of carrying out such studies by virtue of the fact that comorbidity is quite common in adult ADHD and adult ADHD typically goes undetected and untreated even among adults who are in treatment for comorbid adult mental disorders.

The results reported above regarding the adverse effects of adult ADHD on work performance taken together with the results showing that most adult ADHD goes untreated raise the question whether ADHD might be a candidate for targeted workplace screening and treatment. Short screening scales that are both sensitive and specific for adult ADHD exist [103, 129]. But would it be cost-effective from the employer perspective to implement workplace screening programs with such a scale to detect and provide treatment for workers with ADHD? In coming to an answer to this question, it is important to note that ADHD has a nontrivial prevalence in the workplace along with high workplace costs. Therapies that might be cost-effective in reducing these adverse workplace effects exist and have been shown to promote improvements in some objective aspects of role performance [130–132]. It is far from clear, though, whether workplace screening, outreach, and treatment would be cost-effective in reducing the workplace costs of ADHD. Effectiveness trials are needed to evaluate this question.

Although the results reviewed here could be used to make a strong argument that most of the societal burdens of ADHD are associated with adult rather than pediatric cases, the epidemiological literature on adult ADHD is very limited. Only a few epidemiological studies of adult ADHD exist and none of these studies included an assessment of ADHD in partial remission or addressed the fact that uncertainties exist about the appropriate criteria for assessment of adult ADHD. Another methodological challenge that needs to be resolved in future studies concerns the mode of assessing adult ADHD. Childhood ADHD is diagnosed largely on the basis of parent and teacher reports rather than self-reports because parents and teachers are both in good positions to observe child behavior and because children with ADHD often have little insight into the severity of their symptoms [133]. The situation is different for adults, where there is great variability in the extent to which other people observe their behavior and where access to reliable informants varies with the respondent's marital status, occupational status, and social networks, making it necessary as a practical matter to base assessment largely on self-reports [134]. Epidemiological studies of adult ADHD have consequently relied almost entirely on self-reports. This might be problematic, as some methodological studies comparing adult self-reports versus informant reports of ADHD symptoms have documented a similar pattern of disagreement as in studies of child self-reports versus informant reports, with informants reporting higher symptom levels than focal respondents [111, 135]. This suggests that self-report scales might underestimate the true prevalence of adult ADHD. If so, it might be necessary to develop a new paradigm for assessing adult ADHD.

This last issue could be difficult to address because of the practical impossibility of obtaining informant reports on adult emotional functioning in representative community epidemiological surveys other than through reports provided by spouses: a difficulty exacerbated by the fact that a comparatively high proportion of people with adult ADHD are unmarried. This concern is somewhat reduced by the fact that the one methodological study of adult self versus informant ADHD symptom report carried out in a non-clinical sample found fairly strong associations between the two reports and no self versus informant difference in reported symptom severity [136]. This problem is presumably greater in obtaining retrospective adult assessments of childhood ADHD, which are required for a diagnosis of adult ADHD. There is evidence, based on prospective studies that compare adult retrospective reports with baseline evaluations made in childhood, that such retrospective reports can be inaccurate in their particulars even when they are based on clinical interviews, although accuracy can be enhanced through use of structured assessments [78]. It is also important to note that follow-up studies show that the vast majority of adults who were diagnosed with ADHD as children retrospectively report at least some symptoms of childhood ADHD [137]. A more serious problem might be that a meaningful minority of adults known not to have had hyperactivity in childhood retrospectively recalled that they had childhood

symptoms of ADHD [137]. Methodological research is needed to sort out these uncertainties in order to improve the validity of community epidemiological studies of adult ADHD.

An important opportunity for future epidemiological research on adult ADHD lies in studies of workplace prevalence and indirect costs, as it would presumably be more tractable to obtain supervisor and coworker informant reports in such a setting than informant reports in community samples. Furthermore, emerging evidence about the value of objective neurocognitive tests that might be easier to implement in workplace than community samples suggests that these tests might be useful in detecting cases that go undetected by self-report [6]. The enormous costs of ADHD to the workplace would also increase interest in making the workplace a focus of research attention as well as providing opportunities for obtaining unique objective information on the effects of ADHD on role functioning and possibly even information on the effects of treatment on objective measures of role functioning.

Acknowledgments

This chapter was prepared as part of the work of the World Health Organization World Mental Health (WMH) Survey Initiative ADHD workgroup. The centralized activities of WMH are supported by the US National Institute of Mental Health (NIMH; R01 MH070884), the John D. and Catherine T. MacArthur Foundation, the Pfizer Foundation, the US Public Health Service (R13-MH066849, R01-MH069864, and R01 DA016558), the Fogarty International Center (FIRCA R03-TW006481), the Pan American Health Organization, Eli Lilly and Company, Ortho-McNeil Pharmaceutical, GlaxoSmithKline, and Bristol-Myers Squibb. We thank the staff of the WMH Data Collection and Data Analysis Coordination Centres for assistance with instrumentation, fieldwork, and consultation on data analysis.

Portions of this paper appeared previously in: Fayyad J, de Graaf R, Kessler RC, *et al.* Cross-national prevalence and correlates of adult attention-deficit hyperactivity disorder. *Br J Psychiatry.* 2007; **190**(5):402–9. © 2007 The Royal College of Psychiatrists; Kessler RC, Green JG, Adler LA, *et al.* Structure and diagnosis of adult attention-deficit/hyperactivity disorder: Analysis of expanded symptom criteria from the Adult ADHD Clinical Diagnostic

Scale. *Arch Gen Psychiatry.* 2010;**67**(11):1168–78. © 2010 American Medical Association; Lara C, Fayyad J, de Graaf R, *et al.* Childhood predictors of adult attention-deficit/hyperactivity disorder: results from the World Health Organization World Mental Health Survey Initiative. *Biol Psychiatry.* 2009; **65**(1):46–54. © 2009 Elsevier B.V.; de Graaf R, Kessler RC, Fayyad J. The prevalence and effects of adult attention-deficit/hyperactivity disorder (ADHD) on the performance of workers: results from the WHO World Mental Health Survey Initiative. *Occup Environ Med.* 2008;**65**(12):835–42. © 2008 BMJ Publishing Group; and Kessler RC, Adler L, Barkley R. The prevalence and correlates of adult ADHD. In: Buitelaar JK, Kan CC, Asherson P, eds. *ADHD in Adults.* Cambridge: Cambridge University Press. 2011; 9–17. © 2011 Cambridge University Press. All rights reserved. All used with permission.

References

1. Bird HR, Canino G, Rubio-Stipec M, *et al.* Estimates of the prevalence of childhood maladjustment in a community survey in Puerto Rico. The use of combined measures. *Arch Gen Psychiatry.* 1988; **45**(12):1120–6.

2. Shekim WO, Kashani J, Beck N, *et al.* The prevalence of attention deficit disorders in a rural midwestern community sample of nine-year-old children. *J Am Acad Child Psychiatry.* 1985;**24**(6):765–70.

3. Cantwell DP. Hyperactive children have grown up. What have we learned about what happens to them? *Arch Gen Psychiatry.* 1985;**42**(10):1026–8.

4. Mannuzza S, Klein RG, Moulton JL, 3rd. Persistence of attention-deficit/hyperactivity disorder into adulthood: what have we learned from the prospective follow-up studies? *J Atten Disord.* 2003;**7**(2):93–100.

5. Wilens TE, Faraone SV, Biederman J. Attention-deficit/hyperactivity disorder in adults. *JAMA.* 2004;**292**(5):619–23.

6. McGough JJ, Barkley RA. Diagnostic controversies in adult attention deficit hyperactivity disorder. *Am J Psychiatry.* 2004;**161**(11):1948–56.

7. Polanczyk G, de Lima MS, Horta BL, *et al.* The worldwide prevalence of ADHD: a systematic review and metaregression analysis. *Am J Psychiatry.* 2007; **164**(6):942–8.

8. Polanczyk G, Jensen P. Epidemiologic considerations in attention deficit hyperactivity disorder: a review and update. *Child Adolesc Psychiatr Clin N Am.* 2008;**17**(2):245–60, vii.

9. Scahill L, Schwab-Stone M. Epidemiology of ADHD in school-age children. *Child Adolesc Psychiatr Clin N Am.* 2000;**9**(3):541–55, vii.

10. Farah LG, Fayyad JA, Eapen V, *et al.* ADHD in the Arab world: a review of epidemiologic studies. *J Atten Disord.* 2009;**13**(3):211–22.

11. Faraone SV, Sergeant J, Gillberg C, *et al.* The worldwide prevalence of ADHD: is it an American condition? *World Psychiatry.* 2003;**2**(2):104–13.

12. World Health Organization. *International Statistical Classification of Diseases and Related Health Problems, 10th Revision (ICD-10).* Geneva, Switzerland: World Health Organization; 1992.

13. American Psychiatric Association. *Diagnostic and Statistical Manual of Mental Disorders,* 4th edn (DSM-IV). Washington, DC: American Psychiatric Association; 1994.

14. American Psychiatric Association. *Diagnostic and Statistical Manual of Mental Disorders,* 3rd edn, rev (DSM-III-R). Washington, DC: American Psychiatric Association; 1987.

15. Lahey BB, Pelham WE, Loney J, *et al.* Instability of the DSM-IV subtypes of ADHD from preschool through elementary school. *Arch Gen Psychiatry.* 2005;**62**(8): 896–902.

16. Grizenko N, Paci M, Joober R. Is the inattentive subtype of ADHD different from the combined/hyperactive subtype? *J Atten Disord.* 2010;**13**(6): 649–57.

17. Diamond A. Attention-deficit disorder (attention-deficit/hyperactivity disorder without hyperactivity): a neurobiologically and behaviorally distinct disorder from attention-deficit/hyperactivity disorder (with hyperactivity). *Dev Psychopathol.* 2005;**17**(3): 807–25.

18. Baeyens D, Roeyers H, Walle JV. Subtypes of attention-deficit/hyperactivity disorder (ADHD): distinct or related disorders across measurement levels? *Child Psychiatry Hum Dev.* 2006;**36**(4):403–17.

19. Kessler RC, Green JG, Adler LA, *et al.* Structure and diagnosis of adult attention-deficit/hyperactivity disorder: analysis of expanded symptom criteria from the Adult ADHD Clinical Diagnostic Scale. *Arch Gen Psychiatry.* 2010;**67**(11):1168–78.

20. Angold A, Costello EJ, Erkanli A. Comorbidity. *J Child Psychol Psychiatry.* 1999;**40**(1):57–87.

21. Fergusson DM, Horwood LJ, Lynskey MT. Prevalence and comorbidity of DSM-III-R diagnoses in a birth cohort of 15 year olds. *J Am Acad Child Adolesc Psychiatry.* 1993;**32**(6):1127–34.

22. Lahey BB, Rathouz PJ, Van Hulle C, *et al.* Testing structural models of DSM-IV symptoms of common

forms of child and adolescent psychopathology. *J Abnorm Child Psychol*. 2008;**36**(2):187–206.

23. Stein MB, Fuetsch M, Muller N, *et al*. Social anxiety disorder and the risk of depression: a prospective community study of adolescents and young adults. *Arch Gen Psychiatry*. 2001;**58**(3):251–6.

24. McGough JJ, Smalley SL, McCracken JT, *et al*. Psychiatric comorbidity in adult attention deficit hyperactivity disorder: findings from multiplex families. *Am J Psychiatry*. 2005;**162**(9):1621–7.

25. Pliszka SR. Patterns of psychiatric comorbidity with attention-deficit/hyperactivity disorder. *Child Adolesc Psychiatr Clin N Am*. 2000;**9**(3):525–40.

26. Costello EJ, Mustillo S, Erkanli A, *et al*. Prevalence and development of psychiatric disorders in childhood and adolescence. *Arch Gen Psychiatry*. 2003;**60**(8):837–44.

27. Fergusson DM, Boden JM, Horwood LJ. Classification of behavior disorders in adolescence: scaling methods, predictive validity, and gender differences. *J Abnorm Psychol*. 2010;**119**(4):699–712.

28. Taurines R, Schmitt J, Renner T, *et al*. Developmental comorbidity in attention-deficit/hyperactivity disorder. *Atten Defic Hyperact Disord*. 2010;**2**(4): 267–89.

29. Lahey BB, Van Hulle CA, Rathouz PJ, *et al*. Are oppositional-defiant and hyperactive-inattentive symptoms developmental precursors to conduct problems in late childhood?: genetic and environmental links. *J Abnorm Child Psychol*. 2009;**37**(1):45–58.

30. Biederman J. Resolved: mania is mistaken for ADHD in prepubertal children–affirmative. *J Am Acad Child Adolesc Psychiatry*. 1998;**37**(10):1091–3.

31. Klein RG, Pine DS, Klein DF. Resolved: mania is mistaken for ADHD in prepubertal children–negative. *J Am Acad Child Adolesc Psychiatry*. 1998;**37**(10): 1093–6.

32. Biederman J, Faraone S, Mick E, *et al*. Attention-deficit hyperactivity disorder and juvenile mania: an overlooked comorbidity? *J Am Acad Child Adolesc Psychiatry*. 1996;**35**(8):997–1008.

33. Hassan A, Agha SS, Langley K, *et al*. Prevalence of bipolar disorder in children and adolescents with attention-deficit hyperactivity disorder. *Br J Psychiatry*. 2011;**198**(3):195–8.

34. Galanter CA, Leibenluft E. Frontiers between attention deficit hyperactivity disorder and bipolar disorder. *Child Adolesc Psychiatr Clin N Am*. 2008;**17**(2):325–46, viii–ix.

35. Youngstrom EA, Arnold LE, Frazier TW. Bipolar and ADHD comorbidity: both artifact and outgrowth of

shared mechanisms. *Clin Psychol (New York)*. 2010; **17**(4):350–9.

36. Kim EY, Miklowitz DJ. Childhood mania, attention deficit hyperactivity disorder and conduct disorder: a critical review of diagnostic dilemmas. *Bipolar Disord*. 2002;**4**(4):215–25.

37. Sood AB, Razdan A, Weller EB, *et al*. How to differentiate bipolar disorder from attention deficit hyperactivity disorder and other common psychiatric disorders: a guide for clinicians. *Curr Psychiatry Rep*. 2005;**7**(2):98–103.

38. Hack M, Youngstrom EA, Cartar L, *et al*. Behavioral outcomes and evidence of psychopathology among very low birth weight infants at age 20 years. *Pediatrics*. 2004;**114**(4):932–40.

39. Faraone SV, Biederman J, Mennin D, *et al*. Attention-deficit hyperactivity disorder with bipolar disorder: a familial subtype? *J Am Acad Child Adolesc Psychiatry*. 1997;**36**(10):1378–87; discussion 1387–90.

40. Scheffer RE, Kowatch RA, Carmody T, *et al*. Randomized, placebo-controlled trial of mixed amphetamine salts for symptoms of comorbid ADHD in pediatric bipolar disorder after mood stabilization with divalproex sodium. *Am J Psychiatry*. 2005; **162**(1):58–64.

41. Shuai L, Chan RC, Wang Y. Executive function profile of Chinese boys with attention-deficit hyperactivity disorder: different subtypes and comorbidity. *Arch Clin Neuropsychol*. 2011;**26**(2):120–32.

42. Barnett R, Maruff P, Vance A. Neurocognitive function in attention-deficit-hyperactivity disorder with and without comorbid disruptive behaviour disorders. *Aust N Z J Psychiatry*. 2009;**43**(8):722–30.

43. Qian Y, Shuai L, Cao Q, *et al*. Do executive function deficits differentiate between children with attention deficit hyperactivity disorder (ADHD) and ADHD comorbid with oppositional defiant disorder? A cross-cultural study using performance-based tests and the behavior rating inventory of executive function. *Clin Neuropsychol*. 2010;**24**(5):793–810.

44. Geurts HM, Verte S, Oosterlaan J, *et al*. ADHD subtypes: do they differ in their executive functioning profile? *Arch Clin Neuropsychol*. 2005;**20**(4):457–77.

45. Pasini A, Paloscia C, Alessandrelli R, *et al*. Attention and executive functions profile in drug naive ADHD subtypes. *Brain Dev*. 2007;**29**(7):400–8.

46. Barkley RA. Global issues related to the impact of untreated attention-deficit/hyperactivity disorder from childhood to young adulthood. *Postgrad Med*. 2008;**120**(3):48–59.

47. Guevara JP, Mandell DS. Costs associated with attention deficit hyperactivity disorder: overview and

future projections. *Expert Rev Pharmacoecon Outcomes Res.* 2003;**3**(2):201–10.

48. Matza LS, Paramore C, Prasad M. A review of the economic burden of ADHD. *Cost Eff Resour Alloc.* 2005;**3**:5.

49. Minkoff NB. ADHD in managed care: an assessment of the burden of illness and proposed initiatives to improve outcomes. *Am J Manag Care.* 2009;**15** (Suppl 5):S151–9.

50. Pelham WE, Foster EM, Robb JA. The economic impact of attention-deficit/hyperactivity disorder in children and adolescents. *J Pediatr Psychol.* 2007;**32** (6):711–27.

51. Mannuzza S, Klein RG, Bessler A., *et al.* Educational and occupational outcome of hyperactive boys grown up. *J Am Acad Child Adolesc Psychiatry.* 1997;**36**(9):1222–7.

52. Barkley RA. Major life activity and health outcomes associated with attention-deficit/hyperactivity disorder. *J Clin Psychiatry.* 2002;**63**(Suppl 12):10–15.

53. Loe IM, Feldman HM. Academic and educational outcomes of children with ADHD. *J Pediatr Psychol.* 2007;**32**(6):643–54.

54. Fayyad J, De Graaf R, Kessler R, *et al.* Cross-national prevalence and correlates of adult attention-deficit hyperactivity disorder. *Br J Psychiatry.* 2007;**190**(5):402–9.

55. Kessler RC, Adler L, Barkley R, *et al.* The prevalence and correlates of adult ADHD in the United States: results from the National Comorbidity Survey Replication. *Am J Psychiatry.* 2006;**163**(4):716–23.

56. Lahey BB, Pelham WE, Loney J, *et al.* Three-year predictive validity of DSM-IV attention deficit hyperactivity disorder in children diagnosed at 4–6 years of age. *Am J Psychiatry.* 2004;**161**(11):2014–20.

57. Wazana A. Are there injury-prone children? A critical review of the literature. *Can J Psychiatry.* 1997;**42**(6):602–10.

58. McKinlay A, Dalrymple-Alford JC, Horwood LJ, *et al.* Long term psychosocial outcomes after mild head injury in early childhood. *J Neurol Neurosurg Psychiatry.* 2002;**73**(3):281–8.

59. Lynam DR, Miller JD, Miller DJ, *et al.* Testing the relations between impulsivity-related traits, suicidality, and nonsuicidal self-injury: a test of the incremental validity of the UPPS model. *Personal Disord.* 2011;**2**(2):151–60.

60. Karazsia BT, Guilfoyle SM, Wildman BG. The mediating role of hyperactivity and inattention on sex differences in paediatric injury risk. *Child Care Health Dev.* 2012;**38**(3):358–65.

61. Retz W, Rosler M. The relation of ADHD and violent aggression: what can we learn from epidemiological and genetic studies? *Int J Law Psychiatry.* 2009;**32**(4):235–43.

62. Sihvola E, Rose RJ, Dick DM, *et al.* Prospective relationships of ADHD symptoms with developing substance use in a population-derived sample. *Psychol Med.* 2011;**41**(12):2615–23.

63. Oquendo MA, Mann JJ. The biology of impulsivity and suicidality. *Psychiatr Clin North Am.* 2000;**23**(1):11–25.

64. Leibson CL, Long KH. Economic implications of attention-deficit hyperactivity disorder for healthcare systems. *Pharmacoeconomics.* 2003;**21**(17):1239–62.

65. Guevara J, Lozano P, Wickizer T, *et al.* Utilization and cost of health care services for children with attention-deficit/hyperactivity disorder. *Pediatrics.* 2001;**108**(1):71–8.

66. Leibson CL, Katusic SK, Barbaresi, WJ, *et al.* Use and costs of medical care for children and adolescents with and without attention-deficit/hyperactivity disorder. *JAMA.* 2001;**285**(1):60–6.

67. Escobar R, Hervas A, Soutullo C, *et al.* Attention deficit/hyperactivity disorder: burden of the disease according to subtypes in recently diagnosed children. *Actas Esp Psiquiatr.* 2008;**36**(5):285–94.

68. Johnston C, Mash EJ. Families of children with attention-deficit/hyperactivity disorder: review and recommendations for future research. *Clin Child Fam Psychol Rev.* 2001;**4**(3):183–207.

69. Lewis K. Family functioning as perceived by parents of boys with attention deficit disorder. *Issues Ment Health Nurs.* 1992;**13**(4):369–86.

70. Brown RT, Pacini JN. Perceived family functioning, marital status, and depression in parents of boys with attention deficit disorder. *J Learn Disabil.* 1989;**22**(9):581–7.

71. Coghill D, Soutullo C, d'Aubuisson C, *et al.* Impact of attention-deficit/hyperactivity disorder on the patient and family: results from a European survey. *Child Adolesc Psychiatry Ment Health.* 2008;**2**(1):31.

72. Noe L, Hankin C. Health outcomes of childhood attention-deficit/hyperactivity disorder (ADHD): health care use and work status of caregivers. *Value Health.* 2001;**4**(2):142–3.

73. Rucklidge JJ. Gender differences in attention-deficit/hyperactivity disorder. *Psychiatr Clin North Am.* 2010;**33**(2):357–73.

74. Derks EM, Hudziak JJ, Boomsma DI. Why more boys than girls with ADHD receive treatment: a study of Dutch twins. *Twin Res Hum Genet.* 2007;**10**(5):765–70.

75. Weiss G, Hechtman L. *Hyperactive Children Grown Up: ADHD in Children, Adolescents, and Adults*. New York, NY: Guilford Press; 1993.

76. Biederman J. Impact of comorbidity in adults with attention-deficit/hyperactivity disorder. *J Clin Psychiatry*. 2004;**65**(Suppl 3):3–7.

77. Barkley RA. Age dependent decline in ADHD: true recovery or statistical illusion? *ADHD Rep*. 1997;**5**:1–5.

78. Shaffer D. Attention deficit hyperactivity disorder in adults. *Am J Psychiatry*. 1994;**151**(5):633–8.

79. WHO International Consortium in Psychiatric Epidemiology. Cross-national comparisons of the prevalences and correlates of mental disorders. WHO International Consortium in Psychiatric Epidemiology. *Bull World Health Organ*. 2000;**78**(4): 413–26.

80. Weissman MM, Bland RC, Canino GJ, et al. Cross-national epidemiology of major depression and bipolar disorder. *JAMA*. 1996;**276**(4):293–9.

81. Weiss G, Hechtman L, Milroy T, et al. Psychiatric status of hyperactives as adults: a controlled prospective 15-year follow-up of 63 hyperactive children. *J Am Acad Child Psychiatry*. 1985; **24**(2):211–20.

82. Hill JC, Schoener EP. Age-dependent decline of attention deficit hyperactivity disorder. *Am J Psychiatry*. 1996;**153**(9):1143–6.

83. Sawilowsky S, Musial JL. Modeling ADHD exponential decay. *ADHD Rep*. 1988;**6**(1):10–11.

84. Biederman J, Mick E, Faraone SV. Age-dependent decline of symptoms of attention deficit hyperactivity disorder: impact of remission definition and symptom type. *Am J Psychiatry*. 2000;**157**(5):816–18.

85. Faraone SV, Biederman J, Mick E. The age-dependent decline of attention deficit hyperactivity disorder: a meta-analysis of follow-up studies. *Psychol Med*. 2006;**36**(2):159–65.

86. Kessler RC, Adler LA, Barkley R, et al. Patterns and predictors of attention-deficit/hyperactivity disorder persistence into adulthood: results from the national comorbidity survey replication. *Biol Psychiatry*. 2005;**57**(11):1442–51.

87. Faraone SV, Biederman J. What is the prevalence of adult ADHD? Results of a population screen of 966 adults. *J Atten Disord*. 2005;**9**(2):384–91.

88. Kooij JJ, Buitelaar JK, van den Oord EJ, et al. Internal and external validity of attention-deficit hyperactivity disorder in a population-based sample of adults. *Psychol Med*. 2005;**35**(6):817–27.

89. Kessler RC, Üstün TB, eds. *The WHO World Mental Health Surveys: Global Perspectives on the Epidemiology of Mental Disorders*. New York, NY: Cambridge University Press; 2008.

90. Kessler RC, Üstün TB. The World Mental Health (WMH) Survey Initiative Version of the World Health Organization (WHO) Composite International Diagnostic Interview (CIDI). *Int J Methods Psychiatr Res*. 2004;**13**(2):93–121.

91. Adler, L. Cohen J. Diagnosis and evaluation of adults with attention-deficit/hyperactivity disorder. *Psychiatr Clin North Am*. 2004;**27**(2):187–201.

92. Adler L, Spencer T. *The Adult ADHD Clinical Diagnostic Scale (ACDS) V 1.2*. New York, NY: New York University School of Medicine; 2004.

93. DuPaul GJ, Power TJ, Anastopoulos AD, et al. *ADHD Rating Scale-IV: Checklists, Norms, and Clinical Interpretation*. New York, NY: Guilford Press; 1998.

94. Michelson D, Adler L, Spencer T, et al. Atomoxetine in adults with ADHD: two randomized, placebo-controlled studies. *Biol Psychiatry*. 2003;**53**(2):112–20.

95. Spencer T, Biederman J, Wilens T, et al. Efficacy of a mixed amphetamine salts compound in adults with attention-deficit/hyperactivity disorder. *Arch Gen Psychiatry*. 2001;**58**(8):775–82.

96. Lahey BB, Applegate B, McBurnett K, et al. DSM-IV field trials for attention deficit hyperactivity disorder in children and adolescents. *Am J Psychiatry*. 1994; **151**(11):1673–85.

97. Spitzer RL, Davies M, Barkley RA. The DSM-III-R field trial of disruptive behavior disorders. *J Am Acad Child Adolesc Psychiatry*. 1990;**29**(5):690–7.

98. Faraone SV, Biederman J, Spencer T, et al. Attention-deficit/hyperactivity disorder in adults: an overview. *Biol Psychiatry*. 2000;**48**(1):9–20.

99. Wolraich ML, Wibbelsman CJ, Brown TE, et al. Attention-deficit/hyperactivity disorder among adolescents: a review of the diagnosis, treatment, and clinical implications. *Pediatrics*. 2005;**115**(6):1734–46.

100. Barkley RA, Murphy KR, Fischer M. *ADHD in Adults: What the Science Says*. New York, NY: Guilford Press; 2008.

101. Biederman J, Faraone S, Milberger S, et al. Predictors of persistence and remission of ADHD into adolescence: results from a four-year prospective follow-up study. *J Am Acad Child Adolesc Psychiatry*. 1996;**35**(3):343–51.

102. Hart EL, Lahey BB, Loeber R, et al. Developmental change in attention-deficit hyperactivity disorder in boys: a four-year longitudinal study. *J Abnorm Child Psychol*. 1995;**23**(6):729–49.

103. Kessler RC, Adler L, Ames M, et al. The World Health Organization Adult ADHD Self-Report Scale (ASRS):

a short screening scale for use in the general population. *Psychol Med.* 2005;**35**(2):245–56.

104. Lara C, Fayyad J, de Graaf R, *et al.* Childhood predictors of adult attention-deficit/hyperactivity disorder: results from the World Health Organization World Mental Health Survey Initiative. *Biol Psychiatry.* 2009;**65**(1):46–54.

105. Larsson H, Lichtenstein P, Larsson JO. Genetic contributions to the development of ADHD subtypes from childhood to adolescence. *J Am Acad Child Adolesc Psychiatry.* 2006;**45**(8):973–81.

106. Millstein RB, Wilens TE, Biederman J, *et al.* Presenting ADHD symptoms and subtypes in clinically referred adults with ADHD. *J Atten Disord.* 1997;**2**(3): 159–66.

107. Barkley RA. ADHD behavior checklist for adults. *ADHD Rep.* 1995;**3**:16.

108. Ratey JJ, Greenberg MS, Bemporad JR, *et al.* Unrecognized attention-deficit hyperactivity disorder in adults presenting for outpatient psychotherapy. *J Child Adolesc Psychopharmacol.* 1992;**2**(4):267–75.

109. Faraone SV, Biederman J, Spencer T. Diagnostic efficiency of symptom items for identifying adult ADHD. *J ADHD Relat Disord.* 2010;**1**(2):38–48.

110. Ward MF, Wender PH, Reimherr FW. The Wender Utah Rating Scale: an aid in the retrospective diagnosis of childhood attention deficit hyperactivity disorder. *Am J Psychiatry.* 1993;**150**(6):885–90.

111. Gittelman R, Mannuzza S. Diagnosing ADD-H in adolescents. *Psychopharmacol Bull.* 1985;**21**(2):237–42.

112. Mannuzza S, Klein RG, Bessler A, *et al.* Adult outcome of hyperactive boys. Educational achievement, occupational rank, and psychiatric status. *Arch Gen Psychiatry.* 1993;**50**(7):565–76.

113. Wilens TE, Biederman J, Faraone SV, *et al.* Presenting ADHD symptoms, subtypes, and comorbid disorders in clinically referred adults with ADHD. *J Clin Psychiatry.* 2009;**70**(11):1557–62.

114. Nierenberg AA, Miyahara S, Spencer T, *et al.* Clinical and diagnostic implications of lifetime attention-deficit/hyperactivity disorder comorbidity in adults with bipolar disorder: data from the first 1000 STEP-BD participants. *Biol Psychiatry.* 2005;**57**(11): 1467–73.

115. Tamam L, Karakus G, Ozpoyraz N. Comorbidity of adult attention-deficit hyperactivity disorder and bipolar disorder: prevalence and clinical correlates. *Eur Arch Psychiatry Clin Neurosci.* 2008;**258**(7):385–93.

116. Wingo AP, Ghaemi SN. A systematic review of rates and diagnostic validity of comorbid adult attention-deficit/hyperactivity disorder and bipolar disorder. *J Clin Psychiatry.* 2007;**68**(11):1776–84.

117. Goodman DW. The consequences of attention-deficit/hyperactivity disorder in adults. *J Psychiatr Pract.* 2007;**13**(5):318–27.

118. Biederman J, Faraone SV, Spencer TJ, *et al.* Functional impairments in adults with self-reports of diagnosed ADHD: a controlled study of 1001 adults in the community. *J Clin Psychiatry.* 2006;**67**(4):524–40.

119. Able SL, Johnston JA, Adler LA, *et al.* Functional and psychosocial impairment in adults with undiagnosed ADHD. *Psychol Med.* 2007;**37**(1):97–107.

120. Hervey AS, Epstein JN, Curry JF. Neuropsychology of adults with attention-deficit/hyperactivity disorder: a meta-analytic review. *Neuropsychology.* 2004;**18**(3): 485–503.

121. de Graaf R, Kessler RC, Fayyad J, *et al.* The prevalence and effects of adult attention-deficit/hyperactivity disorder (ADHD) on the performance of workers: results from the WHO World Mental Health Survey Initiative. *Occup Environ Med.* 2008;**65**(12):835–42.

122. Birnbaum HG, Kessler RC, Lowe SW, *et al.* Costs of attention deficit-hyperactivity disorder (ADHD) in the US: excess costs of persons with ADHD and their family members in 2000. *Curr Med Res Opin.* 2005;**21**(2):195–206.

123. Swensen AR, Birnbaum HG, Secnik K, *et al.* Attention-deficit/hyperactivity disorder: increased costs for patients and their families. *J Am Acad Child Adolesc Psychiatry.* 2003;**42**(12):1415–23.

124. Barkley RA. Driving impairments in teens and adults with attention-deficit/hyperactivity disorder. *Psychiatr Clin North Am.* 2004;**27**(2):233–60.

125. Weafer J, Camarillo D, Fillmore MT, *et al.* Simulated driving performance of adults with ADHD: comparisons with alcohol intoxication. *Exp Clin Psychopharmacol.* 2008;**16**(3):251–63.

126. Waite R. Women and attention deficit disorders: a great burden overlooked. *J Am Acad Nurse Pract.* 2007;**19**(3):116–25.

127. Bernfort L, Nordfeldt S, Persson J. ADHD from a socio-economic perspective. *Acta Paediatr.* 2008;**97**(2): 239–45.

128. Biederman J, Monuteaux MC, Spencer T, *et al.* Do stimulants protect against psychiatric disorders in youth with ADHD? A 10-year follow-up study. *Pediatrics.* 2009;**124**(1):71–8.

129. Kessler RC, Adler LA, Gruber MJ, *et al.* Validity of the World Health Organization Adult ADHD Self-Report Scale (ASRS) Screener in a representative sample of health plan members. *Int J Methods Psychiatr Res.* 2007;**16**(2):52–65.

130. Schweitzer JB, Lee DO, Hanford RB, *et al.* Effect of methylphenidate on executive functioning in adults

with attention-deficit/hyperactivity disorder: normalization of behavior but not related brain activity. *Biol Psychiatry*. 2004;**56**(8):597–606.

131. Simpson D, Plosker GL. Spotlight on atomoxetine in adults with attention-deficit hyperactivity disorder. *CNS Drugs*. 2004;**18**(6):397–401.

132. Turner DC, Clark L, Dowson J, *et al*. Modafinil improves cognition and response inhibition in adult attention-deficit/hyperactivity disorder. *Biol Psychiatry*. 2004;**55**(10):1031–40.

133. Jensen PS, Rubio-Stipec M, Canino G, *et al*. Parent and child contributions to diagnosis of mental disorder: are both informants always necessary? *J Am Acad Child Adolesc Psychiatry*. 1999;**38**(12):1569–79.

134. Wender PH, Wolf LE, Wasserstein J. Adults with ADHD. An overview. *Ann N Y Acad Sci*. 2001;**931**:1–16.

135. Zucker M, Morris MK, Ingram SM, *et al*. Concordance of self- and informant ratings of adults' current and childhood attention-deficit/hyperactivity disorder symptoms. *Psychol Assess*. 2002;**14**(4):379–89.

136. Murphy P, Schachar R. Use of self-ratings in the assessment of symptoms of attention deficit hyperactivity disorder in adults. *Am J Psychiatry*. 2000;**157**(7):1156–9.

137. Mannuzza S, Klein RG, Klein DF, *et al*. Accuracy of adult recall of childhood attention deficit hyperactivity disorder. *Am J Psychiatry*. 2002;**159**(11):1882–8.

Functional impairment in ADHD

Margaret Weiss

What is meant by functional impairment?

The *Diagnostic and Statistical Manual of Mental Disorders*, fifth edition (DSM-5) [1] has moved our field forward in not only recognizing functional impairment as critical to diagnosis, but also providing tools to define impairment. A significant improvement was use of the World Health Organization Disability Assessment Schedule (WHODAS 2) to evaluate functional impairment in any condition, as opposed to the Global Assessment of Functioning (GAF), which was a measure of severity that mixed different concepts, with different emphasis at the low and high end of the scale. Similar normed scales exist for adaptive life skills (Adaptive Behavior Assessment System – II) [2] and functional impairment (Weiss Functional Impairment Rating Scale, www.caddra.ca) in children. The DSM-5 uses the WHODAS 2 as an empirical and normed measure of impairment as a cross-cutting category across disorders. Barkley has recently published a normed scale for measurement of impairment in attention-deficit hyperactivity disorder (ADHD) in children [3] and in adults [4].

Symptoms, adaptive life skills, functional impairment, quality of life, and development represent overlapping but distinct concepts worth understanding as distinct concepts. A symptom is a behavior that is unique and often seen as part of and an indicator of a diagnostic syndrome. Adaptive life skills are those skills we acquire through development that allow us to do the age-appropriate tasks of routine life: communication, learning, making friends, managing family life, enjoying leisure time. Functional impairment represents one's capacity of lack thereof for meeting the expectations of one's environment: staying out of trouble in school, self-restraint when angry, driving, managing money, exercising, eating well and working to stay in good health, avoiding risk. Quality of life is either measured specific to a particular syndrome (in ADHD, the ADHD Impact Factor [5, 6]) or measured with a single measure designed to be generic enough to measure burden of illness across different conditions. In adults this is often the SF-36 [7], and in children the two most common measures are the Child Health Illness Profile (CHIP) [8–10] or the Child Health Questionnaire (CHQ) [11]. Each stage of the life cycle requires that we negotiate developmental transitions. One of the characteristics of ADHD is that as challenges vary between different developmental stages, symptoms may present new challenges in functioning. The start of elementary school requires sitting still. High school requires the ability to assess and avoid risk. College requires the ability to be self-directed in studying. Adulthood requires the ability to manage life skills or to care for others. There is no measure that identifies the maturity level expected at each age. However, as clinicians, we experience our greatest success when we see a patient who was "stuck" move forward into being able to manage the next stage of the life cycle.

The view presented in this chapter is that the 18 symptoms of ADHD have been, despite their limitations, a reasonably reliable way of identifying those patients who can be identified as having ADHD. The 18 symptoms of ADHD do not describe the breadth of the syndrome, or its manifestation through the life cycle. However, a patient who meets the diagnostic criteria set out by the DSM-5 is going to be likely to have the developmental history, clinical correlates, impairments, and risk factors we associate with ADHD.

Attention-Deficit Hyperactivity Disorder in Adults and Children, ed. Lenard A. Adler, Thomas J. Spencer and Timothy E. Wilens.
Published by Cambridge University Press. © Cambridge University Press 2015.

Studies of outcome of ADHD have in the past focused on symptom response, and as a result we know much more about how symptoms respond to treatment, than we know about how, and to what degree functioning is normalized. For example, Russell Barkley comments that ADHD is, "not a disorder of knowing what to do, but a disorder of doing what you know" (personal communication). ADHD is associated with deficits in social skills, self-care, academic performance, home living, work, self-concept, self-directed activity, executive dysfunction, emotional dysregulation, and multiple high-risk activities (extreme sports, driving, smoking, poor self-care, insomnia, computer addiction, drug use, criminality).

Roizen and Stein noted that impairment in adaptive life skills in ADHD children is at the level of those with developmental delay [12, 13]. Mothers complain: "he does not get ready in the morning; he won't brush his teeth; doing homework is impossible; I can't get him to sleep; he is a picky eater." While symptoms drive many of the difficulties, symptom remission is rarely associated with normalization of adaptive life skills. It is therefore critical to understand that while for years we measured outcome of ADHD in terms of symptoms, symptoms were a proxy for outcome that were more or less effective at actually measuring change in the patient's well-being. Adaptive life skills are often far more severely impaired than suggested by symptom severity or improvement, and do not necessarily improve developmentally. An adult with ADHD may still not be brushing his teeth, paying his bills, or cleaning up his room. While we need to recognize the success in using symptoms as our sole window into outcome, it is particularly important to pay attention to those outcomes that are least sensitive to improvement in symptoms. A teacher may report better handwriting, less disruptive behavior, more on-task work, and better focus, while the parent remains frustrated that their teenager still requires supervision to get ready in the morning.

ADHD is associated with a high burden of illness from early childhood throughout the life cycle [14, 15]. Some children with ADHD seem relatively unperturbed by their circumstances and this has been called a "positive illusory bias." It can be quite striking to interview children who are rejected by teachers, family, and friends, are failing in school and sports, and have no special talents who will nonetheless describe themselves as happy.

The parents of the same child may be devastated that they have never had a play date, a phone call, or been invited to a birthday party, and are a source of great frustration for parents and teachers. From their point of view, if their child says they are fine, this is either a remarkable demonstration of lack of insight or an expression of never having known what to expect from life. Parents consistently describe a devastating burden of illness both for the child, the community, and the family [16]. Even those children who appear relatively immune to rejection grow into adults where the shadow of their childhood experience leads to poor self-esteem, awareness of being different, and disappointment with their situation in life [17].

The real-life outcome of ADHD is only evident if symptoms, functional impairment, adaptive life skills, quality of life, and development are integrated into a holistic understanding. Although we talk about diagnostic criteria as defined by ICD (International Classification of Diseases) or DSM, expert clinicians will often remark that the one aspect of the disorder that is pathognomonic is found in the way in which ADHD has put its stamp on each stage of the life cycle. One does not have cold-induced asthma if you live in the tropics. The nature and presentation of ADHD varies according to the specific demands of each stage of the life cycle. This means that a good clinic history will often reveal specific and familiar patterns that are unique to the condition. For example, a mother comes in with her 27-year-old son who has never been diagnosed. She describes that she suspected this child would be different even whilst he was in utero in that he never stopped moving and kicking. At 8 months he climbed out of his crib, and even at that age – "he did not walk, he ran." She spent the next 2 years never losing sight of him since he could impulsively run across the high way, jump out of the car, or smack his sibling. He was not admitted to any preschool and so remained in her care. She took him to the pediatrician who observed his erratic movement, and destructive play with the tools in his drawers, and suggested he needed a firm hand. She complained she was exhausted. He never napped, would not stay in bed, and was up long before she was, which left her concerned about his safety so that she had him trained to watch cartoons. He did not sit and so she worried about if and when he ate, and feared his diet was poor because he did not seem to notice hunger until it was time for bed. The elementary school could not cope and suggested she have him evaluated, and she saw a psychologist who said his learning was intact, and the pediatrician continued to affirm, "boys will be boys." The school placed him in a social development class with 10 other children and 3 teachers. They saw him as curious, bright, charming, funny, well meaning, but unable to work, focus, write, or sit still. They wondered how it was that he seemed to be learning when they talked with him. In grade 8 he was mainstreamed in a regular high school. At this point he had calmed down but his parents noted they were terrified of what he might do given they could no longer supervise him. He had some teachers he liked and did well in their courses, while failing in other areas. He graduated and was accepted to a trade school, became a contractor, and was now happily married to a woman who took care of his books, and all aspects of daily living. He liked working with his hands in the courses he took, and in his work-study program he shone – enthusiastic, high energy, and fascinated by every aspect of building. He was diagnosed when his 4-year-old son was a "chip off the old block," but times had changed and diagnosis of both of them led to significant improvement for all. While there are many different "ADHD histories," especially for those who are inattentive and sluggish, or for women, the stories all share "the stamp" in which dysregulation of attention, mood, executive function, activity, forced effort, and self-monitoring impact each stage of the life cycle according to what is being demanded. This remains true. A geriatric patient complains that after a life time of being a dare devil, a workaholic, and full of life, he now sits at home with nothing to do and feels useless.

Despite differences in culture, environment, parenting: many aspects of development are consistent across patients. The infant cannot relax to feed. The infant child has colic and never sleeps. The preschool child is sent out for a snack during circle time. In grade three mother and child are spending hours fighting to do 10 minutes of homework. The adolescent finally feels they are fitting in, but with the "bad crowd." The teen insists on being independent; but he shows no signs of self-directed activity and carries the risk of a young child in a pubertal body. The adult with ADHD can have difficulty with any aspect of self-regulation: eating, sleeping, exercise, sex, addiction, managing money, driving, time, mood, and relationships.

The reason patients most often present is that they are faced with a developmental challenge and ADHD stands in the way. An adolescent has been sexually or socially inappropriate. An adult comes in saying, "I know I have ADHD, but my wife says she will leave me if I don't do something about it." A freshman in college had every intention of studying, and never seemed to notice the semester go by before he/she realized he/she was failing. Even more important is that as clinicians, our greatest moments of success are not when we see a normal rating scale, but when a patient comes in and says, "I made my first friend" or "I graduated college" or "I have been in this job a whole year now." When we succeed in moving a patient forward to the next developmental phase, and they see a path open for future growth, they are deeply grateful. Patients are pleased to see that their symptoms have improved on a rating scale, but their world opens up when they are passing college, or able to establish an intimate relationship.

There is literature on remission of ADHD symptoms, adapted from the concept as it is used in mood disorders to predict recurrence. The concept of remission in ADHD has less value if it is viewed as a life long developmental disorder, in which the presentation of symptoms is dependent not on core aspects of the disorder in the patients, but on the match of their skills and developmental expectations. A young man was in a clinical trial of a new medication for ADHD. He had 18 severe symptoms of ADHD. He decided in the trial to drop out of college, which he felt to be beyond his reach, and obtained a job as a gas station attendant. When asked about the same 18 symptoms, he was asymptomatic. He never had to sit. There was nothing to forget or lose, and not much to remember. He was no longer viewed as hyperactive, but enthusiastic in running out the second a car arrived. He did not have to take payment, as this was automated. He said, "This job is a much better cure for my ADHD than the drug was."

This raises the question of "early intervention." The early history of ADHD focused almost exclusively on disruptive, young boys and until the prospective follow-up studies, it was a widespread belief that you "grew out" of ADHD, a misconception that might be attributed instead to the pediatricians growing out of seeing children. This meant that for half a century the focus has been on treatment of children, and most especially children brought in by adults because they were annoying. This "early intervention" was for a long time perceived as dealing with the problem. The longitudinal follow-up of the Multimodal Treatment of ADHD (MTA) study demonstrated quite clearly that there is no early intervention that has lifelong impact. Only in the last 10 years has it really become common knowledge that ADHD can be disabling to a patient, even if they are quiet. ADHD can be most impairing with the organizational and attention demands of higher education or if the complexities of multiple demands in family life overcome a level of skill in these areas that is insufficient to meet increased expectations. This awareness has changed our understanding of the disorder. Remission is a function of demands. Early intervention is not limited to childhood: early intervention is doing work required at each stage of the life cycle to construct the bridge to the next stage.

This chapter will review functional impairment in ADHD through the life cycle. Information is drawn from different types of studies. We have focused our literature review on the following sources:

1. Long-term follow-up studies
2. Cross-sectional studies of functional impairment
3. Studies of functional impairment in a particular age group
4. Studies of a given area of functioning
5. Clinical observation.

Given the enormity of this task we have organized the chapter not by age, but by domain. The measures of functional impairment that currently exist for the most part do not distinguish functional impairment at work or school, or in the family, leisure, self-concept, or risk. These were the empirically validated factors used in the Weiss Functional Impairment Scale for parents and/or self-report, and the items selected were drawn from chart review [18, 19].

Education

ADHD is associated with poor grades [20], poor reading and math standardized test scores [21], and increased grade retention. ADHD is also associated with increased use of school-based services, increased rates of detention and expulsion, relatively low rates of high school graduation and post-secondary education, lower achievement scores, special education placement, and school dropout [22–25]. Children in community samples who show symptoms of inattention, hyperactivity, and impulsivity with or without formal diagnoses of ADHD also show poor academic

and educational outcomes. Pharmacological treatment and behavior management are associated with reduction of the core symptoms of ADHD and increased academic productivity, but not with improved standardized test scores or ultimate educational attainment [26, 27]. The exception is a well-publicized study on the impact of pharmacological treatment on academic outcome in over 500 children followed for 5 years. However, the results of this study need to be viewed in perspective [28]. The authors of this study concluded that "The 2.9-point mathematics and 5.4-point reading score differences are comparable with score gains of 0.19 and 0.29 school years, respectively, but these gains are insufficient to eliminate the test-score gap between children with attention-deficit/hyperactivity disorder and those without the disorder." [28]. A 1 month improvement in academic achievement over 5 years is of questionable clinical significance.

Future research must use conceptually based outcome measures in prospective, longitudinal, and community-based studies to determine which pharmacological, behavioral, and educational interventions can improve academic and educational outcomes of children with ADHD [29].

At the present time it has become standard clinical practice to provide children with ADHD with adaptations to diminish the disparity between their performance and their actual academic potential. These academic adaptations are in widespread use, although there is a relative paucity of direct research to determine if their benefit is specific to ADHD. Whether or not they have been adequately scrutinized by good empirical research, most clinicians will attest that they work, and some adaptations simply "make sense" in leveling the playing field so that the deficits of ADHD do not determine academic success. The central issue behind each one of these specialized interventions is to measure what the student actually has mastered, rather than his or her capacity to demonstrate that knowledge in a task that measures ADHD rather than knowledge.

The most common adaptations are worth reviewing, and carry through all levels of the education system. Children with ADHD are advocating for themselves, and this generation has the opportunity to go to college. If you have slow processing speed, or dream off, and make careless mistakes you need extra time, a quiet setting, and an instructor to insure you have understood and completed all questions. If you cannot read or write, you can be tested orally, be trained in computer programs that perform these functions, or use a reader or a scribe. If you have difficulty with time, organization, and other issues you are far more likely to succeed with fewer courses over a longer time period. This is not a race to the finish line: the issue is getting to the finish line. ADHD students will do much better in a small seminar than a lecture course with hundreds of students, and pre-registration to allow students to take the courses best suited to them makes a difference. ADHD is associated with considerable difficulty with copying: the use of electronic devices, web-based homework assignments, having the teacher slides and lectures on the web for review, mitigates many ADHD symptoms. Diagnosis, treatment, supervision in the student disability service, and access to educational adaptations may mean that the educational attainment of the future is based on actual achievement rather than on performance.

Experience suggests that these interventions, when feasible, make it possible for a child with ADHD to understand the difference between his/her capacity to conceptualize material ("I am not dumb"), and his/her capacity to demonstrate that mastery [30, 31]. Our clinical observations and quick clinical uptake of academic recommendations have yet to be adequately researched [32]. Although there are resilient individuals who go on to achieve academic success, or return to school later to obtain their high school leaving certificate, the educational impairment we have described has profound consequences to self-esteem and to income. Biederman has found that "ADHD is associated with significant educational and occupational underattainments relative to what would have been expected on the basis of intellectual potential" [33] and the opportunity cost of failure to remediate this impairment is profound. Loss of education leads to misemployment and unemployment and becomes a major impact on lifelong impairment as well as the opportunity cost of lost skill to society. The marked discrepancy between studies of the difficulties patients with ADHD have with academic *performance* relative to academic *achievement* on tests is crucial and can be viewed as a major therapeutic opportunity. We are now seeing the first cohort of children with ADHD who received educational accommodations come of age. It is not inconceivable to anticipate a well-researched set of educational adaptations that would allow patients with ADHD to achieve in school at their learning potential. The revolution in education with increasing

use of multi-sensory electronic formats is only going to drive this process further and faster.

Work

Barkley's long-term follow-up study, the "Milwaukee study" provided some of the best data at age 27 we have on occupational outcomes and their relationship to symptoms. Occupational functioning followed by home responsibilities and occupations were the three areas most impaired, whether they were measured by the patient or clinician [34]. The deficits associated with ADHD make the classroom a very particular challenge requiring self-control in multiple dimensions including: talking, appropriate timing, capacity for transitions, attention to detail, accuracy, forced effort, self-regulation, and the capacity to inhibit disruptive behavior. The list of what is required to be "good" at school, reads like the list of symptoms that define ADHD.

The importance of this observation is that it is much easier to find a work environment that is ADHD friendly than the classroom. Some of the qualities associated with ADHD may even be an asset in some professions. Testing motorcycles at high speeds (risk), hyperfocus in areas of interest (computer use), talking too much (radio announcer or DJ), excess friendliness (sales), and oppositional behavior (lawyer) may mean that the very trait that was so annoying at elementary school, allows an adult to define a niche where they excel. The clinician is often in the position of facilitating that process. To do so the clinician needs to be aware that statistical results on populations of individuals with ADHD do not preclude individual success if talent is matched to the demands of a particular workplace. For the first time we are seeing adults with ADHD "coming out," acknowledging their childhood history, and also sharing a new "ADHD culture" in which what has been conceptualized as a form of pathology is reframed to have the potential to enable unusual success. This has created confusion. No one chooses to have ADHD, who has ever suffered the shadow it has cast on their life. Yet it remains true that high profile company chief executive officers, Michael Phelps, and other sports figures showed an energy, drive, persistence, unremitting focus that potentiated success which might have eluded someone else.

It remains true that the majority of adults who were described as underachieving for their potential when they were in school go on as adults to experience the same difficulty as adults. They may be self-employed, but unable to structure their time. They may be disruptive to other workers. They may be late. Paperwork is done last minute, or not at all. In the one excellent current study of treatment of employment using the Endicott Work Productivity Scale (EWPS) with atomoxetine, a profile of work impairments was consistent with what we know about ADHD. If we are to develop success in employment to match that of what is occurring in college, we need to be directing our patients to jobs that are ADHD friendly, and coping strategies that compensate for specific deficits [35].

Clinicians who treat adults with ADHD need to evaluate if the patient is in a suitable work environment for their skills and deficits, review performance evaluations, and work with vocational specialists and on occasion employers to make work, work. If an adult has a delayed sleep phase and sleeps from 2 am to 10 am, perhaps their schedule at work can be adjusted to be 11 am to 8 pm. Patients who have done this often say they also get much more done when the office is quiet. Patients may request work that has a unique interest for them when given a change of posting. Adults with ADHD may thoughtfully turn down a major promotion that moves them out of the field and into management. One patient noted that he was not turning in receipts (or getting the refund), filling out reports, or submitting the detailed summaries required on the nature of what had sold and what had not. He said, "they keep me, despite themselves, because my sales numbers are the top in the country." The employer and the patient would benefit if his excellent sales were paired with a young associate who learned from him while also doing his paperwork.

If clinicians are going to assist patients to find work that suits them, it is helpful to know what professions have been found to be most successful for patients with ADHD. While I do not know of any research on this, years of shared clinical experience have made it apparent that there is a drift towards some types of work and away from others. Individuals with attention deficits do not usually like desk jobs, accounting, or being a bank teller. Individuals whose nature is to be "on the go" seek jobs where they are on their feet and moving, where there is constant change, and for many, take the high-risk jobs no one else is enthused about. Therefore some professions make inherent sense: builder, stockbroker, sales, emergency nursing shifts, extreme sports, waitress. Other professions are common in ADHD although the rationale is harder to come by –

why would their be an excess of ADHD adults who are pilots, cooks, or teachers?

Social functioning

Children with ADHD are often described as too friendly, but often they are either isolated, teased, rejected, or bullied. ADHD is associated with marked impairment in relationships with family, teachers, employers, and peers [36].

It is remarkable to observe a child with ADHD go to a birthday party. Within minutes, a child with no visible disability experiences both almost instant and unanimous rejection. By contrast, a child with Tourette syndrome, an obvious disability, may have no difficulty interacting with peers in the same situation. Social rejection for children with ADHD is often a source of deep grief for their mothers. Saddest of all for some parents has been the experience of organizing a birthday party for the child, inviting the class, and having no one show up.

Parents want to know what their child "is doing wrong," and how they can fix it. They often complain about assessments that focus on teacher reports, history, and rating scales without talking to the child, partly because they feel that the objective of treatment is to remediate the hurt they assume their child feels. Their concern is not unrealistic. In the life of an ADHD child the day starts with a fight with their parents over getting out of bed and getting themselves ready. They go to school where they are bullied on the playground to the delight of other children when they react with explosive rage. It is always the ADHD child, never those who provoked the situation who then lands in trouble. Once they arrive in the classroom, they cannot put their things away, sit down quietly, or copy assignments off the board. Even if they have spent hours getting their homework done, they are in trouble because they do not have it with them. They misbehave on the bus home. The arrive to a household in which they interact with siblings the way other children have interacted with them, and quickly are identified as the "family problem." Dinner is a fight over eating and sitting still. Evenings are a fight over homework. They are put to bed and do not feel sleepy, so bedtime is also a source either of frustration or of continued anger.

The sadness most parents feel is more than justified. There may be things their child loves: LEGO, computer games, skateboarding. However, parents also know that their child is "missing" the social community and companionship that they experienced as one of the joys of human relationships. Parents of autistic children see their aloneness as part of the disorder and are prepared to work with it. Parents of ADHD children are devastated by the social isolation of a child who wants to play, and feel helpless to either understand or remediate it.

The literature on treatment of the social skill deficits of ADHD children is not encouraging. While parents often ask for "therapy" for the child, this is mainly helpful in providing the child with another adult to relate to, not in remediating relationships with peers. Social skills' training has been the source of much effort and research, but the results are at best inconsistent and equivocal. A careful review of this literature suggests that children can "learn" social skills within the group while being monitored, but that this does not generalize to formation of friendships with peers [37].

This does not mean the clinician has no means to alleviate social impairment in youth with ADHD. The recommendations that follow are not "evidence based," but follow the simple principles of what is known about the disorder: treatment must occur at the point of performance, it must be practical and easy to implement by multiple caregivers, and it must draw on the child's strengths. The following is a summary of our clinical practice, describing what we have found "works."

Many, but not all, children with ADHD have what is called a "positive illusory bias," meaning that they are protected by a certain degree of obliviousness to the rejection they receive. Their parents suffer as they watch the lack of companionship, warmth, and positive regard they anticipated from their children. However, they benefit from knowing that the child may be content with how they are.

A second useful strategy is to recognize that it is in the nature of the condition that the one group ADHD children have the most difficulty with is their peers, and that our society is set up such that this is the group they are most often with. The truth is, that, we will spend the rest of our lives in family grouping with different ages. ADHD children often love and show extraordinary patience with animals, a grandparent, one to one with an adolescent, or caring for infants. These are also important types of social engagement, and this success gives them the satisfaction of relating, caring, and mutual compassion. ADHD children may

thrive if given a peer buddy of an older child at school who then receives credit for community service. They may succeed as a mother's helper who is patient and tireless in looking after an infant. ADHD children can be uniquely patient, and infinitely entertained by a pet. Horseback riding, an assistance dog, a pet for company, or volunteering in a shelter can be a source of pride and allow a child to love and be loved by a creature that sees who they are, and not their disability.

Adolescence and early adulthood, far from being what was once believed to be a period in which you outgrow ADHD, are now understood as "the transition years" [38], and the most challenging, and high-risk, period of the life cycle for many patients. During adolescence many patients with ADHD have the appearance of maturity, and the impulse control and behavioral inhibition of a much younger child, but parents lose their involvement opportunities for supervision. This is the age in which ADHD patients are exposed to drugs, parties, dating, driving, sex, self-directed study, moving away from home, and forced independence in self-care.

Could it be more ironic then, that this is when we abandon them? The pediatricians have the knowledge to know and understand their patient with ADHD, but it is the adult clinician who takes over the mandate to treat ADHD at this time. Historically ADHD was born as a disorder of childhood. However, looking at the follow-up findings at 12 years from the MTA study, we have to ask ourselves new questions. There is no early intervention that will preclude impairment in adulthood. We have focused on diagnosis and treatment of ADHD in children, and then abruptly terminated that treatment during their peak period of risk – when they graduate child services. We spend the majority of our lives as adults, and early intervention for developmental disorders is really intervening throughout each stage of the life cycle, to lay the foundation for care in the next stage. This is true right up to treatment of ADHD in the geriatric population. Developmental disorders require not only continuity of care, but when they are more than 80% heritable, they also require family-based care and child and adult clinicians working together. Yet, there are fewer than five life cycle clinics in existence.

The literature shows a decrease in frequency for hyperactivity and impulsivity with time [14, 15]. This does not translate to what is seen in clinical practice. They may be less hyperactive, but the internal restlessness, which the patients still feels, is now ego-dystonic.

A young adult is aware they cannot sit through a class, that they are speeding (on bikes, in cars, or even in their pragmatic speech). They are now aware that they do not meet the "cool" criteria. They interrupt, are annoying, may avoid socializing for fear of failure. They may be impulsive *less often*, but the salience of a single impulsive event: a car accident, quitting school, unprotected sex, or shoplifting, may have ramifications for years afterwards [39]. Most important, the adaptive life skills which were deficient in childhood remain deficient – however, an adult who cannot "do" the simplest things is far more embarrassed and shamed [12, 13].

Adults with ADHD still have problems with people [40]. If oppositional, they will argue with their boss, teacher, or even inside their own head. The "positive illusory bias" observed in children, where they believe they are better liked than they really are, does disappear. In its stead, one of the most pervasive and debilitating attributes that becomes evident in groups or therapy with adults with ADHD is that a life history of rejection and failure is now experienced as a shadow casting unremitting doubt and self-deprecation on their sense of self. This is true whether or not they have succeeded, or in what ways they have succeeded or failed. It is the hallmark of adults with ADHD that their self-esteem eats away at them irrespective of how they are doing. Adults with ADHD evaluated in cross-sectional studies are more likely to be divorced and more dissatisfied with their social relationships [40]. This is consistent with the longitudinal studies: all of which have demonstrated difficulties with work relationships, family, and social isolation [41]. The success of cognitive-behavioral therapy (CBT) for ADHD in adults has been attributed to improvement in executive function, which is typically the focus of the therapy [42–48].

It is to some degree unfortunate that negative outcomes have been so widely emphasized in explaining ADHD to the public. It is as though the profession was so infatuated with the need to make ADHD "a real disorder," that it was assumed that "real" necessarily meant catastrophic. Blindness is real, and not something anyone wishes for, but blind people can make brilliant musicians. The ADHD patient, the clinician, and the public need hope to know those interventions which can be relied on to mitigate harm and to predict success [49, 50].

A mother with three ADHD boys, left to her by her now divorced ADHD ex-husband, was listening to just such a lecture on every outcome of the Milwaukee study, when she turned to me and asked, "and where do I find the good news?" Do we want to teach parents that ADHD is a path to incarceration, substance abuse, welfare, antisocial behavior, school dropout, and isolation. ADHD in childhood is a risk factor, but these negative outcomes are predicted not just by the diagnosis, but individual talent, family pathology, socioeconomic status, conduct disorder, and many other variables. Clinicians need to cushion the burden patients and their families carry with creative alternatives that may bring hope.

Methods for therapeutic intervention in social deficits in adults with ADHD has received relatively scant attention, although it is addressed in the work of Young and Rostain [51, 52]. Support groups, coaching, involvement of family members in treatment, delegation of tasks that are not ADHD friendly, and socialization in areas of strength, such as skiing or racing, are some of the many ways in which continued social impairment can be addressed. Furthermore, there is now a much wider understanding of the impact of ADHD on partners [51]. This work has saved many a marriage: instead of having to live with ADHD and being blamed for it, spouses are now learning to separate the symptoms of the disorder from the relationship, and how to cope with those symptoms.

Summary

This chapter has not attempted to provide a comprehensive perspective on all the functional impairments associated with ADHD. We have not discussed emotional dysregulation [53], executive dysfunction [54], sense of time, sleep [55], quality of life [56], internet addiction [57], driving [58–60], parenting [61, 62]. We have not discussed, and nor is there much research on what aspects of impairment remit with symptom remission and medication, and what aspects of impairment endure [63]. There are areas of impairment we see clinically which have simply never been investigated, such as whether ADHD proffers an increased risk to use of substances in pregnancy and thus fetal alcohol syndrome (FAS) or other disorders in offspring.

What we have been able to demonstrate in this chapter is that there is ample empirical research confirming that ADHD affects almost all aspects of functioning in childhood and adolescence [36] and that this continues in many cases in adulthood [34]. We have demonstrated that this impairment is evidence based and consistent across cross-sectional studies [33, 40] multiple follow-up studies [64–69], and observational studies [70]. Many of these impairments are specific to ADHD over and above other disorders, such as driving, academic performance, and substance abuse. However, the theme of this chapter has been to recognize that with every disability there is also the capacity to succeed, and that the recognition of ADHD as a valid disorder needs to be tempered with recognition that as clinicians we need to focus on research that will identify those factors that permit resilience, and are a source of hope.

References

1. American Psychiatric Association. *Diagnostic and Statistical Manual of Mental Disorders*, 5th edn (DSM-5). Arlington, VA: American Psychiatric Publishing; 2013.

2. Pollack MM, Holubkov R, Glass P, *et al.* Functional Status Scale: new pediatric outcome measure. *Pediatrics.* 2009;**124**(1):e18–28.

3. Barkley R. *Barkley Functional Impairment Scale, Children and Adolescents.* New York, NY and London: Guilford Press; 2012.

4. Barkley R. *Barkley Functional Impairment Scale.* New York, NY and London: Guilford Press; 2012.

5. Frazier TW, Weiss M, Hodgkins P, *et al.* Time course and predictors of health-related quality of life improvement and medication satisfaction in children diagnosed with attention-deficit/hyperactivity disorder treated with the methylphenidate transdermal system. *J Child Adolesc Psychopharmacol.* 2010;**20**(5):355–64.

6. Landgraf JM. Monitoring quality of life in adults with ADHD: reliability and validity of a new measure. *J Atten Disord.* 2007;**11**(3):351–62.

7. Rubin RR, Peyrot M. Psychometric properties of an instrument for assessing the experience of patients treated with inhaled insulin: the inhaled insulin treatment questionnaire (IITQ). *Health Qual Life Outcomes.* 2010;**8**:32.

8. Riley AW, Coghill D, Forrest CB, *et al.* Validity of the health-related quality of life assessment in the ADORE study: Parent Report Form of the CHIP-Child Edition. *Eur Child Adolesc Psychiatry.* 2006;**15**(Suppl 1):I63–71.

9. Riley AW, Forrest CB, Rebok GW, *et al.* The Child Report Form of the CHIP-Child Edition: reliability and validity. *Med Care.* 2004;**42**(3):221–31.

10. Riley AW, Forrest CB, Starfield B, *et al.* The Parent Report Form of the CHIP-Child Edition: reliability and validity. *Med Care.* 2004;**42**(3):210–20.

11. Ruperto N, Ravelli A, Pistorio A, *et al.* Cross-cultural adaptation and psychometric evaluation of the Childhood Health Assessment Questionnaire (CHAQ) and the Child Health Questionnaire (CHQ) in 32 countries. Review of the general methodology. *Clin Exp Rheumatol.* 2001;**19**(4 Suppl 23):S1–9.

12. Roizen NJ, Blondis TA, Irwin M, Stein M. Adaptive functioning in children with attention-deficit hyperactivity disorder. *Arch Pediatr Adolesc Med.* 1994;**148**(11):1137–42.

13. Stein MA, Szumowski E, Blondis TA, Roizen NJ. Adaptive skills dysfunction in ADD and ADHD children. *J Child Psychol Psychiatry.* 1995;**36**(4): 663–70.

14. Faraone SV, Biederman J, Mick E. The age-dependent decline of attention deficit hyperactivity disorder: a meta-analysis of follow-up studies. *Psychol Med.* 2006;**36**(2):159–65.

15. Biederman J, Mick E, Faraone SV. Age-dependent decline of symptoms of attention deficit hyperactivity disorder: impact of remission definition and symptom type. *Am J Psychiatry.* 2000;**157**(5):816–18.

16. Danckaerts M, Sonuga-Barke EJ, Banaschewski T, *et al.* The quality of life of children with attention deficit/hyperactivity disorder: a systematic review. *Eur Child Adolesc Psychiatry.* 2010;**19**(2):83–105.

17. Harpin VA. The effect of ADHD on the life of an individual, their family, and community from preschool to adult life. *Arch Dis Child.* 2005;**90** (Suppl 1):i2–7.

18. Newcorn JH, Stein MA, Childress AC, *et al.* Randomized, double-blind trial of guanfacine extended release in children with attention-deficit/hyperactivity disorder: morning or evening administration. *J Am Acad Child Adolesc Psychiatry.* 2013;**52**(9):921–30.

19. Weiss MD, Brooks BL, Iverson GL, *et al.* Reliability and validity of the Weiss Functional Impairment Rating Scale. 54th Annual Meeting of the American Academy of Child and Adolescent Psychiatry, 2007 October 23–28; Boston, MA; 2007.

20. Barkley RA, Fischer M, Edelbrock CS, Smallish L. The adolescent outcome of hyperactive children diagnosed by research criteria: I. An 8-year prospective follow-up study. *J Am Acad Child Adolesc Psychiatry.* 1990;**29**(4): 546–57.

21. Faraone SV, Biederman J, Lehman BK, *et al.* Intellectual performance and school failure in children with attention deficit hyperactivity disorder and in their siblings. *J Abnorm Psychol.* 1993;**102**(4):616–23.

22. Barkley RA, DuPaul GJ, McMurray MB. Comprehensive evaluation of attention deficit disorder with and without hyperactivity as defined by

research criteria. *J Consult Clin Psychol.* 1990;**58**(6): 775–89.

23. Fischer M, Barkley RA, Edelbrock CS, Smallish L. The adolescent outcome of hyperactive children diagnosed by research criteria: II. Academic, attentional, and neuropsychological status. *J Consult Clin Psychol.* 1990;**58**(5):580–8.

24. Barbaresi WJ, Katusic SK, Colligan RC, Weaver AL, Jacobsen SJ. Modifiers of long-term school outcomes for children with attention-deficit/hyperactivity disorder: does treatment with stimulant medication make a difference? Results from a population-based study. *J Dev Behav Pediatr.* 2007;**28**(4):274–87.

25. Pastura GM, Mattos P, Araujo AP. Academic performance in ADHD when controlled for comorbid learning disorders, family income, and parental education in Brazil. *J Atten Disord.* 2009;**12**(5):469–73.

26. Loe IM, Feldman HM. Academic and educational outcomes of children with ADHD. *J Pediatr Psychol.* 2007;**32**(6):643–54.

27. Hechtman L, Abikoff H, Klein RG, *et al.* Academic achievement and emotional status of children with ADHD treated with long-term methylphenidate and multimodal psychosocial treatment. *J Am Acad Child Adolesc Psychiatry.* 2004;**43**(7):812–19.

28. Scheffler RM, Brown TT, Fulton BD, *et al.* Positive association between attention-deficit/hyperactivity disorder medication use and academic achievement during elementary school. *Pediatrics.* 2009;**123**(5): 1273–9.

29. Mannuzza S, Klein RG. Long-term prognosis in attention-deficit/hyperactivity disorder. *Child Adolesc Psychiatr Clin N Am.* 2000;**9**(3):711–26.

30. Daley D, Birchwood J. ADHD and academic performance: why does ADHD impact on academic performance and what can be done to support ADHD children in the classroom? *Child Care Health Dev.* 2010;**36**(4):455–64.

31. Langberg JM, Molina BS, Arnold LE, *et al.* Patterns and predictors of adolescent academic achievement and performance in a sample of children with attention-deficit/hyperactivity disorder. *J Clin Child Adolesc Psychol.* 2011;**40**(4):519–31.

32. Raggi VL, Chronis AM. Interventions to address the academic impairment of children and adolescents with ADHD. *Clin Child Fam Psychol Rev.* 2006;**9**(2):85–111.

33. Biederman J, Petty CR, Fried R, *et al.* Educational and occupational underattainment in adults with attention-deficit/hyperactivity disorder: a controlled study. *J Clin Psychiatry.* 2008;**69**(8):1217–22.

34. Barkley R, Murphy K, Fischer M. *ADHD in Adults: What the Science Says.* New York, NY: Guilford Press; 2006.

35. Solanto MV, Marks DJ, Wasserstein J, *et al.* Efficacy of meta-cognitive therapy for adult ADHD. *Am J Psychiatry.* 2010;**167**(8):958–68.

36. Barkley RA. *Attention-Deficit/Hyperactivity Disorder: A Handbook for Diagnosis and Treatment*, 3rd edn. New York, NY: Guilford Press; 2006.

37. Antshel KM, Barkley R. Psychosocial interventions in attention deficit hyperactivity disorder. *Child Adolesc Psychiatr Clin N Am.* 2008;**17**(2):421–37, x.

38. Wilens TE, Rosenbaum JF. Transitional aged youth: a new frontier in child and adolescent psychiatry. *J Am Acad Child Adolesc Psychiatry.* 2013;**52**(9):887–90.

39. Barkley RA, Fischer M. The unique contribution of emotional impulsiveness to impairment in major life activities in hyperactive children as adults. *J Am Acad Child Adolesc Psychiatry.* 2010;**49**(5):503–13.

40. Biederman J, Faraone SV, Spencer TJ, *et al.* Functional impairments in adults with self-reports of diagnosed ADHD: a controlled study of 1001 adults in the community. *J Clin Psychiatry.* 2006;**67**(4):524–40.

41. Hechtman L, Weiss G. Long-term outcome of hyperactive children. *Am J Orthopsychiatry.* 1983; **53**(3):532–41.

42. Safren SA, Sprich S, Mimiaga MJ, *et al.* Cognitive behavioral therapy vs relaxation with educational support for medication-treated adults with ADHD and persistent symptoms: a randomized controlled trial. *JAMA.* 2010;**304**(8):875–80.

43. Safren SA, Sprich SE, Cooper-Vince C, Knouse LE, Lerner JA. Life impairments in adults with medication-treated ADHD. *J Atten Disord.* 2010;**13**(5): 524–31.

44. Solanto MV, Marks DJ, Wasserstein J, *et al.* Efficacy of meta-cognitive therapy for adult ADHD. *Am J Psychiatry.* 2010;**167**(8):958–68.

45. Weiss M, Hechtman L, Adult ARG. A randomized double-blind trial of paroxetine and/or dextroamphetamine and problem-focused therapy for attention-deficit/hyperactivity disorder in adults. *J Clin Psychiatry.* 2006;**67**(4):611–19.

46. Weiss M, Safren SA, Solanto MV, *et al.* Research forum on psychological treatment of adults with ADHD. *J Atten Disord.* 2008;**11**(6):642–51.

47. Weiss MD, Gibbins C, Goodman DW, *et al.* Moderators and mediators of symptoms and quality of life outcomes in an open-label study of adults treated for attention-deficit/hyperactivity disorder. *J Clin Psychiatry.* 2010;**71**(4):381–90.

48. Weiss M, Murray C, Wasdell M, *et al.* A randomized controlled trial of CBT therapy for adults with ADHD with and without medication. *BMC Psychiatry.* 2012;**12**:30.

49. Hechtman L. Predictors of long-term outcome in children with attention-deficit/hyperactivity disorder. *Pediatr Clin North Am*. 1999;**46**(5):1039–52.

50. Hechtman L. Resilience and vulnerability in long term outcome of attention deficit hyperactive disorder. *Can J Psychiatry*. 1991;**36**(6):415–21.

51. Young S, Gray K, Bramham J. A phenomenological analysis of the experience of receiving a diagnosis and treatment of ADHD in adulthood: a partner's perspective. *J Atten Disord*. 2009;**12**(4):299–307.

52. Rostain AL, Ramsay JR. A combined treatment approach for adults with ADHD–results of an open study of 43 patients. *J Atten Disord*. 2006;**10**(2):150–9.

53. Surman CB, Biederman J, Spencer T, *et al*. Deficient emotional self-regulation and adult attention deficit hyperactivity disorder: a family risk analysis. *Am J Psychiatry*. 2011;**168**(6):617–23.

54. Barkley RA, Fischer M. Predicting impairment in major life activities and occupational functioning in hyperactive children as adults: self-reported executive function (EF) deficits versus EF tests. *Dev Neuropsychol*. 2011;**36**(2):137–61.

55. Surman CB, Adamson JJ, Petty C, *et al*. Association between attention-deficit/hyperactivity disorder and sleep impairment in adulthood: evidence from a large controlled study. *J Clin Psychiatry*. 2009;**70**(11):1523–9.

56. Weiss MD, Gibbins C, Goodman DW, *et al*. Moderators and mediators of symptoms and quality of life outcomes in an open-label study of adults treated for attention-deficit/hyperactivity disorder. *J Clin Psychiatry*. 2010;**71**(4):381–90.

57. Weiss MD, Baer S, Allan BA, Saran K, Schibuk H. The screens culture: impact on ADHD. *Atten Defic Hyperact Disord*. 2011;**3**(4):327–34.

58. Barkley RA, Guevremont DC, Anastopoulos AD, DuPaul GJ, Shelton TL. Driving-related risks and outcomes of attention deficit hyperactivity disorder in adolescents and young adults: a 3- to 5-year follow-up survey. *Pediatrics*. 1993;**92**(2):212–18.

59. Cox DJ, Madaan V, Cox BS. Adult attention-deficit/hyperactivity disorder and driving: why and how to manage it. *Curr Psychiatry Rep*. 2011;**13**(5):345–50.

60. Richards TL, Deffenbacher JL, Rosen LA, Barkley RA, Rodricks T. Driving anger and driving behavior in adults with ADHD. *J Atten Disord*. 2006;**10**(1):54–64.

61. Whalen CK, Henker B, Jamner LD, *et al*. Toward mapping daily challenges of living with ADHD: maternal and child perspectives using electronic diaries. *J Abnorm Child Psychol*. 2006;**34**(1):115–30.

62. Murray C, Johnston C. Parenting in mothers with and without attention-deficit/hyperactivity disorder. *J Abnorm Psychol*. 2006;**115**(1):52–61.

63. Safren SA, Sprich SE, Cooper-Vince C, Knouse LE, Lerner JA. Life impairments in adults with medication-treated ADHD. *J Atten Disord*. 2010;**13**(5):524–31.

64. Biederman J, Petty CR, O'Connor KB, Hyder LL, Faraone SV. Predictors of persistence in girls with attention deficit hyperactivity disorder: results from an 11-year controlled follow-up study. *Acta Psychiatr Scand*. 2012;**125**(2):147–56.

65. Mannuzza S, Klein RG, Moulton JL, 3rd. Young adult outcome of children with "situational" hyperactivity: a prospective, controlled follow-up study. *J Abnorm Child Psychol*. 2002;**30**(2):191–8.

66. Mannuzza S, Klein RG, Bessler A, Malloy P, LaPadula M. Adult psychiatric status of hyperactive boys grown up. *Am J Psychiatry*. 1998;**155**(4):493–8.

67. Mannuzza S, Klein RG, Bessler A, Malloy P, LaPadula M. Adult outcome of hyperactive boys. Educational achievement, occupational rank, and psychiatric status. *Arch Gen Psychiatry*. 1993;**50**(7):565–76.

68. Fischer M, Barkley RA, Fletcher KE, Smallish L. The stability of dimensions of behavior in ADHD and normal children over an 8-year followup. *J Abnorm Child Psychol*. 1993;**21**(3):315–37.

69. Biederman J, Petty CR, Clarke A, Lomedico A, Faraone SV. Predictors of persistent ADHD: an 11-year follow-up study. *J Psychiatr Res*. 2011;**45**(2):150–5.

70. Molina BS, Hinshaw SP, Swanson JM, *et al*. The MTA at 8 years: prospective follow-up of children treated for combined-type ADHD in a multisite study. *J Am Acad Child Adolesc Psychiatry*. 2009;**48**(5):484–500.

Beyond DSM-IV diagnostic criteria

What changed and what should have changed in DSM-5

Russell A. Barkley

Introduction

New diagnostic criteria for attention-deficit hyperactivity disorder (ADHD) have been introduced in the latest edition of the *Diagnostic and Statistical Manual for Mental Disorders* (fifth edition, DSM-5) that was published in May 2013 [1]. Various changes to DSM-IV were suggested by the committee chosen to revise the criteria which then led to exploration of various large-scale existing datasets to test out the results and discover the implications of many of these proposals. (Note – the author did not serve on this committee but did consult with it and provide datasets to it.) Many of the proposals for change were founded on a number of criticisms that were previously leveled at the extant DSM-IV diagnostic criteria [2–5]. Rather than just discuss the various changes that have occurred in the DSM-5 criteria for ADHD, this chapter places those changes in the context of the larger issues and criticisms they were intended to address. It also discusses several additional issues apparently not planned to be addressed as of this time, yet deserved to be acknowledged and possibly even corrected by clinicians utilizing DSM-5 criteria.

At the outset, it should be understood that the problems with DSM-IV and the need for their correction in no way invalidate those criteria for use in the diagnosis of ADHD in children and adults. Since DSM-III [6], efforts have increased to make the criteria more empirically based, in part, using available scientific evidence as well as testing the proposed criteria in field trials [7, 8]. From a scientific standpoint, existing knowledge (criteria in this case) is always imperfect but can be further refined and made more accurate as a representation of material reality or a truth claim. This occurs through a Darwinian process of testing the existing information against reality and using the

feedback (criticism) received in return from such testing to revise the knowledge base. Subsequent retesting is then carried out through observation and experimentation in a ceaseless process of test–revise-test–revise across generations of such trials. Through such testing one can witness the environment naturally selecting out or culling the features of the information that are not accurate thereby sculpting the existing information into more and more accurate representations of reality [9, 10], in this case the criteria for ADHD. In short, existing science-based diagnostic criteria are useful for identifying cases of the disorder but they can always be refined to be more accurate and hence of even greater utility through further experimentation and subsequent modification. The field has now had 19 years of such testing through clinical and experimental use with DSM-IV. Substantial feedback had accumulated to allow consideration of the likely revisions that needed to be made to improve the accuracy and utility of the next set of diagnostic criteria.

As earlier chapters have noted, the DSM-IV criteria stipulate that individuals must have their symptoms of ADHD for at least 6 months, that these symptoms occur to a degree that is developmentally inappropriate, that symptoms result in impairment in two or more domains of major life activities (home, school, work), and that some symptoms producing impairment have developed by 7 years of age. Two lists of symptoms are specified, each containing nine items. From the Inattention item list, six of nine items must be endorsed as developmentally inappropriate, and/or, six must be endorsed from the nine items on the hyperactive–impulsive item list. The symptoms are all amended with the word "Often" as to their occurrence so as to distinguish the symptom as being excessive or inappropriate rather than merely mild, periodic

Attention-Deficit Hyperactivity Disorder in Adults and Children, ed. Lenard A. Adler, Thomas J. Spencer and Timothy E. Wilens.
Published by Cambridge University Press. © Cambridge University Press 2015.

occurrence. The type of ADHD to be diagnosed depends on whether criteria are met for either or both symptom lists: predominantly inattentive, predominantly hyperactive–impulsive, and combined type, respectively. The problems that have arisen with these criteria will now be considered. The coverage of these issues is not intended to be exhaustive but rather to consider the most salient of the problems with the current criteria and what has been done about them in DSM-5.

The age-appropriateness of diagnostic thresholds

The 18 symptoms used in DSM-IV have remained in DSM-5. DSM-IV had a requirement of having six out of nine symptoms on each list as the threshold for diagnosis and this has remained, at least for children, in DSM-5. This threshold was originally developed from a field trial using only children ages 4–16 years [8]. These symptoms decline significantly with age, particularly those in the hyperactive–impulsive list [11, 12]. This may reflect the possibility that individuals are outgrowing their disorder. Applying the same threshold across such a declining developmental slope, however, could produce a diminishing sensitivity to disorder (false negatives). Studies on large samples of adults aged 17–84 years show just such a problem [11, 13] – the threshold needed to place an individual at the 93rd percentile for his or her age group declined to four of nine inattention items and five of nine hyperactive–impulsive items for ages 17–29 years, then to four of nine on each list for the 30- to 49-year age group, then to three of nine on each list for those 50 years and older. Individuals surpassing these revised thresholds are still highly symptomatic and, just as important, impaired in psychosocial functioning yet they would go undiagnosed if six symptoms remained the threshold for disorder [11, 14, 15]. This shows that adhering to a single symptom cutoff score, regardless of age, could result in increasingly fewer individuals with the disorder meeting that threshold with age. They would outgrow the diagnostic criterion while not actually outgrowing their disorder, as was suggested in at least one longitudinal study [16]. To address this problem, the DSM-5 retained the threshold of six symptoms on each symptom list only for children ages 4–18 years, while requiring a lower threshold of five symptoms on either list for adults. This is certainly an improvement in correcting the original problem with DSM-IV but may not

have gone far enough given that all prior research on the issue had identified four symptoms as a better cutoff for diagnosing adults. Yet a desire not to increase prevalence too much prevailed in the DSM-5 chain of review and so the threshold of five may have been chosen as a compromise. My advice is for clinicians to use well-standardized rating scales of ADHD symptoms for children [17, 18] and adults [17, 19] in addition to the DSM-5 recommended threshold to get a more precise indication of age-inappropriateness of symptoms relative to population samples.

The developmental appropriateness of the symptom content

History shows that the items used to construct the DSM symptom lists were based entirely on research on children [7, 8]. Inspection of the item lists suggests that the items for inattention may have a wider developmental applicability than do the items for hyperactivity across school-age ranges of childhood and possibly into adolescence and young adulthood. Those hyperactive symptoms, in contrast, seem much more applicable to young children and are less appropriate or even not at all applicable to older teens and adults. This is evident in the greater decline in the latter symptoms than those of inattention with age and the findings that hyperactive symptoms are of no diagnostic value by adulthood [11]. Furthermore, the items for impulsivity are few (just three) in number and focus entirely on verbal impulsiveness. Given that poor inhibition is considered a central feature of the disorder in contemporary theories [20–22], one would want more of those symptoms represented in the diagnostic criteria. To partially address these problems, the DSM-5 committee considered adding four new items to the list of impulsive symptoms, these being: act without thinking, being impatient, rushing through activities or tasks or being fast-paced (averse to doing things slowly or systematically), and having difficulty resisting immediate temptations or appealing opportunities while disregarding negative consequences. Further analyses of datasets showed that some of these items were quite useful in identifying cases of ADHD. However, DSM-5 does not contain any of these new items but continues using the original 18 from DSM-IV. Again, a concern about increasing prevalence by including new symptoms may have trumped the logic, rationale, and evidence for expanding the item pool. Therefore, it is strongly suggested that clinicians review these additional symptoms of impulsiveness with their clients to be sure not to rely merely on problems of verbal impulsiveness in making a diagnosis.

This problem leads to a related issue – are all these 18 symptoms really essential for accurate diagnosis of the disorder (to discriminate it from the normal population or other disorders)? Surprisingly, studies indicate that just a single symptom is actually needed to determine if someone has ADHD relative to a general population sample with a high degree of accuracy (98%+) – that item is being easily distracted by extraneous stimuli [11, 23]. But four other symptoms appear to contribute to the discrimination of adult ADHD from adults having other disorders [11]. For instance, in discriminating adults with ADHD, those adults were compared to adults having other outpatient disorders than ADHD but who thought they had ADHD and were seen at the same adult ADHD clinic. The following three symptoms of inattention worked best: Fails to give close attention to details, difficulty sustaining attention to tasks, and fails to follow through on instructions. There were four symptoms of hyperactivity–impulsivity (HI) that contributed to group discrimination when HI symptoms were considered separately. But when analyzed alongside the nine inattention symptoms, only one additional symptom from the HI list proved useful besides the three inattention symptoms already identified above; that HI item was: having difficulty engaging in leisure activities quietly. In sum, just five symptoms (these four symptoms and the item of being easily distracted) would be sufficient for the purposes of diagnosing adults with ADHD. A similar state of affairs probably exists for children.

As noted above, the DSM-IV symptom list was developed on and for children, not adults. It is a fair question to ask if a better item set might be developed for adults with ADHD than the items in DSM-IV. The answer is yes. We used large samples of adults with ADHD, clinical controls, and community control adults, and tested 91 new items for adult ADHD. Those items were based largely on theories of executive functioning (EF) and on a review of the clinical charts of several hundred adults with ADHD [11]. The results showed that six new symptoms along with one from the DSM-IV were all that were needed to accurately discriminate the adults with ADHD from the other groups. None of the hyperactive symptoms proved useful. Adding two more inattention symptoms

from DSM-IV increased the accuracy of discrimination by an additional 1–2%. This new nine-item list is shown below (origin in parentheses: either DSM-IV or EF):

1. Often easily distracted by extraneous stimuli (DSM-IV)
2. Often make decisions impulsively (EF)
3. Often has difficulty stopping activities or behavior when they should do so (EF)
4. Often starts a project or task without reading or listening to directions carefully (EF)
5. Often shows poor follow through on promises or commitments they may make to others (EF)
6. Often has trouble doing things in their proper order or sequence (EF)
7. Often more likely to drive a motor vehicle much faster than others (excessive speeding) (EF)
8. Often has difficulty sustaining attention in tasks or leisure activities (DSM-IV)
9. Often has difficulty organizing tasks and activities (DSM-IV).

Further analyses showed that just four of the initial seven or six out of the entire list of nine symptoms proved to be the best thresholds for the number of symptoms needed to differentiate ADHD from these other groups. It is important to note that these new symptoms load on the same two-dimensional structure of the DSM-IV symptom lists when factor analyzed along with those 18 items – they do not represent some new construct not already reflected in the DSM conceptualization of the disorder [11]. These new items were shared with the DSM-5 committee for consideration. None were adopted as outright new symptoms for adults. Instead, these and other statements have been added in parentheses after each of the 18 symptoms to provide clinicians with some clarification of how that symptom may be expressed in older teens and adults. While clarifying the nature of symptoms as they may be evident in teen and adult age groups may be useful, using the symptoms we tested to do so is not appropriate as they were not evaluated as clarifications of existing items but as outright symptoms in their own right. So clinicians may wish to employ both the above items and DSM-5 items in evaluating adults for ADHD so as to use a more optimum set of symptoms in their evaluations than is the case in DSM-5 alone.

One symptom identified on this list may prove problematic in certain countries, geographic locations, or subcultures and that is the one related to often driving a motor vehicle with excessive speed. An alternative symptom to that item that entered our regression analyses when the driving item was removed was "often has difficulty engaging in leisure activities or doing fun things quietly," which is slightly modified from the original DSM-IV wording so as to be more applicable to adults.

Should emotion be a core feature of ADHD?

Three separate reviews have made a compelling case for the inclusion of symptoms of emotional impulsiveness or mood instability and poor emotional self-regulation as a central feature of ADHD [24–26]. Difficulties with the self-regulation of emotion appear to have been included in the core diagnostic constructs of the disorder throughout much of its history [24] but were not included in the DSM-II or later editions for some reason unknown to this author. Recent studies, however, show that symptoms of impulsive emotion, quickness to anger, low frustration tolerance, impatience, and being emotionally excitable exist in the majority of cases [27, 28], load on the HI dimension of ADHD [24], and most importantly, appear to explain unique variance in predicting various forms of impairment in major life activities in children with ADHD followed to adulthood [27] and in clinic-referred adults newly diagnosed with ADHD [28]. It would therefore seem that some symptoms of emotional impulsiveness ought to be added to the DSM symptom list while also reducing some of those related to hyperactivity so as not to make the list unnecessarily lengthy as noted above. The DSM-5 committee has chosen not to address the issue; as noted above, only the DSM-IV items have been carried forward to DSM-5. Clinicians are advised to pay some attention to these emotional symptoms and not view them as due to some other comorbid disorder but instead to view them as a central feature of ADHD even if not present in DSM-5 criteria.

Are sex-referenced criteria necessary?

Research evaluating the DSM-IV and similar item sets find that male children in the general population display more of these items and to a more severe degree than do females [17, 18, 29]. This is not the case for adults when they report their current symptoms, but it

is true for both adults with ADHD and general population samples when they recall ADHD symptoms from childhood [11,19]. An issue this raises for the diagnosis of children and for the retrospective recall of childhood by adults is whether or not different thresholds for diagnosis should be applied to each sex. Otherwise, the current DSM-IV threshold results in girls having to meet a higher threshold relative to other females to be diagnosed as ADHD than do males relative to other males. The problem is further accentuated by the fact that the majority of individuals in the DSM-IV field trial were males, making the DSM criteria primarily male-referenced. Adjusting the cutoff scores for each gender separately might well result in nullifying the finding that ADHD is more common in males than females by a ratio of roughly 3:1. This is not such a dramatic result given that no sex differences have been identified in ADHD symptoms in adult samples [11, 19]. The DSM-5 does not deal with this potential problem of gender-specific criteria. Clinicians would be wise, however, to use rating scales of ADHD symptoms for children and adults that have separate norms for males and females so as to obtain a more precise evaluation of the inappropriateness of these symptoms relative to same-sex norms.

The problems with the age-of-onset criterion

The age-of-onset criterion (AOC) of age 7 years in DSM-IV was undermined from the results of its own field trial [30] as well as from other longitudinal studies [11, 31] and critical reviews of this issue [4, 5, 32]. The DSM-IV AOC results in more than 35% of children with ADHD not meeting that criterion even though they meet all other requirements. This is especially true for those cases with the predominantly inattentive type. And, up to 50% or more of adults with ADHD who would otherwise meet all other diagnostic criteria do not report an age of onset by 7 years. Moreover, adults who otherwise met all other criteria for ADHD except the AOC do not differ in any important respects from those with onset before age 7 years [11, 14, 15]. Prior reviews suggested that the AOC be generously broadened to include onset of symptoms during childhood or adolescence, with an upper limit being set at between 12 and 16 years of age [4]. Age 16, in fact, would capture virtually all cases of childhood ADHD and over 98% of adult cases. Research also suggests that the recall of any precise age of onset is unreliable and is often 4–5 years after the actual onset of the symptoms in childhood [11, 19]. Given these and other results, the DSM-5 has increased the age of onset to age 12 years for adult cases only. Such a half-measure may address the problem for childhood ADHD cases but does not do so for adult cases; it leaves a substantial minority of adults who do not recall the onset of their symptoms prior to this age [11].

Should there be a lower-bound age limit for diagnosis?

Just how young can the diagnosis of ADHD be reliably and validly made? This is important because research on preschool children shows that a separate dimension of hyperactive–impulsive behavior is not distinguishable from one of aggression or defiant behavior until about 3 years of age [19, 33, 34]. Below this age, these behaviors cluster together to form a dimension known as "behavioral immaturity," or an undercontrolled pattern of temperament or conduct. All this implies that the symptoms of ADHD may be difficult to distinguish from other early behavioral disorders or extremes of temperament until at least 3 years of age. Thus, this age might serve as a lower bound for diagnostic applications. The DSM-5 has no changes in it to address this issue yet it is one that clinicians should be cognizant of in evaluating preschool children or toddlers.

The duration of current symptoms

The duration requirement of 6 months of symptom presence for the diagnosis to be rendered may also be problematic for preschool children. The duration was chosen mainly in keeping with the criteria set forth in earlier DSMs and for consistency with criteria used for other disorders. There is little or no research support for selecting this particular length of time for symptom presence in the case of ADHD. It is undoubtedly important that the symptoms be relatively persistent if we are to view this disorder as arising from intraindividual sources (genetics, neurology) rather than arising purely from context or out of a transient, normal developmental stage. Yet specifying a precise duration is difficult in the absence of research to guide the issue. Research on preschool-age children might prove helpful here, however. The few studies that are pertinent to the issue found that many children aged 3 years (or younger) may have parents or preschool teachers who report concerns about the activity level or attention of the children. Yet these concerns have a high likelihood of remission within 12 months [34–36]. It would seem for preschoolers, then, that the 6-month duration specified in DSM-IV and now held over to DSM-5 may be too brief, resulting in the possibility of over identification of ADHD in children at this age (false positives). However, this same body of research found that for those children whose problems lasted at least 12 months or beyond age 4 years, a persistent pattern of behavior was established that was highly predictive of its continuance into the school-age range. The totality of findings suggests that the duration of symptoms might be better set at 12 months or longer, at least for preschoolers, to improve the rigor of diagnosis in detecting true cases of disorder. The DSM-5 criteria have not changed the ascertainment window of 6 months but clinicians may wish to do so to improve the reliability and accuracy of their diagnoses in this age group.

Cross-setting pervasiveness of symptoms

The DSM-IV requirement that the symptoms be demonstrated in at least two of three settings to establish pervasiveness of symptoms is new to the fourth edition of the DSM and is potentially problematic. Yet it has been carried forward to DSM-5. By stipulating that the symptoms must be present in at least two of three contexts (home, school, work, in the case of DSM-IV), the criteria confound settings with sources of information (parent, teacher, employer, clinician), as noted earlier. The degree of agreement between parents and teacher, for instance, is modest for any dimension of psychological development, often ranging between 0.20 and 0.35 depending on the behavioral dimension being rated [37, 38]. This sets an upper limit on the extent to which parents and teachers can agree on the severity of ADHD symptoms.

Those disagreements among sources certainly reflect in part real differences in the child's behavior in these different settings, probably as a function of true differences in situational demands. School, after all, is quite different in its expectations, tasks, social context, and general demands for public self-regulation than is the home environment. But the disagreements may also reflect differences in the attitudes, experiences, and judgments between different people. At this time there appears to be no scientific basis for viewing one person's opinion (e.g., parents) as more accurate than the others (teachers). Instead, these views should be considered as providing information on the child *in that particular context* and nothing more, rather than as evidence as to whether or not the child really has the disorder. More importantly, the crux of the issue of clinical diagnosis is whether or not impairment exists in children identified by parent-only or teacher-only report that stems from their clinical symptoms of ADHD. If impairment is present, it is to be treated even if the diagnosis is less than certain. Diagnosis is a means to an end (relief of suffering), not the end in itself.

Research is clearly conflicting on the matter of whether pervasiveness of symptoms defines a valid syndrome [39–41]. Indeed, the issue has received scant attention in the past 10 years. Until more research is done to address this issue, the requirement of pervasiveness should probably be interpreted to mean *a history* of symptoms in multiple settings rather than current agreement between parent and teacher on number and severity of symptoms. Clinicians need to keep in mind that the DSM-IV was constructed by blending the reports of parents and teachers so as to count the number of *different* symptoms reported across both sources; they should do likewise. The DSM-5 does not deal with this issue.

The meaning of the term "impairment"

The vast majority of mental disorders listed on Axis I of DSM-IV require that impairment in psychosocial functioning exist as one criterion for the diagnosis of a mental disorder. Yet the manual does not define the meaning of this term and, just as important, does not specify the reference group against which it is to be judged. Though undefined in DSM-IV, the manual does state that mental disorders must produce clinically significant impairment or distress. It illustrates this requirement by the phrase "…causes clinically significant distress or impairment in social, occupational, or other important areas of functioning" [1, p. 7] Often explicit in the other definitions yet only implied here is that impairment is diminished functioning in important psychosocial domains of human life.

The absence of an explicit standard of comparison in defining impairment has led to widespread confusion among clinicians attempting to employ this criterion and to the invention of various specialized reference groups to be used in judging its existence. For instance, some clinicians compare intelligent patients to other high functioning peers as if IQ or equally intelligent peers was an appropriate reference group. Others compare the individual to their peers in highly specialized settings, such as in college education or professional employment settings [42]. In either comparison, the general population is not serving as the standard for judging impairment; a highly intelligent, educated, or specialized peer group is so. But is this what most people would consider to be the meaning of the term?

Various definitions of the term "impairment" exist in dictionaries, such as "A disorder in structure or function resulting from anatomical, physiological, or psychological abnormalities that interfere with normal activities" [43]. The American Medical Association (AMA) defines impairment as "a significant deviation, loss, or loss of use of any body structure or function in an individual with a health condition, disorder or disease" [44]. The US government's definition of the term disability is also worth considering as that term is often used synonymously with that of impairment. For instance, in the Americans with Disabilities Act (ADA), a disability is "an inability to function normally, physically or mentally." It further states that a disability is an "inability to engage in any substantial gainful activity by reason of any medically determinable physical or mental impairment which can be expected to last or has lasted for a continuous period of not less than 12 months." Under the ADA: *The term disability means, with respect to an individual, a physical or mental impairment that substantially limits one or more of the major life activities of such individual, a record of such an impairment; or being regarded as having such an impairment* (P.L. 101–336, 1990).

Embedded in both the AMA and ADA definition of impairment/disability is that the "normal" or average person is to serve as the standard against which the degree of functional ineffectiveness and attendant harm is to be judged [42]. This is implied if not explicitly stated in the foregoing definitions of the terms disorder and impairment. The Equal Employment Opportunity Commission (EEOC), which is responsible for setting forth clarifying regulations regarding the ADA, offered this clarification: "An individual is not substantially limited in a major life activity if the limitation does not amount to a significant restriction when *compared with the abilities of the average person* [italics added]." Impairment or disability is therefore "the inability to function in the normal or usual manner" [43]. The normal or typical human (average person in the general population), not some highly intelligent, high functioning, highly specialized, or highly educated peer group, is the standard against which impairment is judged. It would be clinically helpful if the DSM-5 were to specify that impairment refers to the extent of reduction in functional effectiveness and make it explicit that the general population or average person is to serve as the comparison group for making this determination, consistent with governmental regulations and judicial rulings on the subject [42]. The recently developed Barkley Functional Impairment Scale [45] may prove useful in helping to make this determination. It consists of 15 different major domains of adult life activities with norms for a US adult population (ages 18–89), unlike the subjective clinical ratings of impairment offered in the Global Assessment of Functioning Scale or Social and Occupational Functioning Assessment Scale in DSM-IV that have no norms. A separate scale containing 15 different settings is available for use with children. Although DSM-5 was considering having a separate committee provide recommendations for defining impairment, it is not clear from the published manual that little if any guidance is given to clarify what is meant by this term.

Are there clinically meaningful subtypes of ADHD?

The predominantly inattentive type of ADHD (PI) is a heterogeneous group, many of whom appear to be older individuals who may have previously qualified as combined type (C-type) but who have outgrown enough of their hyperactive symptoms to no longer qualify as such by DSM-IV criteria. Others are subthreshold C-type cases that simply miss the diagnostic threshold for C-type by one or two symptoms. It is difficult to consider either of these groups as having a qualitatively different form of ADHD than those who do qualify for C-type. Some research suggests that a subset of cases now placed in the PI subtype may not actually be a subtype of ADHD [46, 47]. Suffice it to say here that a number of qualitative differences between the sluggish cognitive tempo (SCT) subset of this subtype and those with the C-type are emerging in research that suggest that these subtypes do not have the same deficit in attention [19, 48], the

same risks for comorbid disorders, the same risk for impairments in major life activities, and possibly the same response to various ADHD treatments [46, 47]. Whereas the C-type is associated more with problems of persistence of effort and distractibility, SCT in children is characterized by staring, daydreaming, mental fogginess, being readily confused, lethargy, hypoactivity, and sluggish information processing. For instance, in a recent project collecting norms on ADHD and SCT symptoms [19], the following symptoms of SCT formed a separate factor from the two dimensions that exist in DSM-IV consistent with what has been found for children [48]:

- Prone to daydreaming when I should be concentrating on something or working
- Have trouble staying alert or awake in boring situations
- Easily confused
- Easily bored
- Spacey or "in a fog"
- Lethargic, more tired than others
- Underactive or have less energy than others
- Slow moving
- I don't seem to process information as quickly or as accurately as others.

Should these group differences continue to be confirmed in additional research, it would indicate that the SCT subset of individuals placed in the PI subtype should be made a separate, distinct, and independent disorder or at least an independent subtype of ADHD [47].

The predominantly hyperactive–impulsive type (PHI-type) is also a heterogeneous group. Some cases are really not a separate type from the C-type but are simply an earlier developmental stage of it. The field trial found that PHI cases primarily consisted of preschool-age children whereas C-type cases primarily consisted of school-age children. As noted earlier, this is what one would expect to find given that research previously found hyperactive–impulsive symptoms to appear first in development, followed within a few years by those of inattention [12, 50]. If inattention symptoms are required to be part of the diagnostic criteria, then the C-type will of necessity have a later age of onset than the PHI-type, which seems to be the case [30]. Thus, it seems that some cases of the PHI-type may actually be merely an earlier developmental stage of the C-type of ADHD. Other cases, however, will simply be milder, borderline, or subthreshold cases of the C-type simply because they are one or two symptoms shy of meeting the six required on the inattention list to get into the C-type. There does appear to be, however, a subset of cases in the PHI-type who are simply preschool instances of oppositional defiant disorder (ODD). Parents more readily confuse symptoms of ODD with symptoms of ADHD and thus may tend to rate young ODD children as having ADHD symptoms when they do not. Given that cases where ODD occurs alone have a high remission rate (50% remitting every 2 years) [50], such cases of PHI-type may remit with age and probably never really had the PHI-type at all.

The DSM-5 has eliminated subtyping of ADHD altogether in favor of viewing ADHD as a single disorder varying in its symptoms across the population. Instead of subtypes, it will allow clinicians to specify "presentations" in which inattention or hyperactive–impulsive symptoms are the more predominant yet without signaling that these are different types of disorder. SCT however will not be added as a new disorder in DSM-5; more research on its nature is in order before it can be elevated to the formal status of a mental disorder.

Conclusion

This chapter has raised a number of issues that have proven problematic for the DSM-IV diagnostic criteria in the 19 years since its publication. These have focused on the developmental appropriateness of both the wording of the symptoms and the threshold recommended for the number of symptoms, the restricted item set of impulsive symptoms, overweighting of the criteria with hyperactive symptoms, sex-referenced diagnostic thresholds, the AOC, the nature of the cross-setting occurrence of symptoms as opposed to differences in sources of information (parents, teachers, etc.), the meaning of the term "impairment," and the subtyping of ADHD, among others. Not addressed here were some additional issues, such as that concerning eliminating the statement in DSM-IV that ADHD cannot overlap with a diagnosis of autistic spectrum disorders (it can). The DSM-5 has addressed some of these issues (parenthetical clarification of symptoms for older age groups; a slightly lower diagnostic threshold for adults, an age of onset of 12 years instead of 7, etc.). Others of equal importance appear not to be the object of any changes in DSM-5 to address them. Regardless, clinicians and researchers will find it important to be aware of their

existence and consider ways to deal with the problems they raise in order to better refine the official criteria for the diagnosis of ADHD.

References

1. American Psychiatric Association. *Diagnostic and Statistical Manual of Mental Disorders,* 5th edn (DSM-5). Arlington, VA: American Psychiatric Publishing; 2013.

2. Barkley RA. *Attention Deficit Hyperactivity Disorder: A Handbook for Diagnosis and Treatment,* 2nd edn. New York, NY: Guilford Press; 1998.

3. Barkley RA. *Attention Deficit Hyperactivity Disorder: A Handbook for Diagnosis and Treatment,* 3rd edn. New York, NY: Guilford Press; 2006.

4. Barkley RA, Biederman J. Towards a broader definition of the age-of-onset criterion for attention deficit hyperactivity disorder. *J Am Acad Child Adolesc Psychiatry.* 1997;**36**:1204–10.

5. McGough JJ, Barkley RA. Diagnostic controversies in adult ADHD. *Am J Psychiatry.* 2004;**161**:1948–56.

6. American Psychiatric Association. *Diagnostic and Statistical Manual of Mental Disorders,* 3rd edn (DSM-III). Washington, DC: American Psychiatric Association; 1980.

7. Spitzer RL, Davies M, Barkley RA. The DSM-III-R field trial for the Disruptive Behavior Disorders. *J Am Acad Child Adolesc Psychiatry.* 1990;**29**:690–7.

8. Lahey BB, Applegate B, McBurnett K, *et al.* DSM-IV field trials for attention deficit hyperactivity disorder in children and adolescents. *Am J Psychiatry.* 1994;**151**:1673–85.

9. Barkley RA. *Get Rational: A Framework for Leading an Effective, Moral, Productive, and Satisfying Life.* www.getrational.org, 2010.

10. Popper K. *Objective Knowledge: An Evolutionary Approach.* Oxford: Clarendon Press; 1972.

11. Barkley RA, Murphy KR, Fischer M. *ADHD in Adults: What the Science Says.* New York, NY: Guilford Press; 2008.

12. Hart EL, Lahey BB, Loeber R, *et al.* Developmental changes in attention-deficit hyperactivity disorder in boys: A four-year longitudinal study. *J Abn Child Psychol.* 1995;**23**:729–50.

13. Murphy KR, Barkley RA. Prevalence of DSM-IV symptoms of ADHD in adult licensed drivers: Implications for clinical diagnosis. *J Atten Disord.* 1996;**1**:147–61.

14. Faraone SV, Biederman J, Doyle A, *et al.* Neuropsychological studies of late onset and subthreshold diagnoses of adult attention-deficit

hyperactivity disorder. *Biol Psychiatry*. 2006;**60**: 1081–7.

15. Faraone SV, Biederman J, Spencer T, *et al*. Diagnosing adult attention deficit hyperactivity disorder: are late onset and subthreshold cases valid? *Am J Psychiatry*. 2006;**163**:1720–9.

16. Barkley RA, Fischer M, Smallish L, *et al*. The persistence of attention-deficit/hyperactivity disorder into young adulthood as a function of reporting source and definition of disorder. *J Abnorm Psychol*. 2002; **111**:279–89.

17. DuPaul GJ, Power TJ, Anastopoulos AD, *et al*. *The ADHD Rating Scale-IV: Checklists, Norms, and Clinical Interpretation*. New York, NY: Guilford Press; 1998.

18. Conners CK. *Conners ADHD Rating Scales*. North Tonawanda, NY: Multi-Health Systems, Inc.; 2001.

19. Barkley RA. *The Barkley Adult ADHD Rating Scale-IV*. New York, NY: Guilford Press; 2011.

20. Barkley RA. *ADHD and the Nature of Self-Control*. New York, NY: Guilford Press; 1997.

21. Castellanos FX, Sonuga-Barke EJ, Milham MP, Tannock R. Characterizing cognition in ADHD: Beyond executive dysfunction. *Trends Cogn Sci*. 2006; **10**:117–23.

22. Nigg JT, Casey BJ. An integrative theory of attention-deficit/hyperactivity disorder based on the cognitive and affective neurosciences. *Dev Psychopathol*. 2005;**17**:785–806.

23. Milich R, Widiger TA, Landau S. Differential diagnosis of attention deficit and conduct disorders using conditional probabilities. *J Consult Clin Psychol*. 1987; **55**:762–7.

24. Barkley RA. Deficient emotional self-regulation is a core component of ADHD. *J ADHD Relat Disord*. 2010;**1**:5–37.

25. Martel MM. Research review: A new perspective on attention-deficit/hyperactivity disorder: emotion dysregulation and trait models. *J Child Psychol Psychiatry*. 2009;**50**:1042–51.

26. Skirrow C, McLoughlin G, Kuntsi J, *et al*. Behavioral, neurocognitive and treatment overlap between attention-deficit/hyperactivity disorder and mood instability. *Expert Rev Neurother*. 2009;**9**:489–503.

27. Barkley RA, Fischer M. The unique contribution of emotional impulsiveness to impairment in major life activities in hyperactive children as adults. *J Am Acad Child Adolesc Psychiatry*. 2010;**49**:503–13.

28. Barkley RA, Murphy KR. Deficient emotional self-regulation in adults with ADHD: The relative contributions of emotional impulsiveness and ADHD symptoms to adaptive impairments in major life activities. *J ADHD Relat Disord*. 2010;**1**:5–28.

29. Achenbach TM. *Child Behavior Checklist and Child Behavior Profile – Cross-Informant Version*. Burlington, VT: Author; 1991.

30. Applegate B, Lahey BB, Hart EL, *et al*. Validity of the age of onset criterion for ADHD: A report from the DSM-IV field trials. *J Am Acad Child Adolesc Psychiatry*. 1997;**36**:1211–21.

31. McGee R, Williams S, Feehan M. Attention deficit disorder and age of onset of problem behaviors. *J Abnorm Child Psychol*. 1992;**20**:487–502.

32. Barkley RA. Against the status quo: revising the diagnostic criteria for ADHD. Invited Commentary. *J Am Acad Child Adolesc Psychiatry*. 2010;**49**:205–7.

33. Achenbach TM, Edelbrock CS. *Manual for the Child Behavior Profile and Child Behavior Checklist*. Burlington, VT: Author; 1983.

34. Campbell SB. *Behavior Problems in Preschool Children*. New York, NY: Guilford Press; 1990.

35. Beitchman JH, Wekerle C, Hood J. Diagnostic continuity from preschool to middle childhood. *J Am Acad Child Adolesc Psychiatry*. 1987;**26**:694–9.

36. Palfrey JS, Levine MD, Walker DK, *et al*. The emergence of attention deficits in early childhood: A prospective study. *J Dev Behav Pediatr*. 1985;**6**:339–48.

37. Achenbach TM, McConaughy SH, Howell CT. Child/adolescent behavioral and emotional problems: Implications of cross informant correlations for situational specificity. *Psychol Bull*. 1987;**101**:213–32.

38. Mitsis EM, McKay KE, Schulz KP, *et al*. Parent-teacher concordance for DSM-IV attention-deficit/hyperactivity disorder in a clinic-referred sample. *J Am Acad Child Adolesc Psychiatry*. 2000;**39**:308–13.

39. Cohen NJ, Minde K. The "hyperactive syndrome" in kindergarten children: Comparison of children with pervasive and situational symptoms. *J Child Psychol Psychiatry*. 1983;**24**:443–55.

40. Rapoport JL, Donnelly M, Zametkin A, *et al*. "Situational hyperactivity" in a U.S. clinical setting. *J Child Psychol Psychiatry*. 1986;**27**:639–46.

41. Schachar R, Rutter M, Smith A. The characteristics of situationally and pervasively hyperactive children: Implications for syndrome definition. *J Child Psychol Psychiatry*. 1981;**22**:375–92.

42. Gordon M, Keiser S, eds. *Accommodations in Higher Education under the Americans with Disabilities Act (ADA): A No-Nonsense Guide for Clinicians, Educators, Administrators, and Lawyers*. New York, NY: Guilford Publications and GSI Publications; 1998.

43. *Mosby's Medical Dictionary*. New York, NY: Elsevier; 2009.

44. American Medical Association. *American Medical Association Guide to the Assessment of Permanent*

Impairment. Washington, DC: American Medical Association, 2001.

45. Barkley RA. *The Barkley Functional Impairment Scale.* New York, NY: Guilford Press; 2011.

46. Milich R, Ballentine AC, Lynam DR. ADHD/combined type and ADHD/predominantly inattentive type are distinct and unrelated disorders. *Clin Psychol Sci Pract*. 2001;**8**:463–88.

47. Adams ZW, Milich R, Fillmore MT. A case for the return of attention-deficit disorder in DSM-5. *ADHD Rep*. 2010;**18**(3),1–6.

48. Penny AM, Waschbusch DA, Klein RM, *et al.* Developing a measure of sluggish cognitive tempo for children: content validity, factor structure, and reliability. *Psychol Assess*. 2009;**21**: 380–9.

49. Loeber R, Green SM, Lahey BB, *et al.* Developmental sequences in the age of onset of disruptive child behaviors. *J Child Fam Studies*. 1992;**1**:21–41.

50. Barkley RA. *Defiant Children: A Clinicians Manual for Parent Training,* 3rd edn. New York, NY: Guilford Press; 2013.

Conceptual issues in understanding comorbidity in ADHD

Steven R. Pliszka

Why does comorbidity matter?

Chapters 1–5 have laid out the clinical description of attention-deficit hyperactivity disorder (ADHD), its epidemiology, and functional impairments. It is well established that in a given sample of patients with ADHD, only about 50–60% of the individuals will be free of any other psychiatric disorder, while the remainder will have one or more psychiatric or learning disorders concurrent with their ADHD [1]. From a clinical perspective, these additional disorders often demand concurrent treatment as they may cause more impairment than the ADHD itself; furthermore the presence of comorbidity complicates studies of the life course and etiology of ADHD. Recently, it has been recognized that "reverse comorbidity" is a reality, that is, patients with "primary" diagnosis of another major psychiatric disorder such as affective disorder or autism spectrum disorder (ASD) also meet criteria for ADHD at rates much higher than in the general population. The term "reverse comorbidity" largely reflects the fact that the comorbidity was first recognized and studied in those with ADHD [2] – but its importance is now recognized for all psychiatric disorders; and that excess overlap of ADHD exists in certain other psychiatric disorders.

The usual paradigm in comorbidity research involves comparing at least three groups: those with ADHD alone, those with ADHD who meet criteria for a comorbid disorder (CM), and a sample of controls; ideally a group of patients who have the CM without ADHD should be studied as well, although few studies do this. The psychiatric diagnosis is made via a structured interview according to DSM-IV criteria and groups are examined for differences on a number of variables. First, care must be taken to rule out artificial

comorbidity due to the fact that the DSM criteria for ADHD and some disorders share individual criteria items – for instance poor concentration is a symptom of both ADHD and depressive disorders, while increased activity is common to ADHD and mania. However, most children with comorbidity continue to meet criteria for both disorders even when the overlapping symptoms are subtracted out [3, 4]. Second, while epidemiological studies generally show lower levels of comorbidity than clinical samples, meta-analyses of epidemiological studies clearly show that comorbidity is not purely an artifact of referral bias [5]. Jensen *et al.* have discussed ways in which the CM associated with ADHD is important to study [6].

Distinctive clinical picture. Children with ADHD/CM should differ in substantial ways from children with ADHD on measures other than the diagnostic criteria themselves. For instance, ADHD children with social phobia should be seen as withdrawing from social interactions on the playground by observers blind to the child's diagnostic status. If ADHD children with and without a comorbid diagnosis differ only on the clinician's interview, without any "real world" differences on behavior rating scales, peer interactions, educational achievement, etc., then the validity of the distinction is questionable.

Distinctive demographic factors. The ADHD/CM group may differ from the ADHD children alone in terms of sex, ethnicity, or social class.

Differences in psychosocial factors. The ADHD/CM group may have a differential exposure to major societal stressors such as poverty, crime, urban decay, or exposure to violence.

Differences in biological factors. Are there differences between the ADHD/CM and ADHD groups in terms of genetic markers, brain anatomy,

Attention-Deficit Hyperactivity Disorder in Adults and Children, ed. Lenard A. Adler, Thomas J. Spencer and Timothy E. Wilens.
Published by Cambridge University Press. © Cambridge University Press 2015.

neuroimaging, or physiology? This approach is still in its infancy, but holds great promise for the future.

Distinctive family genetic factors. Does the ADHD/CM condition "breed true?" That is, if a child has ADHD/CM, is there an increased prevalence of both ADHD and CM in his/her relatives? Furthermore, does the ADHD and CM almost always occur in the same relative or does the child have some relatives with CM and others with ADHD? In the former situation, the case for ADHD/CM being a distinct genetic subtype is strengthened. In the latter case, the child most likely inherited two independent disorders from separate relatives and ADHD/CM is not distinct.

Distinctive family environmental factors. Has the ADHD/CM child been exposed to certain family experiences not shared by the child with ADHD alone? Have ADHD children with anxiety disorders experienced more divorce or separation than those with ADHD alone? Are children with ADHD and CD more likely to have been exposed to domestic violence?

Distinctive clinical course and outcome. Are ADHD children with and without CMs different at follow-up? Do ADHD/conduct disorder (CD) children have more criminal convictions? Do ADHD children with depression have a higher rate of adult affective disorder than non-depressed ADHD children? Are there differences in the life course of the ADHD itself for comorbid and non-comorbid children? Does the presence of the CM make continuation of ADHD into adulthood more or less likely?

Unique response to specific treatments. Do ADHD children with and without CMs differ in their response to either psychopharmacological or psychosocial interventions?

Since the early 1990s, a multitude of studies have examined a variety of disorders commonly comorbid with ADHD from the above perspectives. Much of these data will be reviewed in detail in Chapters 7–13; in this chapter a broader view of how our thinking on comorbidity has shifted over the past two decades is presented. Two issues influence thinking on comorbidity: (1) the degree to which the overlap is symmetrical or asymmetrical and (2) whether one looks at categorical diagnoses or dimensional measures of symptoms. For instance oppositional defiant/conduct disorders (ODD/CD) and depressive/anxiety disorders tend to show a symmetrical overlap with their "reverse comorbidities." That is, just as 25–50% of children with ADHD may meet criteria for another disruptive behavior disorder, 25–50% of children with

ODD/CD or mood/anxiety may meet criteria for ADHD [5].

While it gathers less attention, the overlap of ADHD, tic disorders and obsessive–compulsive disorder (OCD) is of considerable theoretical interest [7, 8]. The study of the comorbidity of ASD with ADHD has been limited by the fact that past versions of DSM prohibited these diagnoses to be made concurrently; nonetheless significant numbers of children with ASD have clinically significant symptoms of ADHD [9]. When ASD and OCD are defined categorically, their overlap with ADHD tends to be *asymmetrical*. That is, while the rate of ADHD in those with these disorders exceeds that in the general population, the reverse is not true, patients with ADHD do not suffer from these disorders in rates greatly above normative rates [1, 10]. When the overlap of disorders is asymmetrical, clinicians specializing in the CM may find themselves at cross purposes with those who treat the broad range of ADHD. Specialists may feel that the CM is common among those with ADHD, while the generalist feels the CM is rare. Both types of clinicians need to be aware of the nature of their patient population. When disorders such as ASD are examined dimensionally, however, a different picture emerges. For instance, even excluding patients with formal ASD diagnoses, children with ADHD and their siblings show high rates of autistic-like traits [11, 12]. Thus dimensional approaches may lead to fundamental changes in the way we view comorbidity in ADHD.

Clinical assessment of comorbidity

Chapters 18 and 19 will provide detailed information on the assessment of the adult or child with possible ADHD. Assessment for CMs is a mandatory part of the ADHD workup in both adults and children [13, 14]. Use of broad-range standardized questionnaires can assist the clinician in identifying a wide range of possible comorbid symptoms before and during the clinical interview. Both parents and children can be queried with scales for depression [15, 16], mania [17], anxiety [18–20], and aggression [21–23]. The clinician should review these with the parent and ask detailed questions about areas that stand out. Symptoms regarding OCD, ASD, and tics should be discussed directly since brief screening tools in children for these disorders are less well established. Review of early developmental history is key for detecting possible ASD or signs of possible language/learning delays. The child should be interviewed directly, as children may endorse depressive or anxiety symptoms even when their parents do not report them [24]. Adolescents should be asked about substance abuse, including alcohol and cigarette use.

In adults, a broad range of symptoms can be screened for by using a self-report scale such as the Symptom Checklist 90-Revised [25]. This scale produces nine subscales (Anxious, Phobic, Paranoia, Depression, Somatization, Obsessive-Compulsive, Interpersonal Sensitivity, Psychoticism, Hostility). The clinician can then inquire further as to whether the individual meets DSM criteria for a particular disorder. Substance abuse issues need to be explored. Relative to children, adults are more likely to present to a clinician with a complaint related to mood or anxiety disorder, therefore it is useful to screen these patients with an adult ADHD rating scale [26, 27] and to inquire about the patient's early history in school as well as to whether the patient has children with ADHD. This will assist in identifying the reverse comorbidity of ADHD in the patient with some other presenting complaint.

Overview of comorbidity in childhood ADHD

Biederman *et al.* reviewed studies which examined rates of comorbidity of ODD/CD and ADHD [2], finding that up to 50% of children with ADHD meet criteria for CD, while Pliszka *et al.* found similar results in their review [28]. Pliszka *et al.* noted that in early childhood the overlap with ODD/CD tended to be more asymmetrical [28] – while half of young children with ADHD might meet criteria for ODD/CD, nearly all young children with ODD/CD meet criteria for ADHD [29]. ODD/CD without ADHD is more common in adolescents [30]. Reviewing the vast literature on the comorbidity of ADHD and ODD/CD, Barkley came to several key conclusions [1]: (1) aggressive behavior is a feature primarily of those with ADHD/CD, (2) children with ADHD/CD have a lower verbal IQ than those with ADHD alone, (3) children with ADHD/CD are more likely to show early psychopathic traits and develop antisocial behavior as adults, and (4) children with ADHD/CD show higher levels of family dysfunction. In their review, Pliszka *et al.* noted higher levels of family pathology and risk for substance abuse in those with ADHD/CD relative to those with ADHD alone [28]. ADHD and

CD cosegregate in families, suggesting ADHD/CD is a separate genetic subtype [31, 32]. Interestingly, the comorbidity of ODD/CD does not affect the robustness of stimulant response of the underlying ADHD [33]. Having a comorbid ODD or CD becomes the pathway through which patients with ADHD are at greater risk for substance use disorders [34–38].

Compared to those with ADHD alone, those with comorbid anxiety (without ODD/CD) show lower levels of impulsivity on laboratory measures of attention and a greater tendency to respond to psychosocial interventions [39–41]. Of interest, it is parent report of anxiety, rather than child report that predicts such response. ADHD and anxiety appear to arise from independent genetic contributions [31]. When children with ADHD have the "double" comorbidity of both anxiety and ODD/CD, they tend to resemble children with ADHD + ODD/CD in their cognitive profile [40] yet show an enhanced response to combined medication and psychosocial intervention [39].

The overlap of ADHD with depression is less well studied. In the Multimodality Treatment of ADHD (MTA) study, 11% of the sample also met criteria for major depressive disorder (MDD), a rate similar to that in a large university-clinic-based sample of children with ADHD [14]. Angold *et al.* found the risk of depression in children with ADHD to be increased by a factor of 5.5 relative to the general population [5]. How depression affects the clinical expression of ADHD has not been explored; family studies suggest that ADHD and MDD might share genetic factors [31]. The presence of ADHD alone does not appear to affect treatment response [42] or the long-term course of the depression [43]. The comorbidity of ADHD with mania will be discussed in more detail below and in Chapter 7.

Overview of comorbidity in adult ADHD

Rates of comorbidity in adults with ADHD have been broadly similar to those found in children [44]. The National Comorbidity Survey Replication examined for ADHD and other mental disorders in over 3000 adults [45], finding a prevalence of adult ADHD of 4.4%. Mood, anxiety, substance use, and impulse control disorders were elevated in those with ADHD relative to those without ADHD. The specific rates (ADHD vs. non-ADHD) for each disorder were: major depression (19% vs. 8%), bipolar (19% vs. 3%), any anxiety disorder (47% vs. 20%), any substance use disorder (15% vs. 6%), and intermittent explosive disorder (20% vs. 6%). In contrast to the high rates of bipolar disorder shown in this study, Barkley and Murphy did not find elevated rates of bipolar adults with ADHD in either a cross-sectional or longitudinal study [46], though the latter study did find higher rates of adults with borderline personality disorder, who also show the mood lability seen in patients with mania.

Mood dysregulation and comorbidity

There has been a marked increase in the number of children diagnosed with bipolar disorder. According to the National Ambulatory Medical Care Survey [47], outpatient visits to physicians for youth carrying a diagnosis of bipolar disorder rose from 25 per 100 000 population in 1994–1995 to 1003 per 100 000 in 2002–2003. This is a 40-fold increase compared to a 185% increase in adults. Inpatient admissions of children and adolescents for bipolar disorder showed a near sixfold increase [48]. Most of these children also meet criteria for ADHD. Wozniak *et al.* identified 43 children in a psychiatric outpatient clinic who met their criteria (K-SADS) for mania and all but one of these children also met criteria for ADHD [49]. They were compared to 164 non-manic ADHD children and 84 controls. There was a total of 206 (42 manic and 164 non-manic) ADHD subjects, which yields a prevalence of mania of 20% among the ADHD sample in this study. There were only two children with euphoric mania; and 77% showed "extreme and persistent mania." That is, they did not cycle nor did they have any prolonged periods of euthymia. Eighty-four percent of this group showed mixed mania. Biederman *et al.* studied a second sample of 120 ADHD children and found 29 children (21%) who met criteria for bipolar disorder [50]. Child Behavior Checklist Scores (CBCL) of the ADHD/manic children were elevated over the ADHD-only children on nearly all the subscales. Of note, it was the aggression subscale which most differentiated the manic/ADHD group from the ADHD-only group [51]. The debate over the validity of mania in children with ADHD has focused on two issues: (1) is the absence of inter-episode recovery inconsistent with mania and (2) is the aggressive behavior part of mania ("affective storms") or a sign of CD or another disorder all together [52, 53]?

It is becoming clear that prolonged inter-episode recovery is rare in children and adolescents. In one

study, research nurses questioned the families of 26 children with bipolar disorder closely about the number and length of the manic or depressive episodes [54]. One parent reported that their child had 104 episodes in a year, each of these episodes lasting from 4 hours to a whole day. Another subject had daily episodes of agitation or depression for a whole year. Only two subjects had episodes that lasted longer than 2 weeks as their only episodes. Findling *et al.* identified 90 youth aged 5–17 years with bipolar disorder and used life charting to determine their clinical course [55]. Strikingly, only two of the subjects showed inter-episode recovery, defined as a 2-month period free of symptoms (50% were rapid cyclers). Furthermore, it is becoming clear that inter-episode recovery is rare even in adult patients. Retrospective studies in adults of the age of the first episode of mania clearly show childhood onset in the majority of cases, and such onset is associated with greater severity of illness [56, 57]. Thus if lack of recovery invalidates the diagnosis of bipolar disorder in children with chronically labile mood, then many adult diagnoses would be regarded as suspect as well.

Given that these children show such high rates of negatively reactive mood and aggression, Leibenluft and colleagues proposed a distinction between a narrow phenotype of mania in which it would be required that the child show elated mood (and not irritability) and a broad phenotype they have termed "Severe Mood Dysregulation" (SMD) [58]. While the initial article placed this broad phenotype in the bipolar spectrum, further work by this group and others have suggested that this phenotype is separate from bipolar disorder. This has led to the proposed criteria for temper dysregulation disorder (TDD) in DSM-5. The proposed criteria require that the child *not* show expansive or elated mood accompanied by three or more of DSM "B" criteria of mania (grandiosity, decreased need for sleep, pressured speech, hypersexuality, etc.). The core features are nearly daily temper outbursts (>3 times per week) with irritable mood between outbursts. They must be present in two settings and "severe" in one setting, with an onset by at least 10 years of age. Adoption of such criteria might have profound clinical and research implications for children with comorbid ADHD and bipolar disorder, as the "narrow phenotype" of bipolar disorder (elated, expansive mood, distinct episodes) appears to be quite rare in epidemiological studies [59, 60]. More significantly, children and adolescents with temper/mood dysregulation do not appear to develop manic episodes in longitudinal studies and may show a higher rate of depression instead [61, 62] and show differences from children with narrow phenotype bipolar disorder studies in biological markers [63, 64]. The study of Brotman *et al.* yielded some interesting contrasts between the narrow phenotype bipolar group (n = 43) and the SMD group (n = 29) [63]. The prevalence of ADHD was only 47% in the bipolar group vs. 83% in the SMD group, yet the rate of stimulant treatment was not different (23% vs. 37%). More strikingly, equal proportions of each group were on antipsychotics, lithium, or other mood stabilizers, nor were they distinguished by the prevalence of other CMs (ODD, anxiety, or depression).

Data such as these raise an intriguing question – is TDD vs. "narrow" phenotype bipolar disorder a distinction without a difference? If the patients end up being treated with the same medications will psychiatrists change their practice? They are particularly unlikely to do so if TDD is viewed as just a more severe form of ODD and not viewed worthy of intensive intervention such as antipsychotics and psychiatric hospitalization. Many of these children and adolescents present with life-threatening explosive outbursts. If a clinician reports to a family that their child who carries the diagnosis of bipolar "doesn't have it" but instead has TDD, how will they react, particularly if this new diagnosis does not carry with it any new treatment options? Chapter 7 will delve into these issues further.

Evolving views of comorbidity

The study of comorbidity to this point has involved the comparison of the subjects with ADHD who have or do not have the CM of interest. Both ADHD and the CM under study are defined by clinical interview, without regard to any model of the underlying pathophysiology. This is understandable, as heretofore investigators have not had any means by which to examine the underlying neurobiology of either ADHD or other psychiatric disorders. With the emergence of modern neuropsychology, neuroimaging, and genetics, this is beginning to change. Chapters 14–20 will examine all three of these areas in detail, here we examine their impact on the study of comorbidity.

ADHD has been conceptualized as a disorder of poor inhibitory control, as assessed with measures such as the Go/No-Go and Stop Signal tasks [65]. A meta-analysis of 17 studies involving the Stop Signal task showed that only 45–50% of children with ADHD had a performance level more impaired than the 90th percentile of the control sample [66]. More broadly, ADHD has been viewed as an executive function deficit, yet on any given measure of executive function, only 16–50% of ADHD children are found to be impaired [66, 67]. This has led to the conclusion that other deficits must play a role in ADHD, including the inability to delay response to reward [68, 69], greater intra-individual variability of reaction time which relates to regulation of effort and arousal [70], and problems with sense of time, both in processing time [71] and motor timing [72]. Thus ADHD itself is a heterogeneous disorder from a neuropsychological perspective.

Two recent studies provide some insight into how these new approaches may be relevant to the study of comorbidity. Wahlstedt *et al.* classified 182 school-age children into four groups [73]: controls, high inattention-low impulsivity/hyperactivity, high impulsivity/hyperactivity-low inattention, and combined. They assessed them on several neuropsychological domains: executive dysfunction, poor arousal and effort modulation (reflected by greater reaction time variability), and delay aversion. Most controls (64%) had no deficits in any of the three neuropsychological domains, while the remaining had at least one. In all three ADHD groups, 74% had one or more of the three impairments, but the ADHD was heterogeneous in the types of impairment (44% inhibition problems, 46% arousal regulation issues, 19% delay aversion issues, and 23% working memory problems). A quarter of the ADHD subjects had no deficits in these areas of neuropsychological function. ODD symptoms were related to both hyperactivity and inattention, but only had very low correlations with any of the neuropsychological variables. In contrast, internalizing problems were related only to inattention, with only a very modest relationship to delay aversion. Sonuga-Burke *et al.* used a similar design, comparing children with ADHD to controls and their non-affected siblings on a similar array of neuropsychological domains (executive dysfunction, delay aversion, and time perception) [71]. Similar to Wahlstedt *et al.* [73], Sonuga-Burke *et al.* found that 22 of 77 subjects with ADHD had no deficit in any neuropsychological domain, while the others had some deficits but not others [71]. None of the neuropsychological deficits were associated with ODD. These two studies suggest, surprisingly, that the core neuropsychological deficits of ADHD do not appear to be related to ODD, the most common comorbidity with ADHD! This suggests that other factors (not yet studied or hypothesized) must be involved in the pathway from ADHD to ODD.

A model of how the pathophysiology of ADHD and CMs may overlap is best illustrated by a neuroimaging study of ADHD with and without comorbid CD. Herpetz *et al.* compared 22 adolescents with childhood-onset CD (16 of whom also met criteria for ADHD) to controls on a functional MRI study in which the subjects passively viewed pictures of a negative, positive, or neutral emotional valence [74]. Relative to controls, CD boys had increased amygdala activation when viewing negative pictures vs. neutral pictures. Since so many of the subjects with CD had comorbid ADHD, the authors performed a second experiment using the same neuroimaging task comparing 13 boys with ADHD who had no comorbidity with a second set of 13 controls. There was no difference between the controls and the boys with non-comorbid ADHD in amygdala activation. This study suggests that amygdala dysfunction was related to CD and not to ADHD. The study requires replication via direct comparison of subjects with ADHD, ADHD/CD, CD, and controls, but these studies plus those reviewed above [71, 73] suggest different neuropsychological and neurobiological mechanisms in ADHD and CD which might combine in the CD group. Similar types of studies will be needed to tease out the underlying mechanisms of ADHD and other CMs.

Future directions

Research on comorbidity may be further enhanced by the study of endophenotypes of a variety of psychiatric disorders [75]. An endophenotype is an immediate physiological variable between genes and the expression of a disorder; an endophenotype must be shared by family members who do not express the disorder. For instance, impaired inhibitory control (as assessed by any number of standardized laboratory measures) is present more often in patients with ADHD than controls; it is also present in non-affected siblings of patients with ADHD. It is thought that an endophenotype arises through interaction of the gene with other neurobiological factors (including effects on the neurobiology from the environment). One given endophenotype does not cause the disorder, but multiple endophenotypes may combine to form a given phenotype of ADHD. Impaired inhibitory

control, working memory deficits, poor temporal processing, motor timing, and delay aversion are all hypothesized endophenotypes related to ADHD, but could be related to other disorders as well.

CMs may have their own endophenotypes, such as mood lability (relevant to both aggressive CD and bipolar disorder), exaggerated response to threat (CD, anxiety, depression), poor recognition of facial expression (ASD), and so on. An example of how helpful this approach may be in the future is illustrated by a genetic study of the overlap of ADHD and ASD [76]. The Social Communication Questionnaire was obtained on over 1000 children with ADHD and their siblings (none of the subjects meet formal criteria for ASD). DNA was obtained from the subjects and their parents, and multivariate quantitative trait locus (QTL) linkage was examined for ADHD and ASD symptoms to identify loci in the genome related to ADHD, ASD-like traits, or both. While none of the loci identified reached genome-wide significance, the study suggested separate loci underlying ASD symptoms on chromosomes 7q, 12q, 15q, 16p, and 18p. The loci on chromosomes 12, 16, and 18 were also related to ADHD, suggesting a possible genetic cause for the comorbidity. Much work remains to be done in this area before this work is relevant clinically. Chapters 7–13 are organized categorically, covering the critical comorbidities of bipolar disorder, depression, anxiety, substance use, learning disorders, ODD and CD, and medical issues. In the future, it is conceivable that each of these (as well as ADHD itself) will be related to underlying physiological (and measurable) endophenotypes such as inhibitory control or social communication deficits – and this very wide array of endophenotypes can combine in multiple ways to produce the complex and variable phenotypes encountered in clinical practice.

References

1. Barkley RA. Comorbid disorders, social and family adjustment, and subtyping. *Attention Deficit Hyperactivity Disorder*, 3rd edn. New York, NY; Guilford Press. 2005; 184–218.

2. Biederman J, Newcorn J, Sprich S. Comorbidity of attention deficit hyperactivity disorder with conduct, depressive, anxiety, and other disorders. *Am J Psychiatry*. 1991;**148**:564–77.

3. Biederman J, Faraone S, Mick E, *et al.* Psychiatric comorbidity among referred juveniles with major depression: fact or artifact? *J Am Acad Child Adolesc Psychiatry*. 1995;**34**:579–90.

4. Milberger S, Biederman J, Faraone SV, *et al.* Attention deficit hyperactivity disorder and comorbid disorders: issues of overlapping symptoms. *Am J Psychiatry.* 1995; **152**(12):1793–9.

5. Angold A, Costello EJ, Erkanli A. Comorbidity. *J Child Psychol Psychiatry.* 1999;**40**(1):57–87.

6. Jensen PS, Martin D, Cantwell DP. Comorbidity in ADHD: implications for research, practice, and DSM-V. *J Am Acad Child Adolesc Psychiatry.* 1997; **36**(8):1065–79.

7. Geller D, Petty C, Vivas F, *et al.* Further evidence for co-segregation between pediatric obsessive compulsive disorder and attention deficit hyperactivity disorder: a familial risk analysis. *Biol Psychiatry.* 2007;**61**(12): 1388–94.

8. Pauls DL, Alsobrook JP, Phil M, *et al.* A family study of obsessive-compulsive disorder. *Am J Psychiatry.* 1995;**152**(1):76–84.

9. Goldstein S, Schwebach AJ. The comorbidity of Pervasive Developmental Disorder and Attention Deficit Hyperactivity Disorder: results of a retrospective chart review. *J Autism Dev Disord.* 2004;**34**(3):329–39.

10. Pauls DL, Leckman JF, Cohen DJ. Familial relationship between Gilles de la Tourette's syndrome, attention deficit disorder, learning disabilities, speech disorders, and stuttering. *J Am Acad Child Adolesc Psychiatry.* 1993;**32**:1044–1050.

11. Reiersen AM, Todd RD. Co-occurrence of ADHD and autism spectrum disorders: phenomenology and treatment. *Expert Rev Neurother.* 2008;**8**(4):657–69.

12. Reiersen AM, Constantino JN, Volk HE, *et al.* Autistic traits in a population-based ADHD twin sample. *J Child Psychol Psychiatry.* 2007;**48**(5):464–72.

13. American Academy of Child and Adolescent Psychiatry. Practice parameter for the assessment and treatment of children and adolescents with attention-deficit/hyperactivity disorder. *J Am Acad Child Adolesc Psychiatry.* 2007;**46**(7):894–921.

14. Pliszka SR. Treating ADHD and comorbid disorders. In: *Psychosocial and Psychopharmacological Interventions.* New York, NY: Guilford Press. 2009; 1–25.

15. Kovacs M. *Children's Depression Inventory.* Los Angeles, CA: Multi-Health Systems, Inc.; 1992.

16. Angold A, Costello EJ, Messer SC, *et al.* The development of a short questionnaire for use in epidemiological studies of depression in children and adolescents. *Int J Methods Psychiatr Res.* 1995;**5**: 237–49.

17. Pavuluri MN, Henry DB, Devineni B, *et al.* Child mania rating scale: development, reliability, and

validity. *J Am Acad Child Adolesc Psychiatry.* 2006; **45**(5):550–60.

18. March JS, Parker JDA, Sullivan K, *et al.* The multidimensional anxiety scale for children (MASC): factor structure, reliability, and validity. *J Am Acad Child Adolesc Psychiatry.* 1997;**36**:554–65.

19. Birmaher B, Khetarpal S, Brent D, *et al.* The Screen for Child Anxiety Related Emotional Disorders (SCARED): scale construction and psychometric characteristics. *J Am Acad Child Adolesc Psychiatry.* 1997:**36**(4);545–53.

20. Reynolds CR, Richmond BO. What I Think and Feel: a revised measure of Children's Manifest Anxiety. *J Abnorm Child Psychol.* 1997;**25**(1):15–20.

21. Kronenberger WG, Giauque AL, Dunn DW. Development and validation of the outburst monitoring scale for children and adolescents. *J Child Adolesc Psychopharmacol.* 2007;**17**(4):511–26.

22. Halperin JM, McKay KE, Newcorn JH. Development, reliability, and validity of the children's aggression scale-parent version. *J Am Acad Child Adolesc Psychiatry.* 2002;**41**(3):245–52.

23. Halperin JM, McKay KE, Grayson RH, *et al.* Reliability, validity, and preliminary normative data for the Children's Aggression Scale-Teacher Version. *J Am Acad Child Adolesc Psychiatry.* 2003;**42**(8):965–71.

24. Bird HR, Gould MS, Staghezza B. Aggregating data from multiple informants in child psychiatry epidemiological research. *J Am Acad Child Adolesc Psychiatry.* 1992;**31**(1):78–85.

25. Degrotis LR. *Manual for the Symptom Checklist-90-Revised (SCL-90-R).* San Antonio, TX: PsychCorp; 2010.

26. Adler LA, Kessler RC, Spencer TJ. *The Adult ADHD Self-Report Scale (ASRS v1.1) Symptom Checklist.* Geneva, Switzerland: World Health Organization; 2003.

27. Conners CK, Erhardt D, Sparrow EP. *Conners' Adult ADHD Rating Scales.* North Tonawanda, NY: Multi-Health Systems, Inc.; 1999.

28. Pliszka SR, Carlson CL, Swanson JM. *ADHD with Comorbid Disorders: Clinical Assessment and Management.* New York, NY: Guilford Press; 1999.

29. McArdle P, O'Brien G, Kolvin I. Hyperactivity: prevalence and relationship with conduct disorder. *J Child Psychol Psychiatry.* 1995:**36**(2):279–303.

30. Szatmari P, Boyle M, Offord DR. ADDH and conduct disorder: degree of diagnostic overlap and differences among correlates. *J Am Acad Child Adolesc Psychiatry.* 1989;**28**:865–72.

31. Biederman J, Faraone SV, Keenan K, *et al.* Further evidence for family-genetic risk factors in attention

deficit hyperactivity disorder. Patterns of comorbidity in probands and relatives psychiatrically and pediatrically referred samples. *Arch Gen Psychiatry*. 1992;**49**:728–38.

32. Jain M, Palacio LG, Castellanos FX, *et al*. Attention-deficit/hyperactivity disorder and comorbid disruptive behavior disorders: evidence of pleiotropy and new susceptibility loci. *Biol Psychiatry*. 2007;**61**(12): 1329–39.

33. MTA Cooperative Group. Moderators and mediators of treatment response for children with attention deficit hyperactivity disorder: the MTA study. *Arch Gen Psychiatry*. 1999;**56**:1088–96.

34. Barkley RA, Fischer M, Edelbrock CS, *et al*. The adolescent outcome of hyperactive children diagnosed by research criteria: I. An 8-year prospective follow-up study. *J Am Acad Child Adolesc Psychiatry*. 1990;**29**: 546–57.

35. Fischer M, Barkley RA, Edelbrock CS, *et al*. The adolescent outcome of hyperactive children diagnosed by research criteria: II. Academic, attentional, and neuropsychological status. *J Consult Clin Psychology*. 1990;**58**:580–8.

36. Wilens TE, Biederman J, Spencer TJ, *et al*. Comorbidity of attention-deficit hyperactivity and psychoactive substance use disorders. *Hosp Community Psychiatry*. 1994;**45**:421–3, 435.

37. Biederman J, Wilens T, Mick E, *et al*. Psychoactive substance use disorders in adults with attention deficit hyperactivity disorder (ADHD): effects of ADHD and psychiatric comorbidity. *Am J Psychiatry*. 1995; **152**(11):1652–8.

38. Wilens TE, Biederman J, Millstein RB, *et al*. Risk for substance use disorders in youths with child- and adolescent-onset bipolar disorder. *J Am Acad Child Adolesc Psychiatry*. 1999;**38**(6):680–5.

39. Jensen PS, Hinshaw SP, Kraemer HC, *et al*. ADHD comorbidity findings from the MTA study: comparing comorbid subgroups. *J Am Acad Child Adolesc Psychiatry*. 2001;**40**(2):147–58.

40. Newcorn JH, Halperin JM, Jensen PS, *et al*. Symptom profiles in children with ADHD: effects of comorbidity and gender. *J Am Acad Child Adolesc Psychiatry*. 2001;**40**(20):137–46.

41. March JS, Swanson JM, Arnold LE, *et al*. Anxiety as a predictor and outcome variable in the multimodal treatment study of children with ADHD (MTA). *J Abnorm Child Psychol*. 2000;**28**(6):527–41.

42. Curry J, Rohde P, Simons A, *et al*. Predictors and moderators of acute outcome in the Treatment for Adolescents with Depression Study (TADS). *J Am Acad Child Adolesc Psychiatry*. 2006;**45**(12): 1427–39.

43. Kovacs M, Akiskal HS, Gatsonis C, *et al*. Childhood onset dysthymic disorder: clinical features and prospective naturalistic outcome. *Arch Gen Psychiatry*. 1994;**51**:365–74.

44. Biederman J, Faraone SV, Spencer T, *et al*. Patterns of psychiatric comorbidity, cognition, and psychosocial functioning in adults with attention deficit hyperactivity disorder. *Am J Psychiatry*. 1993;**150**: 1792–8.

45. Kessler RC, Adler L, Barkley R, *et al*. The prevalence and correlates of adult ADHD in the United States: results from the National Comorbidity Survey Replication. *Am J Psychiatry*. 2006;**163**(4):716–23.

46. Barkley RA, Murphy KR, Fischer M. *ADHD in Adults: What the Science Says*. New York, NY: Guilford Press; 2008.

47. Moreno C, Laje G, Blanco C, *et al*. National trends in the outpatient diagnosis and treatment of bipolar disorder in youth. *Arch Gen Psychiatry*. 2007;**64**(9): 1032–9.

48. Blader JC, Carlson GA. Increased rates of bipolar disorder diagnoses among U.S. child, adolescent, and adult inpatients, 1996–2004. *Biol Psychiatry*. 2007; **62**(2):107–14.

49. Wozniak J, Biederman J, Kiely K, *et al*. Mania-like symptoms suggestive of childhood onset bipolar disorder in clinically referred children. *J Am Acad Child Adolesc Psychiatry*. 1995;**34**(7):867–76.

50. Biederman J, Faraone SV, Mick E, *et al*. Attention-deficit hyperactivity disorder and juvenile mania: an overlooked comorbidity? *J Am Acad Child Adolesc Psychiatry*. 1996;**35**(8):997–1008.

51. Biederman J, Wozniak J, Kiely K, *et al*. CBCL clinical scales discriminate prepubertal children with structured interview-derived diagnosis of mania from those with ADHD. *J Am Acad Child Adolesc Psychiatry*. 1995;**34**:464–71.

52. Klein RG, Pine DS, Klein DF. Resolved: mania is mistaken for ADHD in prepubertal children, negative. *J Am Acad Child Adolesc Psychiatry*. 1998;37:1093–6.

53. Biederman J. Resolved: mania is mistaken for ADHD in prepubertal children, affirmative. *J Am Acad Child Adolesc Psychiatry*. 1998;37:1091–3.

54. Geller B, Sun K, Zimmerman B, *et al*. Complex and rapid-cycling in bipolar children and adolescents: a preliminary study. *J Affect Disord*. 1995;34:259–68.

55. Findling RL, Gracious BL, McNamara NK, *et al*. Rapid, continuous cycling and psychiatric co-morbidity in pediatric bipolar I disorder. *Bipolar Disord*. 2001;3(4): 202–10.

56. Perlis RH, Miyahara S, Marangell LB, *et al*. Long-term implications of early onset in bipolar disorder: data

from the first 1000 participants in the systematic treatment enhancement program for bipolar disorder (STEP-BD). *Biol Psychiatry*. 2004;**55**(9):875–81.

57. Sachs GS, Baldassano CF, Truman CJ, *et al.* Comorbidity of attention deficit hyperactivity disorder with early- and late-onset bipolar disorder. *Am J Psychiatry*. 2000;**157**(3):466–8.

58. Leibenluft E, Charney DS, Towbin KE, *et al.* Defining clinical phenotypes of juvenile mania. *Am J Psychiatry*. 2003;**160**(3):430–7.

59. Stringaris A, Santosh P, Leibenluft E, *et al.* Youth meeting symptom and impairment criteria for mania-like episodes lasting less than four days: an epidemiological enquiry. *J Child Psychol Psychiatry*. 2010;**51**(1):31–8.

60. Costello EJ, Angold A, Burns BJ, *et al.* The Great Smokey Mountain study of youth: goals, designs, methods, and the prevalence of DSM-III-R disorders. *Arch Gen Psychiatry*. 1996;**53**:1129–36.

61. Stringaris A, Baroni A, Haimm C, *et al.* Pediatric bipolar disorder versus severe mood dysregulation: risk for manic episodes on follow-up. *J Am Acad Child Adolesc Psychiatry*. 2010;**49**(4):397–405.

62. Stringaris A, Cohen P, Pine DS, *et al.* Adult outcomes of youth irritability: a 20-year prospective community-based study. *Am J Psychiatry*. 2009;**166**(9):1048–54.

63. Brotman MA, Rich BA, Guyer AE, *et al.* Amygdala activation during emotion processing of neutral faces in children with severe mood dysregulation versus ADHD or bipolar disorder. *Am J Psychiatry*. 2010;**167**(1):61–9.

64. Rich BA, Brotman MA, Dickstein DP, *et al.* Deficits in attention to emotional stimuli distinguish youth with severe mood dysregulation from youth with bipolar disorder. *J Abnorm Child Psychol*. 2010;**38**(5):695–706.

65. Barkley RA. Behavioral inhibition, sustained attention, and executive functions: constructing a unifying theory of ADHD. *Psychol Bull*. 1997;**121**(1):65–94.

66. Nigg JT, Willcutt EG, Doyle AE, *et al.* Causal heterogeneity in attention-deficit/hyperactivity

disorder: do we need neuropsychologically impaired subtypes? *Biol Psychiatry*. 2005;**57**(11):1224–30.

67. Willcutt EG, Doyle AE, Nigg JT, *et al.* Validity of the executive function theory of attention-deficit/hyperactivity disorder: a meta-analytic review. *Biol Psychiatry*. 2005;**57**(11):1336–46.

68. Solanto MV, Abikoff H, Sonuga-Barke E, *et al.* The ecological validity of delay aversion and response inhibition as measures of impulsivity in AD/HD: a supplement to the NIMH multimodal treatment study of AD/HD. *J Abnorm Child Psychol*. 2001;**29**(3):215–28.

69. Sonuga-Barke EJ. Psychological heterogeneity in AD/HD–a dual pathway model of behaviour and cognition. *Behav Brain Res*. 2002;**130**(1–2):29–36.

70. Castellanos FX, Sonuga-Barke EJ, Scheres A, *et al.* Varieties of attention-deficit/hyperactivity disorder-related intra-individual variability. *Biol Psychiatry*. 2005;**57**(11):1416–23.

71. Sonuga-Barke E, Bitsakou P, Thompson M. Beyond the dual pathway model: evidence for the dissociation of timing, inhibitory, and delay-related impairments in attention-deficit/hyperactivity disorder. *J Am Acad Child Adolesc Psychiatry*. 2010;**49**(4):345–55.

72. Durston S, Davidson MC, Mulder MJ, *et al.* Neural and behavioral correlates of expectancy violations in attention-deficit hyperactivity disorder. *J Child Psychol Psychiatry*. 2007;**48**(9):881–9.

73. Wahlstedt C, Thorell LB, Bohlin G. Heterogeneity in ADHD: neuropsychological pathways, comorbidity and symptom domains. *J Abnorm Child Psychol*. 2009;**37**(4):551–64.

74. Herpertz SC, Huebner T, Marx I, *et al.* Emotional processing in male adolescents with childhood-onset conduct disorder. *J Child Psychol Psychiatry*. 2008;**49**(7):781–91.

75. Gottesman II, Gould TD. The endophenotype concept in psychiatry: etymology and strategic intentions. *Am J Psychiatry*. 2003;**160**(4):636–45.

76. Nijmeijer JS, Hoekstra PJ, Minderaa RB, *et al.* PDD symptoms in ADHD, an independent familial trait? *J Abnorm Child Psychol*. 2009;**37**(3):443–53.

Bipolar disorder and ADHD
Comorbidity throughout the life cycle

Gagan Joshi and Janet Wozniak

Due to skepticism regarding the childhood and adolescent onset of bipolar disorder (BPD) as well as the continuity of attention-deficit hyperactivity disorder (ADHD) onto the adult years, the comorbid condition of BPD and ADHD has been neglected at both ends of the life cycle. In recent years, however, pediatric-onset BPD has gained acceptance in the clinical and research community as a valid clinical entity [1]. It is not so infrequent as previously reported, with rates of bipolar spectrum disorder reaching an estimated 4% with heightened awareness of the need to screen for its symptoms in youth. One reason for its previous neglect is its high rate of comorbidity: pediatric-onset BPD seldom occurs in the absence of comorbid conditions. Youth with BPD are amongst the most highly impaired individuals with psychiatric illness, with mood swings characterized by severe irritability, euphoria, and depression. The presence of comorbidity compounds disability, complicates treatment, and appears to worsen the prognosis in this population. ADHD in itself is a condition associated with emotional, academic, work, and social disability, and its co-occurrence complicates both the accurate diagnosis and treatment of BPD, especially in pediatric populations in which ADHD is readily and commonly diagnosed. The comorbid condition of BPD and ADHD has remained an "orphan" condition, neglected in adults due to past skepticism regarding the continuity of ADHD into adulthood and neglected in children due to the now debunked concept that BPD does not occur in childhood.

Knowledge of ADHD's comorbid presence with BPD could be informative in determining course, prognosis, and functional and therapeutic outcomes. Early identification and appropriate management may lead to improved functioning, prevention of

impending emergence of comorbid disorders (e.g., oppositional defiant disorder/conduct disorder [ODD/CD], substance use disorders [SUD]), and attenuation of the untreated course of BPD [2, 3]. If the emotional symptoms of BPD are misattributed to demoralization or easy frustration associated with an ADHD diagnosis, increased use of stimulants would expose patients to higher than needed doses, would not help the mood symptoms, and could worsen the course of the mood disorder. On the other hand, if comorbidity with ADHD is not noted in a patient with BPD, inattention, distractibility, and talkativeness from ADHD could be inappropriately attributed to residual symptoms of BPD with unnecessary exposure to neuroleptics, worsening of symptoms, delayed diagnosis, and misuse of mental health resources. Recognition of comorbidity is important as it has therapeutic implications such as increased risk of mood destabilization that is inherent to the therapeutic options for the ADHD comorbidity (i.e., anti-ADHD medications that have manicogenic potential) or less than expected anti-manic response to thymoleptic agents in the presence of comorbid ADHD.

Comorbid disorders may be challenging to diagnose due to overlapping symptoms and complicated, developmentally sensitive patterns of symptom development. Several methods have been applied to scientifically understand comorbidity. Structured diagnostic interviews (for instance, Kiddie-Schedule for Affective Disorders and Schizophrenia-Epidemiological Fifth Version [K-SADS-E] [4] for children and adolescents and the Structured Clinical Interview for DSM [SCID] [5] for adults) are helpful in clinically parsing out the comorbid conditions as they comprehensively assess the spectrum of psychopathologies described in the DSM, including

Attention-Deficit Hyperactivity Disorder in Adults and Children, ed. Lenard A. Adler, Thomas J. Spencer and Timothy E. Wilens.
Published by Cambridge University Press. © Cambridge University Press 2015.

the past and present severity of symptoms. Diagnoses are considered positive only if the diagnostic criteria are met to a degree that would be considered *clinically meaningful*, meaning the data collected from the structured interview indicated the diagnosis should be a clinical concern due to the nature of the symptoms, the associated impairment, and the coherence of the clinical picture. For a given disorder, the overlapping non-specific symptoms contribute to the diagnosis if an adequate number of the respective additional non-overlapping symptoms are present and the disorder is cause for significant impairment. Furthermore, although the DSM criteria often do not permit comorbid presence of certain disorders and assign diagnoses based on a hierarchical system, a non-hierarchical diagnostic approach is taken to assess for comorbid disorders to present a complete clinical picture. In a clinical setting, the use of structured questions for symptoms pertaining to individual disorders is feasible and can help clarify complicated diagnostic clinical pictures. Thus, the approach taken by a structured interview objectively and comprehensively documents symptom presentation and minimizes diagnostic biases.

In a clinical setting, the Child Behavior Checklist (CBCL) [6], an informant-rated instrument, offers a cost-effective and rapid assessment to help identify pediatric cases likely to meet clinical criteria for BPD, especially in youth with ADHD [7–10]. Several studies have shown that children with a deviant profile on the CBCL's attention problems, aggressive behavior, and anxious-depressed subscales (the AAA profile) are more likely to meet criteria for DSM bipolar I disorder (BPD-I) in both epidemiological and clinical samples [6, 10–14]. This profile is also referred to as the CBCL-pediatric bipolar disorder (CBCL-PBD) or CBCL-AAA profile [10]. Faraone *et al.* evaluated the diagnostic efficiency of this CBCL profile in youth with ADHD [8]. They found that the CBCL-AAA profile allowed for the determination of both past and current diagnoses of BPD in ADHD youth and their siblings. In a study of a sample of over 21 000 twins derived from the general population, Hudziak *et al.* [15], found the CBCL-AAA profile to be highly heritable with a population prevalence consistent with epidemiological studies of BPD (~1%) in boys and girls [16]. More recently, in an average 7-year follow-up study of youth with ADHD, Biederman *et al.* reported a positive CBCL-AAA score predicted a subsequent diagnosis of BPD, as well as impaired

psychosocial functioning and a higher risk for psychiatric hospitalization [17]. An intermediate form of this profile with scores elevated by one standard deviation identifies a group of ADHD youth with deficient emotional self-regulation, at greater risk for anxiety and depressive disorders [18]. This suggests the CBCL-AAA profile has the potential to help identify youth at high risk for emotional regulation issues in addition to those at risk of developing BPD.

In a large sample of adults with BPD from the Systematic Treatment Enhancement Program for Bipolar Disorder (STEP-BD) [19], the overall lifetime prevalence of ADHD was 9.5%. This study used the Mini International Neuropsychiatric Interview (MINI version 4.4) [20], which has high reliability with the SCID. This interview was used for both the BPD and the ADHD diagnoses, with the requirement that for the diagnosis of ADHD, adults had to meet 6 out of 10 criteria prior to age 7 years and that during adulthood they needed to meet 9 out of 14 criteria with significant dysfunction in two arenas. In this study, BPD adult patients with comorbid ADHD versus those without had an earlier onset of mood symptoms (by 5 years), shorter periods of wellness, more depression, and higher rates of comorbidity.

Present studies addressing comorbidity generally rely either on cross-sectional observations or on recall of disorders over the whole life course. Both of these approaches pose limitations. Longitudinal studies offer the best possibility for observing the developmental progression and emergence of comorbid conditions. Studies of ADHD in youth with BPD as well as studies of BPD in youth with ADHD have been informative in establishing the comorbidity of these two conditions. Systematic studies of pediatric populations with BPD find rates of comorbid ADHD ranging from 60% to 90% [21–23]. While this very high prevalence of ADHD is reported in youth with BPD, a more modest rate (22%) of comorbid BPD is reported in the reverse situation when examining pediatric populations ascertained for the presence of ADHD, suggesting an asymmetrical bidirectional overlap of these two disorders in youth [24]. Faraone *et al.* found BPD prevalence in children with ADHD ranged from 11% in an outpatient population to 22% in hospitalized patients [25].

Although the rates of ADHD in youth with BPD are universally high, the age at onset modifies the risk for comorbid ADHD. ADHD comorbidity is more often associated with early-onset BPD (<18 years) [26–28]. Rates of ADHD in adolescents with BPD are reported to be greater in childhood-onset BPD ($\leq$12 years) than in adolescent-onset BPD (>13 years) [25, 29]. Among adults with BPD, a history of comorbid ADHD is more evident in those subjects with pediatric onset of BPD ($\leq$18 years) [28]. Sachs *et al.* compared BPD adult subjects with and without comorbid ADHD [26]. Those BPD subjects with ADHD had a mean age at onset of first affective episode that was significantly lower than that of subjects without a history of childhood ADHD.

An additional and compelling report from the adult literature on the subject of comorbidity between BPD and ADHD comes from The National Comorbidity Survey Replication epidemiological study, which documented high bidirectional comorbidity between BPD and ADHD. The survey documented significantly higher rates of BPD in the adult population with ADHD than without ADHD (19.4% vs. 3.1%) and equally higher rates of ADHD in the adult population with BPD compared with adults without BPD (21.2% vs. 3.5%) [30]. Consistent with the documented association of comorbid ADHD almost exclusively with early-onset BPD, a relatively lower lifetime prevalence (9.5%) of comorbid ADHD is reported in an adult research population with BPD [19].

The prevalence of ADHD and BPD comorbidity varies depending on the subtypes of ADHD and BPD involved. Limited information is available regarding the potential for different rates of comorbidity with BPD among the DSM-IV subtypes of ADHD. Based on reported information, the rates of BPD are reported to be highest among youth with combined-type ADHD (26.5%), but also elevated among hyperactive–impulsive (14.3%) and inattentive (8.7%) youth [31]. Wilens and colleagues examined a research population of adults with ADHD where nearly half the population also met the criteria for BPD (47%); the vast majority were BPD-II (88%) [32]. Although ADHD adults with comorbid BPD shared the prototypic characteristics of both the disorders, they had higher rates of combined-type ADHD, with a greater number of DSM-IV ADHD symptoms (especially attentional symptoms) [32].

A high comorbidity with major depressive disorder (MDD) has been documented in both youth and adults with ADHD [33–38]. The risk of having MDD has been found to increase several fold in those with ADHD [39]. Both are coupled by the fact that half of the children with MDD have been documented to develop mania by the age of 21 years [40, 41]. Based on these findings, Biederman and his colleagues examined the

risk for switch from unipolar major depression to BPD in youth with ADHD and non-ADHD controls [42]. They concluded the risk for switches from unipolar major depression to BPD was significantly higher in youth with ADHD (28%) when compared to the risk in youth without ADHD (6%). Furthermore, in subjects with ADHD, the risk of switching from unipolar major depression to BPD was predicted by the presence of comorbid conduct disorder, school behavior problems, and a positive family history of parental mood disorder. In a follow-up to this study, this same group found that switch to BPD-I is also more likely among those ADHD subjects with subthreshold BPD and among those with elevated scores on certain subscales of the CBCL which have been associated with BPD in multiple studies on the subject (the attention, anxiety, and aggression or so-called AAA scales) [43]. Thus, clinicians should monitor ADHD subjects with comorbid MDD closely (especially those with multiple risk factors for bipolar switches).

As ADHD and mania diagnostically share non-specific symptoms (distractibility, motoric hyperactivity, and talkativeness), there is a risk of unintentional over-diagnosis. Several studies have addressed this issue [44]. In an analysis of prepubertal children with BPD and ADHD, Wozniak *et al.* demonstrated correlates of both conditions [45]. Consistent with BPD, affected children had high rates of major depression, psychosis, multiple anxiety disorders, impaired psychosocial function, and hospitalization. Similarly, phenotypic features of ADHD and associated neuropsychiatric correlates (that is, high rates of learning disabilities and need for educational services) have striking homology to the presentation of ADHD in the context of comorbidity with BPD. This suggests ADHD may be a bona fide disorder when comorbid with BPD and vice versa, not due to misdiagnosis from overlapping features [46]. Biederman *et al.* showed the majority of children with the combined condition continued to meet criteria of both mania and ADHD after removing overlapping symptoms [24], suggesting BPD and ADHD comorbidity is not a methodological artifact due to shared diagnostic criteria. In this study, the authors removed the three overlapping symptoms (distractibility, motoric hyperactivity, and talkativeness) from the diagnostic algorithm. Without these symptoms the majority of children continued to meet full or subthreshold criteria for both disorders. This suggested that the overlapping symptoms alone were not accounting for the high rate of comorbidity [44].

The occurrence of comorbid ADHD might have an adverse impact on the clinical correlates of BPD. Most [19, 26, 47–51], but not all [52], studies document earlier onset of BPD in the presence of ADHD. In fact, in the presence of comorbid ADHD, individuals with BPD experience mania symptoms, on average, 3–5 years earlier than typically expected [19, 49]. Additional findings show that, in general, the comorbid condition is associated with a more severe course of the mood disorder [19, 48, 51–54]. Furthermore, comorbid patients' first BPD episode is more likely to be of a depressive nature (71% in an ADHD + BPD population vs. 22% in a BPD-only group). Subsequently, they are more frequently depressed with shorter duration of wellness [19, 52]. For instance, 40.7% of patients with ADHD/BPD reported more than 20 lifetime manic episodes whereas this proportion decreased to 29.6% in BPD patients without comorbid ADHD [19]. In the presence of ADHD, individuals with BPD have poorer global functioning, lower education, fewer partnerships, more suicide attempts, more legal problems (violence), and a greater burden of additional comorbid psychiatric disorders, especially anxiety disorders and SUD [19, 28, 32, 53–56]. In addition, BPD patients with comorbid ADHD have lower attentional resources [57], working memory, and executive functions [58]. Taken together, these findings suggest that the comorbid condition has considerable negative impact on patients' quality of life and overall functioning. Therefore, this comorbidity may prevent patients from reaching their full potential.

Perhaps the most compelling scientific method to examine comorbidity is a familial risk analysis, which addresses uncertainties regarding complex phenotypes in probands by examining the transmission of comorbid disorders in families [59, 60]. While the mechanisms that mediate the association between BPD and ADHD are not entirely clear, other data suggest that subforms of these disorders share genes in common [61]. Both ADHD and BPD individually are known to have strong familial links. Higher rates of adult ADHD have been documented in relatives of BPD adults compared to relatives of controls [62]. Similarly, children of bipolar parents have an elevated risk for ADHD and relatives of ADHD children have an increased risk for BPD [63–65]. Furthermore, in children of bipolar parents, the risk of ADHD is higher in children with versus without BPD [66]. The cosegregation of this comorbidity in families of ADHD and/or BPD patients has been demonstrated in studies and

a meta-analysis [45, 63, 67, 68] in which relatives of ADHD/BPD patients showed increased risks for the combined condition, suggesting these two disorders are transmitted together and not independently. The transmission of these disorders has been studied in families ascertained through pediatric BPD patients, ADHD boys [63] and ADHD girls [69]. In each of these reports, the pattern of transmission supported the hypothesis that a comorbid condition could represent a distinct condition.

Finally, issues of complex comorbidity can also be addressed by applying neurobiological probes to seek the existence of underlying biological attributes commensurate with each comorbid disorder, either disorder, or neither disorder indicating a unique subtype with distinct neurobiological attributes. Despite ample evidence of a bidirectional overlap of these two disorders, neuroimaging data addressing this comorbidity is sparse. One of the first functional neuroimaging studies to account for ADHD comorbidity in BPD patients found significantly different activation patterns in the inferior frontal cortical (IFC)-striatal network between BPD adults with and without ADHD, highlighting the need for imaging data that account for this comorbidity [70]. A volumetric MRI study found that BPD and BPD + ADHD were associated with a significantly smaller orbital prefrontal cortex and larger right thalamus, while ADHD and ADHD + BPD were associated with significantly less neocortical gray matter, smaller overall frontal lobe and superior prefrontal cortex volumes, a smaller right anterior cingulate cortex (ACC), and less cerebellar gray matter. The authors concluded that ADHD and BPD independently contributed to volumetric changes [71]. These findings were extended in the same sample to cortical thickness findings [72]. A different set of investigators concluded that stratification of BPD neuroimaging samples by the presence of ADHD may help in the interpretation of MRI studies of cortical thickness, as some of the brain abnormalities attributed to BPD may actually be due to the presence of ADHD [73]. The emerging proton magnetic resonance spectroscopic (^{1}HMRS) imaging intervention research in youth with BPD suggests a profile of cerebral metabolites in a specific region of the brain. This may facilitate an understanding of neurochemical correlates of BPD in the context of comorbidity. For instance, the ^{1}HMRS profile of cerebral metabolites in the ACC region of the brain in children with ADHD appears to have a significantly higher ratio of glutamate plus glutamine to myo-inositol-containing compounds than does the profile of children with comorbid BPD and ADHD [74]. These differences in ^{1}HMRS profile based on the ADHD comorbidity with BPD could be useful in distinguishing ADHD with and without BPD.

Therapeutic response has also provided evidence of the existence of separate conditions. For instance, in a review of clinical records of manic children, Biederman et al. reported that whereas mood stabilizers significantly improved mania-like symptoms, antidepressants and stimulants did not and, conversely, tricyclic antidepressants and not mood stabilizers were associated with improvement of ADHD symptoms [46]. Additionally, although empirical evidence for the psychopharmacological response in this comorbid condition is limited, the majority of clinically referred youth with BPD receive treatment for ADHD. In a recent chart review addressing the psychopharmacological interventions in clinically referred populations of youth with BPD, 60% of the youth with BPD were treated for ADHD with stimulants or the selective norepinephrine reuptake inhibitor atomoxetine and only 56% of the youth improved on ADHD [75].

Indicative of the growing recognition of combined BPD and ADHD in both youth and adults, the Canadian Network for Mood and Anxiety Treatments published treatment guidelines specifically targeting management of mood disorders in the presence of ADHD [76]. Treatment guidelines for pediatric and adult BPD suggest that comorbid conditions can and should be attended to once the BPD is stabilized [76]. Such a treatment plan may become a complex process of trial and error to find the most effective combination of medications [77]. Guidelines further recommend that in the absence of treatment trials specifically studying a population of children with BPD and specific comorbid disorders, clinicians should use those psychopharmacological and psychosocial treatments generally recommended for each comorbid disorder when that disorder occurs as the primary problem. As ADHD may require treatment with agents that have manicogenic potential, caution with this treatment is reasonably indicated. Available empirical evidence and clinical acumen dictate treatment of ADHD can be addressed only after the symptoms of BPD are stabilized [76, 78]. In mood-stabilized youth with BPD, ADHD symptoms with social, academic, and emotional morbidity often become the second most severe presenting complaint [78]. A decision to treat

comorbid ADHD following stabilization of mania should be guided by clinically determining the level of impairment associated with ADHD, balanced versus the risk of triggering mood destabilization.

Anti-ADHD effects of mood-stabilizing agents have been documented in the recent literature on the treatment trials of youth with BPD. The anti-manic agents carbamazepine and risperidone are suggested to be effective in treating ADHD symptoms in youth with BPD [79, 80]. However, the response in ADHD symptoms reported in these trials could partially be attributed to the response in the overlapping symptoms shared between ADHD and mania (for instance, distractibility, motoric hyperactivity, and talkativeness). In a recent controlled trial of youth with BPD (n = 43), aripiprazole was not found to be superior to placebo in improving ADHD symptoms [81]. Nevertheless, clinical acumen dictates that in youngsters with comorbid BPD and ADHD, the ADHD diagnosis could be addressed selectively with the anti-ADHD armamentarium, only if significant ADHD symptoms persist following mood stabilization.

Currently, limited studies have investigated the response to anti-manic treatment of individuals with comorbid ADHD and BPD. The response to the mood stabilizers lithium and divalproex sodium has been reported to be less robust in the presence of ADHD comorbidity in youth with BPD [82, 83]. This suggests that this subgroup of BPD may constitute a unique genetic subtype with a different treatment response. State et al. [83], in a chart review of the medical records of adolescents with BPD (n = 42) who were treated with either lithium (n = 29) or divalproex sodium (n = 13), observed BPD youth with comorbid ADHD (34.1%) had significantly lower response rates to both treatments compared to BPD youth without ADHD (57.1% vs. 80.9% respectively; p = 0.007).

A few small reports have indicated that stimulants may be efficacious in treating comorbid ADHD without precipitating (hypo)mania in mood-stabilized youth with BPD. A controlled trial of stimulants as an adjunctive therapy for ADHD in BPD youth with manic symptoms stabilized on divalproex found mixed amphetamine salts to be safe and efficacious for the treatment of ADHD in the context of BPD, but this study is limited by the small sample size of 30, flexible entry point into bipolar stabilization (Young Mania Rating Scale [YMRS] 14) and therefore likely lower morbidity from mania, and low dose of amphetamine salts used (5 mg BID) [84]. The role of methylphenidate (MPH) as an adjunctive anti-ADHD agent in mood-stabilized youth with BPD has been studied through two controlled trials with conflicting results. In a sample of youth with BPD stabilized on a steady dose of at least one thymoleptic agent, Findling *et al.* reported that concomitant treatment with MPH improved symptoms of ADHD in a dose-dependent manner without destabilization of mood [85]. MPH adjunctive therapy for the treatment of ADHD in youth stabilized on aripiprazole was not superior to placebo though it was well tolerated with the exception of one youth who developed severe mood destabilization on MPH [86].

Few trials of non-stimulant anti-ADHD agents have been conducted in comorbid BPD and ADHD populations. There is only one treatment trial of ADHD in adult BPD. In this 6-week open-label trial of buproprion in 36 euthymic bipolar adults, 89% of whom were medication free, ADHD symptoms improved, and only one patient developed hypomania [87]. Chang and colleagues examined the role of atomoxetine as an adjunctive therapy for the treatment of ADHD in a small sample (n = 12) of BPD youth with comorbid ADHD who were stabilized and euthymic on anti-manic agent(s) [88]. The authors concluded from their 8-week uncontrolled trial of atomoxetine at a mean dose of 60 mg/day that adjunctive treatment was well tolerated and effective in treating the symptoms of ADHD. None of the participants experienced (hypo)mania switch during the course of the trial. While these aggregate studies indicate that ADHD treatment can be initiated in stabilized bipolar patients, treatment for BPD always needs to precede ADHD treatment and BPD should be stabilized prior to using adjunctive ADHD treatment. Furthermore, given the small evidence base for combined treatment (especially in the adult population), clinical caution and close monitoring is indicated when using ADHD treatments in mood-stabilized bipolar individuals of any age, given that ADHD treatments can destabilize the course of BPD.

The scientific interface between BPD and ADHD remains unclear. Comorbidity may represent an important genetic and clinical subtype with distinct psychopathology, familiality, and cognitive, neural, and genetic underpinnings. Future longitudinal studies addressing the impact of comorbidity on the clinical presentation, course, and response to treatment as well as the cognitive correlates, genetic-candidate genes, and neurobiological overlap would assist in further clarifying the relationship of BPD and ADHD comorbidity.

References

1. Wozniak J. Pediatric bipolar disorder: the new perspective on severe mood dysfunction in children. *J Child Adolesc Psychopharmacol.* 2003;**13**(4):449–51.

2. Campbell M, Cueva JE. Psychopharmacology in child and adolescent psychiatry: A review of the past seven years. part II. *J Am Acad Child Adolesc Psychiatry.* 1995;**34**(10):1262–72.

3. Tarter R. Evaluation and treatment of adolescent substance abuse: a decision tree method. *J Am Acad Child Adolesc Psychiatry.* 1990;**42**:1486.

4. Ambrosini PJ. Historical development and present status of the schedule for affective disorders and schizophrenia for school-age children (K-SADS). *J Am Acad Child Adolesc Psychiatry.* 2000;**39**(1):49–58.

5. First MB, Spitzer RL, Gibbon M, Williams JBW. *Structured Clinical Interview for DSM-IV Axis I Disorders-Clinician Version (SCID-CV).* Washington, DC: American Psychiatric Press; 1997.

6. Achenbach TM. *Manual for the Child Behavior Checklist/4–18 and the 1991 Profile.* Burlington, VT: University of Vermont, Department of Psychiatry; 1991.

7. Althoff RR, Rettew DC, Faraone SV, Boomsma DI, Hudziak JJ. Latent class analysis shows strong heritability of the CBCL-juvenile bipolar phenotype. *Biol Psychiatry.* 2006;**60**(9):903–11.

8. Faraone SV, Althoff RR, Hudziak JJ, Monuteaux MC, Biederman J. The CBCL predicts DSM bipolar disorder in children: A receiver operating characteristic curve analysis. *Bipolar Disord.* 2005;**7**(6):518–24.

9. Hudziak JJ, Althoff RR, Derks EM, Faraone SV, Boomsma DI. Prevalence and genetic architecture of Child Behavior Checklist-juvenile bipolar disorder. *Biol Psychiatry.* 2005;**58**(7):562–8.

10. Mick E, Biederman J, Pandina G, Faraone SV. A preliminary meta-analysis of the Child Behavior Checklist in pediatric bipolar disorder. *Biol Psychiatry.* 2003;**53**(11):1021–7.

11. Wals M, Hillegers MH, Reichart CG, *et al.* Prevalence of psychopathology in children of a bipolar parent. *J Am Acad Child Adolesc Psychiatry.* 2001;**40**(9):1094–102.

12. Carlson GA, Kelly KL. Manic symptoms in psychiatrically hospitalized children – what do they mean? *J Affect Disord.* 1998;**51**(2):123–35.

13. Geller B, Warner K, Williams M, Zimerman B. Prepubertal and young adolescent bipolarity versus ADHD: assessment and validity using the

WASH-U-KSADS, CBCL and TRF. *J Affect Disord.* 1998;**51**:93–100.

14. Hazell P, Lewin T, Carr V. Confirmation that Child Behavior Checklist clinical scales discriminate juvenile mania from attention deficit hyperactivity disorder. *J Paediatr Child Health.* 1999;**35**:199–203.

15. Hudziak J, Althoff RR, Rettew DC, Derks EM, Faraone SV. The prevalence and genetic architecture of CBCL-juvenile bipolar disorder. *Biol Psychiatry.* 2005;**58**(7): 562–8.

16. Lewinsohn P, Klein D, Seeley J. Bipolar disorders in a community sample of older adolescents: prevalence, phenomenology, comorbidity, and course. *J Am Acad Child Adolesc Psychiatry.* 1995;**34**(4):454–63.

17. Biederman J, Petty CR, Monuteaux MC, *et al.* The child behavior checklist-pediatric bipolar disorder profile predicts a subsequent diagnosis of bipolar disorder and associated impairments in ADHD youth growing up: a longitudinal analysis. *J Clin Psychiatry.* 2009;**70**(5):732–40.

18. Spencer T, Faraone SV, Surman C, *et al.* Towards defining deficient emotional self regulation in youth with attention deficit hyperactivity disorder using the CBCL: a controlled study. *Postgrad Med.* 2011;**123**(5): 50–9.

19. Nierenberg AA, Miyahara S, Spencer T, *et al.* Clinical and diagnostic implications of lifetime attention-deficit/hyperactivity disorder comorbidity in adults with bipolar disorder: data from the first 1000 STEP-BD participants. *Biol Psychiatry.* 2005;**57**(11):1467–73.

20. Sheehan DV, Lecrubier Y, Sheehan KH, *et al.* The Mini-International Neuropsychiatric Interview (M.I.N.I.): the development and validation of a structured diagnostic psychiatric interview for DSM-IV and ICD-10. *J Clin Psychiatry.* 1998; **59**(Suppl 20):22–33; quiz 34–57.

21. Wilens T, Biederman J, Forkner P, *et al.* Patterns of comorbidity and dysfunction in clinically referred preschoolers with bipolar disorder. *J Child Adolesc Psychopharmacol.* 2003;**13**(4):495–505.

22. Geller B, Sun K, Zimmerman B, *et al.* Complex and rapid-cycling in bipolar children and adolescents: A preliminary study. *J Affect Disord.* 1995;**34**:259–68.

23. West S, McElroy S, Strakowski S, Keck P, McConville B. Attention deficit hyperactivity disorder in adolescent mania. *Am J Psychiatry.* 1995;**152**(2):271–3.

24. Biederman J, Faraone S, Mick E, *et al.* Attention-deficit hyperactivity disorder and juvenile mania: an overlooked comorbidity? *J Am Acad Child Adolesc Psychiatry.* 1996;**35**(8):997–1008.

25. Faraone SV, Biederman J, Wozniak J, *et al.* Is comorbidity with ADHD a marker for juvenile onset mania? *J Am Acad Child Adolesc Psychiatry.* 1997; **36**(8):1046–55.

26. Sachs GS, Baldassano CF, Truman CJ, Guille C. Comorbidity of attention deficit hyperactivity disorder with early- and late-onset bipolar disorder. *Am J Psychiatry.* 2000;**157**(3):466–8.

27. Chang KD, Steiner H, Ketter TA. Psychiatric phenomenology of child and adolescent bipolar offspring. *J Am Acad Child Adolesc Psychiatry.* 2000; **39**(4):453–60.

28. Karaahmet E, Konuk N, Dalkilic A, *et al.* The comorbidity of adult attention-deficit/hyperactivity disorder in bipolar disorder patients. *Compr Psychiatry.* 2013;**54**:549–55.

29. Biederman J, Petty C, Faraone SV, *et al.* Moderating effects of major depression on patterns of comorbidity in referred adults with panic disorder: a controlled study. *Psychiatry Res.* 2004;**126**(2):143–9.

30. Kessler RC, Adler L, Barkley R, *et al.* The prevalence and correlates of adult ADHD in the United States: results from the National Comorbidity Survey Replication. *Am J Psychiatry.* 2006;**163**(4): 716–23.

31. Faraone SV, Biederman J, Mennin D, Russell RL. Bipolar and antisocial disorders among relatives of ADHD children: parsing familial subtypes of illness. *Am J Med Genet.* 1998;**81**(1):108–16.

32. Wilens T, Biederman J, Wozniak J, *et al.* Can adults with attention-deficit hyperactivity disorder be distinguished from those with comorbid bipolar disorder: findings from a sample of clinically referred adults. *Biol Psychiatry.* 2003;**54**(1):1–8.

33. Anderson JC, Williams S, McGee R, Silva PA. DSM-III disorders in preadolescent children: Prevalence in a large sample from the general population. *Arch Gen Psychiatry.* 1987;**44**:69–76.

34. Biederman J, Newcorn J, Sprich S. Comorbidity of attention deficit hyperactivity disorder with conduct, depressive, anxiety, and other disorders. *Am J Psychiatry.* 1991;**148**(5):564–77.

35. Bird HR, Canino G, Rubio-Stipec M, *et al.* Estimates of the prevalence of childhood maladjustment in a community survey in Puerto Rico: the use of combined measures. *Arch Gen Psychiatry.* 1988;**45**: 1120–6.

36. Jensen JB, Burke N, Garfinkel BD. Depression and symptoms of attention deficit disorder with hyperactivity. *J Am Acad Child Adolesc Psychiatry.* 1988;**27**(6):742–7.

37. Munir K, Biederman J, Knee D. Psychiatric comorbidity in patients with attention deficit disorder: a controlled study. *J Am Acad Child Adolesc Psychiatry.* 1987;**26**(6):844–8.

38. Woolston JL, Rosenthal SL, Riddle MA, *et al*. Childhood comorbidity of anxiety/affective disorders and behavior disorders. *J Am Acad Child Adolesc Psychiatry*. 1989;**28**(5):707–13.

39. Angold A, Costello J, Erkanli A. Comorbidity. *J Child Psychol Psychiatry*. 1999;**40**(1):57–87.

40. Geller B, Fox L, Clark K. Rate and predictors of prepubertal bipolarity during follow-up of 6- to 12-year-old depressed children. *J Am Acad Child Adolesc Psychiatry*. 1994;**33**(4):461–8.

41. Geller B, Zimmerman B, Williams M, Bolhofner K, Craney JL. Bipolar disorder at prospective follow-up of adults who had prepubertal major depressive disorder. *Am J Psychiatry*. 2001;**158**(1):125–7.

42. Biederman J, Petty CR, Byrne D, *et al*. Risk for switch from unipolar to bipolar disorder in youth with ADHD: a long term prospective controlled study. *J Affect Disord*. 2009;**119**(1–3):16–21.

43. Biederman J, Wozniak J, Tarko L, *et al*. Re-examining the risk for switch from unipolar to bipolar major depressive disorder in youth with ADHD: A long term prospective longitudinal controlled study. *J Affect Disord*. 2014;**152–154**:347–51.

44. Milberger S, Biederman J, Faraone SV, Murphy J, Tsuang MT. Attention Deficit Hyperactivity Disorder and comorbid disorders: issues of overlapping symptoms. *Am J Psychiatry*. 1995;**152**(12): 1793–9.

45. Wozniak J, Biederman J, Mundy E, Mennin D, Faraone SV. A pilot family study of childhood-onset mania. *J Am Acad Child Adolesc Psychiatry*. 1995; **34**(12):1577–83.

46. Biederman J, Mick E, Bostic J, *et al*. The naturalistic course of pharmacologic treatment of children with manic-like symptoms: a systematic chart review. *J Clin Psychiatry*. 1998;**59**(11):628–37; quiz 338.

47. Kent L, Craddock N. Is there a relationship between attention deficit hyperactivity disorder and bipolar disorder? *J Affect Disord*. 2003;**73**(3):211–21.

48. Wingo AP, Ghaemi SN. A systematic review of rates and diagnostic validity of comorbid adult attention-deficit/hyperactivity disorder and bipolar disorder. *J Clin Psychiatry*. 2007;**68**:1776–84.

49. Masi G, Perugi G, Toni C, *et al*. Attention deficit-hyperactivity disorder – bipolar comorbidity in children and adolescents. *Bipolar Disord*. 2006;**8**: 373–81.

50. Jaideen T, Reddy Y, Srinath S. Comorbidity of attention deficit-hyperactivity disorder in juvenile bipolar disorder. *Bipolar Disord*. 2006;**8**:182–7.

51. Masi G, Mucci M, Pfanner C, *et al*. Developmental pathways for different subtypes of early-onset

bipolarity in youths. *J Clin Psychiatry*. 2012;**73**(10): 1335–41.

52. Tamam L, Tulu C, Karatas G, Ozcan S. Adult attention-deficit hyperactivity disorder in patients with bipolar I in remission: Preliminary Study. *Psychiatry Clin Neurosci*. 2006;**60**:480–5.

53. Klassen LJ, Katzman MA, Chokka P. Adult ADHD and its comorbidities, with a focus on bipolar disorder. *J Affect Disord*. 2010;**124**(1–2):1–8.

54. Perugi G, Ceraudo G, Vannuchi G, *et al*. Attention deficit/hyperactivity disorder symptoms in Italian bipolar adult patients: a preliminary report. *J Affect Disord*. 2013;**149**:430–4.

55. Ryden E, Thase M, Straht D, *et al*. A history of childhood attention-deficit hyperactivity disorder (ADHD) impacts clinical outcome in adult bipolar patients regardless of current ADHD. *Acta Psychiatr Scand*. 2009;**120**(3):239–46.

56. Sentissi O, Navarro J, Oliveira H, *et al*. Bipolar disorders and quality of life: The impact of attention deficit/hyperactivity disorder and substance abuse in euthymic patients. *Psychiatry Res*. 2008;**161**:36–42.

57. Biederman J, Wilens TE, Mick E, *et al*. Is ADHD a risk factor for psychoactive substance use disorders? Findings from a four-year prospective follow-up study. *J Am Acad Child Adolesc Psychiatry*. 1997;**36**(1):21–9.

58. Brown TE. Executive functions and attention deficit hyperactivity disorder: Implications of two conflicting views. *Int J Disabil Dev Educ*. 2006;**53**(1):35–46.

59. Faraone SV, Tsuang MT. Methods in psychiatric genetics. In: Tohen M, Tsuang MT, Zahner GEP, eds. *Textbook in Psychiatric Epidemiology*. New York, NY: John Wiley. 1995; 81–134.

60. Faraone SV, Tsuang MT, Tsuang D. *Genetics and Mental Disorders: A Guide for Students, Clinicians, and Researchers*. New York, NY: Guilford Press; 1999.

61. Faraone S, Glatt S, Tsuang M. The genetics of pediatric onset bipolar disorder. *Biol Psychiatry*. 2003;**53**(11): 970–7.

62. Turkyilmaz E, Yavuz BG, Karamustafalioglu O, Ozer OA, Bakim B. Prevalence of adult attention deficit hyperactivity disorder in the relatives of patients with bipolar disorder. *Int J Psychiatry Clin Pract*. 2012; **16**(3):223–8.

63. Faraone SV, Biederman J, Mennin D, Wozniak J, Spencer T. Attention-deficit hyperactivity disorder with bipolar disorder: a familial subtype? *J Am Acad Child Adolesc Psychiatry*. 1997;**36**(10):1378–87; discussion 1387–90.

64. Birmaher B, Axelson D, Goldstein B, *et al*. Psychiatric disorders in preschool offspring of parents with

bipolar disorder: the Pittsburgh Bipolar Offspring Study (BIOS). *Am J Psychiatry*. 2010;**167**(3):321–30.

65. Garcia-Amador M, de la Serna E, Vila M, *et al.* Parents with bipolar disorder: are disease characteristics good predictors of psychopathology in offspring? *Eur Psychiatry*. 2013;**28**(4):240–6.

66. Goldstein B, Shamseddeen W, Axelson D, *et al.* Clinical, demographic, and familial correlates of bipolar spectrum disorders among offspring of parents with bipolar disorder. *J Am Acad Child Adolesc Psychiatry*. 2010;**49**(4):388–96.

67. Faraone SV, Biederman J, Wozniak J. Examining the comorbidity between attention deficit hyperactivity disorder and bipolar I disorder: a meta-analysis of family genetic studies. *Am J Psychiatry*. 2012;**169**(12): 1256–66.

68. Biederman J, Faraone SV, Petty C, *et al.* Further evidence that pediatric-onset bipolar disorder comorbid with ADHD represents a distinct subtype: results from a large controlled family study. *J Psychiatr Res*. 2013;**47**(1):15–22.

69. Faraone SV, Biederman J, Monuteaux MC. Attention deficit hyperactivity disorder with bipolar disorder in girls: further evidence for a familial subtype? *J Affect Disord*. 2001;**64**(1):19–26.

70. Townsend JD, Sugar CA, Walshaw PD, *et al.* Frontostriatal neuroimaging findings differ in patients with bipolar disorder who have or do not have ADHD comorbidity. *J Affect Disord*. 2013;**147**(1–3):389–96.

71. Biederman J, Makris N, Valera EM, *et al.* Towards further understanding of the co-morbidity between attention deficit hyperactivity disorder and bipolar disorder: a MRI study of brain volumes. *Psychol Med*. 2008;**38**(7):1045–56.

72. Makris N, Seidman LJ, Brown A, *et al.* Further understanding of the comorbidity between attention-deficit/hyperactivity disorder and bipolar disorder in adults: An MRI study of cortical thickness. *Psychiatry Res*. 2012;**202**(1):1–11.

73. Hegarty CE, Foland-Ross LC, Narr KL, *et al.* ADHD comorbidity can matter when assessing cortical thickness abnormalities in patients with bipolar disorder. *Bipolar Disord*. 2012;**14**(8):843–55.

74. Moore CM, Biederman J, Wozniak J, *et al.* Differences in brain chemistry in children and adolescents with attention deficit hyperactivity disorder with and without comorbid bipolar disorder: a proton magnetic resonance spectroscopy study. *Am J Psychiatry*. 2006;**163**(2):316–18.

75. Potter MP, Liu HY, Monuteaux MC, *et al.* Prescribing patterns for treatment of pediatric bipolar disorder in a specialty clinic. *J Child Adolesc Psychopharmacol*. 2009;**19**(5):529–38.

76. Bond DJ, Hadjipavlou G, Lam RW, *et al.* The Canadian Network for Mood and Anxiety Treatments (CANMAT) task force recommendations for the management of patients with mood disorders and comorbid attention-deficit/hyperactivity disorder. *Ann Clin Psychiatry*. 2012;**24**(1):23–7.

77. Kowatch RA, Fristad M, Birmaher B, *et al.* Treatment guidelines for children and adolescents with bipolar disorder. *J Am Acad Child Adolesc Psychiatry*. 2005; **44**(3):213–35.

78. Wozniak J, Biederman J. A pharmacological approach to the quagmire of comorbidity in juvenile mania. *J Am Acad Child Adolesc Psychiatry*. 1996;**35**(6):826–8.

79. Biederman J, Hammerness P, Doyle R, *et al.* Risperidone treatment for ADHD in children and adolescents with bipolar disorder. *Neuropsychiatr Dis Treat*. 2008;**4**(1):203–7.

80. Joshi G, Wozniak J, Mick E, *et al.* A prospective open-label trial of extended-release carbamazepine monotherapy in children with bipolar disorder. *J Child Adolesc Psychopharmacol*. 2010;**20**(1):7–14.

81. Tramontina S, Zeni CP, Ketzer CR, *et al.* Aripiprazole in children and adolescents with bipolar disorder comorbid with attention-deficit/hyperactivity disorder: a pilot randomized clinical trial. *J Clin Psychiatry*. 2009;**70**(5):756–64.

82. Strober M, DeAntonio M, Schmidt-Lackner S, *et al.* Early childhood attention deficit hyperactivity disorder predicts poorer response to acute lithium therapy in adolescent mania. *J Affect Disord*. 1998; **51**:145–51.

83. State RC, Frye MA, Altshuler LL, *et al.* Chart review of the impact of attention-deficit/hyperactivity disorder comorbidity on response to lithium or divalproex sodium in adolescent mania. *J Clin Psychiatry*. 2004; **65**(8):1057–63.

84. Scheffer RE, Kowatch RA, Carmody T, Rush AJ. Randomized, placebo-controlled trial of mixed amphetamine salts for symptoms of comorbid ADHD in pediatric bipolar disorder after mood stabilization with divalproex sodium. *Am J Psychiatry*. 2005;**162**(1): 58–64.

85. Findling RL, Short EJ, McNamara NK, *et al.* Methylphenidate in the treatment of children and adolescents with bipolar disorder and attention-deficit/hyperactivity disorder. *J Am Acad Child Adolesc Psychiatry*. 2007;**46**(11):1445–53.

86. Zenia C, Tramontina S, Ketzer C, Pheula G, Rohde L. Methylphenidate combined with aripiprazole in children and adolescents with bipolar and attention-deficit/hyperactivity disorder: a randomized crossover trial. *J Child Adolesc Psychopharmacol*. 2009;**19**(5): 553–61.

87. Wilens T, Prince J, Spencer T, *et al.* An open trial of bupropion for the treatment of adults with attention deficit hyperactivity disorder and bipolar disorder. *Biol Psychiatry.* 2003;**54**(1): 9–16.

88. Chang K, Nayar D, Howe M, Rana M. Atomoxetine as an adjunct therapy in the treatment of co-morbid attention-deficit/hyperactivity disorder in children and adolescents with bipolar I or II disorder. *J Child Adolesc Psychopharmacol.* 2009;**19**(5):547–51.

Assessment and treatment of depressive disorders in adults with ADHD

Jefferson B. Prince

Introduction

Attention-deficit hyperactivity disorder (ADHD) and depressive spectrum disorders frequently co-occur. Adults presenting for treatment of depression experience increased rates of ADHD, while those with ADHD suffer with higher rates of depression than their non-ADHD peers. Unfortunately despite the commonness of their occurrence, ADHD in adults with depressive spectrum disorders is often overlooked and therefore not found or treated. Likewise, despite their well-documented increased risk, many adults with ADHD suffer with untreated depression. Adults with ADHD experience significant interpersonal difficulties in relationships with family, friends, colleagues, and themselves. Adults with ADHD are often variably effective, or at least inefficient, in modulating the outflow from their body, mouth, and mind; and may be unaware of how their behavior impacts others. Over the course of development these adults frequently "bump into the walls of life," enduring repeated recriminations and assaults to their self-esteem, which are often experienced as both "stressed and stressful." Although not explicitly included in the diagnostic criteria of the current *Diagnostic and Statistical Manual of Mental Disorders* (DSM-5) [1], adults with ADHD are frequently perceived as "impatient," "hot tempered," and "irritable" [2–4].

Living with ADHD is difficult; and can be disheartening to patients, their loved ones, and their colleagues. Researchers and clinicians from around the globe recognize that adults with ADHD suffer with a variety of depressive spectrum disorders. As clinicians it is crucial to keep both aspects in mind; namely, that many adults with ADHD exhibit frequent affective symptoms (i.e., low frustration tolerance, dysphoria, and excessive emotional reactivity) and that these behaviors may reflect either dejection resulting from their ADHD and/or as an aspect of a clinically significant depression [5–8]. The clinical challenge is to differentiate their affective dysregulation related to ADHD from depressive spectrum disorders such as major depression, dysthymia, seasonal affective disorder, recurrent brief depression as well as the depressive phase of bipolar disorder. Over the course of the past 20 years a variety of researchers have enhanced our understanding of the relationship between depression and ADHD and their work informs our clinical practice. In this chapter I will review these data, paying special attention to the overlap between ADHD in adults, depression, executive function deficits, and emotional dysregulation, and conclude by discussing data about the psychosocial and medical treatments of both conditions.

Epidemiology of depressive disorders

"Depression" may describe a variety of conditions including: major depressive disorder (MDD), dysthymia, bipolar depression, recurrent brief depression, seasonal affective disorder, and depressive personality disorder. Depression frequently occurs among persons with chronic medical conditions, including obesity, cardiovascular disease, diabetes, asthma, arthritis, and cancer and/or psychiatric conditions including anxiety, addictions, trauma (i.e., physical, emotional, sexual abuse, or neglect), personality disorders, and eating disorders. Moreover, people who smoke cigarettes, are physically inactive, and binge-drinking experience increased rates of depression. A recent population-based study among 235 067 US adults, using the

Attention-Deficit Hyperactivity Disorder in Adults and Children, ed. Lenard A. Adler, Thomas J. Spencer and Timothy E. Wilens.
Published by Cambridge University Press. © Cambridge University Press 2015.

Patient Health Questionnaire 8 (PHQ-8), found that 9.0% met the criteria for current depression, including 3.4% who met the criteria for major depression [9]. In this cohort, the prevalence of MDD occurred more often in women than men (4.0% vs. 2.7%) and increased with age, from 2.8% in 18- to 24-year-olds to 4.6% in 45- to 64-year-olds. The authors did not comment on rates of comorbid disorders, including ADHD.

What have we learned from population-based studies of adults about the prevalence of ADHD in adults and about the relationship between ADHD and depression?

The National Comorbidity Survey Replication (NCS-R) [10, 11], a large community-based survey, estimated the point prevalence of ADHD in the United States as 4.4%; however, only approximately 10% of these adults were currently being treated for ADHD. The World Health Organization (WHO) supported population-based study of adults aged 18–44 years old from seven "developed" (Belgium, France, Germany, Italy, the Netherlands, Spain, and the United States) and three "less developed" (Colombia, Lebanon, and Mexico) countries estimated the prevalence of ADHD in adults as 3.4% [12]. Both of these studies observed that ADHD and depressive disorders commonly co-occur. In the NCS-R sample of 3199 US adults aged 19–44 years, 9.4% of respondents with MDD met criteria for ADHD compared to 3.7% of respondents without MDD; while 18.6% of respondents with ADHD met criteria for MDD compared to 7.8% of respondents without ADHD ($p < 0.05$; odds ratio 2.7; 95% confidence interval [CI] 1.5–4.9). Moreover, 22.6% of respondents with dysthymia met criteria for ADHD compared to 3.7% without dysthymia; and dysthymia occurred in 12.8% of respondents with ADHD compared to 1.9% of respondents without ADHD ($p < 0.05$; OR = 7.5; 95% CI 3.8–15.0). Similarly, the WHO study found that, compared to adults without ADHD, mood disorders occurred significantly more frequently (11.1%; OR = 3.9; 95% CI 3.0–5.1) in adults with ADHD; and usually developed after the onset of ADHD (85.6%). Similarly, ADHD occurred in significantly more adults with Mood Disorders (24.8%). In addition, a population-based sample of

middle-aged Australian adults (n = 2091; 47% male) indicated strong positive correlations between symptoms of ADHD and depression/anxiety [13].

A number of recent studies provide helpful insights into the relationship between ADHD and Depression from clinical samples from around the world. First, in a large representative sample of the German population (n = 1655) investigators recently estimated the prevalence of ADHD in adults as 4.7% [14]. In this cohort ADHD was associated with an increased likelihood of screening positive for depression. These investigators also screened for comorbid disorders and used the 2-item Patient Health Questionnaire (PHQ-2), a screening tool for depression that asks respondents; in the last 2 weeks "Do you have little interest in doing things?" and "Are you feeling down, depressed or hopeless?" ranked on a scale from 0 ("not at all") to 3 ("nearly everyday"). Using a cutoff score ≥ 3, the PHQ-2 has a sensitivity of 87% and a specificity of 78% for MDD and a sensitivity and specificity of 79% and 86% respectively for any depressive disorder. Using the PHQ-2 these investigators found that adults with ADHD were about three times (OR = 2.9; 95% CI 1.3–6.4; χ^2 6.87; $p < 0.01$) more likely to report symptoms of depression than those without ADHD. In this population subjects who screened positive on the PHQ-2 had a significantly higher rate of ADHD than those who screened negative (17.4% vs. 3.6% respectively) and those with ADHD were significantly more likely to report a positive PHQ-2 screen compared to subjects without ADHD (29.5% vs. 6.9%).

Second, over a 5-year period and from a catchment area of approximately 90 000, Norwegian investigators described the characteristics of the 45 adults diagnosed with ADHD and treated with stimulant medication [15]. In this cohort 86.7% (n = 39) had lifetime comorbidity for at least one other Axis I disorder, with MDD (n = 24; 53%) the most common. However, within the past year, Substance Use Disorders were most common (approximately 33%) while MDD occurred in 9%.

Third, in a large sample (n = 447; 266 men; 335 diagnosed with ADHD) of adults evaluated at an Adult ADHD Research Clinic in Montreal, investigators found that diagnosis of current (8 vs. 64; $\chi^2 = 8.548$, $p < 0.002$) and lifetime (24 vs. 112; $\chi^2 = 5.264$, $p < 0.01$) MDD occurred significantly more frequently in subjects with ADHD; especially those with ADHD, combined type compared to inattentive type [16].

Fourth, in a sample of 80 adults with ADHD (43 men and 37 women) from Melbourne, Australia, 54 suffered with ADHD + Learning Disabilities (LD) [17]. In this sample, women with ADHD + LD experienced significantly more cognitive symptoms of depression; including thoughts of worthlessness, hopelessness, and personal failure compared to men and/or women with ADHD only, as well as to men with ADHD + LD. It is useful for clinicians to recognize that women with ADHD + LD may suffer with particular malicious cognitive symptoms of depression, and therefore connect these patients with the proper treatments and supports.

Fifth, in a large clinical sample (n = 320) of outpatients with ADHD treated at a tertiary care hospital in Brazil, Fischer and colleagues found significant differences in the clinical picture of ADHD in adults with MDD, compared to adults with ADHD but "free of MDD" [18]. Adults with ADHD + MDD had increased rates of generalized anxiety disorder (GAD), Social Phobia, and Panic Disorder. Surprisingly, in this cohort no differences were observed in externalizing disorders such as oppositional defiant disorder, conduct disorder, and drug dependence, or in ADHD severity as measured by a revised Swanson, Nolan, and Pelham (SNAP) Questionnaire (SNAP-IV). In this sample, MDD (n = 81; 25.31%) occurred more often in women (n = 48; 32.4%) than men (n = 33; 19.2%) ($\chi^2 = 7.83$; p < 0.01) and occurred equally in all three subtypes of ADHD. Although subjects with ADHD + MDD sought treatment with psychotherapy and medications more frequently, the co-occurrence of MDD was not associated with an earlier diagnosis of ADHD, therefore losing an opportunity for earlier intervention and treatment. This is not surprising given that empirical data suggest that when ADHD is not identified in childhood it often remains unidentified [19, 20].

Sixth, utilizing the Adult ADHD Self-Report Scale Version 1.1 Screener [21], Able and colleagues surveyed a large sample (n = 21 000) of patients in a managed care plan, identifying 752 adults "undiagnosed" with ADHD, 199 "non-ADHD" controls and 198 "diagnosed" with ADHD [22]. Compared to the control group, adults with "undiagnosed" ADHD were significantly more likely to be female and to experience more interpersonal difficulties, characterized by emotional symptoms that disrupted their work, social, and family relationships. These subjects achieved lower levels of education, earned less income, and reported a lower quality of life. Moreover, they were significantly more likely to have a lifetime history of depression (31% vs. 12.9%; p < 0.001), anxiety (19.8% vs. 7.3%; p < 0.001), or bipolar disorder (5.9% vs. 0.9%; p < 0.001); and were significantly more likely to screen positive for a current episode of depression (46.4% vs. 21%; p < 0.001). Likewise, ADHD in adults treated for MDD is often under recognized. Analysis of claims data from one large Health Maintenance Organization (HMO) found that of 17 792 adults coded for MDD, only 454 (0.2%) were also diagnosed with ADHD [23]. Similarly, another HMO reported ADHD in 1.7% of patients diagnosed with MDD and Anxiety [24].

Clinical presentation and course of ADHD in adults with ADHD + depression

Adults with ADHD + MDD experience an earlier onset of depression, more severe symptoms of depression, more frequent episodes, more suicide attempts, and an earlier onset of depression. Regardless of mood state, adults with depression + ADHD may manifest restlessness, psychomotor agitation, difficulty concentrating, increased distractibility, and decreased attention. However, symptoms such as depressed mood, changes in appetite or weight, loss of interest in usual activities, and hopelessness/thoughts of death/suicide occur during an episode of depression. Family studies of subjects with ADHD + MDD suggest a familial link and shared genetic risks between ADHD and depression. These studies find elevated rates of depression in relatives of individuals with ADHD as well as increased rates of ADHD in relatives of subjects with MDD [25]. In addition, a family history of mood disorders was associated with persistence of ADHD [26]. In a study of adolescents with ADHD, longer onset of pharmacotherapy with stimulant medication for ADHD was associated with increased likelihood of MDD [27]. Several clinical studies document that adults referred for ADHD [6, 8, 28] display the "classic triad" of ADHD symptoms seen in youth with ADHD, namely inattention, impulsivity, and hyperactivity, as well as symptoms of stubbornness, low tolerance for frustration, anger outbursts, and conflicted relationships with peers, family members, and authorities. On the other hand, ADHD does not appear to influence the symptoms of depression. Depressive disorders appear similar in patients with and without ADHD as demonstrated by a similar age of onset of MDD, gender distribution, symptom constellation and course (similar number, duration, and severity of episodes). In addition, MDD appears to respond equally well to usual treatments in patients with ADHD [29]. Recently, investigators studied large employer-sponsored health plans, comparing adults without ADHD (n = 95 256) to those with ADHD (n = 31 752) or depression (n = 29 965) [30]. In this large cohort, subjects with ADHD were significantly more likely to experience depression than matched non-ADHD controls (14% vs. 3.2%; p ≤ 0.0001). Moreover, patients with ADHD + depression were significantly more likely to have comorbid medical conditions such as diabetes, hypertension, asthma, irritable bowel syndrome as well as psychiatric conditions such as bipolar disorder, anxiety, alcohol abuse, and substance abuse (p ≤ 0.0001). These subjects also experienced significantly more lost work productivity and had higher healthcare costs.

ADHD and depressive disorders have a number of symptoms in common, including reduced ability to concentrate, an inner feeling of restlessness or physical agitation, low self-esteem, and sleep disturbances. These overlapping symptoms make it challenging to diagnose ADHD in the presence of an ongoing depressive episode. However, the longitudinal course of each condition provides clinically useful information. Namely, symptoms related to depression diminish in periods between episodes, whereas symptoms of ADHD may vary based on context but are nonetheless continuous. Furthermore, medication used in the treatment of ADHD may both mimic and exacerbate symptoms of depression [31]. A recent investigation of neurocognition found that adults with ADHD and depression performed significantly worse on tasks involving processing speed, delayed recall of conceptual verbal information, and shifting [32].

Recurrent brief depression (RBD) and ADHD

Recognized by both DSM-5 and *International Classification of Diseases*, 10th edition (ICD-10), RBD is characterized by "brief" (from 1 or 2 to 13 days) episodes of depressive symptoms. A large epidemiological study estimates the 1-year and lifetime prevalence of RBD to be 5% and 16% respectively [33]. In a group of 40 adult outpatients with ADHD from Germany treated

in a University Hospital setting, 28 (70%) met criteria for a lifetime diagnosis of RBD; and 5 of these 28 adults also experienced MDD [34]. These authors speculate that adults with ADHD and RBD may respond to adrenergic antidepressants, with or without a stimulant.

Seasonal affective disorder (SAD) and ADHD

An understudied area in adults with ADHD is the seasonal pattern of affective disturbances. To date such data have not been collected in most studies of adults with ADHD, with or without mood disorders. SAD commonly known as "winter depression" is defined as two or more consecutive episodes of major depression in autumn or winter with spontaneous remission in the spring or summer. Patients often experience daytime sleepiness, hypersomnia, increased appetite, carbohydrate craving, and weight gain. Patients with either/both ADHD or/and SAD experience poor concentration, sleep disturbances, forgetfulness, and irritability. In an adult ADHD clinic in Toronto, Ontario, Canada investigators found that SAD occurred in 19% of their sample; a rate the authors report that was significantly higher than the rate of SAD expected at their latitude [35]. These patients with ADHD + SAD were women and manifest a lot of impulsivity. A more recent study from the Netherlands of 259 adults with ADHD, estimates the prevalence of SAD at 27%. Of the 115 patients with ADHD and an identified mood disorder (primarily various forms of depressive spectrum as there were only 2 patients with bipolar disorder) 70 (61%) demonstrated a "seasonal pattern" of affective worsening [36]. The SAD+ patients were significantly more likely to be female and have the ADHD, combined type. These authors encourage clinicians to consider SAD in adults with ADHD and if present consider bright light therapy [37]. Patients and clinicians may find a lot of useful information about SAD, assessment, and treatment at www.cet.org.

ADHD in patients presenting for treatment of depressive or bipolar disorder

In a cohort of 116 adult patients with MDD, Alpert and colleagues found that 16% met full or subthreshold criteria for a DSM-III-R diagnosis of childhood ADHD and that 12% had clinically meaningful persistence of ADHD symptoms into adulthood [29]. These investigators found no differences in the clinical picture of depression in the group with ADHD + MDD (n = 19) to that of the group with MDD alone (n = 97), including gender distribution, age of onset of depression, number of depressive episodes, or response to the pharmacological treatment for depression.

In a recent report of the first 399 subjects enrolled in the International Mood Disorders Collaborative Project, investigators found that 5.4% (n = 11) of 203 diagnosed with MDD meet criteria for lifetime diagnosis of ADHD; however, no one was being treated for ADHD [38]. Although no differences were noted in sex distribution in subjects with MDD + ADHD, subjects with MDD + ADHD experienced their initial affective episode almost 10 years earlier that those with MDD without ADHD (16.10 ± 12.44 years vs. 25.99 ± 15.49 years respectively; p = 0.049) and those with MDD meeting Adult ADHD Self-Report Scale (ASRS) Version 1.1 criteria for ADHD experienced significantly more severe symptoms as measured by the Hamilton Depression Rating Scale and the Montgomery–Asberg Depression Rating Scale. In addition, no differences were noted between groups in the frequency of affective episodes or in the severity of their apparent risk of suicide.

The National Institute for Mental Health sponsored the Systematic Treatment Enhancement Program for Bipolar Disorder (STEP-BD), which greatly enhanced our understanding of the relationship between ADHD and Bipolar Disorder in adults [39]. In this large multicenter study, 9.5% of the first 1000 adult subjects treated for bipolar disorder were comorbid for ADHD. In this cohort, subjects with ADHD + bipolar disorder experienced an earlier onset of their mood disorder (5 years earlier), a more severe course of their mood disorder, were more likely to be depressed currently, and 41.2% suffered more than 20 episodes of depression. These subjects frequently had comorbidity with several anxiety disorders and substance abuse and/or dependence. While the severity of depressive symptoms is often similar in adults with unipolar and bipolar disorders other symptoms may be useful to distinguish these conditions. Those with bipolar depression appear more likely to have psychomotor retardation, melancholic features, mood reactivity, reversed sleep as well as appetite disturbances [40]. In a cohort of youth with ADHD, compared to unipolar depression, those with bipolar depression were more severely

impaired, suicidal, irritable, and sad. These subjects had high levels of comorbidity with disruptive behavior disorders, alcohol abuse, and agoraphobia [41].

Special considerations in adults with ADHD and depressive disorders

Relationship between ADHD, depressive disorders, and deficits of executive function, emotional impulsivity, and deficit of emotional regulation

Adults with ADHD are frequently emotionally impulsive and deficits of emotional self-regulation cause significant dysfunction in adults with ADHD and represent a distinct familial subtype [42]. These difficulties clinically manifest as being significantly more impulsive, quick to anger, easily frustrated, lose temper, be easily annoyed, and emotional overreaction [2]. Emotional impulsivity contributes to impairments in relationships of all kinds (social, marital, dating, work), driving, leisure activities, and managing money. These symptoms may be confused with and must be distinguished from an "irritable" or "agitated" depression, and often manifest as impatience, low frustration tolerance, hot-temperedness, quickness to anger, irritability, and easily emotionally excitable. These symptoms were described as part of ADHD in adults earlier by Paul Wender and Hans Huessy [3, 43]. Emotional self-control involves inhibiting emotional reactions provoked by life circumstances and events and then self-regulating the emotional state in order to be socially appropriate and consistent with longer-term goals. Emotional impulsivity can be understood as a part of the difficulties arising from hyperactivity–impulsivity symptoms. The substrates for deficits of this type appear to be the "hot" executive functions modulated and monitored by orbital and medial prefrontal cortex and implicated in the regulation of emotions. Zelazo and Cunningham suggest that these "hot" executive function areas are well connected to the amygdala and other parts of the limbic system, therefore making this circuit well suited to regulate emotionally related information and regulation of approach and withdrawal responses [44]. Difficulties with self-regulation may arise out of deficits in the "cool" executive which may be part of the attention network, the "what" and/or "when" executive network. The "cool" executive function system is modulated and monitored by the dorsolateral prefrontal cortex and implicated in non-emotive, abstract, decontextualized problem solving.

Moreover, regardless of levels of anxiety or depression, adults with ADHD often have more difficulties recognizing emotional expressions, which appear improved during treatment with methylphenidate [45].

Obesity

In a meta-analysis of 17 community-based studies comprising 204 507 subjects, de Wit *et al.* report a significant association between obesity and depression in the general population (OR = 1.26; 95% CI 1.17–1.36; p ≤ 0.001), especially for women [46]. Recent data suggest a linear relationship between increase in risk of obesity and increasing ADHD symptoms, especially hyperactive/impulsive symptoms [47]. At this time there are no studies of obesity in patients with ADHD and depression; and the impact of obesity on the clinical presentation, severity, and treatment of ADHD and depression remains unclear. Therefore, the wisest approach to such patients takes each condition into consideration and builds a treatment plan addressing each of these difficult conditions.

Suicide

It is clear that several factors increase the likelihood of completing suicide; depression, previous suicide attempts, antisocial behaviors, substance use/misuse/abuse and personality traits of impulsivity and aggression. Preliminary results in adolescents suggest a significant association between ADHD and suicide. A review of the literature between 1966 and 2003 by James *et al.* found a modest elevated risk ratio of completed suicide compared to US national suicide rates (relative risk [RR] 2.91; 95% CI 1.47–5.7, χ^2 = 9.3, df = 1). In this review the group at most increased risk were adolescent males with ADHD, depression and conduct disorder. The authors suggest this grouping of conditions may alert clinicians to those at increased risk [48]. In a small (n = 23; 18 females) group of Israeli adolescents admitted to a Psychiatric Emergency Room due to suicidal behaviors, structured interviews revealed that 65% had ADHD (66% with Inattentive subtype and 34% with combined subtype), 43.5% with major depression and 39% with Cluster B personality disorders. Only 22% of these suicidal subjects had been previously diagnosed with ADHD, and only 13% were being treated for it [49]. These results support the importance of considering unrecognized/untreated ADHD as a significant contributing factor in suicidal adolescents. More recently, using data from the NCS-R, ADHD

alone was not strongly associated with probability of attempting suicide. However, in those ADHD adults with one or more comorbid disorder, the risk of suicidal behaviors was elevated 4- to 12-fold [50]. These authors encourage early treatment of ADHD and comorbid disorders.

Personality development, ADHD and depression: borderline, antisocial

Recently, investigators reported a significant overlap between borderline personality disorder (BPD) and the seven symptom clusters in the Wender Utah Rating Scale (WURS): inattentiveness, hyperactivity, mood lability, irritability/hot tempered, impaired stress tolerance, disorganization, and impulsivity [51]. Other investigators identified ADHD in 38% of subjects with BPD; with ADHD, combined type occurring most commonly [52]. Compared with the BPD-only group those subjects with BPD + ADHD were observed to be more impulsive as evidenced by higher rates of cannabis abuse, non-specific anxiety disorders, and suicidal behaviors (but not in self-harming behaviors or emergency room visits). The BPD-only group was observed to have increased rates of MDD, benzodiazepine abuse, and panic disorder. Recognition that patients with BPD comorbid with ADHD are at increased risk of impulsivity may be helpful in clarifying etiological pathways and development and implementation of an appropriate treatment plan to address the full range of biopsychosocial needs of these patients. Since patients with ADHD and BPD may manifest similar symptoms, including impulsivity, affective instability, anger outbursts, and feelings of boredom, it is important for clinicians to distinguish these symptoms. In the ADHD patient, impulsivity and anger is usually short-lived and thoughtless, rather than driven; conflict relationships, suicidal preoccupation, self-mutilation, identity disturbances, and feelings of abandonment are usually less intense than in BPD.

Treatments for ADHD and depressive disorders

As yet, no formal guidelines have been developed for the treatment of adults with ADHD in the United States. However, guidelines for the treatment of ADHD in children and adolescents, as well as international guidelines for the treatment of adult ADHD, offer recommendations that can be extrapolated to adults in the USA. Considerable concordance exists among the guidelines established by the Canadian Network for Mood and Anxiety Treatments (CANMET) task force [53], the American Academy of Child and Adolescent Psychiatry (AACAP) [54], the National Institute for Health and Care Excellence (NICE) (please see http://www.nice.org.uk/CG72), and the European Network Adult ADHD [55]. These guidelines endorse similar multimodal approaches to the care of adults with ADHD; building upon a foundation of education about ADHD, an overview of possible non-pharmacological interventions (i.e., coaching, cognitive-behavioral therapy (CBT), problem solving, and training in time management skills), and moving towards pharmacotherapy for ADHD and its common comorbidities. While comprehensive, it remains unclear how these guidelines are best implemented in each patient.

Prior to treating patients with ADHD and depressive disorders, it is important and necessary to complete a thorough clinical evaluation including a complete history of symptoms, differential diagnosis, review of prior assessments/treatments, medical history, and current physical symptoms (including questions about the physical history including either a personal or family history of cardiovascular symptoms or problems). When assessing for depression, it is important to consider the following conditions: anxiety/stress/sadness, grief, trauma, abuse, neglect, attachment disorders, bipolar disorder (especially mixed states), ADHD and/or ODD/CD, learning disorders, substance use disorders, developmental disorders (e.g., Asperger's, non-verbal learning disorder), eating disorders, medical/neurological disorders (e.g., head injury, endocrine disorders of thyroid or glucose metabolism, and seizure), and/or medications.

Having made the diagnosis of ADHD and a depressive disorder, it is necessary to discuss your clinical impression, including the primary diagnosis, with the patient/family and develop a treatment plan. Patients/families need to be familiarized with the risks and benefits of pharmacotherapy, the availability of alternative treatments, likely adverse effects and how to manage them. Patient expectations need to be explored and realistic goals of treatment clearly delineated. In regards to medications, the clinician should review with the patient the various pharmacological options available, including not using medications, and that each will require a systematic trial for reasonable durations of time and at clinically meaningful doses. It

is recommended that treating or consulting clinicians directly communicate with other clinicians involved in the care of the patient (e.g., primary care physician and/or therapist). Prior to treatment with medications, it is usually important to measure baseline height, weight, blood pressure, and pulse and to monitor them over the course of treatment. While there are a myriad of factors to be considered in each patient, it is important for the clinician and patients/families to agree on the diagnoses, aims of treatment, and initial treatment(s) selected. With medications it is essential to discuss options, select an initial medication, understand how to titrate and how to measure outcome (i.e., anchor points of functional change and/or changes in rating scale), and anticipate expected/common side effects. In adults with ADHD and depressive disorders, a common factor to monitor for is if the pharmacological treatment for ADHD (stimulants and non-stimulants) are worsening mood.

Despite frequently overlapping, there are no double-blind placebo-controlled randomized trials and few clinical trials comparing the safety, tolerability, and efficacy of treatments for adults with both conditions. In fact, there are almost as many "expert guidelines" as there are clinical studies. Recently several different groups have reviewed the literature and offered guidance about treating adults with ADHD and depression [53, 54]. The clinical approach is that depressive disorders trump ADHD. This method involves two important organizing steps; first to withdraw medications/treatments that may be aggravating/causing/contributing to depressive disorder and second, to put into place treatments that help with treating depression. While the components of each patient's system vary, the "bottom line" is to join with the patient/family in a collaborative investigative process with a clear common aim. The use of medications is largely guided by the answers to three questions; how well are you (the patient) tolerating the medication(s)? How helpful are these medications? In which contexts do I need to take the medications? I summarize the application of this approach as *"RAPS": Recognize, Assess, Prioritize, and Sequence*. In my experience patients with ADHD and depression most often benefit from treatment that draws from elements of education, psychosocial treatments, and pharmacotherapy. Depressive symptoms in adults with ADHD + MDD appear to respond well to usual pharmacological treatments for depression; however, during an episode of depression the efficacy of stimulants for ADHD symptoms appears to diminish [29, 56, 57].

Trials in youth with ADHD + MDD

TADS subgroup

In the Treatment for Adolescents with Depression Study (TADS), 377 adolescents were randomized for treatment of MDD, and 62 (14.1%) had comorbid ADHD [58, 59]. Recently Kratochvil and colleagues investigated the impact of the comorbid ADHD on the treatment of depression [60]. Interestingly, in this trial youth with MDD and ADHD presented with similar levels of global impairments due to depression and similar rates of suicidality. Moreover, these investigators found no differences in age of onset, duration, or rate of recurrence of depression in these adolescents with MDD and ADHD. In fact, the depressed subjects with comorbid ADHD responded similarly to treatment with CBT, fluoxetine or the combination, whereas in adolescents without ADHD the combination treatment was more effective than either CBT or fluoxetine alone, both of which were superior to placebo. Based on their results, the authors suggest that any of these three treatments may be appropriate in the initial treatment of adolescents with MDD and ADHD. These results may be applied to the care of adults with ADHD and comorbid depression, namely that there are increasing data supporting the use of combinations of treatments with these patients.

Medications

Four medications are currently US Food and Drug Administration (FDA) approved for treatment of ADHD in adults, including Strattera, Concerta, Adderall XR, and Vyvanse. However, as with youth, all formulations of stimulants and non-stimulants may be useful in adults with ADHD. A recent meta-analysis of 18 clinical trials with stimulants and non-stimulants demonstrated that both of these treatments are effective in reducing ADHD symptoms [61]. These studies found an effect size of 0.86 for short-acting stimulants, 0.76 for extended delivery stimulants, and 0.39 for non-stimulants. While these authors do not comment on the impact of depression on the effect size of stimulants or non-stimulants, it is important to recognize that in these studies, a current depressive episode is an exclusion criterion.

Stimulants in ADHD and depression

Gammon and Brown report excellent tolerability and efficacy when adding fluoxetine to stimulant for the treatment of depression or dysthymia [62]. Recently Weiss and Hechtman demonstrated the efficacy of dextroamphetamine (maximum dose 40 mg/day) and paroxetine (maximum dose 40 mg/day) together to help improve ADHD as well as mood/anxiety symptoms [63].

Non-stimulants in ADHD and depression

Atomoxetine (ATMX) is reported to reduce symptoms of anxiety and depression in ADHD youth [64, 65]. Compared with placebo (n = 70), ATMX (n = 72) significantly reduced ADHD, but did not significantly reduce symptoms of depression. In another trial 173 (7- to 17-year-old) youth with ADHD (75% combined type) and depression (Childhood Depression Rating Scale [CDRS-R] score >36) or anxiety (Manifest Anxiety Scale for Children [MASC] score ≥1 SD above norm) were randomized in an unbalanced blinded fashion to 8 weeks of treatment with ATMX + fluoxetine (n = 127) or ATMX + placebo (n = 46). After randomization fluoxetine or placebo were given as a single dose of 20 mg each morning for 2 weeks and then ATMX was added. ATMX was initiated at 0.5 mg/kg/day dosed evenly BID and titrated to a mean of 1.36 ± 0.55 mg/kg/day in ATMX + fluoxetine and 1.52 ± 0.41 mg/kg/day in ATMX + placebo groups respectively. Both treatment arms led to significant reductions in symptoms of ADHD, depression, and anxiety. CDRS-R scores decreased by approximately 20 points in each group; those subjects with ATMX peak plasma concentrations over the median had significantly greater reductions in CDRS-R scores. Subjects treated with both ATMX and fluoxetine experienced greater increases in blood pressure and pulse. These results suggest ATMX may be helpful in patients with symptoms of anxiety and depression, as well as in emotional dysregulation manifesting as mood lability, mild depression, irritability, difficulty controlling temper, over reactivity to stress, and feeling frequently frustrated [66].

Emslie and colleagues employed an algorithm-based treatment of youth with depression (n = 24) and ADHD plus depression (n = 15) [67]. Following the algorithm, youth with ADHD were initially treated with a stimulant for 2 weeks. After 2 weeks, if ADHD symptoms improved and depressive symptoms remained, a selective serotonin reuptake inhibitor (SSRI) antidepressant was added; if ADHD symptoms worsened or did not respond, then the stimulant was discontinued and the SSRI started. Four of the 15 subjects with ADHD + depression were treated with an antidepressant, 3 with SSRI, and 1 with bupropion. Improvements were noted in ADHD, depression, and global functioning. In light of the limited evidence base, clinicians should generally assess severity of ADHD and depression and direct initial treatment towards the most impairing condition. In treating patients up to the age of 24 with depression (with or without ADHD), clinicians must keep in mind black box warnings about antidepressants and risk of suicidality. Excellent reliable information for professionals, patients, and families can be found at http://www.fda.gov/Drugs/DrugSafety/InformationbyDrugClass/UCM096273 or www.parentsmedguide.org.

Role of antidepressants (non-FDA approved for treatment of ADHD)

Bupropion, a novel-structured antidepressant, has been reported to be moderately helpful in reducing ADHD symptoms in adults [68–70] and may be particularly helpful when ADHD is comorbid with depression [71, 72]. Dosing of bupropion in adults with ADHD and depression usually ranges from 200 to 450 mg daily (75–150 mg TID of immediate-release formulation or 100–200 mg sustained-release formulation BID or 300–450 mg of the extended delivery formulation) and, while not formally studied, is often used with stimulant medication. Side effects of bupropion include insomnia, edginess, agitation, increased motor activity, insomnia, tremor, and tics. Bupropion appears to be more stimulating than other antidepressants, and it is associated with a higher rate of drug-induced seizures than other antidepressants [73]. These seizures appear to be dose-related (>450 mg/day) and to be elevated in patients with bulimia nervosa or a previous seizure history.

Although their use has decreased considerably since the availability of ATMX, tricyclic antidepressants (TCAs) have been used as alternatives to the stimulants for ADHD in adults [74, 75]. Compared to the stimulants, TCAs have negligible abuse liability, single daily dosing, and efficacy for comorbid anxiety and depression. However, given concerns about potential cardiotoxicity, use of the TCAs has been significantly curtailed. A controlled trial of desipramine with a target dose of 200 mg/day resulted in significant reductions in ADHD symptoms in adults [76]. In that study, response was noted during the initial titration at 2 weeks, and this continued to improve at the 6-week end point. Whereas a minority of subjects responded to <100 mg/day, the majority required more robust dosing (mean of 150 mg/day) for efficacy. Generally, TCA daily doses of 50–250 mg are required, with a relatively rapid response to treatment (i.e., 2 weeks) when the appropriate dose is reached. TCAs should be initiated at 25 mg and slowly titrated upward within dosing and serum level parameters until an acceptable response or intolerable adverse effects are reported. Common side effects of the TCAs include dry mouth, constipation, blurred vision, weight gain, and sexual dysfunction. Although cardiovascular effects (reduced cardiac conduction, elevated blood pressure, and heart rates) are not infrequent, if monitored they rarely prevent treatment. As serum TCA levels are variable, they are best used as guidelines for efficacy and to reduce central nervous system and cardiovascular toxicity.

The monoamine oxidase inhibitor (MAOI) antidepressants have also been studied for the treatment of ADHD in adults. Whereas open studies with pargyline and deprenyl in adult ADHD showed moderate improvements [77, 78] a controlled trial of selegiline (deprenyl) yielded less promising findings [79]. Data for the reversible MAOI moclobemide on its effectiveness for adult ADHD are limited to case reports [80]. The MAOIs may have a role in the management of non-impulsive adults with treatment-refractory ADHD and comorbid depression and anxiety who are able to comply with the stringent requirements of these agents (tryramine-free diet and no stimulants). The concerns about diet- or medication-induced hypertensive crisis limit the usefulness and safety of these medications, however, especially in those patients with ADHD who are vulnerable to impulsivity. Other adverse effects associated with the MAOIs include agitation or lethargy, orthostatic hypotension, weight gain, sexual dysfunction, sleep disturbances, and edema, often leading to the discontinuation of these agents.

While SSRIs do not appear to be effective for ADHD [81], venlafaxine, an antidepressant which may inhibit both serotonergic and noradrenergic reuptake, may have a role in the treatment of patients with ADHD and depression. In three open studies with a total of 41 adults, 75% of adults who tolerated venlafaxine had a measurable reduction in their ADHD at doses of 75–150 mg daily [82–84]. Although further controlled trials are necessary to determine its optimal dosing and efficacy, venlafaxine is generally titrated from 25 mg/day to more typical antidepressant dosing of between 150 and 225 mg/day for ADHD control. Side effects of venlafaxine in adults include nausea and other gastrointestinal distress; there are concerns about elevated blood pressure at relatively higher dosing. Venlafaxine is often used conjointly with stimulants for control of ADHD in adults. Along the same lines, Niederhofer recently described the use of the "dual action" antidepressant duloxetine in two adolescent patients with ADHD but without depression [85].

Psychosocial treatments

CBT is an attractive intervention for adults with ADHD + depression for several reasons. First, CBT is an effective treatment for many forms of depression [86]. Second, many adults with ADHD seeking treatment have some awareness that their primarily self-evolved coping skills are not working "well enough" and they are open to skill-based treatments that help them develop effective compensatory strategies and improve other functional impairments typically associated with ADHD. Many clinicians recommend CBT or other forms of psychotherapy once the patient has been stabilized on pharmacotherapy. CBT and other interventions can help the patient address organization skills and self-efficacy that have evolved over many years of insufficient treatment for ADHD. CBT may also help the subset of patients who choose not to use medications (or for whom medications are not appropriate or intolerable), as well as the large proportion of patients who have comorbid conditions. A number of recent trials and a meta-analysis suggest that CBT may enhance the response to and benefits of pharmacological treatments [87–89]. Although it may be effective, CBT appears to work well when an engaged and creative clinician and accepting, motivated patient collaborate as informed allies to manage the residual symptoms of negative emotions and distorted cognitions. Excellent clinical manuals include those by Ramsay and Rostain [90] and Safren *et al.* [91].

Metacognitive therapy (MCT) uses principles and methods of CBT to teach time management, organization, and planning skills, and to address depressive and anxious thoughts that undermine effective self-management. Solanto and colleagues compared a 12-week course of group MCT (n = 41; 13 reported with "any mood disorder") with supportive therapy (including non-specific group support and validation, psychoeducation, and therapist attention; n = 38; 15 [35%] reported with "any mood disorder") in adults with ADHD [92]. Although approximately one-third of this sample was reported to have "any mood disorder," baseline scores on the Beck Depression Inventory (BDI) were in the clinically normal range. Although, the overall scores did not change significantly, an analysis of variance (ANOVA) showed that subjects with a concurrent Axis I mood disorder experienced a significant decrease in mean BDI scores from 17 to 13; yielding a significant main effect of time (pre- to post-treatment assessment; F = 4.99, df = 1, 24, p = 0.035) but no interaction with treatment condition. The authors conclude that MCT provided significantly more benefit in adults with ADHD "with respect to inattention symptoms that reflect the specific functions of time management, organization, and planning." These benefits were seen in patients who were receiving medication treatment as well as those who were not.

What is the role of mindfulness-based cognitive therapy (MBCT) in these patients? While MBCT is an exciting treatment, to date one study has demonstrated the tolerability and short-term positive effects of a mindfulness group-training program on behavioral and neurocognitive impairments in adolescents and adults with ADHD [93]. This program may have an additional favorable impact on the development of inhibitory control and self-regulation. While experience may increase the benefits of meditation, short-term training also appears to promote observable effects. By promoting a heightened state of concentration that triggers activity of the attentional networks, meditative practices such as mindfulness training may improve behavior [94] and prove useful – at least as ancillary treatment – for individuals with attention-specific deficits.

Problem-focused therapy, ADHD and depression

Recently Weiss and Hechtman demonstrated the efficacy of dextroamphetamine (maximum dose 40 mg/day) and paroxetine (maximum dose 40 mg/day) together to help improve ADHD as well as symptoms of mood/anxiety [63].

Traditional psychotherapies

These may help differentiate problematic behaviors due to ADHD (capacity issues) or depressive disorders or the combination from those that are due to one's particular psychodynamics (motivational issues) [95].

Role for couples and families

When appropriate, patients may also benefit from couples or family counseling or both, and life-skills training or coaching. A review of studies of group and individual psychosocial treatments for adult ADHD found that various psychosocial therapies, including skills training and psychoeducation, improved motivation and reduced residual symptoms in adults with ADHD.

Role of self-help and other supports

When treating adults with ADHD and depression it is wise to discuss wellness/lifestyle changes including: playing to their strengths, to "what is still right with them" by making time to be with things/people/activities that make them feel positive; investigating their "diet" of food, media, and social contacts; regular physical activity; smiling and laughing; improving sleep hygiene; decreasing caffeine (especially too many "energy drinks"), nicotine, alcohol, marijuana, and other substances; investigating their motivation (i.e., what is really really really important to them and as Larry James said, "The main thing is to keep the main thing the main thing.") and practicing the relaxation response and/or stress reduction. Other supports such as coaching may be clinically useful. While not studied in the same way as medications and psychosocial treatments, coaching is often well received, helpful but not usually supported by insurance. Local coaching can be found through http://www.adhdcoaches.org/ and a helpful description of "receiving coaching" is available at http://www.additudemag.com/adhd/article/4002.html. Additional support is available through national organizations such as Children and Adults with ADD (www.CHADD.org) and Adults with ADD (www.add.org). This support is generally free, up to date, innovative, practical, enthusiastic, and empathic. Some patients benefit from adjunctive strategies to address executive function deficits and improve organization. Patients with ADHD and depression may also find it useful to maintain a mood diary; a useful example can be found at http://www.psychiatry24x7.com/bgdisplay.jhtml?itemname=mooddiary.

Table 8.1. Strength of evidence for the treatment of ADHD in adults with MDD + ADHD

Level of evidence*	Treatment	Data from
1	None	None
2	Atomoxetine	Youth
3	Bupropion	Youth and adults
3	SSRIs	Youth and adults
4	SSRIs + stimulants	Youth and adults
4	CBT	Adults
4	Modafinil	Adults
4	Venlafaxine	Adults
4	Desipramine	Adults
4	Nortriptyline	Adults
4	Lisdexamfetamine	Adults

* 1 = ≥2 placebo-controlled trials or meta-analysis; 2 = 1 randomized controlled trial with placebo or active comparator; 3 = open-label trial >10; 4 = anecdotal or expert opinion.
Source: Adapted from Bond *et al.* [53].

Table 8.2. Treatment recommendations for the management of ADHD in adults with MDD + ADHD

Lines of evidence	Treatment recommendation
First line	Bupropion Antidepressant + extended delivery stimulant Antidepressant + CBT
Second line	Venlafaxine Nortriptyline Desipramine
Third line	Antidepressant + short-acting stimulant Antidepressant + ATMX Antidepressant + lisdexamfetamine

Source: Adapted from Bond *et al.* [53].

Clinical guidance based on type of depressive disorder (Tables 8.1 and 8.2)

Demoralization due to previously untreated symptoms of ADHD occurs often in transition to college or from college to graduate school or when changing jobs within a company; usually, treating patients with these difficulties consists of optimizing medical and psychosocial treatments and supports for the adult with ADHD.

Brief reactive depression: usually follow the guidance as described above; close monitoring that brief reactive depression does not morph into Dysthymia or an episode of Depression.

Seasonal depression: monitor using a mood chart; pay close attention to sleep patterns; often first choice is to use light therapy and supplement with vitamin D (if the patient's level is low); often use melatonin to regulate sleep–wake cycle. Please see www.cet.org for additional excellent information about implementing these treatments.

Major depressive episode or disorder: if the major depressive episode is of at least moderate severity (often not brought to clinician in situations where it is "only minor") then it is usually important to prioritize treatment of depression first. Once depression is responding, then reconsider treatment for ADHD.

Dysthymia: usual approach is to tailor treatment with full menu of options including medications to reduce symptoms of depression and ADHD as well as psychosocial treatments aimed to enhance and maintain response as well as education/training in ways the patient may enhance their own well-being.

Depressed phase of a bipolar disorder: means enhancing all treatments that support and bring about stabilization of the mood first. Then once mood has stabilized reconsider treatments for ADHD, remembering to monitor for worsening of mood.

Personality disorders: clinically it is important to recognize that ADHD, trauma, and personality disorders may co-occur. The usual approach is to collaboratively differentiate relational difficulties from core symptoms of ADHD and usually to offer a combination of evidence-based psychosocial and medical treatments.

Substance-induced mood disorders: usually will address the substance use disorder first; once it is stable then prioritize the mood component; addressing it sufficiently with a combination of psychosocial and medications treatments; once the patient has earned 2–3 months of sobriety and his/her mood is improved and he/she is actively engaged in treatments to sustain these improvements then it is reasonable to reassess ADHD and if present to treat it; usually the pharmacotherapy will consist of either non-stimulants, or, if stimulants are used, a form of stimulant that is less likely to be abused or misused such as Daytrana or Vyvanse; there may also be a role for Wellbutrin.

Conclusion

While there is increasing recognition of the comorbidity between ADHD and depressive disorders, the evidence base remains largely empirical. The general clinical approach is to recognize that various forms of depression occur in adults with ADHD (as well as ADHD occurring in adults with depression), to prioritize the treatment of depression with psychosocial and pharmacological treatments and then to address the ADHD. A variety of other psychiatric and medical conditions occur in adults with ADHD and depression.

References

1. American Psychiatric Association. *Diagnostic and Statistical Manual of Mental Disorder*, 5th edn (DSM-5). Arlington, VA: American Psychiatric Publishing; 2013.

2. Barkley RA. Differential diagnosis of adults with ADHD: the role of executive function and self-regulation. *J Clin Psychiatry*. 2010;**71**(7):e17.

3. Wender PH, Reimherr FW, Wood DR. Attention deficit disorder ('minimal brain dysfunction') in adults: a replication study of diagnosis and drug treatment. *Arch Gen Psychiatry*. 1981;**38**:449–56.

4. Shekim WO, Asarnow RF, Hess E, Zaucha K, Wheeler N. A clinical and demographic profile of a sample of adults with attention deficit hyperactivity disorder, residual state. *Compr Psychiatry*. 1990;**31**:416–25.

5. Milberger S, Biederman J, Faraone S, Murphy J, Tsuang M. Attention deficit hyperactivity disorder and comorbid disorders: issues of overlapping symptoms. *Am J Psychiatry*. 1995;**152**(12):1793–9.

6. Biederman J. Impact of comorbidity in adults with attention-deficit/hyperactivity disorder. *J Clin Psychiatry*. 2004;**65**(Suppl 3):3–7.

7. Biederman J, Faraone S, Mick E, Lelon E. Psychiatric comorbidity among referred juveniles with major depression: fact or artifact? *J Am Acad Child Adolesc Psychiatry*. 1995;**34**(5):579–90.

8. Wilens TE, Biederman J, Faraone SV, *et al.* Presenting ADHD symptoms, subtypes, and comorbid disorders in clinically referred adults with ADHD. *J Clin Psychiatry*. 2009;**70**(11):1557–62.

9. Centers for Disease Control & Prevention. Current depression among adults – United States 2006–2008. *MMWR Morb Mortal Wkly Rep*. 2010;**59**(38):1230–5.

10. Kessler RC, Adler L, Barkley R, *et al.* The prevalence and correlates of adult ADHD in the United States: results from the National Comorbidity Survey Replication. *Am J Psychiatry*. 2006;**163**(4):716–23.

11. Kessler RC, Adler LA, Barkley R, *et al.* Patterns and predictors of attention-deficit/hyperactivity disorder persistence into adulthood: results from the national

comorbidity survey replication. *Biol Psychiatry*. 2005;**57**(11):1442–51.

12. Fayyad J, De Graaf R, Kessler R, *et al*. Cross-national prevalence and correlates of adult attention-deficit hyperactivity disorder. *Br J Psychiatry*. 2007;**190**: 402–9.

13. Das D, Cherbuin N, Anstey KJ, Easteal S. ADHD symptoms and cognitive abilities in the midlife cohort of the PATH through life study. *J Atten Disord*. 2012.

14. de Zwaan M, Gruss B, Muller A, *et al*. The estimated prevalence and correlates of adult ADHD in a German community sample. *Eur Arch Psychiatry Clin Neurosci*. 2012;**262**(1):79–86.

15. Torgersen T, Gjervan B, Rasmussen K. ADHD in adults: a study of clinical characteristics, impairment and comorbidity. *Nord J Psychiatry*. 2006;**60**(1): 38–43.

16. Cumyn L, French L, Hechtman L. Comorbidity in adults with attention-deficit hyperactivity disorder. *Can J Psychiatry*. 2009;**54**(10):673–83.

17. McGillivray JA, Baker KL. Effects of comorbid ADHD with learning disabilities on anxiety, depression, and aggression in adults. *J Atten Disord*. 2009;**12**(6): 525–31.

18. Fischer AG, Bau CH, Grevet EH, *et al*. The role of comorbid major depressive disorder in the clinical presentation of adult ADHD. *J Psychiatr Res*. 2007; **41**(12):991–6.

19. Biederman J, Faraone SV, Spencer T, *et al*. Patterns of psychiatric comorbidity, cognition, and psychosocial functioning in adults with attention deficit hyperactivity disorder. *Am J Psychiatry*. 1993;**150**: 1792–8.

20. Weiss M, Murray C. Assessment and management of attention-deficit hyperactivity disorder in adults. *CMAJ*. 2003;**168**(6):715–22.

21. Adler LA, Spencer T, Faraone SV, *et al*. Validity of pilot Adult ADHD Self-Report Scale (ASRS) to rate adult ADHD symptoms. *Ann Clin Psychiatry*. 2006; **18**(3):145–8.

22. Able SL, Johnston JA, Adler LA, Swindle RW. Functional and psychosocial impairment in adults with undiagnosed ADHD. *Psychol Med*. 2007;**37**(1): 97–107.

23. Fishman PA, Stang PE, Hogue SL. Impact of comorbid attention deficit disorder on the direct medical costs of treating adults with depression in managed care. *J Clin Psychiatry*. 2007;**68**(2):248–53.

24. Adler LA, Sutton VK, Moore RJ, *et al*. Quality of life assessment in adult patients with attention-deficit/ hyperactivity disorder treated with atomoxetine. *J Clin Psychopharmacol*. 2006;**26**(6):648–52.

25. Faraone SV, Biederman J. Do attention deficit hyperactivity disorder and major depression share familial risk factors? *J Nerv Ment Dis*. 1997;**185**(9): 533–41.

26. Biederman J, Petty CR, Monuteaux MC, *et al*. Adult psychiatric outcomes of girls with attention deficit hyperactivity disorder: 11-year follow-up in a longitudinal case-control study. *Am J Psychiatry*. 2010;**167**(4):409–17.

27. Daviss WB, Birmaher B, Diler RS, Mintz J. Does pharmacotherapy for attention-deficit/hyperactivity disorder predict risk of later major depression? *J Child Adolesc Psychopharmacol*. 2008;**18**(3):257–64.

28. Milberger S, Biederman J, Faraone SV, Murphy J, Tsuang MT. Attention deficit hyperactivity disorder and comorbid disorders: issues of overlapping symptoms. *Am J Psychiatry*. 1995;**152**(12):1793–9.

29. Alpert JE, Maddocks A, Nierenberg AA, *et al*. Attention deficit hyperactivity disorder in childhood among adults with major depression. *Psychiatry Res*. 1996;**62**(3):213–19.

30. Hodgkins P, Montejano L, Sasane R, Huse D. Cost of illness and comorbidities in adults diagnosed with attention-deficit/hyperactivity disorder: a retrospective analysis. *Prim Care Companion CNS Disord*. 2011;**13**(2).

31. Haavik J, Halmoy A, Lundervold AJ, Fasmer OB. Clinical assessment and diagnosis of adults with attention-deficit/hyperactivity disorder. *Expert Rev Neurother*. 2010;**10**(10):1569–80.

32. Larochette AC, Harrison AG, Rosenblum Y, Bowie CR. Additive neurocognitive deficits in adults with attention-deficit/hyperactivity disorder and depressive symptoms. *Arch Clin Neuropsychol*. 2011;**26**(5):385–95.

33. Angst J, Hochstrasser B. Recurrent brief depression: the Zurich Study. *J Clin Psychiatry*. 1994;**55** (Suppl):3–9.

34. Hesslinger B, Tebartz van Elst L, Mochan F, Ebert D. A psychopathological study into the relationship between attention deficit hyperactivity disorder in adult patients and recurrent brief depression. *Acta Psychiatr Scand*. 2003;**107**(5):385–9.

35. Levitan RD, Jain UR, Katzman MA. Seasonal affective symptoms in adults with residual attention-deficit hyperactivity disorder. *Compr Psychiatry*. 1999;**40** (4):261–7.

36. Amons PJ, Kooij JJ, Haffmans PM, Hoffman TO, Hoencamp E. Seasonality of mood disorders in adults with lifetime attention-deficit/hyperactivity disorder (ADHD). *J Affect Disord*. 2006;**91**(2–3):251–5.

37. Golden RN, Gaynes BN, Ekstrom RD, *et al*. The efficacy of light therapy in the treatment of mood

disorders: a review and meta-analysis of the evidence. *Am J Psychiatry*. 2005;**162**(4):656–62.

38. McIntyre RS, Kennedy SH, Soczynska JK, *et al*. Attention-deficit/hyperactivity disorder in adults with bipolar disorder or major depressive disorder: results from the international mood disorders collaborative project. *Prim Care Companion J Clin Psychiatry*. 2010;**12**(3).

39. Nierenberg AA, Miyahara S, Spencer T, *et al*. Clinical and diagnostic implications of lifetime attention-deficit/hyperactivity disorder comorbidity in adults with bipolar disorder: data from the first 1000 STEP-BD participants. *Biol Psychiatry*. 2005;**57**(11): 1467–73.

40. Mitchell PB, Wilhelm K, Parker G, *et al*. The clinical features of bipolar depression: a comparison with matched major depressive disorder patients. *J Clin Psychiatry*. 2001;**62**(3):212–16; quiz 217.

41. Wozniak J, Spencer T, Biederman J, *et al*. The clinical characteristics of unipolar vs. bipolar major depression in ADHD youth. *J Affect Disord*. 2004;**82**(Suppl 1): S59–69.

42. Surman CB, Biederman J, Spencer T, *et al*. Deficient emotional self-regulation and adult attention deficit hyperactivity disorder: a family risk analysis. *Am J Psychiatry*. 2011;**168**(6):617–23.

43. Huessy HR. Letter: The adult hyperkinetic. *Am J Psychiatry*. 1974;**131**:724–5.

44. Zelazo PD, Cunningham WA. Executive function: mechanisms underlying emotion regulation. In: Gross JJ, ed. *Handbook of Emotion Regulation* New York, NY: Guilford Press. 2007; 135–58.

45. Williams LM, Hermens DF, Palmer D, *et al*. Misinterpreting emotional expressions in attention-deficit/hyperactivity disorder: evidence for a neural marker and stimulant effects. *Biol Psychiatry*. 2008; **63**(10):917–26.

46. de Wit L, Luppino F, van Straten A, *et al*. Depression and obesity: a meta-analysis of community-based studies. *Psychiatry Res*. 2010;**178**(2):230–5.

47. Fuemmeler BF, Ostbye T, Yang C, McClernon FJ, Kollins SH. Association between attention-deficit/hyperactivity disorder symptoms and obesity and hypertension in early adulthood: a population-based study. *Int J Obes (Lond)*. 2011;**35**(6):852–62.

48. James A, Lai FH, Dahl C. Attention deficit hyperactivity disorder and suicide: a review of possible associations. *Acta Psychiatr Scand*. 2004;**110**(6): 408–15.

49. Manor I, Gutnik I, Ben-Dor DH, *et al*. Possible association between attention deficit hyperactivity disorder and attempted suicide in adolescents – a pilot study. *Eur Psychiatry*. 2010;**25**(3):146–50.

50. Agosti V, Chen Y, Levin FR. Does Attention Deficit Hyperactivity Disorder increase the risk of suicide attempts? *J Affect Disord*. 2011;**133**(3):595–9.

51. Ferrer M, Andion O, Matali J, *et al*. Comorbid attention-deficit/hyperactivity disorder in borderline patients defines an impulsive subtype of borderline personality disorder. *J Pers Disord*. 2010;**24**(6):812–22.

52. Philipsen A, Limberger MF, Lieb K, *et al*. Attention-deficit hyperactivity disorder as a potentially aggravating factor in borderline personality disorder. *Br J Psychiatry*. 2008;**192**(2):118–23.

53. Bond DJ, Hadjipavlou G, Lam RW, *et al*. The Canadian Network for Mood and Anxiety Treatments (CANMAT) task force recommendations for the management of patients with mood disorders and comorbid attention-deficit/hyperactivity disorder. *Ann Clin Psychiatry*. 2012;**24**(1):23–37.

54. Pliszka S. Practice parameter for the assessment and treatment of children and adolescents with attention-deficit/hyperactivity disorder. *J Am Acad Child Adolesc Psychiatry*. 2007;**46**(7):894–921.

55. Kooij SJ, Bejerot S, Blackwell A, *et al*. European consensus statement on diagnosis and treatment of adult ADHD: The European Network Adult ADHD. *BMC Psychiatry*. 2010;**10**:67.

56. Sobanski E. Psychiatric comorbidity in adults with attention-deficit/hyperactivity disorder (ADHD). *Eur Arch Psychiatry Clin Neurosci*. 2006;**256**(Suppl 1): i26–31.

57. Wender PH, Reimherr FW, Wood D, Ward M. A controlled study of methylphenidate in the treatment of attention deficit disorder, residual type, in adults. *Am J Psychiatry*. 1985;**142**:547–52.

58. Glass RM. Fluoxetine, cognitive-behavioral therapy, and their combination for adolescents with depression: Treatment for Adolescents with Depression Study (TADS) randomized controlled trial. *J Pediatr*. 2005;**146**(1):145.

59. March J, Silva S, Petrycki S, *et al*. Fluoxetine, cognitive-behavioral therapy, and their combination for adolescents with depression: Treatment for Adolescents with Depression Study (TADS) randomized controlled trial. *JAMA*. 2004;**292**(7): 807–20.

60. Kratochvil CJ, May DE, Silva SG, *et al*. Treatment response in depressed adolescents with and without co-morbid attention-deficit/hyperactivity disorder in the Treatment for Adolescents with Depression Study. *J Child Adolesc Psychopharmacol*. 2009;**19**(5):519–27.

61. Faraone SV, Glatt SJ. A comparison of the efficacy of medications for adult attention-deficit/hyperactivity disorder using meta-analysis of effect sizes. *J Clin Psychiatry*. 2010;**71**(6):754–63.

62. Gammon GD, Brown TE. Fluoxetine and methylphenidate in combination for treatment of attention deficit disorder and comorbid depressive disorder. *J Child Adolesc Psychopharmacol.* 1993;3(1):1–10.

63. Weiss M, Hechtman L. A randomized double-blind trial of paroxetine and/or dextroamphetamine and problem-focused therapy for attention-deficit/ hyperactivity disorder in adults. *J Clin Psychiatry.* 2006;67(4):611–19.

64. Kratochvil CJ, Newcorn JH, Arnold LE, *et al.* Atomoxetine alone or combined with fluoxetine for treating ADHD with comorbid depressive or anxiety symptoms. *J Am Acad Child Adolesc Psychiatry.* 2005;44(9):915–24.

65. Bangs ME, Emslie GJ, Spencer TJ, *et al.* Efficacy and safety of atomoxetine in adolescents with attention-deficit/hyperactivity disorder and major depression. *J Child Adolesc Psychopharmacol.* 2007;17(4): 407–20.

66. Reimherr FW, Marchant BK, Strong RE, *et al.* Emotional dysregulation in adult ADHD and response to atomoxetine. *Biol Psychiatry.* 2005;58(2):125–31.

67. Emslie GJ, Hughes CW, Crismon ML, *et al.* A feasibility study of the childhood depression medication algorithm: the Texas Children's Medication Algorithm Project (CMAP). *J Am Acad Child Adolesc Psychiatry.* 2004;43(5):519–27.

68. Wender PH, Reimherr FW. Bupropion treatment of attention deficit hyperactivity disorder in adults. *Am J Psychiatry.* 1990;147:1018–20.

69. Wilens T, Prince J, Biederman J, *et al.* An open trial of bupropion for the treatment of adults with attention-deficit hyperactivity disorder and bipolar disorder. *Biol Psychiatry.* 2003;54(1):9–16.

70. Wilens TE, Haight BR, Horrigan JP, *et al.* Bupropion XL in adults with attention-deficit/hyperactivity disorder: a randomized, placebo-controlled study. *Biol Psychiatry.* 2005;57(7):793–801.

71. Daviss WB. A review of co-morbid depression in pediatric ADHD: etiology, phenomenology, and treatment. *J Child Adolesc Psychopharmacol.* 2008;18(6):565–71.

72. Daviss WB, Bentivoglio P, Racusin R, *et al.* Bupropion SR in adolescents with combined attention-deficit/ hyperactivity disorder and depression. *J Am Acad Child Adolesc Psychiatry.* 2001;40:307–14.

73. Gelenberg AJ, Bassuk EL, Schoonover SC. *The Practitioner's Guide to Psychoactive Drugs*, 3rd edn. New York, NY: Plenum Medical Book Company; 1991.

74. Wilens TE, Morrison NR, Prince J. An update on the pharmacotherapy of attention-deficit/hyperactivity disorder in adults. *Expert Rev Neurother.* 2011;11(10): 1443–65.

75. Wilens TE, Biederman J, Milberger S, *et al.* Is bipolar disorder a risk for cigarette smoking in ADHD youth? *Am J Addict.* 2000;9(3):187–95.

76. Wilens T, Biederman J, Prince J, *et al.* Six-week, double blind, placebo-controlled study of desipramine for adult attention deficit hyperactivity disorder. *Am J Psychiatry.* 1996;153:1147–53.

77. Wender PH, Wood DR, Reimherr FW, Ward M. An open trial of pargyline in the treatment of attention deficit disorder, residual type. *Psychiatry Res.* 1983;9: 329–36.

78. Wender PH, Wood DR, Reimherr FW. Pharmacological treatment of attention deficit disorder, residual type (ADD,RT, "minimal brain dysfunction," "hyperactivity") in adults. *Psychopharmacol Bull.* 1985;21(2):222–31.

79. Ernst M, Liebenauer L, Jons P, *et al.* Selegiline in adults with attention deficit hyperactivity disorder: Clinical efficacy and safety. *Psychopharmacol Bull.* 1996;32:327–34.

80. Myronuk LD, Weiss M, Cotter L. Combined treatment with moclobemide and methylphenidate for comorbid major depression and adult attention-deficit/ hyperactivity disorder. *J Clin Psychopharmacol.* 1996;16(6):468–9.

81. Spencer T, Biederman J, Wilens T. Nonstimulant treatment of adult attention-deficit/hyperactivity disorder. *Psychiatr Clin North Am.* 2004;27(2): 373–83.

82. Adler LA, Resnick S, Kunz M, Devinsky O. Open label trial of venlafaxine in adults with attention deficit disorder. *Psychopharmacol Bull.* 1995;31:785–8.

83. Reimherr FW, Hedges DW, Strong RE, Wender PH, eds. An open trial of venlafaxine in adult patients with attention deficit hyperactivity disorder. Annu Meet New Clin Drug Evaluation Unit Program, 35th; 1995; Orlando, Florida.

84. Findling RL, Schwartz MA, Flannery DJ, Manos MJ. Venlafaxine in adults with attention-deficit/ hyperactivity disorder: an open clinical trial. *J Clin Psychiatry.* 1996;57(5):184–9.

85. Niederhofer H. Duloxetine may improve some symptoms of attention-deficit/hyperactivity disorder. *Prim Care Companion J Clin Psychiatry.* 2010;12(2).

86. Tolin DF. Is cognitive-behavioral therapy more effective than other therapies? A meta-analytic review. *Clin Psychol Rev.* 2010;30(6):710–20.

87. Safren SA, Sprich S, Mimiaga MJ, *et al.* Cognitive behavioral therapy vs relaxation with educational support for medication-treated adults with ADHD and

persistent symptoms: a randomized controlled trial. *JAMA*. 2010;**304**(8):875–80.

88. Weiss M, Murray C, Wasdell M, *et al*. A randomized controlled trial of CBT therapy for adults with ADHD with and without medication. *BMC Psychiatry*. 2012;**12**:30.

89. Mongia M, Hechtman L. Cognitive behavior therapy for adults with attention-deficit/hyperactivity disorder: a review of recent randomized controlled trials. *Curr Psychiatry Rep*. 2012;**14**(5):561–7.

90. Ramsay RJ, Rostain AL. *Cognitive-Behavioral Therapy for Adult ADHD: An Integrative Psychosocial and Medical Approach (Practical Clinical Guidebooks)*. New York, NY: Routledge; 2008.

91. Safren SA, Perlman CA, Sprich S, Otto MW. *Mastering Your Adult ADHD: A Cognitive-Behavioral Treatment*

Program Therapist Guide (Treatments That Work). Oxford: Oxford University Press; 2005.

92. Solanto MV, Marks DJ, Wasserstein J, *et al*. Efficacy of meta-cognitive therapy for adult ADHD. *Am J Psychiatry*. 2010;**167**(8):958–68.

93. Zylowska L, Ackerman DL, Yang MH, *et al*. Mindfulness meditation training in adults and adolescents with ADHD: a feasibility study. *J Atten Disord*. 2008;**11**(6):737–46.

94. Jha AP, Krompinger J, Baime MJ. Mindfulness training modifies subsystems of attention. *Cogn Affect Behav Neurosci*. 2007;7(2):109–19.

95. Bemporad J, Zambenedetti M. Psychotherapy of adults with attention deficit disorder. *J Psychother Pract Res*. 1996;**5**:228–37.

Comorbidity of ADHD and anxiety disorders
Diagnosis and treatment across the lifespan

Beth Krone and Jeffrey H. Newcorn

Descriptive and clinical features

Prevalence

Although anxiety disorders and ADHD are distinct classes of disorders with different developmental trajectories across the lifespan, the disorders have very high rates of comorbidity and may share common symptom presentations [1–3]. Anxiety disorders can present very early in life, with several forms of anxiety disorders differentiating by age 2 years [4–7]. However, the prevalence of anxiety increases with age and many individuals diagnosed in youth will experience ongoing anxiety problems, often experiencing multiple anxiety disorders across the lifespan [8–10]. Among adults in the US population, 18.1% meet criteria for an anxiety disorder in any given year; nearly three-quarters of these individuals experienced their first episode by age 21 [9, 11]. The overall lifetime prevalence of 28.8% makes anxiety disorders one of the most commonly diagnosed classes of disorders [9, 11]. Within the population of individuals with anxiety disorders, nearly one-quarter experience clinically significant attention problems as a feature of their disorder [9, 12]. Individuals with anxiety disorders are also at double the risk for meeting full criteria for ADHD than the general population [3].

The lifetime prevalence of ADHD is lower; early age of onset is also characteristic, although later than the earliest onset anxiety disorders [4, 10, 13, 14]. The population-wide prevalence of ADHD in the United States is approximately 8% among youth ages 4 to 18 years [13, 14]. That number declines to 4.4% among adults [2]. The trend of declining diagnosis with age is in accordance with etiological theories describing ADHD as a neurobiological disorder characterized by a delayed developmental trajectory – as suggested by the finding of delayed cortical thickening in youth with ADHD vs. healthy controls [2, 15–17]. Continued symptom impairment during adulthood would then be associated with developmental differences, rather than delay [17].

Among the population of individuals with ADHD, between one-fourth to one-half of youth and one-half of adults meet diagnostic criteria for at least one anxiety disorder. The clinical manifestations of these anxiety disorders can be quite distinct, as exemplified by the pervasive anxiety characteristic of generalized anxiety disorder (GAD), performance anxiety which is restricted to situations requiring task completion, and physiological over-arousal seen in panic disorder and post-traumatic stress disorder (PTSD) [2, 12, 18, 19]. For all individuals, anxiety increases in prevalence across the lifespan, but the magnitude of increase in anxiety disorder diagnoses among individuals with ADHD is larger than among those without ADHD. The population-wide prevalence of at least one diagnosable anxiety disorder among individuals with ADHD is approximately 4% among preschool-aged youth, 18% among school-aged youth, and 47% among adults [2, 13, 14].

In clinical practice, it is quite common to encounter individuals who meet criteria for both ADHD and one or more anxiety disorders. Among clinically treated youth, between 31% and 34% meet criteria for at least one anxiety disorder comorbid with ADHD [20, 21]. Despite the marked increase in anxiety across the lifespan and the increased prevalence of anxiety disorders among these diverse samples, the comorbidity rates in diverse samples of clinically treated adults with ADHD are similar to those (approximately 34%) of youth [3, 11, 13, 22]. A recent longitudinal study that followed affluent white males with and without ADHD, many of whom no longer sought clinical care as adults,

Attention-Deficit Hyperactivity Disorder in Adults and Children, ed. Lenard A. Adler, Thomas J. Spencer and Timothy E. Wilens.
Published by Cambridge University Press. © Cambridge University Press 2015.

found no greater lifetime prevalence of anxiety among the ADHD cohort [23]; however, another large longitudinal study found an increased rate of anxiety disorders in adulthood [24].

Developmental perspective

Typically developing youth experience anxiety for adaptive purposes, and normal childhood fears can be mapped for age of onset and resolution. Infants and toddlers typically exhibit fear on separation from their caregivers, with individual differences dependent upon both the child's temperament and sensitivity of the caregiver to the child's needs [5, 6, 10]. As children develop through toddlerhood, preschool, and early elementary school years, the fear of separation resolves. Separation anxiety disorder (SAD) is diagnosed in children who continue to experience significant and impairing fears of separation (4.1% of the population; [7]). Among youth diagnosed with ADHD, 3.5% of preschool children also have SAD, making it the most often reported co-occurring anxiety disorder among preschoolers with or without ADHD [14].

Typically developing children also develop specific fears during infancy, such as the fear of animals or ghosts [25]. These fears can be distressing; they often remain relatively stable until later in childhood, declining slightly over this period [25]. A second developmental trajectory can be identified among approximately 2% of youth in the general population [25], in whom fears increase sharply in severity, and reach a higher level of distress at approximately 8 years old, then decline sharply throughout preadolescence [25]. This roughly concurs with the early onset of phobic disorders at age 7 years among individuals with ADHD, although the mean age of onset for phobias among individuals without ADHD is 13 years [11]. Social phobias tend to emerge in adolescence, with a population-wide mean age of onset at 15.1 years, and median age of onset at 13 years [8, 26]. The majority of individuals with social phobia experience the disorder as a manifestation of performance anxiety, consisting of the fear of observation and meeting with disapproval or failure [26]. Approximately 5–7% of individuals with social phobia meet criteria for ADHD, although social phobia occurs at higher rates among individuals with ADHD [27]. Symptoms of social phobia occur earlier and with more severity among youth diagnosed with ADHD,

and are associated with greater impairment from both disorders [28].

Obsessive–compulsive disorder (OCD) has a population-wide prevalence of between 2% and 3% and a mean age of onset at 19 years. However, 8–10% of youth with ADHD are diagnosed with comorbid OCD during preadolescence, and more develop OCD as adults [29–31]. Thirty percent of children and adolescents with OCD have comorbid ADHD, and these youth have an earlier onset with poorer prognosis as compared to youth with OCD alone [29, 30, 32]. The comorbid condition is also associated with higher prevalence of oppositional defiant disorder (ODD) and more severe symptoms of ADHD [30, 32]. The strong association between ADHD and OCD has prompted speculation that this particular comorbidity represents a subtype of OCD [29, 32–34]. The increased prevalence of the comorbid condition among family members has also prompted speculation regarding heritability, and candidate genes common to both disorders have been identified [29, 32, 34].

Despite its general onset in adolescence among youth with ADHD, panic disorder has a later mean age of onset of 24 years within the general population. Approximately one-third of adults with panic disorder (0.8% of the population) develop agoraphobia with a median onset at age 20 years, suggesting that the younger onset of panic disorder is associated with more serious and complicated trajectory of disorder.

Approximately 3.5% of the adult population meets diagnostic criteria for PTSD, with a median age of onset of 23 years [3, 35]. Although the onset of PTSD is dependent on environmental trauma, the mean age of onset tends to be lower and the prevalence greater among individuals with ADHD. In addition, the prevalence of ADHD is greater than the prevalence of other disorders in the presence of PTSD – leading some to speculate that ADHD may represent a risk factor for PTSD [36, 37]. Among the population with ADHD, 13.4% meet criteria for current or lifetime PTSD, as compared to the 3.5–3.8% found in non-ADHD samples [2]. Others have speculated that the diagnostic criteria for these disorders are not sufficiently specific; in some studies, youth with ADHD are not more likely to suffer trauma or develop PTSD [38, 39]. However, disrupted arousal is common to both disorders; and, it is thought by some that disrupted arousal may be the mechanism by which ADHD predisposes individuals to develop PTSD in response to trauma [40].

Most divergent between individuals with and without ADHD is the onset and prevalence of GAD [11]. Although early-onset cases may be diagnosed in infancy, GAD which occurs without ADHD typically has its onset either in adolescence (early onset) or adulthood (late onset), with an overall median age of onset of 31 years and a mean onset age of 48.8 years with increasing prevalence over time [9, 11, 41, 42]. The majority of early-onset cases begin in early adolescence, and are characterized by both the temperamental characteristic of behavioral inhibition and exposure to family problems [25, 41, 42]. Approximately 11% of early-onset cases are characterized by a sharp increase in symptoms that rise to a peak at age 7 to 8 years, and then decline throughout preadolescence [25]. Among individuals with ADHD, the anxiety symptoms preceding the onset of GAD are pronounced, and often present as symptoms of SAD which give way to GAD prior to age 14 years [13, 41, 43]. Among individuals with ADHD, the prevalence of GAD varies from 12% among youth with ADHD combined subtype to 22% among youth with Inattentive Subtype [43]. Thus, the prevalence of GAD is higher among youth with ADHD, the onset is earlier, and the clinical presentation is characterized by greater symptom severity than is typical of the general population. Further, the prevalence may differ between the different ADHD phenotypes.

Primary anxiety and ADHD: shared neurobiological and endocrinological features

The clinical presentation of anxiety disorders is thought to occur in the context of environmental influences on genetic, neurobiological, and physiological processes. Fear-inducing stimuli in the environment are processed along dual pathways: through the sensory-limbic system governing instinctive reflex and conditioned responses, and through the cortical-processing executive functioning system governing coping and reasoned responses. Among individuals with anxiety disorders, dysregulation of healthy neurobiological correlates of fear processing is evident, and can be seen in functional MRI studies that involve processing of fearful stimuli [44–46]. This dysregulation is congruent with developmental differences and changes in symptom presentation. While anxiety often exists without ADHD and vice versa, shared neurobiological features may account for some cases of comorbidity.

Dysregulation of the temporal lobes occurs in both healthy and pathological anxiety, and also in ADHD. State and trait anxiety are characterized by increased temporal lobe activity associated with hypervigilance [47]. The temporal lobes are less well developed and functionally different among boys with ADHD as compared to those without ADHD, corresponding to problems with selecting and maintaining attention to environmental stimuli [48]. Observed differences in functioning of the temporal lobes between boys and girls with ADHD could potentially contribute to the symptomatic differences often described between males and females with the disorder [48]. However, associations between brain function and symptom presentation have yet to be delineated [49].

Among both youth with GAD and youth with ADHD, ventrolateral prefrontal cortex (VLPFC) activity appears to moderate symptom presentation [50–54]. Among youth with GAD, underactivation of the VLPFC results in greater anxiety [50–52], while in youth with ADHD, underactivation results in an inability to sustain attention [54]. While greater activity of the VLPFC is associated with better response to stressors and reduced anxiety symptoms, it also correlates with greater impulsivity and less successful ability to inhibit responses in ADHD [55]. The ventromedial prefrontal cortex is known to regulate amygdala activity and may stimulate hyperarousal of the autonomic nervous system in both pathological and healthy anxiety. Specific functions may include regulation of fear and pain perception, fear extinction, mood, rejection sensitivity, anticipatory and reactive anxiety, and perception of traumatic content [56]. In ADHD, the VLPFC is associated with pathological reward processing and distractibility [57, 58].

Regulation of the amygdala via the medial prefrontal cortex is considered to be dopamine dependent [59], which could provide a basis for shared pathophysiology in ADHD and anxiety disorders. Activity at D_2 receptors within the amygdala establishes connectivity between the anterior cingulate cortex and the amygdala, leading to positive coping behaviors and decreased anxiety [59, 60]. Within the amygdala itself, activation of D_1 receptors is believed to induce anxiety for purposes of fear conditioning [60]. Insufficient burst firing in response to a stimulus is associated with the development of generalized anxiety due to the inability to appropriately encode the cues necessary for predicting an aversive condition [61]. This pattern of dopamine burst firing among healthy individuals, and attenuated dopamine release among individuals with social anxiety disorder, has been noted in response to acute social stress [62].

Deficient stress reactivity in ADHD and anxiety disorders is also likely attributable to dysregulation of the noradrenergic system [63]. Noradrenergic regulation of attention and motor activity via alpha-2 (α_2)-adrenergic receptors in the locus coeruleus results in initiation and maintenance of alertness, as well as cognitive-affective processing, modulation of sensory input, and both cognitive and physiological hyperarousal in ADHD [63–65]. Among patients with GAD, synaptic norepinephrine is generally high, due to hypoactivity of α_2 receptors [66]. Thus noradrenergic mechanisms are associated with both ADHD symptoms and anxiety through dysregulated arousal mechanisms and poorly mediated stress responses, to which individuals with both ADHD and anxiety may be genetically predisposed.

Diagnostic criteria for ADHD and anxiety disorders: disentangling interrelated constructs

ADHD and anxiety disorders are defined by behavioral criteria that are intended to capture distinct constructs; but these conditions are also partially overlapping – raising important questions regarding attribution. The core symptoms of ADHD, which include being easily distractible, having difficulty concentrating, being fidgety and restless, and needing to be in constant motion, can potentially be misattributed to conditions other than ADHD, including oppositional, mood, and anxiety disorders [12]. The marked procrastination and avoidance characteristic of motivation deficits in ADHD or the active defiant avoidance seen in oppositional defiant disorder can be misattributed by parents or other adult reporters as behavioral avoidance characteristic of anxiety, as well. A large minority of youth with anxiety disorders report attention problems either as a core symptom of anxiety, or due to comorbidity with ADHD [12]. While these behaviors may appear to be indistinguishable to untrained or emotionally invested observers, the cognitive and emotional processes associated with the different conditions are distinct and readily distinguished [12].

Excessive, uncontrolled worry and attentional biases toward threatening stimuli help to inform proper diagnosis of anxiety disorders [67]. These may be observed by a well-trained observer, self-reported, or assessed through direct measures of attention and cognitive control. Therefore, a battery consisting of observer report, self-report, and direct measures is considered optimal.

Comorbidity of ADHD and anxiety disorders likely increases in adolescence, although it can be hard to clearly distinguish the different disorders. Among youth with ADHD, psychomotor hyperactivity decreases, but complaints related to attention problems increase in adolescence. Increasing demands for independent organization, self-directed activity, task completion, and other factors that correspond to symptoms of inattention stress the adolescent's capacity to perform [68]; this is especially true of adolescents with ADHD. These symptoms may persist into adulthood, so that up to 90% of adults with unresolved ADHD seek treatment for inattentive symptoms and cognitive impairments [69, 70]. Among youth with ADHD, symptoms of irritability, impatience, difficulty sleeping due to physical and mental restlessness, tiredness or distress, overreacting to frustration, and mood instability may be seen with greater frequency and severity [68]. The occurrence of comorbidity between ADHD and anxiety disorders may increase during adolescence for three reasons. First, the inherent developmental stressors of adolescence may induce heightened anxiety – as adolescents face increasing responsibilities and challenges that tax their abilities, and increase risk of failure and exposure to negative consequences of the disorder. Second, the resolution of psychomotor activity may make symptom tracking and diagnosis more difficult because symptoms of inattention may be less obviously related to ADHD and more easily confounded with anxiety. Third, the prevalence of anxiety disorders increases with age, making comorbidity with other disorders such as ADHD more likely to occur.

Gender

Males are diagnosed with impulse control disorders at a lifetime prevalence rate of 13.5% as compared with 5.6% among females; however, only half of diagnosed individuals in the USA (6.9% of males and 2.5% of females) will receive treatment [9, 11]. This is also the case in the United Kingdom; treatment rates were found to be disproportionate to prevalence, with 9 males treated for every 1 female [69]. The apparent gender bias in ADHD appears to exceed that of other impulse control disorders, with a 3:1 male-to-female ratio of ADHD diagnoses seen in most large clinical samples, and females tending to remain undiagnosed until their symptoms are more severe than those of their male counterparts [71, 72]. Gender role expectations influence how symptoms are manifested, whether the manifestations are attributed to mental health problems by self (patient) or others (family, clinician), and care-seeking behaviors among those who believe there may be a problem, which, in turn, influences the likelihood of being diagnosed with a disorder. This makes it difficult to determine whether gender or actual sex-based differences exist in distribution of the disorders among the population. Whichever the cause, females are more often viewed as exhibiting emotional lability and emotional comorbidities such as depression, bipolar disorder, and anxiety [73]. In contrast, males are more often considered to have disruptive behaviors problems and are diagnosed with aggression, conduct problems, and oppositional defiance [73].

ADHD subtype

It is frequently said that anxiety occurs more often among individuals with the inattentive subtype of ADHD [74]. Consistent with this view, youth with ADHD and co-occurring anxiety in the Multimodal Treatment of ADHD (MTA) study achieved relatively lower ratings of impulsivity and relatively greater ratings of inattention on direct neuropsychological measures [75]. However, prevalence data do not fully support the contention that anxiety disorders are more frequently seen in individuals with inattentive subtype ADHD. Youth with inattentive subtype ADHD experience the least severe symptoms of anxiety compared with youth with the combined or hyperactive–impulsive subtypes [21]. Symptoms of anxiety are associated with greater ADHD symptom severity, which might explain why they are more often reported among youth with combined type ADHD [21]. This may be consistent with the finding that comorbidity is generally associated with greater ADHD symptom severity, since combined type ADHD is often associated with ODD, and this comorbidity often presents with anxiety as well [1, 76]. Yet, other studies find no difference

in prevalence of anxiety disorder between ADHD subtypes [77].

ADHD + anxiety + ODD

Although we often speak about comorbidity of ADHD and individual disorders, the occurrence of multiple comorbid disorders among youth and adults with ADHD is quite common. Forty percent of youth with ADHD also meet diagnostic criteria for ODD. Both youth with ADHD and youth with ODD experience anxiety at higher rates than typically developing peers, and are at risk for continued social, emotional, and behavioral problems [75, 78, 79]. In one large-scale study, parents reported that youth with this triad of disorders exhibited increased impulsivity and hyperactivity beyond that which is experienced in ADHD alone [75]. Another large study found increased severity of ODD symptoms among youth with subclinical trait anxiety, but only when comorbid with ADHD combined subtype [76]. This is consistent with teacher reports that the presence of ODD negates the inhibitory effects of anxiety on impulsivity associated with ADHD, so that symptoms of the triad are characterized by hyperactivity and impulsivity as well as inattention [75].

Secondary anxiety in association with ADHD

When individuals with ADHD are unable to meet situational demands, fear of consequences may manifest. Individuals with self-regulatory deficits associated with ADHD, particularly those with autonomic hyperarousal or executive functioning deficits, may lack the ability to effectively cope with situational performance anxiety. Repeated exposure to fear- and anxiety-producing situations with little internal control, in the context of a lifelong, pervasive pattern of impairment due to untreated or poorly managed symptoms, can generalize across situations and result in problems with self-efficacy or self-esteem. By this rationale, symptoms of school avoidance due to emotional distress at the thought of an upcoming test, classroom punishments for misplaced books and incomplete assignments, or teasing by classmates might best be conceptualized as a secondary consequence of ADHD rather than as manifestations of primary anxiety disorders [80].

Treatment of ADHD + anxiety disorders

Treatment of ADHD and comorbid anxiety disorders necessarily depends upon the specifics of the case formulation, which will differ across individuals; however, several professional organizations have established guidelines for best practices that advocate a multimodal approach [81, 82]. Guidelines from both the American Academy of Pediatrics (AAP) and the American Academy of Child and Adolescent Psychiatry (AACAP) highlight that ADHD is best conceptualized as a chronic illness that may be treated as early as age 3 or 4 years [81, 82], and recommend that preschool children with the disorder first be treated using behavioral parent-training techniques to manage distressing symptoms of the disorder, and to prevent or alleviate additional anxiety and mood problems stemming from relational difficulties [82, 83]. Due to evidence that behavioral interventions are insufficient to treat core symptoms of ADHD among youth, but that they provide additive value in treating both comorbidity and sequelae of ADHD, medication treatments have been the recommended standard of care for children and adolescents with moderately to severely impairing ADHD symptoms [81, 84]. Several studies support the efficacy of psychotherapy as a specific treatment for ADHD among adults, and one has found that CBT combined with placebo is equally effective as dextroamphetamine [85, 86]. However, medication treatments are a primary modality in this age group as well.

Pharmacological intervention for anxiety disorders among youth is not universally embraced, owing to concerns that medication treatments may interfere with fear extinction processes, thereby making therapy more difficult and prolonging the course of the disorder [87–91]. However, several medication options are approved for youth and adults with anxiety disorders, and can be considered. Psychosocial treatment is highly effective in treating anxiety disorders, although the specific modality of treatment differs as a function of diagnoses [92]. These treatments require time and effort, and may be distressing for the patient until the fear processes have been extinguished. For chronic conditions such as PTSD, symptomatic management often requires medication intervention. Taken together, the combination of medication treatment for ADHD and psychosocial treatments for anxiety disorders (and possibly ADHD as well) is likely to be the most effective approach in many individuals with comorbid ADHD + anxiety disorders. However, combining different medication or psychosocial treatments which target the different conditions may also be an effective strategy.

Although comorbidity of ADHD and anxiety disorders is relatively common there are only a handful of well-designed treatment studies [12]. Existing research shows that the core symptoms of inattention and hyperactivity in ADHD are non-responsive to behavioral treatment, although related impairment can be reduced through use of behavioral techniques [93]. The MTA study [22] found that children with ADHD combined subtype and anxiety disorders responded equally well to medication and behavioral treatments on core symptoms of ADHD, with benefits seen at follow-up 14 months later, although medication outperformed behavior therapy for all other youth. In subsequent studies, anxiety symptoms were shown to decline with behavioral treatment, but ADHD symptoms did not [93, 94].

Both youth with ADHD and youth with ADHD + anxiety often have academic and/or behavioral problems that are best treated with appropriate academic supports such as behavioral classroom management [81, 82, 92, 95]. Parent behavioral training techniques also appear to improve functioning and augment improvement beyond that achieved through medication treatment for ADHD among youth with ADHD and anxiety [81, 82, 92, 95]. While several manualized programs exist to guide treatment of youth with ADHD, modifications to these approaches are not yet available for youth with ADHD + anxiety. Consequently, pieces of interventions developed for anxiety disorders are used together with interventions for ADHD. Anxious youth benefit from positive contingency reinforcement – which is a critical component of behavior therapy to promote graded exposure to anxiety triggers, but also can effectively shape child behavior to promote compliance [92]. While response cost is often used as punishment in behavior plans for youth with ADHD, this may exacerbate preexisting anxiety [92]. Anxiety-specific behavioral treatments also employ somatic symptom management skills training, which can be readily incorporated into a behavioral treatment plan for youth with ADHD [92]. Among youth with school-related anxiety, academic support, supportive therapy, and psychoeducation may be as effective as CBT, although the core symptoms of ADHD do not respond to supportive therapies

[92]. While there is not strong evidence of efficacy for social skills training programs among youth with ADHD, these programs are effective for treating social anxiety and may benefit youth with comorbid ADHD + anxiety disorders [82, 92].

Findings from studies examining staging of treatment for ADHD and anxiety disorders have been mixed. Some recommend treating comorbid ADHD and anxiety disorders concurrently [92]. Others propose treating anxiety as the primary disorder, and then reassessing the degree of ADHD-related impairments [3, 93, 96]. However, while the latter approach may be appropriate in individuals with high levels of anxiety, it may delay treatment of core symptoms of ADHD and result in poorer response to behavioral interventions for anxiety than would be the case for concurrent therapy. The case for primary treatment of ADHD or concurrent therapy of ADHD and anxiety disorders is supported by a review of likely clinical outcomes. Treatment for anxiety disorders rarely results in complete resolution of symptoms, and partial response to behavioral treatment may necessitate use of selective serotonin reuptake inhibitors (SSRIs) or other anxiolytic medications. However, primary or concurrent treatment of ADHD core symptoms may have secondary effects on anxiety symptoms, and could therefore minimize the need for or reduce the dose of additional medications for anxiety.

Stimulant medications are the recommended first-line pharmacological treatment for child and adolescent ADHD, and although there are not yet guidelines for adults, stimulants are considered the most effective medication class in this age group as well [97]. Although the majority of early studies showed lower efficacy and poorer tolerability of stimulants (primarily methylphenidate) among youth with ADHD and anxiety comorbidity, more recent studies have shown stimulants to be no less effective for improving core symptoms of ADHD and no more likely to increase severity of anxiety among youth with comorbidity [22, 92, 98, 99]. However, when used alone, stimulants such as methylphenidate may not resolve anxiety symptoms without concurrent behavior therapy or pharmacotherapy for anxiety [98].

In cases where stimulant treatment is ineffective for treating ADHD without comorbidity, the AAP guidelines recommend using the non-stimulants guanfacine or clonidine to augment stimulant treatment – based on the fact that the α_2 agonists are approved for combined treatment with stimulants for ADHD [82].

However, this face valid approach has not been formally assessed in youth with comorbid ADHD and anxiety disorders. Use of atomoxetine alone or in combination with stimulants would also seem to be worthy of consideration, based on positive findings of atomoxetine on anxiety symptoms in youth and adults with comorbid ADHD and anxiety disorders. Finally, combined treatment with stimulants and SSRIs may be appropriate.

Several well-controlled studies have examined the use of the non-stimulant atomoxetine among youth and adults with comorbid ADHD and anxiety disorders, based on preliminary findings that suggested improvement in both ADHD and anxiety symptoms [100, 101]. A large-scale, placebo-controlled study in 176 youth with well-documented ADHD + anxiety disorders [33, 34] found an effect size (ES) of 1.0 for ADHD symptoms, substantially larger than the ES for atomoxetine in youth without ADHD (generally around 0.7) – which raises the question of whether atomoxetine is *more effective* in the presence of comorbid anxiety. Additionally, the ES for anxiety symptoms (as measured using the Pediatric Anxiety Rating Scale [PARS]) was 0.5, which is approximately the same as that for SSRIs in anxiety disorders in youth. Findings of improved efficacy on both ADHD and anxiety symptoms was also demonstrated in adults. Adler *et al.* conducted a randomized double-blind study of atomoxetine in over 400 adults with ADHD and social anxiety disorder, using well-standardized scales for both conditions [102]. Atomoxetine produced greater improvement than placebo in the Conners' Adult ADHD Rating Scale total score, as expected, indicating that the presence of social anxiety does not moderate ADHD response. In addition, atomoxetine produced significant improvement in the Liebowitz Social Anxiety Scale, indicating incremental improvement in comorbid anxiety symptoms.

Investigating a related but somewhat different question, Kratochvil *et al.* examined the combined use of atomoxetine and SSRIs with the idea of incrementally improving ADHD symptoms [100]. The rationale for this approach is that atomoxetine is metabolized via CYP2D6, and approximately 7% of the population are poor metabolizers – resulting in increased plasma level and half-life of atomoxetine. Similarly, the plasma level and half-life of atomoxetine may be greatly enhanced by SSRIs, which are also metabolized by CYP2D6 (e.g., paroxetine; fluoxetine) – which could theoretically be beneficial in enhancing ADHD treatment response.

Based on this thinking, Kratochvil *et al.* compared the effects of atomoxetine alone and atomoxetine plus fluoxetine on ADHD, mood, and anxiety symptoms [100]. The overall response was not different between the two treatments, although the effects were numerically slightly (though not significantly) larger with the combined treatment. While the combined treatment was not titrated to optimize improvement of mood and anxiety symptoms (it is conceivable that higher dose treatment would have produced greater improvement), it was well tolerated – providing at least some safety basis for off-label combined use, should this be entertained.

Another approach to combining medication treatment is to use different medications for ADHD and anxiety together. This is often necessary, because the SSRIs (the most widely used antidepressants) do not produce improvements in ADHD symptoms, and the stimulants (most widely used treatment for ADHD) do not produce adequate improvement in anxiety symptoms [98]. Results of clinical studies in adults indicating that the combination of stimulants and SSRIs is generally well tolerated and can be effective [70] provide initial support for this approach.

A variety of other face-valid treatment approaches have not been studied sufficiently to inform clinical recommendations. Despite the links between noradrenergic functioning and anxiety disorders, guanfacine was not found to be effective for treating anxiety disorder characterized by hypervigilance and autonomic arousal without the presence of ADHD [103]. Clonidine has been used off-label to treat anxiety disorders, but further research is required to determine whether unresolved anxiety symptoms in the context of comorbid ADHD and anxiety disorders can be successfully treated with clonidine or guanfacine.

Summary and future directions

Comorbidity of ADHD and anxiety disorders represents a frequently occurring condition in both youth and adults. The importance of properly assessing and diagnosing this condition is based on the unique aspects of its clinical presentation, high level of impairment in functional status, and often incomplete treatment response to monotherapy. However, proper assessment and diagnosis are complicated by the subjective nature of evaluating symptoms, the fact that symptoms of inattention and hyperactivity are often seen in individuals with anxiety disorders, and anxiety is a frequent associated feature in individuals with persistent ADHD. Therefore, there is considerable potential for misattribution or under-identification of symptoms of the two conditions. The importance of recognizing comorbid ADHD and anxiety disorders is further highlighted by the elevated level of symptom severity and impairment in youth with this comorbid presentation, and the increasing prevalence of anxiety disorders in the developmental course of youth with ADHD. Whether there is a common underlying neurobiological basis for the frequent co-occurrence of ADHD and anxiety disorders has not been fully established; however, this conclusion is suggested by studies indicating shared neurobiological features of ADHD and anxiety disorders. It is hoped that translational studies will provide greater clarity on the nature of shared risk, and also help in directing future treatment approaches.

There has been animated discussion in the field as to whether comorbid anxiety disorders portend a less satisfactory treatment course among youth with ADHD, as suggested by initial studies indicating decreased efficacy and poorer tolerability of stimulants in youth with comorbid ADHD + anxiety. However, more recent studies suggest this is not the case. The development of non-stimulant medications (such as atomoxetine) that can successfully target both ADHD and anxiety symptoms in individuals with comorbidity is a welcome event. It is hoped that other non-stimulant medications either currently available or in development will similarly prove to be useful.

Despite the potential for parsimonious monotherapy with non-stimulants, combined treatment is required for many patients with comorbid ADHD + anxiety disorders. Fortunately, approved medications for the different conditions can be used together without compromising efficacy, and there is reason to hope that some of the medications could be more effective when used together. However, for most individuals, medication treatment will only partially provide symptom amelioration. There are several psychosocial treatments for youth and adults with anxiety disorders with a well-established evidence base, and these have an important role in the treatment armamentarium. There are also emerging treatments for symptoms of inattention and executive function deficits in adolescents and adults with ADHD, and these symptom domains are frequently seen in individuals with ADHD + anxiety disorders. Consequently, there are many different options for combined treatment, and these approaches should be strongly considered.

A final clinical consideration is whether to treat one disorder or the other first, or treat both simultaneously. The answer to this question will necessarily vary as a function of individual circumstances. As a rule, it is important to treat the most impairing condition first, using the best available treatment approach.

Unfortunately, despite the high prevalence and clinical importance of comorbid ADHD and anxiety disorders, the database supporting our understanding of the clinical presentation, pathophysiology and treatment of this condition is relatively sparse. Given the intuitive appeal and initial positive findings regarding models positing common underlying neurobiological features and potentially parsimonious treatments, it is hoped that future research will better inform the understanding, evaluation and treatment of ADHD + comorbid anxiety disorders.

References

1. Adler L, Spencer T, Stein M, Newcorn J. Best practices in adult ADHD: epidemiology, impairments and differential diagnosis. *CNS Spectr.* 2008;**13** (10 Suppl 15):4.

2. Kessler RC, Adler L, Barkley R, *et al.* The prevalence and correlates of adult ADHD in the United States: results from the National Comorbidity Survey Replication. *Am J Psychiatry.* 2006;**163**(4):716–23.

3. Kooij JJ, Huss M, Asherson P, *et al.* Distinguishing comorbidity and successful management of adult ADHD. *J Atten Disord.* 2012;**16**(5 Suppl):3S–19S.

4. Costello EJ, Egger HL, Angold A. The developmental epidemiology of anxiety disorders: phenomenology, prevalence, and comorbidity. *Child Adolesc Psychiatr Clin N Am.* 2005;**14**(4):631–48, vii.

5. Edme R, Egger H, Fenichel E, Guedeney A, Wise B, Wright H. Introducing DC:0–3R2005. Available from: http://main.zerotothree.org/site/DocServer/vol26–1a. pdf?docID=2201&AddInterest=1221.

6. ZERO TO THREE. *Diagnostic Classification of Mental Health and Developmental Disorders in Infancy and Early Childhood,* rev. ed. Washington, DC: ZERO TO THREE; 2005.

7. Shear K, Jin R, Ruscio AM, Walters EE, Kessler RC. Prevalence and correlates of estimated DSM-IV child and adult separation anxiety disorder in the National Comorbidity Survey Replication. *Am J Psychiatry.* 2006;**163**(6):1074–83.

8. Kessler RC, Chiu WT, Demler O, Merikangas KR, Walters EE. Prevalence, severity, and comorbidity of 12-month DSM-IV disorders in the National Comorbidity Survey Replication. *Arch Gen Psychiatry.* 2005;**62**(6):617–27.

9. Lenze EJ, Mulsant BH, Mohlman J, *et al.* Generalized anxiety disorder in late life: lifetime course and comorbidity with major depressive disorder. *Am J Geriatr Psychiatry.* 2005;**13**(1):77–80.

10. Rapee RM, Schniering CA, Hudson JL. Anxiety disorders during childhood and adolescence: origins and treatment. *Annu Rev Clin Psychol.* 2009;**5**:311–41.

11. Kessler RC, Berglund P, Demler O, *et al.* Lifetime prevalence and age-of-onset distributions of DSM-IV disorders in the National Comorbidity Survey Replication. *Arch Gen Psychiatry.* 2005;**62**(6):593–602.

12. Jarrett MA, Ollendick TH. A conceptual review of the comorbidity of attention-deficit/hyperactivity disorder and anxiety: implications for future research and practice. *Clin Psychol Rev.* 2008;**28**(7):1266–80.

13. Larson K, Russ SA, Kahn RS, Halfon N. Patterns of comorbidity, functioning, and service use for US children with ADHD, 2007. *Pediatrics.* 2011; **127**(3):462–70.

14. Lavigne JV, Lebailly SA, Hopkins J, Gouze KR, Binns HJ. The prevalence of ADHD, ODD, depression, and anxiety in a community sample of 4-year-olds. *J Clin Child Adolesc Psychol.* 2009;**38**(3):315–28.

15. Giedd JN, Rapoport JL. Structural MRI of pediatric brain development: what have we learned and where are we going? *Neuron.* 2010;**67**(5):728–34.

16. Shaw P, Eckstrand K, Sharp W, *et al.* Attention-deficit/hyperactivity disorder is characterized by a delay in cortical maturation. *Proc Natl Acad Sci USA.* 2007;**104**(49):19649–54.

17. Shaw P, Gilliam M, Liverpool M, *et al.* Cortical development in typically developing children with symptoms of hyperactivity and impulsivity: support for a dimensional view of attention deficit hyperactivity disorder. *Am J Psychiatry.* 2011; **168**(2):143–51.

18. Adler LA, Barkley RA, Newcorn JH. ADHD and comorbid disorders in adults. *J Clin Psychiatry.* 2008;**69**(8):1328–35.

19. Adler LA. Diagnosing and treating adult ADHD and comorbid conditions. *J Clin Psychiatry.* 2008; **69**(11):e31.

20. Jensen PS, Hinshaw SP, Kraemer HC, *et al.* ADHD comorbidity findings from the MTA study: comparing comorbid subgroups. *J Am Acad Child Adolesc Psychiatry.* 2001;**40**(2):147–58.

21. Tsang TW, Kohn MR, Efron D, *et al.* Anxiety in young people with ADHD: clinical and self-report outcomes. *J Atten Disord.* 2012; in press.

22. Moderators and mediators of treatment response for children with attention-deficit/hyperactivity disorder: The multimodal treatment study of children with attention-deficit/hyperactivity disorder. *Arch Gen Psychiatry*. 1999;**56**(12):1088–96.

23. Klein RG, Mannuzza S, Olazagasti MA, *et al.* Clinical and functional outcome of childhood attention-deficit/hyperactivity disorder 33 years later. *Arch Gen Psychiatry*. 2012;**69**(12):1295–303.

24. Biederman J, Petty CR, Woodworth KY, *et al.* Adult outcome of attention-deficit/hyperactivity disorder: a controlled 16-year follow-up study. *J Clin Psychiatry*. 2012;**73**(7):941–50.

25. Broeren S, Muris P, Diamantopoulou S, Baker JR. The course of childhood anxiety symptoms: developmental trajectories and child-related factors in normal children. *J Abnorm Child Psychol*. 2013;**41**(1): 81–95.

26. Grant BF, Hasin DS, Blanco C, *et al.* The epidemiology of social anxiety disorder in the United States: results from the National Epidemiologic Survey on Alcohol and Related Conditions. *J Clin Psychiatry*. 2005;**66**(11): 1351–61.

27. Mörtberg E, Tilfors K, Bejerot S. Screening for ADHD in an adult social phobia sample. *J Atten Disord*. 2012;**16**(8):645–9.

28. Ollendick TH, Jarrett MA, Grills-Taquechel AE, Hovey LD, Wolff JC. Comorbidity as a predictor and moderator of treatment outcome in youth with anxiety, affective, attention deficit/hyperactivity disorder, and oppositional/conduct disorders. *Clin Psychol Rev*. 2008;**28**(8):1447–71.

29. Geller DA. Obsessive-compulsive and spectrum disorders in children and adolescents. *Psychiatr Clin North Am*. 2006;**29**(2):353–70.

30. Masi G, Millepiedi S, Mucci M, *et al.* Comorbidity of obsessive-compulsive disorder and attention-deficit/hyperactivity disorder in referred children and adolescents. *Compr Psychiatry*. 2006;**47**(1):42–7.

31. Petersen C. The Child Advocate 2010 [cited 2010]. Available from: http://www.childadvocate.net/divorce_effects_on_children.htm.

32. Walitza S, Zellmann H, Irblich B, *et al.* Children and adolescents with obsessive-compulsive disorder and comorbid attention-deficit/hyperactivity disorder: preliminary results of a prospective follow-up study. *J Neural Transm*. 2008;**115**(2):187–90.

33. Geller D, Petty C, Vivas F, *et al.* Examining the relationship between obsessive-compulsive disorder and attention-deficit/hyperactivity disorder in children and adolescents: a familial risk analysis. *Biol Psychiatry*. 2007;**61**(3):316–21.

34. Geller D, Petty C, Vivas F, *et al.* Further evidence for co-segregation between pediatric obsessive compulsive disorder and attention deficit hyperactivity disorder: a familial risk analysis. *Biol Psychiatry*. 2007;**61**(12): 1388–94.

35. Moss SB, Nair R, Vallarino A, Wang S. Attention deficit/hyperactivity disorder in adults. *Prim Care*. 2007;**34**(3):445–73, v.

36. Adler LA, Kunz M, Chua HC, Rotrosen J, Resnick SG. Attention-deficit/hyperactivity disorder in adult patients with posttraumatic stress disorder (PTSD): is ADHD a vulnerability factor? *J Atten Disord*. 2004;**8**(1):11–16.

37. Famularo R, Fenton T, Kinscherff R, Augustyn M. Psychiatric comorbidity in childhood post traumatic stress disorder. *Child Abuse Negl*. 1996;**20**(10): 953–61.

38. Weinstein D, Staffelbach D, Biaggio M. Attention-deficit hyperactivity disorder and posttraumatic stress disorder: differential diagnosis in childhood sexual abuse. *Clin Psychol Rev*. 2000;**20**(3):359–78.

39. Wozniak J, Crawford MH, Biederman J, *et al.* Antecedents and complications of trauma in boys with ADHD: findings from a longitudinal study. *J Am Acad Child Adolesc Psychiatry*. 1999;**38**(1): 48–55.

40. Harrington KM, Miller MW, Wolf EJ, *et al.* Attention-deficit/hyperactivity disorder comorbidity in a sample of veterans with posttraumatic stress disorder. *Compr Psychiatry*. 2012;**53**(6):679–90.

41. Beesdo K, Pine DS, Lieb R, Wittchen HU. Incidence and risk patterns of anxiety and depressive disorders and categorization of generalized anxiety disorder. *Arch Gen Psychiatry*. 2010;**67**(1):47–57.

42. Hoehn-Saric R, Hazlett RL, McLeod DR. Generalized anxiety disorder with early and late onset of anxiety symptoms. *Compr Psychiatry*. 1993;**34**(5):291–8.

43. Elia J, Ambrosini P, Berrettini W. ADHD characteristics: I. Concurrent co-morbidity patterns in children & adolescents. *Child Adolesc Psychiatry Ment Health*. 2008;**2**(1):15.

44. Shin LM, Liberzon I. The neurocircuitry of fear, stress, and anxiety disorders. *Neuropsychopharmacology*. 2010;**35**(1):169–91.

45. Sylvester CM, Corbetta M, Raichle ME, *et al.* Functional network dysfunction in anxiety and anxiety disorders. *Trends Neurosci*. 2012;**35**(9):527–35.

46. van Well S, Visser RM, Scholte HS, Kindt M. Neural substrates of individual differences in human fear learning: evidence from concurrent fMRI, fear-potentiated startle, and US-expectancy data. *Cogn Affect Behav Neurosci*. 2012;**12**(3):499–512.

47. Bruhl AB, Rufer M, Delsignore A, *et al.* Neural correlates of altered general emotion processing in social anxiety disorder. *Brain Res.* 2011;**1378**:72–83.

48. Wang J, Jiang T, Cao Q, Wang Y. Characterizing anatomic differences in boys with attention-deficit/hyperactivity disorder with the use of deformation-based morphometry. *AJNR Am J Neuroradiol.* 2007; **28**(3):543–7.

49. Qiu MG, Ye Z, Li QY, *et al.* Changes of brain structure and function in ADHD children. *Brain Topogr.* 2011;**24**(3–4):243–52.

50. Etkin A, Prater KE, Hoeft F, Menon V, Schatzberg AF. Failure of anterior cingulate activation and connectivity with the amygdala during implicit regulation of emotional processing in generalized anxiety disorder. *Am J Psychiatry.* 2010;**167**(5):545–54.

51. McClure EB, Monk CS, Nelson EE, *et al.* Abnormal attention modulation of fear circuit function in pediatric generalized anxiety disorder. *Arch Gen Psychiatry.* 2007;**64**(1):97–106.

52. Monk CS, Telzer EH, Mogg K, *et al.* Amygdala and ventrolateral prefrontal cortex activation to masked angry faces in children and adolescents with generalized anxiety disorder. *Arch Gen Psychiatry.* 2008;**65**(5):568–76.

53. Schulz KP, Newcorn JH, Fan J, Tang CY, Halperin JM. Brain activation gradients in ventrolateral prefrontal cortex related to persistence of ADHD in adolescent boys. *J Am Acad Child Adolesc Psychiatry.* 2005; **44**(1):47–54.

54. Rubia K, Smith AB, Halari R, *et al.* Disorder-specific dissociation of orbitofrontal dysfunction in boys with pure conduct disorder during reward and ventrolateral prefrontal dysfunction in boys with pure ADHD during sustained attention. *Am J Psychiatry.* 2009; **166**(1):83–94.

55. Schulz KP, Fan J, Bedard AC, *et al.* Common and unique therapeutic mechanisms of stimulant and non-stimulant treatments for ADHD. *Arch Gen Psychiatry.* 2012;**69**(9):952–61.

56. Myers-Schulz B, Koenigs M. Functional anatomy of ventromedial prefrontal cortex: implications for mood and anxiety disorders. *Mol Psychiatry.* 2012;**17**(2): 132–41.

57. Godefroy O, Rousseaux M. Divided and focused attention in patients with lesion of the prefrontal cortex. *Brain Cogn.* 1996;**30**(2):155–74.

58. Miller EK, Cohen JD. An integrative theory of prefrontal cortex function. *Annu Rev Neurosci.* 2001;**24**:167–202.

59. Kienast T, Hariri AR, Schlagenhauf F, *et al.* Dopamine in amygdala gates limbic processing of aversive stimuli in humans. *Nat Neurosci.* 2008;**11**(12):1381–2.

60. de la Mora MP, Gallegos-Cari A, Arizmendi-Garcia Y, Marcellino D, Fuxe K. Role of dopamine receptor mechanisms in the amygdaloid modulation of fear and anxiety: structural and functional analysis. *Prog Neurobiol.* 2010;**90**(2):198–216.

61. Zweifel LS, Fadok JP, Argilli E, *et al.* Activation of dopamine neurons is critical for aversive conditioning and prevention of generalized anxiety. *Nat Neurosci.* 2011;**14**(5):620–6.

62. Nagano A, Dagher A, Booij L, *et al.* Stress-Induced Dopamine Release in mPFC: An 18F-Fallypride/PET Study in Healthy Volunteers. *Scandinavian Neuropsychopharmacology.* 2009;**2**(1).

63. Arnsten AF, Pliszka SR. Catecholamine influences on prefrontal cortical function: Relevance to treatment of attention deficit/hyperactivity disorder and related disorders. *Pharmacol Biochem Behav.* 2011;**99**(2): 211–16.

64. Berridge CW, Waterhouse BD. The locus coeruleus-noradrenergic system: modulation of behavioral state and state-dependent cognitive processes. *Brain Res Rev.* 2003;**42**(1):33–84.

65. Pliszka SR. Effect of anxiety on cognition, behavior, and stimulant response in ADHD. *J Am Acad Child Adolesc Psychiatry.* 1989;**28**(6):882–7.

66. Kalk NJ, Melichar J, Holmes RB, *et al.* Central noradrenergic responsiveness to a clonidine challenge in generalized anxiety disorder: a single photon emission computed tomography study. *J Psychopharmacol.* 2012;**26**(4): 452–60.

67. Weissman AS, Chu BC, Reddy LA, Mohlman J. Attention mechanisms in children with anxiety disorders and in children with attention deficit hyperactivity disorder: implications for research and practice. *J Clin Child Adolesc Psychol.* 2012;**41**(2): 117–26.

68. Asherson P, Akehurst R, Kooij JJ, *et al.* Under diagnosis of adult ADHD: cultural influences and societal burden. *J Atten Disord.* 2012;**16**(5 Suppl): 20s–38s.

69. McCarthy S, Asherson P, Coghill D, *et al.* Attention-deficit hyperactivity disorder: treatment discontinuation in adolescents and young adults. *Br J Psychiatry.* 2009;**194**(3):273–7.

70. Wilens TE, Zusman RM, Hammerness PG, *et al.* An open-label study of the tolerability of mixed amphetamine salts in adults with attention-deficit/hyperactivity disorder and treated primary essential hypertension. *J Clin Psychiatry.* 2006;**67**(5): 696–702.

71. Robinson R, Cartwright-Hatton S. Maternal disciplinary style with preschool children: associations

with children's and mothers' trait anxiety. *Behav Cogn Psychother*. 2008;**36**(01):49–59.

72. Robinson M, Oddy WH, Li J, *et al.* Pre- and postnatal influences on preschool mental health: a large-scale cohort study. *J Child Psychol Psychiatry*. 2008;**49**(10): 1118–28.

73. Robinson OJ, Sahakian BJ. Recurrence in major depressive disorder: a neurocognitive perspective. *Psychol Med*. 2008;**38**(3):315–18.

74. Faraone SV, Mick E. Molecular genetics of attention deficit hyperactivity disorder. *Psychiatr Clin North Am*. 2010;**33**(1):159–80.

75. Newcorn JH, Halperin JM, Jensen PS, *et al.* Symptom profiles in children with ADHD: effects of comorbidity and gender. *J Am Acad Child Adolesc Psychiatry*. 2001;**40**(2):137–46.

76. Humphreys KL, Aguirre VP, Lee SS. Association of anxiety and ODD/CD in children with and without ADHD. *J Clin Child Adolesc Psychol*. 2012;**41**(3): 370–7.

77. Lubke GH, Hudziak JJ, Derks EM, van Bijsterveldt TC, Boomsma DI. Maternal ratings of attention problems in ADHD: evidence for the existence of a continuum. *J Am Acad Child Adolesc Psychiatry*. 2009;**48**(11): 1085–93.

78. Bubier JL, Drabick DA. Co-occurring anxiety and disruptive behavior disorders: the roles of anxious symptoms, reactive aggression, and shared risk processes. *Clin Psychol Rev*. 2009;**29**(7): 658–69.

79. McKay KE, Halperin JM. ADHD, aggression, and antisocial behavior across the lifespan. Interactions with neurochemical and cognitive function. *Ann N Y Acad Sci*. 2001;**931**:84–96.

80. Pliszka SR. Tricyclic antidepressants in the treatment of children with attention deficit disorder. *J Am Acad Child Adolesc Psychiatry*. 1987;**26**(2):127–32.

81. Pliszka S. Practice parameter for the assessment and treatment of children and adolescents with attention-deficit/hyperactivity disorder. *J Am Acad Child Adolesc Psychiatry*. 2007;**46**(7):894–921.

82. Wolraich M, Brown L, Brown RT, *et al.* ADHD: clinical practice guideline for the diagnosis, evaluation, and treatment of attention-deficit/ hyperactivity disorder in children and adolescents. *Pediatrics*. 2011;**128**(5):1007–22.

83. Charach A, Dashti B, Carson P, *et al.* AHRQ *Comparative Effectiveness Reviews. Attention Deficit Hyperactivity Disorder: Effectiveness of Treatment in At-Risk Preschoolers; Long-Term Effectiveness in All Ages; and Variability in Prevalence, Diagnosis, and Treatment*. Rockville (MD): Agency for Healthcare Research and Quality (US); 2011.

84. Clinical practice guideline: diagnosis and evaluation of the child with attention-deficit/hyperactivity disorder. American Academy of Pediatrics. *Pediatrics*. 2000; **105**(5):1158–70.

85. Weiss M, Murray C, Wasdell M, *et al.* A randomized controlled trial of CBT therapy for adults with ADHD with and without medication. *BMC Psychiatry*. 2012;**12**:30.

86. Weiss M, Safren SA, Solanto MV, *et al.* Research forum on psychological treatment of adults with ADHD. *J Atten Disord*. 2008;**11**(6):42–51.

87. Barlow DH, Gorman JM, Shear MK, Woods SW. Cognitive-behavioral therapy, imipramine, or their combination for panic disorder: a randomized controlled trial. *JAMA*. 2000;**283**(19):2529–36.

88. Davis M, Ressler K, Rothbaum BO, Richardson R. Effects of D-cycloserine on extinction: translation from preclinical to clinical work. *Biol Psychiatry*. 2006;**60**(4):369–75.

89. Foa EB, Franklin ME, Moser J. Context in the clinic: how well do cognitive-behavioral therapies and medications work in combination? *Biol Psychiatry*. 2002;**52**(10):987–97.

90. Kodish I, Rockhill C, Varley C. Pharmacotherapy for anxiety disorders in children and adolescents. *Dialogues Clin Neurosci*. 2011;**13**(4):439–52.

91. Smits JAJ, O'Cleirigh CM, Otto MW. Combining cognitive-behavioral therapy and pharmacotherapy for the treatment of panic disorder. *J Cogn Psychother*. 2006;**20**(1):75–84.

92. Connolly SD, Bernstein GA. Practice parameter for the assessment and treatment of children and adolescents with anxiety disorders. *J Am Acad Child Adolesc Psychiatry*. 2007;**46**(2):267–83.

93. Jarrett MA, Ollendick TH. Treatment of comorbid attention-deficit/hyperactivity disorder and anxiety in children: a multiple baseline design analysis. *J Consult Clin Psychol*. 2012;**80**(2):239–44.

94. Verreault M, Berthiaume C, Turgeon L, Lageix P, Guay MC. Efficiency of a cognitive-behavioral treatment addressing anxiety symptoms in children with comorbid ADHD and anxiety disorder. World Congress of Behavioral and Cognitive Therapies; Barcelona, Spain 2007.

95. March JS, Swanson JM, Arnold LE, *et al.* Anxiety as a predictor and outcome variable in the multimodal treatment study of children with ADHD (MTA). *J Abnorm Child Psychol*. 2000;**28**(6): 527–41.

96. Philipsen A, Hesslinger B, Tebartz van Elst L. Attention deficit hyperactivity disorder in adulthood: diagnosis, etiology and therapy. *Dtsch Arztebl Int*. 2008;**105**(17):311–17.

97. National Collaborating Centre for Mental Health. National Institute for Health and Clinical Excellence. *Guidance. Attention Deficit Hyperactivity Disorder: Diagnosis and Management of ADHD in Children, Young People and Adults.* Leicester (UK): British Psychological Society (UK), The British Psychological Society & The Royal College of Psychiatrists; 2009.

98. Abikoff H, McGough J, Vitiello B, *et al.* Sequential pharmacotherapy for children with comorbid attention-deficit/hyperactivity and anxiety disorders. *J Am Acad Child Adolesc Psychiatry.* 2005;**44**(5): 418–27.

99. Tannock R, Ickowicz A, Schachar R. Differential effects of methylphenidate on working memory in ADHD children with and without comorbid anxiety. *J Am Acad Child Adolesc Psychiatry.* 1995;**34**(7): 886–96.

100. Kratochvil CJ, Newcorn JH, Arnold LE, *et al.* Atomoxetine alone or combined with fluoxetine for treating ADHD with comorbid depressive or anxiety symptoms. *J Am Acad Child Adolesc Psychiatry.* 2005;**44**(9):915–24.

101. Weiss MD, Weiss JR. A guide to the treatment of adults with ADHD. *J Clin Psychiatry.* 2004;**65**(Suppl 3): 27–37.

102. Adler LA, Liebowitz M, Kronenberger W, *et al.* Atomoxetine treatment in adults with attention-deficit/hyperactivity disorder and comorbid social anxiety disorder. *Depress Anxiety.* 2009;**26**(3):212–21.

103. Neylan TC, Lenoci M, Samuelson KW, *et al.* No improvement of posttraumatic stress disorder symptoms with guanfacine treatment. *Am J Psychiatry.* 2006;**163**(12):2186–8.

Chapter 10

Attention-deficit hyperactivity disorder and the substance use disorders in ADHD

Timothy E. Wilens and Nicholas R. Morrison

Synopsis

There has been increasing interest in the overlap between attention-deficit hyperactivity disorder (ADHD) and substance use disorders (SUD). In this chapter, we discuss the developmental relationship between ADHD and SUD and associated concurrent disorders. Recent data shed light on the role of treatment of ADHD in children on subsequent cigarette smoking and SUD in adolescence and adulthood. Studies in patients with ADHD and SUD suggest that SUD treatment needs to be sequenced initially with ADHD treatment quickly thereafter. Diagnostic and treatment strategies for adolescents and adults with ADHD plus SUD are discussed.

Introduction

The overlap between attention-deficit hyperactivity disorder (ADHD) and alcohol or drug abuse or dependence (referred to here as substance use disorders [SUD]) in adolescents and adults has been an area of increasing clinical, research, and public health interest. ADHD onsets in early childhood and affects from 6% to 9% of children and adolescents and up to 5% of adults worldwide [1, 2]. Longitudinal data suggest that childhood ADHD persists in 75% of cases into adolescence and in approximately one-half of cases into adulthood (for review see Mick *et al.* [3] and Wilens and Spencer [4]). SUD usually onsets in adolescence or early adulthood and affect up to 30% of US adults [5, 6] with approximately 9% of adolescents manifesting a drug use disorder and 6% an alcohol use disorder [6]. The study of comorbidity between SUD and ADHD is relevant to both research and clinical practice in developmental pediatrics, psychology, and psychiatry, with implications for diagnosis, prognosis, treatment, and healthcare delivery.

Overlap between ADHD and SUD

Studies incorporating structured psychiatric diagnostic interviews assessing ADHD and other disorders in substance abusing groups have indicated that from one-quarter to one-half of adolescents and adults with SUD have ADHD (for review see Wilens [7] and Frodl [8]). For example, aggregate data from government-funded studies of mainly cannabis abusing youth indicate that ADHD is the second most common comorbidity with 40–50% of both girls and boys manifesting full criteria for ADHD. Data ascertained from adult groups with SUD also show a higher risk for ADHD, as well as earlier onset and more severe SUD associated with ADHD [9, 10]. ADHD is under identified in the setting of addiction treatment. For example, recent work in an addiction treatment center indicates that while 3% of youth were identified in the records as having ADHD, systematic assessment of ADHD identified a rate of 44% [11].

ADHD as a risk factor for SUD

The association of ADHD and SUD is particularly compelling from a developmental perspective as ADHD manifests itself earlier than SUD; therefore, SUD as a risk factor for ADHD is unlikely. Thus, it is important to evaluate to what extent ADHD is a precursor of SUD. Studies indicate that ADHD is a risk factor for later SUD. For example, a recent meta-analysis of 13 studies showed a clinically and statistically significant increase in SUD associated with ADHD [12]. However, prospective studies of ADHD children have provided evidence that the groups with conduct or bipolar disorders co-occurring with ADHD have the poorest outcome with respect to developing SUD and major morbidity [13–17]. For instance, as part of a prospective study of ADHD, we

Attention-Deficit Hyperactivity Disorder in Adults and Children, ed. Lenard A. Adler, Thomas J. Spencer and Timothy E. Wilens. Published by Cambridge University Press. © Cambridge University Press 2015.

found differences in the risk for SUD in ADHD adolescents (mean age 15 years) compared to non-ADHD controls which were accounted for by comorbid conduct or bipolar disorders [13]; however, the age of risk for SUD onset in non-comorbid ADHD was approximately 17 years in girls and 19 years in boys [7]. Moreover, as part of a 10-year follow-up through adolescence, we failed to find any features within ADHD such as family history of SUD, cognitive impairment, socialization, or family environment that predicted later SUD [16]. Likewise, it has been speculated that the executive functioning deficits related to ADHD may be the most pernicious component of the disorder that result in subsequent SUD. Yet, we examined this issue longitudinally and failed to find that adolescents with neuropsychologically defined executive functioning deficits manifested SUD 5 years later [18].

ADHD treatment and later SUD

Controversy continues in the lay and scientific literature and media about the effects of ADHD treatment and later SUD. Clarification of the critical influence of ADHD treatment in youth on later SUD remains hampered by methodological issues. Since prospective studies in ADHD youth are naturalistic, and hence not randomized for treatment, attempts to disentangle positive or deleterious effects of treatment from the severity of the underlying condition(s) are hampered by serious confounds. Whereas concerns of the abuse liability and potential kindling of specific types of abuse (i.e., cocaine) secondary to early stimulant exposure in ADHD children have been raised [19], the preponderance of clinical data does not appear to support such a contention.

To reconcile findings in this important area, we completed previously a meta-analysis of the literature [20] and reported that stimulant pharmacotherapy did not increase the risk for later SUD. In fact, we found that stimulant pharmacotherapy protected against later SUD (odds ratio [OR] of 1.9); and that the effect was stronger in adolescents relative to adults [20]. Recent work has shed more light on this issue. Katusic et al. [21] reported a protective effect of stimulants into young adulthood whereas Biederman et al. [22] and Mannuzza et al. [23] simultaneously reported that early stimulant treatment did not increase nor decrease the risk for subsequent SUD in young adulthood. Two prospective single-site studies examining the prevention of cigarette smoking in ADHD has also

suggested that stimulant treatment may protect against the onset of cigarette smoking during adolescence [24]. For instance, in a recent open study of up to 2 years duration (mean of 10 months), Hammerness and colleagues reported that treatment with up to 72 mg of osmotic-release oral system methylphenidate (OROS MPH) in 154 adolescents with ADHD resulted in rates of new-onset cigarette smoking that were similar to matched groups of non-ADHD controls and of ADHD adolescents treated for their ADHD [25]. We reported in a sample of adolescent girls with ADHD that stimulant treatment resulted in an almost twofold reduction in cigarette smoking and SUD [26]. Of interest, we did not find that the onset or duration of stimulant treatment was related to the risk for SUD, in distinction to Mannuzza et al. [23].

In the largest study to date that has examined the issue of longer-term outcomes with ADHD treatment, Lichtenstein et al. reported on a national registry of 25 656 adolescents/young adults with ADHD by examining the "criminality" of roughly one half of registrants who were both receiving medications for ADHD and followed for five years [27]. Approximately 40% of convictions were related to drug offenses – thus serving as a proxy of drug use outcome. In this study, treatment with either stimulants or non-stimulants resulted in a 32% (men) to 41% (women) reduction in crimes – with a significant reduction specifically on drug-related offenses (OR = 0.6). No differences emerged when comparing outcomes between stimulant and non-stimulant medications. Given this recent report, the aggregate of the literature seems to suggest that early stimulant treatment reduces or delays the onset of SUD and cigarette smoking into adolescence and can facilitate more general improvement of serious drug-related issues into adulthood. The protective effect of early medication treatment on cigarette smoking and alcohol in adulthood remains unclear. The loss of the protective effect in adults that has been reported in smaller samples may be a reflection of findings in adolescents not spanning through the full age of risk of SUD or that many adolescents discontinue their ADHD treatment during later adolescence and young adulthood, thus losing the protective effect of stimulants.

SUD pathways associated with ADHD

An increasing body of literature shows an intriguing association between ADHD and cigarette smoking [28]. We have previously reported that ADHD was a significant predictor of early initiation of cigarette smoking (before age 15) and that conduct and mood disorders coupled with ADHD put youth at particularly high risk for early-onset smoking [29]. Data also suggest that one-half of ADHD smokers go on to later SUD [30]. This is not surprising given that smoking leads to peer group pressures and availability of illicit substances and that biologically, nicotine exposure may affect brain plasticity, increasing susceptibility to later behavioral problems and SUD [31]. Interestingly, nicotinic modulating agents are increasingly being evaluated for the treatment of ADHD [32].

The precise mechanism(s) mediating the expression of SUD in ADHD populations remains to be seen. The self-medication hypothesis is compelling in ADHD considering that the disorder is chronic and often associated with demoralization and failure, factors frequently associated with SUD in adolescents. Studies indicate a linear relationship between ADHD symptoms and risk for cigarette smoking [28, 33]. Moreover, we found that among substance abusing adolescents with and without ADHD, ADHD adolescents reported using substances more frequently to attenuate their mood and to help them sleep [34]. No evidence of differences in types of substances has emerged between ADHD and non-ADHD substance abusing teens [13]. Other important links include family/genetic contributions [35] and exposure to parental SUD during vulnerable developmental phases [36].

Diagnosis and treatment guidelines

Evaluation and treatment of comorbid ADHD and SUD should be part of a plan in which consideration is given to all aspects of the individual's life. Any intervention in this group should follow a careful assessment of the adolescent, including psychiatric, addiction, social, cognitive, educational, and family evaluations. A thorough history of substance use should be obtained, including past and current usage and treatments. Although no specific guidelines exist for evaluating the patient with active SUD, our experience suggests that at least 1 month of abstinence is useful in accurately and reliably assessing for ADHD symptoms. Semi-structured psychiatric interviews or validated rating scales of ADHD are invaluable

aids for the systematic diagnostic assessments of this group [11, 37].

There has been much debate on the age-of-onset criteria currently used for diagnosing older adolescents and adults with ADHD. Barkley and Biederman have previously proposed that requiring child-based symptoms for adults to meet the diagnosis of ADHD is too stringent [38]. A limited literature has shed important light on establishing the diagnosis of ADHD in adults with SUD who fail to have clear recollection of ADHD symptom onset in childhood. Faraone et al. have examined differences between groups of adults with ADHD based on age of onset of symptoms [39]. These researchers investigated whether differences existed between 79 adults who had full current criteria for ADHD but did not have a clear track of symptoms prior to age 7 years and 127 adults who had their ADHD onset prior to age 7 years [39, 40]. Interestingly, no differences in rates of psychiatric comorbidity, SUD, family history of ADHD, or impairment were found between groups of adults with full criteria ADHD and those who had a longitudinal track of ADHD without clear onset in youth. This finding highlights the potential problems associated with using the current onset of symptoms prior to age 7 years stringently, particularly in adults with SUD [41].

There are no studies examining psychotherapy exclusively for the treatment of individuals with ADHD and SUD. However, recent studies have demonstrated efficacy of cognitive-behavioral therapies (CBT) for ADHD and related problems in adults with ADHD using both individual [42] and adapted group therapies [43]. It appears that effective psychotherapy for this comorbid group combines the following elements: motivational-enhancement, structured and goal-directed sessions, proactive therapist involvement, and knowledge of SUD and ADHD [44]. Often, SUD and ADHD therapeutics are completed in tandem with other addiction modalities (e.g., alcoholics and narcotics anonymous, rational recovery) including pharmacotherapy.

The treatment needs of individuals with SUD and ADHD should be considered simultaneously; however, if possible, the SUD should be addressed initially [45]. If the SUD is active, immediate attention needs to be paid to *stabilization of the addiction(s)*. Depending on the severity and duration of the SUD, individuals may require full or partial inpatient treatment. Self-help groups offer a helpful treatment modality for many with SUD. In tandem with addiction treatment,

SUD individuals with ADHD require intervention(s) for the ADHD (and if applicable, comorbid psychiatric disorders).

Medication serves an important role in reducing the symptoms of ADHD and other concurrent psychiatric disorders. Effective agents for ADHD include the stimulants, alpha agonists, noradrenergic agents, and catecholaminergic antidepressants.

In general, while open studies are more encouraging, results from controlled trials with stimulants and/or bupropion suggest that ADHD pharmacotherapy used in adults with ADHD plus SUD has meager effects on the ADHD and substance use or cravings (see Tables 10.1 and 10.2). Schubiner and colleagues reported the results of a prospective, double-blind, randomized trial of methylphenidate (MPH) in cocaine abusing subjects with ADHD [46]. Of 48 enrolled, 52% of subjects completed the 13-week trial. While significant reductions in symptoms of ADHD were reported, no changes in cocaine use (self-report or urine toxicologies) or cocaine craving were found in the MPH group. Similarly, in two well-conducted studies of MPH and/or bupropion in adults with cocaine addiction ($\pm$ opioid replacement with methadone) Levin et al. found only small to no improvements in ADHD and SUD outcomes [47, 48]. It is noteworthy that worsening of cocaine or other drug use was not observed by these investigators in relation to MPH or bupropion administration. A pilot, placebo-controlled 12-week study of OROS MPH (72 mg) in 24 adults with amphetamine abuse and ADHD indicated no significant differences in outcome for either ADHD or SUD [49]. A multisite, National Institutes of Health (NIH)-funded placebo-controlled study of stimulants in adult smokers with ADHD was recently reported [50]. In this 11-week study, OROS MPH/placebo was dosed to 72 mg/day in 255 adults with ADHD who were also treated with a nicotine patch to examine the effects on cigarette cessation and ADHD. The results of this trial showed improved ADHD but no effects on rates of cigarette cessation [50]. Of interest, there was no increased cigarette smoking in the medicated group and side effects in these adults were similar to those noted in previous stimulant trials. Data from another NIH multisite study of treatment of adolescents with ADHD and SUD were also reported [51]. In this 16-week placebo-controlled study, 300 adolescents with ADHD and mixed SUD received OROS MPH/placebo to 72 mg/day along with weekly individual CBT. Both treatment arms resulted in significant

improvement compared to baseline; however, there was no significant improvement in ADHD (investigator/parent) or SUD (adolescent self-report) between treatment groups. Side effects were reminiscent of adolescent studies and the medication was reported to be of low abuse liability. Interestingly, the authors speculated that the therapy utilized in this treatment may have been beneficial for the ADHD and SUD [51].

Of interest, no evidence exists that treating ADHD pharmacologically through an active SUD worsens the SUD – consistent with work of Grabowski et al. who have used stimulants to block cocaine and amphetamine abuse [52]. Not surprisingly, older work by Volkow et al. has demonstrated important differences between MPH and cocaine when binding at the dopamine transporter, resulting in very different abuse liabilities [53]. In ADHD adults with recent SUD, the non-stimulant agents (atomoxetine) and antidepressants (bupropion) with low abuse liability and diversion potential are preferable. Due to the broad spectrum of activity in ADHD and lack of abuse liability of atomoxetine [54], results from a controlled multisite study of atomoxetine in adults with alcohol use disorders are of interest and promising [55]. In this 12-week multisite study in recently abstinent alcoholics, atomoxetine (compared with placebo) was effective in treating ADHD and in reducing recurrent episodes of heavy drinking but not relapse to heavy drinking [55]. Similarly, in a small 10-week, open-label study, atomoxetine treated ADHD symptoms and reduced the intensity, frequency, and length of cravings in recently abstinent adults with SUD and comorbid ADHD [56]. Atomoxetine administration in heavy relative to light or non-drinkers was associated with more side effects; yet, no serious adverse events nor evidence of impaired liver functioning emerged in the heavy drinkers in these relatively short-term trials [57]. These promising data in abstinent alcoholics need to be tempered against a recent study in currently using adolescents with SUD. Thurstone et al. studied 70 adolescents with ADHD and at least one active non-nicotine SUD who received 12 weeks of atomoxetine or placebo in addition to motivational interviewing/CBT [58]. There were no differences between ADHD scores or in use of substances between treatment groups that emerged during the study [58]. The authors speculated that the psychotherapy may have contributed to a larger than expected placebo response.

Table 10.1. Representative studies of pharmacological efficacy in adults with ADHD and SUD

Author and year	N	Mean age (yrs)	Design	Sample description	Medication	Duration	Daily dose (range)	Retention	Outcome	Concurrent treatment	Comments
Levin et al., 1998 [78]	12	34	Open	ADHD and cocaine dependence	MPH	12 weeks	68 mg (40–80 mg)	8/12	Improvements in ADHD; decrease in self-reported cocaine use and positive urines	Individual weekly relapse prevention therapy	Mild AEs
Upadhyaya et al., 2001 [79]	10	35	Open	ADHD and alcohol and/or cocaine ab/dep	Venlafaxine	12 weeks	300 mg	4/10	Significant improvements in ADHD and in alcohol craving and frequency	Weekly and then monthly psychotherapy	± effect on cocaine; 4/10 patients with mood disorder
Levin et al., 2002 [80]	11	31	Open	Outpatients with cocaine dependence and adult ADHD	BPR	12 weeks	250–400 mg	10/11	Reductions in ADHD and cocaine cravings (p's < 0.01)	Individual weekly relapse prevention therapy	No subjects dropped out due to AEs
Schubiner et al., 2002 [46]	48	37	Double-blind, placebo-controlled	Cocaine use and some evidence of ADHD	MPH	13 weeks	90 mg	25/48	Trend to improved hyperactive–impulsive sxs; no difference in cocaine use (self-reported or urines)	Twice weekly group CBT for SUD; weekly individual CBT for ADHD	55% of the MPH group dropped out of the study
Somoza et al., 2004 [81]	41		Open	Adults with ADHD and cocaine dependence	MPH Cocaine	10 weeks	60 mg MPH	29/41	Subjective measures showed improvement in cocaine use and ADHD	Individual substance use therapy	MPH was well tolerated
Carpentier et al., 2005 [82]	25	31.9	Double-blind, placebo-controlled	Adults with ADHD receiving substance use disorder tx	MPH	8 weeks	0.6 mg/kg	19/25	Positive response to active treatment (36%) was not significantly higher than that of placebo (20%)	One subject was using benzodiazepine	24% of subjects dropped out of the study
Levin et al., 2006 [47]	98	39 – placebo 40 – MPH 38 – BPR	Double-blind, placebo-controlled	Methadone-maintained patients with ADHD, 53% with cocaine ab/dep	MPH and BPR	12 weeks	MPH 10–80 mg BPR 100–400 mg	69/98 75% – placebo 65% – MPH 29% – BPR	Significant reduction of ADHD sxs in all three groups; no significant difference in outcome between treatments	Methadone, individual CBT	

(cont.)

Table 10.1. (cont.)

Author and year	N	Mean age (yrs)	Design	Sample description	Medication	Duration	Daily dose (range)	Retention	Outcome	Concurrent treatment	Comments
Levin et al., 2007 [48]	106	37	Double-blind, placebo-controlled	Adults with ADHD, currently seeking treatment for cocaine dependence	MPH	14 weeks	10–60 mg	47/106	Both groups showed >30% improvement in their ADHD sxs, with no significant difference b/t groups	Weekly individual CBT	High drop out rates in both groups; ADHD responders showed reduction in cocaine use
Wilens et al., 2008 [55]	147	≥18	Double-blind, placebo-controlled	Adults with ADHD and alcohol ab/dep	Atomoxetine	12 weeks	25–100 mg	80/147	Significant improvement in ADHD; reduced heavy drinking, no effect on relapse	No additional tx	Heavy drinkers had higher rates of decreased appetite and increased irritability
Wilens et al., 2010 [83]	32	32	Open	Outpatients with ADHD and mixed SUD	BPR SR	6 weeks	326 mg (100–400 mg)	19/32	Improvements in ADHD (46%) and substance use severity (22%, $p < 0.01$)	No additional tx	Low retention; 3 subjects dropped due to AEs; no drug interactions
Adler et al., 2010 [56]	18	36.8	Open	Adults with SUD meeting ADHD criteria	Atomoxetine	10 weeks	25–120 mg	12/18	Significant improvement in ADHD; reduced intensity, length, and frequency of cravings	No additional tx	All AEs were mild/moderate; no AEs resulted in discontinued participation
Winhusen et al., 2010 [50]	255	38	Double-blind, placebo-controlled	Adults with ADHD who smoke cigarettes	OROS MPH	11 weeks	≤72 mg/day	204/255	Significant improvements in ADHD; no differences in cigarette cessation rates between groups	Brief office based manualized counseling; no worsening of cigarettes with MPH	Trends to fewer cigarettes in smoking group; medication well tolerated
Konstenius et al., 2010 [49]	24	37.4	Double-blind, placebo-controlled	Abstinent adults with amphetamine dependence and ADHD	OROS MPH	13 weeks	18–72mg	84% – placebo 59% – MPH	Both groups significantly reduced self-rated ADHD symptoms, but no difference between treatment arms	Weekly sessions of a skills training program	No difference on craving for amphetamine
TOTAL (n = 13)	827	34 (18–55)	Double-blind = 7 Open = 6	ADHD and mixed SUD	MPH = 8 BPR = 3 Atomoxetine = 2 Venlafaxine = 1	6–14 weeks	Moderate doses		Overall significant reduction in ADHD symptoms; mild reduction of SUD	The majority of subjects received concurrent treatment	Moderate adverse events

Abbreviations: ab = abuse, ADHD = attention-deficit hyperactivity disorder, AE = adverse event, BPR = bupropion, CBT = cognitive-behavioral therapy, dep = dependence, MPH = methylphenidate, OROS MPH = osmotic-release oral system methylphenidate, SR = sustained release, SUD = substance use disorder, sx = symptom, tx = treatment.

Table 10.2. Representative studies of pharmacological efficacy in adolescents with ADHD and SUD

Author and year	N	Mean age (yrs)	Design	Sample description	Medication	Duration	Daily dose (range)	Retention	Outcome	Concurrent treatment	Comments
Riggs et al., 1996 [84]	15	15	Open	Boys with ADHD, SUD, and CD in Res Tx	Pemoline	1 month	112.5–185.5 mg (1.2–3.3 mg/kg)	13/15	Significant reductions in activity (7%) and hyperactivity (14%) ($p \leq 0.002$)	All subjects in a Res Tx program; 3 were taking other medications	2 subjects dropped out because of side effects; no change in CPT
Riggs et al., 1998 [85]	13	16	Open	Boys with ADHD, SUD, and CD in Res Tx	Bupropion	5 weeks	300 mg (3.9–5.6 mg/kg)	13/13	Hyperactivity declined 13%, severity of ADHD 39% ($p < 0.002$)	All subjects in a Res Tx program	Side effects mild and transient, one developed hypomania
Riggs et al., 2004 [86]	69	13–19	Double-blind, placebo-controlled	Outpatients with ADHD, SUD, and CD	Pemoline	12 weeks	(75–112 mg)	36/69	Reduced hyperactivity, inattention; no change in SUD	No additional tx	No hepatic dysfunction, three adverse events were reported
Solhkhah et al., 2005 [87]	14	15	Open	Outpatients with ADHD, SUD, and a mood disorder	Bupropion SR	6 months	315 mg (100–400 mg)	13/14	Significant reductions in DUSI (39%), ADHD (43%), HAM-D (76%), SUD by CGI	21% of subjects on concurrent medication; 57% had concurrent counseling	Naturalistic tx; no significant adverse events
Szobot et al., 2008 [88]	16	15–21	Single-blind, placebo-controlled	Adolescents with ADHD/SUD	Methylphenidate (MPH-SODAS)	6 weeks	0.3–1.2 mg/kg	14/16	Improved global functioning (SNAP-IV and CGI); no effect on SUD	No additional tx	Med well tolerated
Riggs, 2011 [51]	300	16.5	Double-blind, placebo-controlled	Adolescents with ADHD/SUD	OROS MPH	16 weeks	≤72 mg/day	72%–placebo 76%–OROS MPH	Both groups improved in ADHD and SUD; no significant differences between groups on SUD and ADHD outcomes	Cognitive-behavioral therapy in all subjects	11-site study, high level of adherence to protocol; med well tolerated; no evidence of med abuse
Thurstone et al., 2010 [58]	70	16	Double-blind, placebo-controlled	Adolescents with ADHD/SUD	Atomoxetine	12 weeks	<70 kg: 0.5–1.5 mg/kg >70 kg: 50–100 mg	65/70	No difference in change in ADHD scores or change in SUD vs. placebo	All received motivational interviewing and cognitive behavioral-therapy	Mild adverse events
TOTAL (n = 7)	497	13–21	Double-blind = 3 Open = 3 Single-blind = 1	ADHD and mixed SUD; some comorbid disorders	MPH = 2 Bupropion = 2 Pemoline = 2 Atomoxetine = 1	1 month–16 weeks	Moderate doses		Reduction in ADHD symptoms; mild reduction of SUD	The majority of subjects received concurrent treatment	Mild adverse events

Abbreviations: ADHD = attention-deficit hyperactivity disorder, CD = conduct disorder, CPT = continuous performance task, CGI = Clinical Global Impression, DUSI = Drug Use Screening Inventory, HAM-D = Hamilton Depression Rating Scale, MPH = methylphenidate, MPH-SODAS = methylphenidate spheroidal oral drug absorption system, OROS MPH = osmotic-release oral system methylphenidate, Res Tx = residential treatment, SNAP-IV = Swanson, Nolan, and Pelham Questionnaire, SR = sustained release, SUD = substance use disorder, tx = treatment.

The above findings linked with an older meta-analysis of 10 studies suggest that medications used in adolescents and adults with ADHD plus active SUD have only a meager effect on the ADHD and have little effect on cigarette or substance use or cravings [59]. It may be that even some abstinence may result in improved outcomes for both ADHD and SUD [55]. In individuals with SUD and ADHD, frequent monitoring of pharmacotherapy should be undertaken, including evaluation of compliance with treatment, questionnaires, random toxicology screens as indicated, and coordination of care with addiction counselors and other caregivers.

Issues of misuse and diversion

There is increasing interest in misuse and diversion of stimulants prescribed for ADHD (for review see Wilens *et al.* [60]). The majority of individuals treated for their ADHD use their medications appropriately [60–63], although they also report being pressured into giving away or selling their medication to others [64]. Survey studies have indicated that approximately 5% of college students have misused stimulants [62, 63]. This practice is more common in competitive colleges where the stimulants are more often misused for their pro-cognitive effects than euphoria [63]. Interestingly, in a secondary analysis of an internet-based survey, young adults with higher Adult ADHD Self-Report Scale (ASRS) scores were significantly more likely to engage in non-medical use of ADHD medications, while young adults with lower scores were significantly less likely to engage in non-medical use [65]. The majority of college students who misuse stimulants obtain them from friends, with only a minority reporting "scamming" local practitioners to obtain stimulants [66].

Data from children are similar to data from adults [67]. Poulin surveyed 13 549 students in grades 7–12 and found that 8.5% had used non-prescribed stimulants in the year prior to the survey [68]. Of those students who were receiving prescribed stimulants, 15% had given their medication and 7% had sold their medication to other students. Stimulant misuse was generally in context with other substances of abuse [67] and psychopathology such as depression [69], ADHD [65, 70], and conduct disorder [61].

Recent basic work suggests that the preparations of stimulants may have an impact on misuse and diversion [71]. For instance, less misuse of extended-

compared to immediate-release stimulants has been reported in clinical [61, 72] and epidemiological reports [73]. Likewise, using simultaneous neuroimaging and self-report queries, less likeability has been reported with extended-release MPH than equipotent doses of immediate-release MPH [74, 75]. In one study, despite similar overall serum concentrations of MPH, extended release was associated with a slower binding and less saturation of the dopamine transporter corresponding to less effect or likeability on the drug use questionnaire [74]. Differences in likeability are even evident between different extended-release compounds [76]. Work with lisdexamfetamine, a prodrug stimulant that is metabolized in vivo to d-amphetamine, indicates less likelihood for intravenous or intranasal abuse than equipotent d-amphetamine [77]. Hence, a growing literature suggests the consideration of extended-release stimulant preparations rather than their immediate-release counterparts in populations at higher risk of misusing or diverting their stimulants [8].

Summary

In summary, practitioners are increasingly recognizing the overlap between ADHD and SUD. ADHD is a risk factor for SUD, particularly in context to comorbidity. Likewise, relatively high rates of ADHD exist in adolescents and adults with SUD. Both family-genetic and self-medication influences may be operational in the development and continuation of SUD in ADHD. Adolescents and adults with ADHD and SUD require multimodal intervention incorporating addiction and mental health treatment. CBT appear to be effective in both ADHD and SUD. If possible, the data suggest that an individual's SUD should be stabilized prior to starting medication. Pharmacotherapy in ADHD and SUD individuals needs to take into consideration timing, misuse and diversion liability, potential drug interactions, and compliance concerns. Choice of non-stimulants or extended-release stimulants should be considered to treat those with recent addictions or those at high risk of misusing or diverting their medications.

While the existing literature has provided important information on the relationship of ADHD and SUD, it also points to a number of areas in need of further study. The mechanism by which untreated ADHD leads to SUD, as well as the specificity of risk reduction of ADHD treatment on cigarette smoking and SUD at apparent developmental time points needs to be better understood. The long-term outcomes for alcohol and cigarette use in adherent samples of ADHD youth who are treated throughout their life need be undertaken. Given the prevalence and major morbidity of SUD and ADHD, as well as the impairment so frequently generated by these disorders, prevention and treatment strategies for these adolescents and adults need to be further developed and evaluated.

Acknowledgments

This research was supported by NIH K24 DA016264 to TW. Dr. Wilens over the past 3 years has received grant support from NIH (NIDA) and Shire; and has been a consultant for Euthymics and Shire. Mr. Morrison has no conflicts of interest to report.

References

1. Kessler RC, Adler L, Barkley R, *et al*. The prevalence and correlates of adult ADHD in the United States: results from the National Comorbidity Survey Replication. *Am J Psychiatry*. 2006;**163**(4):716–23.

2. Polanczyk G, de Lima MS, Horta BL, Biederman J, Rohde LA. The worldwide prevalence of ADHD: a systematic review and metaregression analysis. *Am J Psychiatry*. 2007;**164**(6):942–8.

3. Mick E, Faraone SV, Biederman J, Spencer T. The course and outcome of ADHD. *Primary Psychiatry*. 2004;**11**(7):42–8.

4. Wilens TE, Spencer TJ. Understanding attention-deficit/hyperactivity disorder from childhood to adulthood. *Postgrad Med*. 2010;**122**(5):97–109.

5. Kessler RC. The epidemiology of dual diagnosis. *Biol Psychiatry*. 2004;**56**(10):730–7.

6. Merikangas KR, He JP, Burstein M, *et al*. Lifetime prevalence of mental disorders in U.S. adolescents: results from the National Comorbidity Survey Replication–Adolescent Supplement (NCS-A). *J Am Acad Child Adolesc Psychiatry*. 2010;**49**(10):980–9.

7. Wilens T. Attention-deficit/hyperactivity disorder and the substance use disorders: the nature of the relationship, subtypes at risk and treatment issues. *Psychiatr Clin North Am*. 2004;**27**(2):283–301.

8. Frodl T. Comorbidity of ADHD and Substance Use Disorder (SUD): a neuroimaging perspective. *J Atten Disord*. 2010;**14**(2):109–20.

9. Carroll KM, Rounsaville BJ. History and significance of childhood attention deficit disorder in treatment-seeking cocaine abusers. *Compr Psychiatry*. 1993;**34**: 75–82.

10. Levin FR, Evans SM. Diagnostic and treatment issues in comorbid substance abuse and adult attention-deficit hyperactivity disorder. *Psychiatr Ann*. 2001; **31**(5):303–12.

11. McAweeney M, Rogers NL, Huddleston C, Moore D, Gentile JP. Symptom prevalence of ADHD in a community residential substance abuse treatment program. *J Atten Disord*. 2010;**13**(6):601–8.

12. Charach A, Yeung E, Climans T, Lillie E. Childhood attention-deficit/hyperactivity disorder and future substance use disorders: comparative meta-analyses. *J Am Acad Child Adolesc Psychiatry*. 2011;**50**(1):9–21.

13. Biederman J, Wilens T, Mick E, *et al*. Is ADHD a risk for psychoactive substance use disorder? Findings from a four year follow-up study. *J Am Acad Child Adolesc Psychiatry*. 1997;**36**:21–9.

14. Katusic SK, Barbaresi WJ, Colligan RC, *et al.*, eds. Substance abuse among ADHD cases: A population-based birth cohort study. Pediatric Academic Society; 2003 April; Seattle, WA.

15. Molina B, Pelham W. Childhood predictors of adolescent substance use in a longitudinal study of children with ADHD. *J Abnorm Child Psychol*. 2003;**112**(3):497–507.

16. Wilens T, Martelon M, Joshi G, *et al*. Does ADHD predict substance use disorders? A 10-year follow-up study of young adults with ADHD. *J Am Acad Child Adolesc Psychiatry*. 2011;**50**(6):543–53.

17. Brook DW, Brook JS, Zhang C, Koppel J. Association between attention-deficit/hyperactivity disorder in adolescence and substance use disorders in adulthood. *Arch Pediatr Adolesc Med*. 2010;**164**(10):930–4.

18. Wilens TE, Martelon M, Fried R, *et al*. Do executive function deficits predict later substance use disorders among adolescents and young adults? *J Am Acad Child Adolesc Psychiatry*. 2011;**50**(2):141–9.

19. Vitiello B. Long-term effects of stimulant medications on the brain: possible relevance to the treatment of attention deficit hyperactivity disorder. *J Child Adolesc Psychopharmacol*. 2001;**11**(1):25–34.

20. Wilens T, Faraone S, Biederman J, Gunawardene S. Does stimulant therapy of ADHD beget later substance abuse? A meta-analytic review of the literature. *Pediatrics*. 2003;**11**(1):179–85.

21. Katusic SK, Barbaresi WJ, Colligan RC, *et al.* Psychostimulant treatment and risk for substance abuse among young adults with a history of attention-deficit/hyperactivity disorder: a population-based, birth cohort study. *J Child Adolesc Psychopharmacol*. 2005;**15**(5):764–76.

22. Biederman J, Monteaux MC, Spencer T, *et al*. Stimulant therapy and risk for subsequent substance use disorders in male adults with ADHD: a naturalistic

controlled 10-year follow-up study. *Am J Psychiatry.* 2008;**165**(5):597–603.

23. Mannuzza S, Klein RG, Truong NL, *et al.* Age of methylphenidate treatment initiation in children with ADHD and later substance abuse: prospective follow-up into adulthood. *Am J Psychiatry.* 2008; **165**(5):553–5.

24. Monuteaux MC, Spencer TJ, Faraone SV, Wilson AM, Biederman J. A randomized, placebo-controlled clinical trial of bupropion for the prevention of smoking in children and adolescents with attention-deficit/hyperactivity disorder. *J Clin Psychiatry.* 2007;**68**(7):1094–101.

25. Hammerness P, Joshi G, Doyle R, *et al.* Do stimulants reduce the risk for cigarette smoking in youth with attention-deficit hyperactivity disorder? A prospective, long-term, open-label study of extended-release methylphenidate. *J Pediatr.* 2013;**162**(1):22–7.e2.

26. Wilens TE, Adamson J, Monuteaux MC, *et al.* Effect of prior stimulant treatment for attention-deficit/hyperactivity disorder on subsequent risk for cigarette smoking and alcohol and drug use disorders in adolescents. *Arch Pediatr Adolesc Med.* 2008;**162**(10): 916–21.

27. Lichtenstein P, Halldner L, Zetterqvist J, *et al.* Medication for attention deficit-hyperactivity disorder and criminality. *N Engl J Med.* 2012;**367**(21):2006–14.

28. Kollins SH, McClernon FJ, Fuemmeler BF. Association between smoking and attention-deficit/hyperactivity disorder symptoms in a population-based sample of young adults. *Arch Gen Psychiatry.* 2005;**62**(10): 1142–7.

29. Milberger S, Biederman J, Faraone S, Chen L, Jones J. ADHD is associated with early initiation of cigarette smoking in children and adolescents. *J Am Acad Child Adolesc Psychiatry.* 1997;**36**:37–44.

30. Biederman J, Monuteaux M, Mick E, *et al.* Is cigarette smoking a gateway drug to subsequent alcohol and illicit drug use disorders? A controlled study of youths with and without ADHD. *Biol Psychiatry.* 2006;**59**: 258–64.

31. Trauth JA, Seidler FJ, Slotkin TA. Persistent and delayed behavioral changes after nicotine treatment in adolescent rats. *Brain Res.* 2000;**880**(1–2): 167–72.

32. Wilens T, Verlinden MH, Adler LA, Wozniak PA, West SA. ABT-089, a neuronal nicotinic receptor partial agonist, for the treatment of attention-deficit/hyperactivity disorder in adults: results of a pilot study. *Biol Psychiatry.* 2006;**59**(11):1065–70.

33. Wilens TE, Vitulano M, Upadhyaya H, *et al.* Cigarette smoking associated with attention deficit hyperactivity disorder. *J Pediatr.* 2008;**153**(3):414–19.

34. Wilens T, Adamson J, Sgambati S, *et al.* Do individuals with ADHD self-medicate with cigarettes and substances of abuse? Results from a controlled family study of ADHD. *Am J Addict.* 2007;**16**(Suppl 1):14–23.

35. Biederman J, Petty CR, Wilens TE, *et al.* Familial risk analyses of attention deficit hyperactivity disorder and substance use disorders. *Am J Psychiatry.* 2008;**165**(1): 107–15.

36. Yule AM, Wilens TE, Martelon M, Simon A, Biederman J, eds. Impact of exposure to parental substance use disorders (SUD) on SUD risk in girls and their siblings. 57th Annual Meeting of the American Academy of Child and Adolescent Psychiatry, 2010 October 26–31; New York, NY; 2010.

37. Adler L, Cohen J. Diagnosis and evaluation of adults with ADHD. *Psychiatr Clin North Am.* 2004;**27**(2): 187–201.

38. Barkley RA, Biederman J. Toward a broader definition of the age-of-onset criterion for attention-deficit hyperactivity disorder. *J Am Acad Child Adolesc Psychiatry.* 1997;**36**(9):1204–10.

39. Faraone SV, Biederman J, Spencer TJ, *et al.* Diagnosing adult attention deficit hyperactivity disorder: Are late onset and subthreshold diagnoses valid? *Am J Psychiatry.* 2006;**163**(10):1720–9.

40. Faraone SV, Wilens TE, Petty C, *et al.* Substance use among ADHD adults: implications of late onset and subthreshold diagnoses. *Am J Addict.* 2007; **16**(Suppl 1):24–32; quiz 33–4.

41. Levin FR, Evans S, Kleber HD. Prevalence of adult attention-deficit/hyperactivity disorder among cocaine abusers seeking treatment. *Drug Alcohol Depend.* 1998;**52**:15–25.

42. Safren SA, Sprich S, Mimiaga MJ, *et al.* Cognitive behavioral therapy vs relaxation with educational support for medication-treated adults with ADHD and persistent symptoms: a randomized controlled trial. *JAMA.* 2010;**304**(8):875–80.

43. Solanto MV, Marks DJ, Wasserstein J, *et al.* Efficacy of meta-cognitive therapy for adult ADHD. *Am J Psychiatry.* 2010;**167**(8):958–68.

44. McDermott SP, Wilens TE. Cognitive therapy for adults with ADHD. In: Brown T, ed. *Subtypes of Attention Deficit Disorders in Children, Adolescents, and Adults.* Washington, DC: American Psychiatric Press, Inc. 2000; 569–606.

45. Wilens T, Biederman J. Alcohol, drugs, and attention-deficit/hyperactivity disorder: A model for the study of addictions in youth. *J Psychopharmacol.* 2006;**20**(4): 580–8.

46. Schubiner H, Saules KK, Arfken CL, *et al.* Double-blind placebo-controlled trial of methylphenidate in

the treatment of adult ADHD patients with comorbid cocaine dependence. *Exp Clin Psychopharmacol.* 2002;**10**(3):286–94.

47. Levin FR, Evans SM, Brooks DJ, *et al.* Treatment of methadone-maintained patients with adult ADHD: Double-blind comparison of methylphenidate, bupropion and placebo. *Drug Alcohol Depend.* 2006; **81**:137–48.

48. Levin FR, Evans SM, Brooks DJ, Garawi F. Treatment of cocaine dependent treatment seekers with adult ADHD: double-blind comparison of methylphenidate and placebo. *Drug Alcohol Depend.* 2007;**87**(1):20–9.

49. Konstenius M, Jayaram-Lindstrom N, Beck O, Franck J. Sustained release methylphenidate for the treatment of ADHD in amphetamine abusers: a pilot study. *Drug Alcohol Depend.* 2010;**108**(1–2):130–3.

50. Winhusen TM, Somoza EC, Brigham GS, *et al.* Impact of attention-deficit/hyperactivity disorder (ADHD) treatment on smoking cessation intervention in ADHD smokers: a randomized, double-blind, placebo-controlled trial. *J Clin Psychiatry.* 2010;**71**(12): 1680–8.

51. Riggs P, ed. Multi-site of OROS-MPH for ADHD in substance abusing adolescents. Scientific Proceedings of the 56th Annual Meeting for the American Academy of Child and Adolescent Psychiatry, Honolulu HI, American Academy of Child and Adolescent Psychiatry; 2009.

52. Grabowski J, Shearer J, Merrill J, Negus SS. Agonist-like, replacement pharmacotherapy for stimulant abuse and dependence. *Addict Behav.* 2004;**29**(7):1439–64.

53. Volkow N, Wang G, Fowler J, *et al.* Dopamine transporter occupancies in the human brain induced by therapeutic doses of oral methylphenidate. *Am J Psychiatry.* 1998;**155**(10):1325–31.

54. Heil SH, Holmes HW, Bickel WK, *et al.* Comparison of the subjective, physiological, and psychomotor effects of atomoxetine and methylphenidate in light drug users. *Drug Alcohol Depend.* 2002;**67**(2): 149–56.

55. Wilens TE, Adler LA, Weiss MD, *et al.* Atomoxetine treatment of adults with ADHD and comorbid alcohol use disorders. *Drug Alcohol Depend.* 2008;**96**(1–2): 145–54.

56. Adler L, Guida F, Irons S, Shaw D. Open label pilot study of atomoxetine in adults with ADHD and substance use disorder. *J Dual Diagn.* 2010;**6**(3–4): 196–207.

57. Adler L, Wilens T, Zhang S, *et al.* Retrospective safety analysis of atomoxetine in adult ADHD patients with or without comorbid alcohol abuse and dependence. *Am J Addict.* 2009;**18**(5):393–401.

58. Thurstone C, Riggs PD, Salomonsen-Sautel S, Mikulich-Gilbertson SK. Randomized, controlled trial of atomoxetine for attention-deficit/hyperactivity disorder in adolescents with substance use disorder. *J Am Acad Child Adolesc Psychiatry.* 2010;**49**(6): 573–82.

59. Wilens T, Monuteaux M, Snyder L, Moore H, Gignac M. The clinical dilemma of using medications in substance abusing adolescents and adults with ADHD: What does the literature tell us? *J Child Adolesc Psychopharmacol.* 2005;**15**(5):787–98.

60. Wilens TE, Adler LA, Adamson J, *et al.* Misuse and diversion of stimulants prescribed for ADHD: a systematic review of the literature. *J Am Acad Child Adolesc Psychiatry.* 2008;**47**(1):21–31.

61. Wilens TE, Gignac M, Swezey A, Monuteaux MC, Biederman J. Characteristics of adolescents and young adults with ADHD who divert or misuse their prescribed medications. *J Am Acad Child Adolesc Psychiatry.* 2006;**45**(4):408–14.

62. McCabe SE, Knight JR, Teter CJ, Wechsler H. Non-medical use of prescription stimulants among US college students: prevalence and correlates from a national survey. *Addiction.* 2005;**99**(1):96–106.

63. Teter CJ, McCabe SE, LaGrange K, Cranford JA, Boyd CJ. Illicit use of specific prescription stimulants among college students: prevalence, motives, and routes of administration. *Pharmacotherapy.* 2006;**26**(10): 1501–10.

64. Janusis GM, Weyandt LL. An exploratory study of substance use and misuse among college students with and without ADHD and other disabilities. *J Atten Disord.* 2010;**14**(3):205–15.

65. Upadhyaya HP, Kroutil LA, Deas D, *et al.* Stimulant formulation and motivation for nonmedical use of prescription attention-deficit/hyperactivity disorder medications in a college-aged population. *Am J Addict.* 2010;**19**(6):569–77.

66. McCabe SE, Boyd CJ. Sources of prescription drugs for illicit use. *Addict Behav.* 2005;**30**(7):1342–50.

67. McCabe SE, Teter CJ, Boyd CJ. The use, misuse and diversion of prescription stimulants among middle and high school students. *Subst Use Misuse.* 2004;**39**(7): 1095–116.

68. Poulin C. Medical and nonmedical stimulant use among adolescents: from sanctioned to unsanctioned use. *CMAJ.* 2001;**165**(8):1039–44.

69. Poulin C. From attention-deficit/hyperactivity disorder to medical stimulant use to the diversion of prescribed stimulants to non-medical stimulant use: connecting the dots. *Addiction.* 2007;**102**(5):740–51.

70. Arria AM, Garnier-Dykstra LM, Caldeira KM, *et al.* Persistent nonmedical use of prescription stimulants

among college students: possible association with ADHD symptoms. *J Atten Disord*. 2011;**15**(5): 347–56.

71. Kollins SH. ADHD, substance use disorders, and psychostimulant treatment: current literature and treatment guidelines. *J Atten Disord*. 2008;**12**(2): 115–25.

72. Bright GM, Delphia B, Wildberger B, eds. Survey evaluation of the abuse potential of prescription stimulants among patients with ADHD. The 160th Annual Meeting of the American Psychiatric Association, May 19–24, 2007; San Diego, CA; 2007.

73. Kroutil LA, Van Brunt DL, Herman-Stahl MA, *et al.* Nonmedical use of prescription stimulants in the United States. *Drug Alcohol Depend*. 2006;**84**: 135–43.

74. Spencer TJ, Biederman J, Ciccone PE, *et al.* PET study examining pharmacokinetics, detection and likeability, and dopamine transporter receptor occupancy of short- and long-acting oral methylphenidate. *Am J Psychiatry*. 2006;**163**(3):387–95.

75. Parasrampuria D, Schoedel K, Schuller R, *et al.*, eds. Abuse potential of OROS methylphenidate versus immediate-release methylphenidate and placebo. The American Academy of Child and Adolescent Psychiatry/Canadian Academy of Child and Adolescent Psychiatry Joint Annual Meeting; 2005 Oct. 20; Toronto, Canada: AACAP; 2005.

76. Spencer TJ, Bonab AA, Dougherty DD, *et al.* A PET study examining pharmacokinetics and dopamine transporter occupancy of two long-acting formulations of methylphenidate in adults. *Int J Mol Med*. 2010;**25**(2):261–5.

77. Jasinski DR, Krishnan S. Abuse liability and safety of oral lisdexamfetamine dimesylate in individuals with a history of stimulant abuse. *J Psychopharmacol*. 2009; **23**(4):419–27.

78. Levin FR, Evans SM, McDowell DM, Kleber HD. Methylphenidate treatment for cocaine abusers with adult attention-deficit/hyperactivity disorder: a pilot study. *J Clin Psychiatry*. 1998;**59**(6):300–5.

79. Upadhyaya HP, Brady KT, Sethuraman G, Sonne SC, Malcolm R. Venlafaxine treatment of patients with comorbid alcohol/cocaine abuse and attention-deficit/ hyperactivity disorder: a pilot study. *J Clin Psychopharmacol*. 2001;**21**(1):116–18.

80. Levin FR, Evans SM, McDowell DM, Brooks DJ, Nunes E. Bupropion treatment for cocaine abuse and adult attention-deficit/hyperactivity disorder. *J Addict Dis*. 2002;**21**(2):1–16.

81. Somoza EC, Winhusen TM, Bridge TP, *et al.* An open-label pilot study of methylphenidate in the treatment of cocaine dependent patients with adult attention deficit/hyperactivity disorder. *J Addict Dis*. 2004;**23**(1):77–92.

82. Carpentier PJ, de Jong CA, Dijkstra BA, Verbrugge CA, Krabbe PF. A controlled trial of methylphenidate in adults with attention deficit/hyperactivity disorder and substance use disorders. *Addiction*. 2005;**100**(12): 1868–74.

83. Wilens T, Prince JB, Waxmonsky JG, *et al.* An open trial of sustained release bupropion for attention-deficit/hyperactivity disorder in adults with ADHD plus substance use disorders. *J ADHD Relat Disord*. 2010;**1**(3):25–35.

84. Riggs PD, Thompson LL, Mikulich SK, Whitmore EA, Crowley TJ. An open trial of pemoline in drug dependent delinquents with attention deficit hyperactivity disorder. *J Am Acad Child Adolesc Psychiatry*. 1996;**35**:1018–24.

85. Riggs P, Leon S, Mikulich S, Pottle L. An open trial of bupropion for ADHD in adolescents with substance use disorders and conduct disorder. *J Am Acad Child Adolesc Psychiatry*. 1998;**37**(12):1271–8.

86. Riggs PD, Hall SK, Mikulich-Gilbertson SK, Lohman M, Kayser A. A randomized controlled trial of pemoline for attention-deficit/hyperactivity disorder in substance-abusing adolescents. *J Am Acad Child Adolesc Psychiatry*. 2004;**43**(4):420–9.

87. Solhkhah R, Wilens TE, Daly J, *et al.* Bupropion SR for the treatment of substance-abusing outpatient adolescents with attention-deficit/hyperactivity disorder and mood disorders. *J Child Adolesc Psychopharmacol*. 2005;**15**(5):777–86.

88. Szobot CM, Rohde LA, Katz B, *et al.* A randomized crossover clinical study showing that methylphenidate-SODAS improves attention-deficit/hyperactivity disorder symptoms in adolescents with substance use disorder. *Braz J Med Biol Res*. 2008;**41**(3):250–7.

ADHD and learning disorders

Lisa G. Hahn and Joel E. Morgan

Introduction

Learning disorders ("disabilities;" LD) are one of the most common comorbid conditions with ADHD [1–4], with prevalence estimates ranging from 20% to 25% [5]. Conceptually, a LD refers to the presumed presence of cognitive dysfunction that impedes a child's ability to learn knowledge and skills at an appropriate level of expectation relative to age and grade standards [6, 7]. A "learning disability" represents the legal standard for the construct of a LD [8], essentially defined as a discrepancy of a specific magnitude between aptitude/ability and achievement, or unexpectedly low academic achievement [9].

The range of abnormalities of cognition underlying LD are many and represent cognitive dysfunction that spans all domains of cognition, including verbal and language processing, perceptual functions, memory, abstract reasoning, sensorimotor skills, and attention and executive functions. From this perspective it would not be unexpected that a child with ADHD, with deficits in the normal ability to attend, concentrate, control impulses, sit still, and/or stay on task, would demonstrate low academic achievement compared to normative standards. This makes the rather high prevalence rate of ADHD and LD quite understandable.

Readers of this volume know that ADHD is a chronic psychiatric disorder typically diagnosed in childhood that is manifested behaviorally by core symptoms of deficits in attention, impaired impulse control, and hyperactivity, among others. The disorder was initially recognized in the early 1900s by physicians and educational professionals who noticed that some children appeared to have problems with fidgeting, being inattentive and controlling their impulses. The disorder was formally included in the *Diagnostic*

and Statistical Manual of Mental Disorders (DSM) in 1968 [10]. At that time it was named "hyperkinetic reaction of childhood" based on the primary symptom of hyperactivity. In the 1970s research conducted by Virginia Douglas [11] and Susan Campbell [12] led to the term attention deficit disorder (ADD) to describe children who appeared to be inattentive. The disorder was included in the 1980 version of the DSM and was diagnosed as ADD with hyperactivity or ADD without hyperactivity. The current nomenclature is attention-deficit hyperactivity disorder (ADHD) and has three subtypes: inattentive (I), hyperactive/impulsive (HI) or combined (C) [13]. These three subtypes share some commonalities and some differences. For instance the hyperactive/impulsive and combined groups share an externalizing dimension – specifically in terms of increased motoric activity and disinhibition of impulsive behaviors, while the inattentive type may manifest sluggish cognitive tempo (SCT), reflecting more internalized aspects of behavior such as withdrawal, daydreaming, mental fogginess, confusion, slowed motor and processing speed, and quiet inattentiveness [14, 15].

Neurobiology of ADHD

Frontal systems and associated neural networks involving the striatum and cerebellum largely subserve attention and executive functions in man [16–19]. Executive functions refer to a set of higher functions of a self-regulatory nature, aspects of human behavior at the highest levels, and include such essentially human activities as planning, organization, initiating task behavior/getting started, transitioning or changing gears, using feedback, inhibiting impulses, and regulation of emotions and behavior [20]. Executive functions govern abstract reasoning

Attention-Deficit Hyperactivity Disorder in Adults and Children, ed. Lenard A. Adler, Thomas J. Spencer and Timothy E. Wilens.
Published by Cambridge University Press. © Cambridge University Press 2015.

and problem solving, as well [16]. Individuals with ADHD also may exhibit any number of executive function abnormalities.

ADHD is a disorder of abnormal attention and executive functions, characterized by structural cerebral abnormalities and imbalances of dopaminergic and noradrenergic neurotransmitter systems [21–23]. The disorder is associated with abnormalities of the prefrontal cortex (PFC), particularly in the right hemisphere [23, 24], and include the anterior cingulate, dorsolateral PFC, inferior PFC, and regions of the basal ganglia, thalamus, and parietal lobe systems [25]. Patients with ADHD typically have symptoms similar to those with documented acute lesions of the right PFC [26]. ADHD patients with hyperactivity are often said to look "frontal," that is, inattentive, impulsive, disorganized, disinhibited, and emotionally labile [27–29]. Imaging studies have documented disrupted white matter tracks emanating from the PFC in ADHD patients [30] and reduced PFC volume [31].

Neurobiology of LD

As noted above, clinical experience informs that cognitive impairment of almost any nature may contribute to unexpectedly low educational performance, attention deficits being one among them. Children with visual-spatial, memory, language, sensorimotor, and attention and executive dysfunction may, and do, manifest LD.

Since reading disability (sometimes referred to as dyslexia or "developmental dyslexia" to differentiate it from acquired dyslexia, such as may occur in stroke) represents over 80% of those identified as having a learning disability [32, 33], discussion of the neurobiological aspects of LD in this chapter will focus on reading disorders.

There is a very large literature documenting that reading is dependent on the integrity of primarily three neural systems in the left hemisphere (for the vast majority of right-handed individuals, see Chapter 17) and that abnormality of one or more of these systems is associated with reading disorder. These include two posterior brain regions: (1) the parietotemporal system, encompassing portions of the supramarginal gyrus in the inferior parietal lobule, the posterior aspect of the superior temporal gyrus, and portions of the angular gyrus of the parietal lobe; and (2) the occipitotemporal system involving the left occipitotemporal and fusiform gyri [32, 34, 35]. (3) The

third neural system involved in reading is an anterior system, the inferior frontal gyrus, known as Broca's area, a very well-understood system serving the motor aspects of speech and involved in reading, silent reading, and naming [16, 32, 36]. These neural systems of the left hemisphere subserve cognitive functions crucial to reading that promote fluency and automaticity for efficient reading [37]. Note that an efficient reader is one who "automatically" recognizes the words (grapheme-phoneme) without applying much cognitive effort. The more a child does this automatically, without thinking, the more fluent a reader he is.

Children with comorbid ADHD and reading disorders may have multiple neural system abnormalities, including of the aforementioned PFC. Literature is emerging linking attention, the inferior parietal cortex, and reading [38], suggesting that attentional systems of the PFC activate the more posterior reading systems, producing distributed activation of the fronto-temporo-parietal network. From the treatment perspective, clinical evidence supports these findings in that stimulant medication in children with comorbid ADHD and reading disorders may improve reading [39].

ADHD and LD comorbidity

Research has clearly established the deleterious effects of attentional problems on the normal acquisition of academic knowledge and skills [40–43]. If a child is inattentive or hyperactive he/she is unable to readily take advantage of the teaching opportunities in the classroom. It stands to reason that if one is not attending to the lesson that little of the material will be retained. When a student is unable to sustain his attention for the length of a math or reading lesson then important information is missed, which can result in difficulty understanding and building on skills base. Research has shown that a child's ability to control and sustain attention, coupled with participation in the classroom, predicts achievement test scores during the early educational years (i.e., preschool and elementary grades) and later achievement in general [32, 44–63]. Studies examining older children diagnosed with ADHD have shown that such children tend to earn lower scores on standardized achievement tests relative to their neurotypical peers [7, 9, 64–78].

In turn, children with ADHD often earn poorer grades and are more likely to be retained. It is not surprising then that rates of school failure are higher for students with ADHD [50, 62, 79–84]. Similarly, poor attention often results in inadequate independent work habits and the inability to manage one's behaviors [85]. Consequently, a common comorbidity of ADHD is LD.

One study noted that children diagnosed with ADHD and a comorbid learning disability evidenced reduced motor dominance and slowed reading speed, which may suggest anomalies of cerebral lateralization. The results also revealed that when a comorbid learning disability is present these children tend to be less organized than their counterparts who suffer only from ADHD [86].

Some research has identified differences between the inattentive and hyperactive subtypes of ADHD related to learning disabilities. Children diagnosed with ADHD – Inattentive type are more likely to have a concomitant learning disability, have a family history of LD, and generally exhibit slowed speed of cognitive processing [87–92]. It appears that inattention is more significantly related to poor academic achievement than hyperactivity [90, 93, 94]. Furthermore, parents and teachers tend to report greater homework problems and school difficulties in children with the inattentive subtype of ADHD [71].

Merrell and Tymms conducted a study using teacher rating scales that revealed significantly greater inattentive behaviors in children with poor performance on reading and math tests [95]. Another study using the Conners' Continuous Performance Test-II [96], CPT-II, a neuropsychological measure of sustained attention and inhibition, reported a relationship between sustained attention and academic achievement in children with ADHD [97].

In general, most studies conducted have shown that children with ADHD and executive dysfunction tend to experience greater academic problems than those with ADHD alone [98, 99]. Preston and colleagues examined three aspects of attention (i.e., sustained, selective, and attentional control/switching) and their effect on academic achievement tests in children with ADHD [100]. The findings revealed that academic achievement was significantly related to performance on measures of attentional control/switching. The higher-order executive function of attentional control/switching requires the child to use working memory, inhibition, and set-shifting simultaneously. The researchers concluded that the results indicate symptoms of inattention are most strongly related to learning problems rather than hyperactivity.

Furthermore, studies have shown that academic difficulties continue into the teens, college, and adult years regardless of age at diagnosis [101, 102]. A relationship between poor academic achievement in teens with ADHD and delinquency has also been reported [103]. A longitudinal study revealed that children diagnosed with ADHD and LD at baseline had increased rates of school dysfunction compared to those diagnosed only with ADHD [104].

Defining LD

A learning disability is defined as a developmental disorder that affects cognition and is related to brain dysfunction. There are several learning disabilities identified in the DSM-IV and these include: reading disorder, mathematics disorder, disorder of written expression, and learning disorder, not otherwise specified (NOS) [13]. A LD is identified by administering a test of aptitude (intellectual function) and a test of academic achievement. The following criteria are set forth by the DSM-IV for each disorder.

A reading disorder is defined based on the following DSM-IV criteria:

1. Reading achievement, as measured by individually administered standardized tests of reading accuracy or comprehension, is substantially below that expected given the person's chronological age, measured intelligence, and age-appropriate education.
2. The disturbance in criterion 1 significantly interferes with academic achievement or activities of daily living that require reading skills.
3. If a sensory deficit is present, the reading difficulties are in excess of those usually associated with it.

A mathematics disorder is similarly defined as a reading disorder.

1. Mathematical ability, as measured by individually administered standardized tests, is substantially below that expected given the person's chronological age, measured intelligence, and age-appropriate education.
2. The disturbance in criterion 1 significantly interferes with academic achievement or activities of daily living that require mathematical ability.
3. If a sensory deficit is present, the difficulties in mathematical ability are in excess of those usually associated with it.

A disorder of written expression is defined as:

1. Writing skills, as measured by individually administered standardized tests (or functional assessments of writing skills), are substantially below those expected given the person's chronological age, measured intelligence, and age-appropriate education.

2. The disturbance in criterion 1 significantly interferes with academic achievement or activities of daily living that require the composition of written texts (e.g., writing grammatically correct sentences and organized paragraphs).

3. If a sensory deficit is present, the difficulties in writing skills are in excess of those usually associated with it.

The term "substantially below the person's chronological age, measured intelligence, and age-appropriate education" is rather vague, which allows each state to interpret this as they see fit. It is the state's decision to decide specifically how a LD will be defined and what will be acceptable for a student to receive academic accommodations.

The most common model utilized to diagnose LD is the discrepancy model [105]. This is based on the difference between the child's aptitude (i.e., intellectual functioning or IQ) and academic achievement, which is not due to lack of adequate instruction or exposure. The most common discrepancy model uses a difference of 1.5 standard deviations to diagnose a LD.

Measuring aptitude and achievement

The gold standard of aptitude measurement is the Wechsler scales. This set of tests is the Wechsler Intelligence Scale for Children – Fourth Edition (WISC-IV; [106]) and the Wechsler Adult Intelligence Scale – Fourth Edition (WAIS-IV; [107]). The WISC-IV consists of 10 core and four optional subtests that measure four domains or indices. Indices and IQs appear as Standard Scores with a mean of 100 and a standard deviation of 15. The first index is the Verbal Comprehension Index (VCI). The VCI measures language expression, comprehension, listening, and the ability to apply these skills to solving problems. The examiner gives the question orally, and a spoken response is required. The second index is the Perceptual Reasoning Index (PRI), which assesses non-verbal problem solving, perceptual organization, and visual-motor proficiency. The directions are given orally and

the answers can be provided verbally or pointing to stimuli or manipulating stimuli. The third index measures working memory (WMI) or the ability to briefly hold and manipulate information. The answers are provided verbally. Finally, the fourth index measures processing speed (PSI), which is achieved through tasks of visual scanning that are completed through a paper and pencil task. The Full Scale IQ provides a comprehensive composite of the subtests. Similar to the WISC-IV, the WAIS-IV also consists of the same four indices. There are 10 core subtests and five optional subtests.

The most common measures of academic achievement are the Woodcock-Johnson Tests of Achievement – Third Edition (WJ-III; [108] and the Wechsler Individual Achievement Test – Third Edition (WIAT-III; [109]). Both tests measure reading, mathematics, writing, academic fluency, and oral language.

Based on the discrepancy model, the most common diagnostic approach, a child with a Standard Score of 100 in verbal comprehension on the WISC-IV whose reading comprehension is a Standard Score of 78 meets criterion 1 and would be diagnosed with a reading disorder. States and school districts may differ in the criteria used to establish the presence of a discrepancy, however (i.e., 1.5 standard deviations or other).

The discrepancy model is often termed the "wait to fail" approach given the necessity of allowing time to pass to see if the child is able to achieve at grade level within the mainstream classroom before providing services. It is not until the child's achievement is significantly below expectation that interventions are then implemented. To reduce the likelihood of the child failing before an evaluation is provided or services are placed, another model called response to intervention (RTI) [9] has been proposed that may alleviate the necessity of the student experiencing failure. This model focuses on a brief screening once teachers recognize the child may be struggling. After the screening is completed then additional instruction is provided thereby circumventing the necessity of allowing the child to fail. After the services have been implemented for a period of time, then a screening is completed again to measure progress. This newer model, however, is not instituted as frequently as the IQ-achievement discrepancy approach. Therefore, the clinical cases, which are presented later in this chapter, will utilize the discrepancy model for diagnostic purposes.

Reading disorder

Research has shown that a reading disorder is often associated with ADHD. Prevalence studies have revealed significantly higher rates of reading disorder in children diagnosed with ADHD, falling between 15% and 50% [56, 110–115]. There are fewer studies examining rates of ADHD in teens diagnosed with reading disorder but of those available the reported rates have been between 15% and 26%, which is rather significant [116–118].

Furthermore, there are reported gender differences with each disorder independently. While reading disorder is approximately equal in gender in community samples, clinic samples (children/teens who present at clinics) have shown that the disorder is roughly four times more prevalent in boys [119–121]. Most clinicians are aware that ADHD tends to be diagnosed more often in boys versus girls but the ratio is again substantially higher in clinic samples when compared to community and school-based samples [122–125].

One study examined children diagnosed with ADHD without a learning disability compared to a sample of children with ADHD and a reading disorder compared to a typically developing comparison group. The results revealed the ADHD-only group exhibited deficits in visual-spatial storage and verbal and visual-spatial functions. The sample of ADHD/learning disordered children performed poorly on both verbal and spatial storage and working memory tasks. The study found that symptoms of inattention were more strongly related to poor executive function performance compared to hyperactivity impairments [126].

Children with ADHD have also evidenced slower reading speeds which can significantly affect their ability to keep up with the classroom instructional pace [86]. Furthermore, when a student's reading speed is slow it becomes more difficult to complete exams and homework assignments in the required time frame. This can have far-reaching consequences because without extended time, the student then may be evaluated on the limited material he/she completed rather than his/her actual knowledge base.

Mathematics disorder

The research examining the relationship between ADHD and mathematics LD compared to a reading disorder is not as vast. The available studies indicate a prevalence rate of 24–60% for math LD in children with ADHD [56, 111, 115].

It appears that in children diagnosed with ADHD, weak working memory is responsible for arithmetic learning problems. When a sample of children with ADHD who had average reading abilities was compared to age- and ability-matched controls, one study found that performance on only working memory was significantly related to poor mathematic performance [127].

Another study reported a relationship between poor math ability and ADHD due to slower speed and less accuracy. The researchers noted that students with ADHD were off-task (i.e., out of their seat, talking, looking away from the board or their work) more often than their non-ADHD peers. This resulted in reduced speed and accuracy [128].

Disorder of written expression

Studies have shown that writing problems are rather common in children [129] and specifically, children with a math or reading disability encounter difficulty with writing [130–133]. However, studies specifically examining writing disorder are rather limited.

Mayes and colleagues found in a sample of children diagnosed with ADHD, 27% met criteria for a reading disorder and 31% for a mathematics disorder [93]. There is a striking difference, however, noted when written expression was assessed. In this particular study, 65% of the ADHD sample also suffered from a disorder of written expression.

Case examples

In order to provide a better idea of how a neuropsychological evaluation informs the professional of the presence of neurocognitive and psychiatric disorders, we present several cases.

Case 1: ADHD and reading disorder

Referral

At the time of the evaluation, K.M. was a 13-year, 6-month-old female adolescent who was referred for a comprehensive neuropsychological evaluation by her parents to evaluate her cognitive abilities and academic skills in order to determine her strengths and weaknesses. Her parents noted that she had a history of difficulty acquiring grade level reading skills.

Brief background information

K.M. was a seventh grade student and was classified as communication impaired. Her mother noted a long-standing history of academic problems and difficulty keeping up with the pace of the classroom. She was not a fluent reader and also had difficulty with math. Her mother stated that even though K.M. learns better in a small group, she has failed to acquire grade level reading skills. Ms. M. reported her daughter's reading resource room class originally had five students, but several months prior to the evaluation the size was increased to reportedly more than 20 students. She received resource room instruction for language arts and mathematics as well as in-class support for science and social studies. She participated in speech and language therapy twice a week in school. Ms. M. reported her daughter failed to make adequate progress in her current program despite the academic interventions.

K.M. was the youngest child of parents who both obtained post-graduate degrees. Her mother reported age-appropriate social skills although she noted K.M. had trouble keeping up with the pace of conversation with her peers. Her medical history was notable for a febrile seizure at age five. She achieved her developmental milestones within normal limits, although they reportedly were at the lower end of the normal range. Family medical history was notable for cancer, hypertension, diabetes, heart disease, stroke, ADHD, and depression.

With regard to emotional and behavioral history, Ms. M. noted her daughter easily and frequently became frustrated and angry because she had trouble keeping up with the pace of conversations. But she recovered quickly and preferred not to talk about it.

Previous evaluations

An educational evaluation was completed 6 months prior to the neuropsychological evaluation. At that time, K.M.'s WIAT-II Reading Composite score fell in the severely impaired range (1st percentile), Math Composite score fell in the average range (27th percentile), and Written Language Composite score fell in the borderline range (5th percentile). K.M.'s word reading was at the 6th percentile (3.8 grade level), reading comprehension was below the 1st percentile (2.9 grade level), and pseudoword decoding was at the 2nd percentile (1.5 grade level). Her spelling skills fell at the 14th percentile (4.5 grade level) and written expression was at the 2nd percentile (3.0 grade level).

A psychological evaluation was also completed in a similar time frame. The results indicated a WISC-IV

Full Scale IQ of 87, VCI score of 99, PRI score of 88, WMI score of 68, and PSI score of 100.

A neuropsychological evaluation was completed 5 years earlier and revealed that K.M.'s WISC-IV Full Scale IQ, PRI and PSI were all average. Her VCI was low average and her WMI was in the borderline range. Her academic achievement based on the WJ-III indicated Broad Reading fell in the borderline range while Math and Written Language were normal. Her Academic Fluency was low average. Visual-spatial skills and motor functions were intact. K.M. was diagnosed with a reading disorder.

Behavioral observations

K.M. easily separated from her mother and transitioned to the examining room. She was a timid and shy young lady; however, she readily answered the examiner's questions. She was very pleasant and cooperative throughout the evaluation, even when certain tasks were quite difficult for her. She appeared embarrassed if she did not know the answer to a question but usually with encouragement she would attempt to answer. She was very responsive to praise. Aside from these observations, her spontaneous speech was fluent, grammatical, and free of paraphasic errors. There was no evidence for clinically significant aphasia or an underlying thought disorder during testing. Further, there was no evidence of frank neurobehavioral anomalies such as dysphasia, dystaxia, or gait or balance disturbance.

Test results

K.M.'s overall Full Scale IQ fell at the 14th percentile, which is low average. Her verbal comprehension and processing speed were intact (34th and 58th percentiles). However, her perceptual organization was low average (12th percentile) while her working memory was moderately impaired (2nd percentile).

Review of K.M.'s academic achievement revealed significant weakness in reading including fluency with scores in the low average to severely impaired range. Her math abilities were average. The discrepancy between K.M.'s overall Full Scale IQ and Broad Reading noted on the WJ-III revealed a difference of 15 points.

In addition, K.M.'s performance on a measure of sustained attention revealed significant inattention with mild impulsivity. Her auditory attention was very poor as was her selective inhibition (both falling in the borderline range). Her divided attention or ability to shift set was low average and letter fluency was severely impaired.

K.M.'s fine motor dexterity was borderline for her dominant right hand and severely impaired for her non-dominant hand.

Language skills revealed intact verbal abstract reasoning, vocabulary, and comprehension. However, visual object naming was severely impaired.

Her learning and memory was variable. When presented with a list of unrelated words (rote learning/memory), her recall was in the low average range. Her ability to learn and retrieve stories was in the borderline range. Her recall of complex visual information and pictures was severely impaired.

K.M.'s ability to copy a complex figure was reduced, falling in the low average range. Her judgment of line orientations fell in the borderline range.

Summary

K.M. completed comprehensive neuropsychological testing that revealed weaknesses in numerous cognitive areas including executive function (sustained attention, inhibition, selective inhibition, auditory attention, letter fluency, fine motor dexterity, working memory, and retrieval of visual stimuli). Furthermore, significant language and reading impairments were noted. This profile was consistent with areas of severe weakness in the dominant (left) hemisphere, given the poor reading and fine motor skills, and bilateral frontal region, given the executive dysfunction. In addition, weakness of the fronto-tempo-parietal system was also present given poor visual-spatial and visual learning skills. She also struggled to complete reading and writing tasks quickly and accurately. In sum, the following diagnoses were warranted: reading disorder, ADHD – inattentive type, and impaired academic fluency.

At the age of 13, the severity of K.M.'s reading disability was striking. Research indicates that remediation of reading impairment becomes more difficult with increasing age. She required immediate, intensive, one-on-one reading instruction to bring her up to age/grade expectations and ensure that she did not continue to fall further behind her peers.

Recommendations

Despite its efforts, the school district failed to adequately remediate K.M.'s severe disabilities, particularly her reading disability. The potential negative consequences of carrying such a severe reading disability into later grades is increased frustration, further deterioration of academic skills development, failure to keep up with instructional demands and pacing, further erosion of her self-esteem and the probable development of an emotional disorder such as anxiety and/or depression. As time goes on in middle school and high school, if left un-remediated, the demands placed on her reading ability will heighten, as textbooks will all be well beyond her capacity. She will struggle even more and become more frustrated. Her potential for achievement in all classes, so dependent as it is on fundamental reading skills, will plummet.

Keeping K.M. in the public school atmosphere with most all neurotypical students will increase her sense of being different, of being "stupid" and not like everyone else. Further, at her age, and with many normal abilities, placing her in a self-contained program will be equally deleterious and destructive to her self-esteem, emotionality, social relations, and sense of belongingness. She needed an atmosphere where the students were more similar to her, not more different.

It was strongly recommended that K.M. be placed in an out of district school specifically for students with severe learning disabilities. Because K.M.'s reading skills were seriously deficient and grossly behind her peers, she needed a small, supportive academic atmosphere of like-peers to assist with basic reading and writing, reading comprehension, spelling, punctuation, phonemic awareness, and other academic language domains, as they were all severely affected and sadly District had been unable to address her needs.

K.M. also needed to work with a professional trained in a multi-sensory reading instruction method such as Lindamood-Bell, Orton Gillingham, or the Wilson Method. These methods of reading instruction have a research track record and are indicated for reading disordered students. It was imperative that this type of training be immediately initiated in order to provide K.M. with the intense therapy she needed as well as consistency in teaching/learning style. She required at least 1 hour of individual reading instruction by a reading specialist 5 days per week. Clearly, K.M. had failed to make adequate gains in her current program and was almost 6 years behind her peers in reading comprehension. The small group instruction in her current academic setting, which originally consisted of 5 students, had grown to 20 students. Classes of 5 students would likely be too large for K.M. given her severe reading disorder. K.M. was entering the eighth grade in the fall yet was reading at the 3.9 grade level. Since K.M.'s current academic placement had not provided the necessary intensive reading training program to bring her skills up to an appropriate level, a specialty out of district placement for students with severe reading disabilities was strongly recommended. Such a placement would provide an extended school year with intensive reading instruction in an atmosphere where all teachers and staff were experienced in providing the emotional support and encouragement such students need. K.M. should be placed in an academic environment that was small, structured, and provides multi-sensory instruction. She required a slow paced instructional method that was repetitive, given her attention and memory disorders. Given her array of learning disabilities, specifically the severity of the Reading disorder along with the presence of ADHD, she required intense academic instruction. In order to meet her emotional needs, she required a supportive and nurturing environment. It was imperative that K.M. be placed in an environment with other children with learning challenges such as hers. This was considered necessary in order to foster a feeling of acceptance and belonging rather than isolation or even being ostracized due to her different learning needs. Specifically, because K.M. was painfully aware of her disabilities she was at risk for consequent emotional disorder.

Given the presence of ADHD, several accommodations should be provided to reduce K.M.'s distractibility. First, preferential seating should be provided and directions/instructions should be repeated and provided in written format. Her teachers should review her homework assignments with her prior to her leaving the classroom. These accommodations are fully a part of the type of out of district placement recommendations, as are the following.

To adequately meet K.M.'s unique learning needs she required training in metacognitive strategies. This training should be implemented in each subject so that she was instructed in varied ways to approach the different activities that required organization and integration of self-monitoring techniques to improve attention. Assisting her with creating a plan or breaking down projects into small steps was optimal. In addition, working with K.M. on study skills to help improve her visual and verbal learning/memory was suggested. For example, teaching K.M. how to create note cards and rehearse would assist her with memorization of rote material.

In addition, K.M.'s parents should consult with their physician about the possibility of pharmacological treatment for ADHD. K.M.'s poor attention would interfere with her ability to adequately attend during academic instruction. The greater concern was her severe reading disorder and the affect her ADHD had on her ability to attend during remediation lessons. Without medication, she was at-risk of continuing to encounter significant difficulty paying attention and gaining academic skills.

It was strongly suggested that K.M. undergo a repeat neuropsychological evaluation in approximately 1 year. This was considered helpful because assessing her cognitive abilities after the above recommendations had been implemented would provide information on the efficacy of the interventions.

If K.M.'s mood and behavior appeared to change, a consultation with a pediatric psychologist was recommended to assess for depression or other emotional disorder.

Case 2: ADHD, major depression, and mixed receptive-expressive disorder and prenatal drug addiction

Referral question

B.W. was a 10-year, 6-month-old boy who was referred for a comprehensive neuropsychological evaluation by his Division of Youth and Family Services (DYFS) caseworker as he was a ward of the state. B.W. was currently enrolled in the fourth grade and was diagnosed with ADHD. He had a history of aggressive as well as sexually inappropriate behaviors. His caseworker and the DYFS nurse were interested in obtaining a better understanding of B.W.'s current cognitive functioning and to provide recommendations for educational planning.

Background information

At birth, B.W. tested positive for opiates. He was removed from his mother's care when she was arrested and incarcerated for burglarizing vehicles when he was 5 years old. He reportedly witnessed his mother using illegal substances and also obtained illicit drugs for her. He also witnessed his mother being physically abused by boyfriends.

Although the records indicate he was diagnosed with ADHD, a formal neuropsychological evaluation had not been conducted. He was prescribed Vyvanse but the medication was discontinued at age 9 due to poor growth. He was prescribed Atarax 50 mg for sleep. A medical evaluation noted lack of growth, allergies, and possible signs of physical abuse "due to parallel linear marks" on B.W.'s forearm and upper back. B.W. had a history of aggressive and defiant behavior including fire setting. He had on several occasions required physical restraints because he was physically aggressive toward staff and residents at his group home. B.W. was granted weekend visits with a great-aunt until he began to display sexually inappropriate behavior and draw sexually explicit pictures. A psychosocial evaluation resulted in a diagnosis of impulse control disorder, NOS and ADHD – combined type.

Educational history revealed B.W. was enrolled in the third grade and had been retained twice. He was classified as emotionally disturbed. He was reportedly reading at the 4.1 grade level and his math skills fell at the 2.8 grade level. He engaged in many acting out behaviors in school. He was aggressive, hyperactive, inattentive, defiant, and argumentative.

Behavioral observations and mental status examination

When testing began the patient evidenced a low frustration tolerance and poor self-esteem. He quickly gave up on tasks and required a significant amount of verbal encouragement. He was responsive to using a sticker system to earn time to use his PSP but again required reminders that he needed to cooperate to earn stickers. When verbally praised for completing a difficult task he attempted to hide a smile. He was impulsive and easily distracted by external stimuli. For example, a fly was in the room and he watched the bug fly around the room. He needed to be reminded to focus on the task at hand. Surprisingly, he was not distracted by people walking in and out of the dining room. After testing in the dining room for an hour, however, the examiners decided it was not conducive to testing and were able to move to a private office. Although B.W. appeared less distracted in this environment he continued to engage in impulsive behavior and required a great deal of prompting to remain on task. His affect and mood were appropriate to the testing situation. He appeared to enjoy making comments that would get the attention of the examiners. Aside from these observations, his spontaneous speech was fluent, grammatical, and free of paraphasic errors. His speech was notable for mild articulation problems. There was no evidence for clinically significant aphasia or an underlying thought

disorder. Further, there was no evidence of frank neurobehavioral anomalies such as dysphasia, dystaxia, or gait or balance disturbance.

Test results

B.W.'s overall intellectual functioning fell at the 37th percentile, which is average. While his vocabulary was weak (16th percentile), abstract reasoning and comprehension were average (37th and 63rd percentiles). His visual-motor integration and non-verbal abstract reasoning were average to high average (63rd and 84th percentiles). His digit span and letter-number sequencing were average (63rd percentiles) and his visual scanning with motor integration was intact (37th percentile). His ability to draw increasingly complex designs and category fluency were average.

His academic achievement was below expectation with respect to word reading and math calculation. However, his reading comprehension, spelling, and phoneme awareness were intact. His academic fluency was average.

B.W.'s sustained visual attention was very poor and he scored in the inattentive range on five out of eight indicators. His selective inhibition fell at the 6th percentile and divided attention was at the 5th percentile. B.W.'s letter fluency was in the borderline range. His fine motor dexterity was impaired.

His verbal learning and memory for stories was below expectation (low average range) and his rote (lists) learning and memory was borderline. His recall of complex visual information was poor. However, his picture learning and memory was average.

Summary

B.W. completed comprehensive neuropsychological testing that revealed deficits in the area of executive function, namely attention, inhibition/impulse control, word retrieval, retrieval of complex visual information, and motor planning and organization. Clinical observations were consistent with the neuropsychological findings warranting a diagnosis of ADHD – combined type. A mathematics disorder and receptive and expressive language disorder were also present. Vocabulary was weak, as was verbal fluency. In addition, weakness in fine motor skills/dyspraxia and verbal memory were noted. B.W. also has significant difficulty retrieving verbal information. A diagnosis of cognitive disorder, NOS was also warranted. All other areas – intellectual functioning, academic achievement, visual learning and memory, and visual-perceptual skills were average or better.

There was convergent evidence of dysfunction of bilateral frontal cerebral systems with the presence of inattentiveness, impulsivity, verbal initiation, retrieval of complex visual information, and fine motor deficits, consistent with ADHD. Evidence of weakness of the dominant (left) hemisphere was found with the presence of language difficulties and math weakness. Furthermore, weakness of the dominant fronto-temporal region is noted given the poor verbal memory abilities.

Personality/emotional implications

Based on our clinical observations and historical information gleaned from the available records, B.W.'s acting out behavior was likely related to his feelings of abandonment. He wanted to be accepted by adults and was eager to please them as was evident during the neuropsychological evaluation. Unfortunately, he had been let down by his family members on numerous occasions, specifically his own mother, whom he should have been able to rely on to provide a safe and caring home and emotional support. When these feelings of abandonment surfaced he was filled with anger and resentment. For example, he expected his family to visit him on his tenth birthday but no one did. He strongly desired to be like any other child who had a family that cared about him and accepted him. When his expectations of his family were not fulfilled he was unable to contain his negative feelings and an emotional outburst results. This coupled with his poor emotional controls and low frustration tolerance related to ADHD all come to the forefront. Children with ADHD already struggle to adequately control their emotions and inhibitions. For a child who also had a background of neglect and abandonment with a resultant superimposed emotional disorder, it was not surprising that B.W. acted out in a physically aggressive manner. His coping skills were very poor.

Recommendations

The following recommendations were to be included in B.W.'s Individualized Education Plan (IEP) to assist with helping to increase B.W.'s academic development given the diagnosis of ADHD – combined type, mathematics disorder, receptive-expressive language disorder, and cognitive disorder, NOS.

B.W.'s educational setting should integrate accommodations typically used for children with attention and impulsivity problems. Some simple accommodations would be especially helpful to reduce distractibility and improve attention. For example, preferential seating should be provided in that B.W. should be seated closest to the teacher. Directions should be given in verbal and written format. Any handouts provided by the teacher should be simple and clearly written to avoid distractions. In addition, copies of teachers' notes would help B.W. review the material he may have missed during class due to ADHD (i.e., inattentiveness). B.W.'s teachers needed to repeat and then review instructions with him to ensure that he was able to process the directions. They also needed to review his homework assignments with him prior to him leaving the classroom and to provide written instructions.

B.W.'s teachers should provide positive feedback to B.W. when he was on task, turned in work on-time, and followed directions. He needed to experience a positive environment, especially at school, where he felt accepted regardless of his learning disabilities. His teachers should work on having his peers encourage him as well.

An aide needs to work with B.W. to provide individual attention in order to ensure he remained on task. This additional support would also help to reduce B.W.'s frustration with academic tasks and would likely result in less frequent outbursts in the classroom.

A behavior modification program was strongly suggested for the classroom. B.W. was responsive to a sticker chart that allowed him to work for time playing his PSP. While he required reminders about the chart and his goal, the chart was successful in helping him cooperate and complete the 4 hours of challenging testing.

Given B.W.'s unique learning needs he required training in metacognitive strategies. He needed guidance in learning different ways to approach activities/school work that required organization. He would also benefit from learning to integrate self-monitoring techniques to improve his attention and impulsivity. Training provided by a speech and language therapist or cognitive remediation therapist to show him how to create a plan or break down projects into small steps was strongly suggested so that he learned this vital tool to academic success. His sessions should also provide instruction in mnemonic devices to help him learn to retain verbal information.

Because of B.W.'s slowed processing speed and academic fluency, he required extended time on all academic tasks including standardized testing.

Based on the available records it seemed at the time of the evaluation, B.W. was not prescribed any pharmacological medications to treat ADHD. He required a consultation with a pediatric psychiatrist to review potential medications. His ADHD symptoms were moderate to severe and without the assistance of medication B.W. was likely to continue to struggle both academically as he would miss out on important information/lessons and emotionally as he would continue to encounter difficulty controlling his emotional outbursts.

B.W. required intense one-on-one math instruction to assist with learning math skills. He failed to master basic math facts and was performing at the second grade level.

Intense speech/language therapy was also needed to address B.W.'s expressive/receptive language deficits, specifically in the areas of word naming, vocabulary, and retrieval.

B.W. was easily overwhelmed with complex information and he would likely experience difficulty if given academic work with too many options. For example, multiple choice tasks with four or more options were too many for B.W. He would do best with two options or true/false formats. In addition when evaluating his academic skills, he would benefit from cueing to assist with recall.

In addition to the recommendations for B.W.'s academic setting several other suggestions were equally important to assist with B.W.'s emotional development.

Given B.W.'s background of neglect and abandonment as well as the recent question of possible sexual and physical abuse, it was very important that he participated in counseling with a trained professional. Quite often children who are abused do not readily reveal this information until a strong therapeutic relationship has been established. In order to provide B.W. with the best opportunity to come to terms with his early childhood he needed therapy.

While B.W. was socially appropriate with the examiners, the records indicated significant social problems with peers. It was strongly recommended that he be enrolled in a social skills program within the school setting as soon as possible. This was an additional means of support for him and would provide the opportunity to create positive friendships under the guidance of a trained educational provider. It was also suggested that the sessions included lessons on how he could appropriately express his feelings, specifically when feeling frustrated or angry with others.

B.W. also would benefit from a mentor program. Establishing a long-term healthy relationship with an adult that was a positive role model would serve to help to teach B.W. how to have an appropriate relationship with adults. This would also provide emotional stability for B.W. beyond his therapeutic relationship with his therapist.

Discussion

In this chapter we presented research evidence documenting the comorbidity of ADHD and LD. Underlying neurobiological abnormalities of both disorders were also presented, as well as in their combined state. The range of comorbidities in ADHD is very broad, encompassing numerous Axis I and II disorders and LD is perhaps among the most common. Children and teens diagnosed with ADHD do not only have to learn to handle the associated symptoms of this disorder but they also frequently suffer from many school-related problems and learning disabilities, which the reader will recognize appear in various manifestations. Appropriate treatment for the management of attention and executive functions is a first step of intervention, as well as appropriate accommodations for educational planning. Patients appropriately treated for ADHD perform better in school as they can take better advantage of the interventions for their learning disabilities.

References

1. Stefanatos GA, Baron IS. Attention-deficit/hyperactivity disorder: a neuropsychological perspective towards DSM-V. *Neuropsychol Rev.* 2007;**17**:5–38.

2. Seager MC, O'Brien G. Attention deficit hyperactivity disorder: review of ADHD in learning disability: the *Diagnostic Criteria for Psychiatric Disorders for Use with Adults with Learning Disabilities/Mental Retardation* [DC-LD] criteria for diagnosis. *J Intellect Disabil Res.* 2003;**47**(Suppl 1):26–31.

3. Barry TD, Lyman RD, Klinger LG. Academic underachievement and attention-deficit/hyperactivity disorder: the negative impact of symptom severity on school performance. *J Sch Psychol.* 2002;**40**(3):259–83.

4. Willicut EG, Pennington BF, Olson RK, Chhabildas N, Hulslander J. Neuropsychological analyses of

comorbidity between reading disability and attention deficit hyperactivity disorder: in search of the common deficit. *Dev Neuropsychol.* 2005;**27**(1):35–78.

5. Pliska SR. Patterns of psychiatric comorbidity with attention-deficit hyperactivity disorder. *Child Adolesc Psychiatry Clin North Am.* 2000;**9**:525–40.

6. Pennington BF. *Diagnosing Learning Disorders: A Neuropsychological Framework,* 2nd edn. New York, NY: Guilford Press; 2009.

7. Fletcher JM, Lyon GR, Fuchs LS, Barnes MA. *Learning Disabilities: From Identification to Intervention*. New York, NY: Guilford Press; 2007.

8. Individuals with Disabilities Education Improvement Act of 2004 (IDEIA). P.L. 108–446; 2004.

9. Fletcher JM, Vaughn S. Response to intervention: preventing and remediating academic difficulties. *Child Dev Perspect.* 2009;**3**:30–7.

10. American Psychiatric Association. *Diagnostic and Statistical Manual of Mental Disorders*, 2nd edn (DSM-II). Washington, DC: American Psychiatric Association; 1968.

11. Douglas VI. Stop, look and listen: the problem of sustained attention and impulse control in hyperactive and normal children. *Can J Behav Sci.* 1972;**4**:259–82.

12. Campbell SB. Mother-child interaction in reflective, impulsive and hyperactive children. *Dev Psychol.* 1973;**8**:341–9.

13. American Psychiatric Association. *Diagnostic and Statistical Manual of Mental Disorders*, 4th edn (DSM-IV). Washington, DC: American Psychiatric Association; 2000.

14. Bauermeister JJ, Barkley RA, Bauermeister JA, Martinez JV, McBurnett, K. Validity of the sluggish cognitive tempo, inattention, and hyperactivity symptom dimensions: neuropsychological and psychosocial correlates. *J Abnorm Child Psychol.* 2012;**40**:683–97.

15. Milich R, Balentine AC, Lynam DR. ADHD/combined type and ADHD/predominantly inattentive type are distinct and unrelated disorders. *Clin Psychol Sci Pract.* 2001;**8**:463–88.

16. Lezak MD, Howieson DB, Bigler ED, Tranel D. *Neuropsychological Assessment,* 5th edn. New York, NY: Oxford University Press; 2012.

17. Blumenfeld H. *Neuroanatomy through Clinical Cases,* 2nd edn. Sunderland, MA: Sinauer Associates, Inc. 2010.

18. Heilman KM, Valenstein E. *Clinical Neuropsychology,* 5th edn. New York, NY: Oxford University Press; 2011.

19. Darby D, Walsh K. *Walsh's Neuropsychology: A Clinical Approach,* 5th edn. Edinburgh: Churchill Livingstone; 2005.

20. Biederman J, Seidman LJ, Petty CR, *et al.* Effects of stimulant medication on neuropsychological functioning in young adults with attention-deficit/hyperactivity disorder. *J Clin Psychiatry.* 2008;**69**(7):1150–6.

21. Seidman LJ, Valera EM, Makris N. Structural brain imaging of attention-deficit/hyperactivity disorder. *Biol Psychiatry.* 2005;**57**(11):1263–72.

22. Spencer TJ, Biederman J, Mick E. Attention-deficit/hyperactivity disorder: diagnosis, lifespan, comorbidities, and neurobiology. *J Pediatr Psychol* 2007;**32**(6):631–42.

23. Arnsten AFT. The emerging neurobiology of attention deficit hyperactivity disorder: the key role of the prefrontal association cortex. *J Pediatr.* 2009; **154**(5):I-S43.

24. Clark L, Blackwell A, Aron A, *et al.* Association between response inhibition and working memory in adult ADHD: a link to right frontal cortex pathology? *Biol Psychiatry.* 2007;**61**:1395–401.

25. Makris N, Biederman J, Valera EM, *et al.* Cortical thinning of the attention and executive function networks in adults with attention-deficit/hyperactivity disorder. *Cereb Cortex.* 2007;**17**(6): 1364–75.

26. Rubia K, Smith A, Taylor E. Performance of children with attention deficit hyperactivity disorder (ADHD) on a test battery of impulsiveness. *Child Neuropsychol.* 2007;**13**(3):276–304.

27. Aron AR, Robbins TW, Poldrack RA. Inhibition and the right inferior frontal cortex. *Trends Cogn Sci.* 2004;**8**(4):170–7.

28. Davidson RJ, Putnam KM, Larson CL. Dysfunction in the neural circuitry of emotion regulation – a possible prelude to violence. *Science.* 2000;**289**(5479): 591–4.

29. Stuss DT, Gow CA, Hetherington CR. "No longer Gage": frontal lobe dysfunction and emotional changes. *J Consult Clin Psychol.* 1992;**60**(3): 349–59.

30. Makris N, Buka SL, Biederman J, *et al.* Attention and executive systems abnormalities in adults with childhood ADHD: a DT-MRI study of connections. *Cereb Cortex.* 2007;**18**(5):1210–20.

31. Seidman LJ, Valera EM, Makris N, *et al.* Dorsolateral prefrontal and anterior cingulate cortex volumetric abnormalities in adults with attention-deficit/hyperactivity disorder identified by magnetic resonance imaging. *Biol Psychiatry.* 2006;**60**(10):1071–80.

32. Shaywitz SE, Shaywitz BA. Paying attention to reading: the neurobiology of reading and dyslexia. *Dev Psychopathol.* 2008;**20**(4):1329–49.

33. Lerner J. Educational interventions in learning disabilities. *J Am Acad Child Adolesc Psychiatry*. 1989;**28**:326–31.

34. Fiebach CJ, Friederici AD, Muller K, Cramon DYV. fMRI evidence for dual routes to the mental lexicon in visual word recognition. *J Cogn Neurosci*. 2002; **14**:11–23.

35. Brambati S, Termine C, Ruffino M, *et al.* Neuropsychological deficits and neural dysfunction in familial dyslexia. *Brain Res*. 2006;**1113**:174–85.

36. Frackowiak R, Friston K, Frith C, *et al. Human Brain Function,* 2nd edn. San Diego, CA: Academic Press/Elsevier Science; 2004.

37. Shaywitz SE, Shaywitz BA. Psychopathology of dyslexia and reading disorders. In: *Psychopathology of Childhood and Adolescence: A Neuropsychological Approach* New York, NY: Springer Publishing Company. 2013; 109–26.

38. Nakamura K, Dehaene S, Jobert A, Le Bihan D, Kouider S. Subliminal convergence of Kanji and Kana words: further evidence for functional parcellation of the posterior temporal cortex in visual word perception. *J Cogn Neurosci*. 2005;**17**:954–68.

39. Grizenko N, Bhat M, Schwartz G, Ter-Sttepanian M, Joober R. Efficacy of methylphenidate in children with attention-deficit hyperactivity disorder and learning disabilities: a randomized crossover trial. *J Psychiatry Neurosci*. 2006:**31**:46–51.

40. Halperin JM, Marks DJ, Schulz KP. Neuropsychological perspectives on ADHD. In: Morgan JE, Ricker JH, eds. *Textbook of Clinical Neuropsychology*. New York, NY: Psychology Press. 2008; 333–45.

41. Mapou RL. Learning disabilities in adults. In: Morgan JE, Ricker JH, eds. *Textbook of Clinical Neuropsychology*. New York, NY: Psychology Press; 2008.

42. Rapport MD, Scanlan SW, Denney CB. Attention deficit hyperactivity disorder and scholastic achievement: A model of dual developmental pathways. *J Child Psychol Psychiatry*. 1999;**40**: 1169–83.

43. Silver LB. Psychological and family problems associated with learning disabilities: assessment and intervention. *J Am Acad Child Adolesc Psychiatry*. 1989;**28**:319–25.

44. Alexander KL, Entwisle DR, Dauber SL. First grade classroom behavior: its short- and long-term consequences for school performance. *Child Dev*. 1993;**64**:801–14.

45. Barriga AQ, Doran JW, Newell SB, *et al.* Relationships between problem behaviors and academic achievement in adolescents: the unique role of

46. Cantwell DP. Hyperactive children have grown up: What have we learned about what happens to them? *Arch Gen Psychiatry*. 1985;**4**:1026–8.

47. DeShazo BT, Lyman RD, Klinger LG. Academic underachievement and attention-deficit/hyperactivity disorder: the negative impact of symptom severity on school performance. *Journal of School Psychology*, 2002;**40**(3):259–83.

48. Douglas VI. Stop, look and listen: the problem of sustained attention and impulse control in hyperactive and normal children. *Can J Behav Sci*. 1972;4259–282.

49. Douglas VI. Perceptual and cognitive factors as determinants of learning disabilities: a review chapter with special emphasis on attentional factors. In: Knights RM, Bakker DJ, eds. *The Neuropsychology of Learning Disorders: Theoretical Approaches*. Baltimore: University Park Press. 1976.

50. Faraone SV, Biederman J, Krifcher Lehman B, *et al.* Intellectual performance and school failure in children with attention deficit hyperactivity disorder and in their siblings. *J Abnorm Psychol*. 1993;**102**;616–23.

51. Hinshaw SP. Externalizing behavior problems and academic underachievement in childhood and adolescence: causal relationships and underlying mechanisms. *Psychol Bull*. 1992;**111**:127–55.

52. Holborow PL, Berry PS. Hyperactivity and learning difficulties. *J Learn Disabil*. 1986;**19**:426–31.

53. Kamphaus RW, Frick PJ. *Clinical Assessment of Child and Adolescent Personality and Behavior*. Needham Heights, MA: Allyn & Bacon; 1996.

54. Konold TR, Pianta RC. Empirically-derived, person-oriented patterns of school readiness in typically-developing children: Description and prediction to first-grade achievement. *Appl Dev Sci*. 2005;**9**:174–87.

55. Ladd GW, Birch SH, Buhs ES. Children's social and scholastic lives in kindergarten: related spheres of influence? *Child Dev*. 1999;**70**:1373–400.

56. Lambert NM, Sandoval JH. The prevalence of learning disabilities in a sample of children considered hyperactive. *J Abnorm Child Psychol*. 1980;**8**:33–50.

57. Levine MD, Busch B, Aufseeser C. The dimension of inattention among children with school problems. *Pediatrics*. 1982;**70**:387–95.

58. Normandeau S. Preschool behavior and first-grade achievement: the mediational role of cognitive self-control. *J Educ Psychol*. 1998;**90**:111–21.

59. Raver CC, Smith-Donald R, Hayes T, Jones SM. Self-regulation across differing risk and sociocultural contexts: preliminary findings from the Chicago

attention problems. *J Emot Behav Disord*. 2002;**10**:233–40.

School Readiness Project. Paper presented at the biennial meeting of the Society for Research in Child Development, Atlanta, GA; 2005, April.

60. Silver LB, Brunstetter RW. Attention deficit disorder in adolescents. *Hosp Community Psychiatry*. 1986; **37**:608–13.

61. Trzesniewski KH, Moffitt TE, Caspi A, Taylor A, Maughan B. Revisiting the association between reading achievement and antisocial behavior: new evidence of an environmental explanation from a twin study. *Child Dev*. 2006;**77**:72–88.

62. Weiss G, Hechtman L, Perlman T, Hopkins J, Wener A. Hyperactives as young adults: A controlled prospective ten-year follow-up of 75 children. *Arch Gen Psychiatry*. 1979;**3**:675–81.

63. Wilson J, Marcotte AC. Psychosocial adjustment and educational outcome in adolescents with a childhood diagnosis of attention-deficit disorder. *J Am Acad Child Adolesc Psychiatry*. 1996;**35**(5):579–87.

64. Abikoff H, Courtney ME, Szeibel PJ, Koplewicz HS. The effects of auditory stimulation on the arithmetic performance of children with ADHD and nondisabled children. *J Learn Disabil*. 1996;**29**:238–46.

65. Carlson CL, Tamm L. Responsiveness of children with attention deficit–hyperactivity disorder to reward and response cost: differential impact on performance and motivation. *J Consult Clin Psychol*. 2000;**68**: 73–83.

66. Carter CS, Krener P, Chaderjian M, Northcutt C, Wolfe V. Abnormal processing of irrelevant information in attention deficit hyperactivity disorder. *Psychiatry Res*. 1995;**56**:59–70.

67. Frankenberger W, Cannon C. Effects of Ritalin on academic achievement from first to fifth grade. *Int J Disabil Dev Educ*. 1999;**46**:199–221.

68. Gaub M, Carlson CL. Behavioral characteristics of *DSM-IV* ADHD subtypes in a school-based population. *J Abnorm Child Psychology*. 1997; **25**:103–11.

69. Halperin JM, Newcorn JH, Matier K, *et al.* Discriminant validity of attention-deficit hyperactivity disorder. *J Am Acad Child Adolesc Psychiatry*. 1993;**32**:1038–43.

70. Hoza B, Pelham WE, Dobbs J, Owens JS, Pillow DR. Do boys with attention-deficit/hyperactivity disorder have positive illusory self-concepts? *J Abnorm Psychol*. 2002;**111**:268–78.

71. Lahey BB, Willcutt EG. Validity of the diagnosis and dimensions of attention-deficit/hyperactivity disorder. Paper presented at the National Institutes of Health Consensus Development Conference on the Diagnosis and Treatment of Attention-Deficit/Hyperactivity Disorder, Washington, DC; 1998, November.

72. Purvis KL, Tannock R. Language abilities in children with attention deficit hyperactivity disorder, reading disabilities, and normal controls. *J Abnorm Child Psychol*. 1997;**25**:133–44.

73. Purvis KL, Tannock R. Phonological processing, not inhibitory control, differentiates ADHD and reading disability. *J Am Acad Child Adolesc Psychiatry*. 2000;**39**:485–94.

74. Seidman LJ, Biederman J, Faraone SV, *et al.* A pilot study of neuropsychological function in girls with ADHD. *J Am Acad Child Adolesc Psychiatry*. 1997;**33**:366–73.

75. Semrud-Clikeman M, Guy K, Griffin JD, Hynd GW. Rapid naming deficits in children and adolescents with reading disabilities and attention deficit hyperactivity disorder. *Brain Lang*. 2000;**74**:70–83.

76. Semrud-Clikeman M, Steingard RJ, Filipek M, *et al.* Using MRI to examine brain–behavior relationships in males with attention deficit disorder with hyperactivity. *J Am Acad Child Adolesc Psychiatry*. 2000;**39**:477–84.

77. Tannock R, Martinussen R, Frijters J. Naming speed performance and stimulant effects indicate effortful, semantic processing deficits in attention deficit/ hyperactivity disorder. *J Abnorm Child Psychol*. 2000;**28**:237–52.

78. Zametkin AJ, Liebenauer LL, Fitzgerald GA, *et al.* Brain metabolism in teenagers with attention deficit hyperactivity disorder. *Arch Gen Psychiatry*. 1993;**50**:333–40.

79. Edelbrock C, Costello AJ, Kessler MD. Empirical corroboration of attention deficit disorder. *J Am Acad Child Adolesc Psychiatry*. 1984;**23**(3): 285–90.

80. Gittelman R, Mannuzza S, Shenker R., Bonagura N. Hyperactive boys almost grown up: I. Psychiatric status. *Arch Gen Psychiatry*. 1985;**42**:937–47.

81. Lahey BB, Schaughency EA, Strauss CC, Frame CL. Are attention deficit disorders with and without hyperactivity similar or dissimilar disorders? *J Am Acad Child Adolesc Psychiatry*. 1984;**23**:302–9.

82. Silver LB. The relationship between learning disabilities, hyperactivity, distractibility, and behavioral problems. *J Am Acad Child Adolesc Psychiatry*. 1981;**20**:385–97.

83. Weiss G. Follow up studies on outcome of hyperactive children. *Psychopharmacol Bull*. 1985;**21**: 169–77.

84. Weiss G, Hechtman L, Milroy T, Perlman T. Psychiatric status of hyperactives as adults: a controlled prospective 15-year follow-up of 63 hyperactive children. *J Am Acad Child Adolesc Psychiatry*. 1985;**24**:211–20.

85. Hughes CA, Ruhl KL, Misra A. Self-management with behaviorally disordered students in school settings: a promise unfulfilled? *Behav Disord.* 1989;**14**:250–62.

86. Seidman LJ, Biederman J, Faraone S, *et al.* Effects of family history and comorbidity on the neuropsychological performance of ADHD children: preliminary findings. *J Am Acad Child Adolesc Psychiatry.* 1995;**34**:1015–24.

87. Barkley RA, DuPaul GJ, McMurray MB. A comprehensive evaluation of attention deficit disorder with and without hyperactivity. *J Consult Clin Psychol.* 1990;**58**:775–89.

88. Goodyear P, Hynd GW. Attention-deficit disorder with (ADD/H) and without (ADD/WO) hyperactivity: behavioral and neuropsychological differentiation. *J Clin Child Psychol.* 1992;**21**:273–305.

89. Hynd GW, Lorys AR, Semrud-Clikeman M, *et al.* Attention deficit disorder without hyperactivity: A distinct behavioral and neurocognitive syndrome. *J Child Neurol.* 1991;**6**:S37–43.

90. Lahey BB, Pelham WE, Stein MA, *et al.* Validity of DSM-IV attention-deficit/hyperactivity disorder for young children. *J Am Acad Child Adolesc Psychiatry.* 1998;**37**:695–702.

91. Lahey BB, Schaughency EA, Frame C, Strauss C. Teacher ratings of attention problems in children experimentally classified as exhibiting attention deficit disorder with and without hyperactivity. *J Am Acad Child Adolesc Psychiatry.* 1985;**24**:613–16.

92. Marshall R, Hynd GW, Handwerk M, Hall J. Academic underachievement in ADHD subtypes. *J Learn Disabil.* 1997;**30**:635–42.

93. Mayes SD, Calhoun SL, Crowell EW. Learning disabilities and ADHD: overlapping spectrum disorders. *J Learn Disabil.* 2000;**33**:417–24.

94. Willcutt EG. A twin study of the internal and external validity of DSM-IV attention-deficit/hyperactivity disorder. Unpublished doctoral dissertation, University of Denver, 1998.

95. Merrell C, Tymms PB. Inattention, hyperactivity, and impulsiveness: their impact on academic achievement and progress. *Br J Educ Psychol.* 2001;**71**(1):43–56.

96. Conners CK. *Conners' Continuous Performance Test – Second Edition (CPT- II).* Minneapolis, MN: Pearson Assessments; 2004.

97. Aylward GP, Gordon M., Verhulst SJ. Relationships between continuous performance task scores and other cognitive measures: Causality or commonality? *Assessment.* 1997;**4**(4):325–36.

98. Biederman J, Monuteaux MC, Doyle AE. Impact of executive function deficits and attention-deficit/hyperactivity disorder (ADHD) on academic outcomes in children. *J Consult Clin Psychol.* 2004;**72**(5):757–66.

99. Willcutt EG, Doyle AE, Nigg JT, Faraone SV, Pennington BF. Validity of the executive function theory of attention deficit/hyperactivity disorder: a meta-analytic review. *Biol Psychiatry.* 2005;**57**:1336–46.

100. Preston AS, Heaton SC, McCann SJ, Watson WD, Selke G. The role of multidimensional attentional abilities in academic skills of children with ADHD. *J Learn Disabil.* 2009;**42**:240–9.

101. Faraone SV, Biederman J, Mennin D, Gershon J, Tsuang MG. A prospective four-year follow-up study of children at risk for ADHD: Psychiatric, neuropsychological, and psychosocial outcomes. *J Am Acad Child Adolesc Psychiatry.* 1996;**35**:1449–59.

102. Frazier TW, Demaree HA, Youngstrom EA. A meta-analysis of intellectual and neuropsychological test performance in attention-deficit/hyperactivity disorder. *Neuropsychology.* 2004;**18**:543–55.

103. Pisecco S, Wristers K, Swank P, Silva PA, Baker DB. The effect of academic self-concept on ADHD and antisocial behaviors in early adolescence. *J Learn Disabil.* 2001;**34**:450–61.

104. Faraone SV, Biederman J, Monuteaux JC, Doyle AE, Seidman LJ. A psychometric measure of learning disability predicts educational failure four years later in boys with attention deficit/hyperactivity disorder. *J Atten Disord.* 2001;**4**:220–30.

105. Sattler J. *Psychological Assessment,* 4th edn. New York, NY: McGraw-Hill; 1988.

106. Wechsler D. *Manual for the Wechsler Intelligence Scale for Children – Fourth Edition.* New York, NY: Psychological Corporation; 2008.

107. Wechsler D. *Manual for the Wechsler Adult Intelligence Scale – Fourth Edition.* New York, NY: Psychological Corporation; 2003.

108. Mather N, Woodcock RW. *Woodcock-Johnson III Tests of Achievement Examiner's Manual.* Itasca, IL; Riverside Publishing; 2001.

109. Wechsler D. *Manual for the Wechsler Individual Achievement Test – Third Edition.* New York, NY: Psychological Corporation; 2009.

110. August GJ, Garfinkel BD. Comorbidity of ADHD and reading disability among clinic-referred children. *J Abnorm Child Psychol.* 1990;**18**:29–45.

111. Barkley RA. Associated problems, subtyping, and etiology. In: Barkley RA, ed. *Attention-Deficit Hyperactivity Disorder: A Handbook for Diagnosis and Treatment.* New York, NY: Guilford Press. 1990; 74–105.

112. Dykman RA, Ackerman PT. ADD and specific reading disability: separate but often overlapping disorders. *J Learn Disabil*. 1991;**24**:96–103.

113. Livingston RL, Dykman RA, Ackerman PT. The frequency and significance of additional self-reported psychiatric diagnoses in children with attention deficit disorder. *J Abnorm Child Psychol*. 1990;**18**:465–78.

114. McGee R, Share D. Attention deficit disorder-hyperactivity and academic failure: which comes first and which should be treated? *J Am Acad Child Adolesc Psychiatry*. 1988;**27**:318–25.

115. Semrud-Clikeman M, Biederman J, Sprich-Buckminster S, *et al.* Comorbidity between ADDH and LD: a review and report in a clinically referred sample. *J Am Acad Child Adolesc Psychiatry*. 1992;**31**:439–48.

116. Gilger JW, Pennington BF, De-Fries JC. A twin study of the etiology of comorbidity: attention deficit hyperactivity disorder and dyslexia. *J Am Acad Child Adolesc Psychiatry*. 1992;**31**:343–8.

117. Shaywitz BA, Fletcher JM, Holahan JM, *et al.* Interrelationships between reading disability and attention deficit/hyperactivity disorder. *Child Neuropsychol*. 1995;**1**:170–86.

118. Shaywitz BA, Fletcher JM, Shaywitz SE. Defining and classifying learning disabilities and attention deficit/hyperactivity disorder. *J Child Neurol*. 1995;**10**:S50–7.

119. Pennington BF. *Diagnosing Learning Disabilities*. New York, NY: Guilford Press; 1991.

120. Shaywitz SE, Shaywitz BA, Fletcher JM, Escobar MD. Prevalence of reading disability in boys and girls. *J Am Med Assoc*. 1990;**264**:998–1002.

121. Wadsworth S, DeFries J, Stevenson J, Gilger J, Pennington B. Gender ratios among reading-disabled children and their siblings as a function of parental impairment. *J Child Psychol Psychiatry*, 1992;**7**:1229–39.

122. Barkley RA. *Attention-Deficit Hyperactivity Disorder*. New York, NY: Guilford Press; 1998.

123. Lewinsohn PM, Hops H, Roberts RE, Seeley JR, Andrews JA. Adolescent psychopathology: I. Prevalence and incidence of depression and other DSM-III-R disorders in high school students. *J Abnorm Psychology*. 1993;**102**:133–44.

124. McGee R, Feehan M, Williams S, *et al.* DSM-III disorders in a large sample of adolescents. *J Am Acad Child Adolesc Psychiatry*. 1990;**29**:611–19.

125. Szatmari P, Offord DR, Boyle MH. Correlates, associated impairments, and patterns of service utilization of children with attention-deficit disorders: findings from the Ontario Child Health Study. *J Child Psychol Psychiatry*. 1989;**30**:205–17.

126. Martinussen R, Tannock R. Working memory impairments in children with attention-deficit hyperactivity disorder with and without comorbid language learning disorders. *J Clin Exp Neuropsychol*. 2006;**28**:1073–94.

127. McLean F, Hitch GJ. Working memory impairments in children with specific arithmetic learning difficulties. *J Exp Child Psychol*. 1999;**74**:240–60.

128. Zentall SS, Smith YN, Lee YB, Wieczorek C. Mathematical outcomes of attention-deficit hyperactivity disorder. *J Learn Disabil*. 1994;**27**(8):510–19.

129. Hooper SR, Swartz CW, Wakely MB, de Kruif RE, Montgomery JW. Executive functions in elementary school children with and without problems in written expression. *J Learn Disabil*. 1993;**35**:57–68.

130. Bruck M. The adult outcome of children with learning disabilities. *Ann Dyslexia*. 1985;**37**:252–63.

131. Keefe CH, Candler AC. LD students and word processors: questions and answers. *Learn Disabil Focus*. 1989;**4**:78–83.

132. Kerchner LB, Kistinger BJ. Language processing/word processing: written expression, computers and learning disabled students. *Learn Disabil Quart*. 1984;**7**:329–35.

133. Poplin M, Gray R, Larsen S, Banikowski A, Mehring T. A comparison of written expression abilities in learning disabled and non-learning disabled students at three grade levels. *Learn Disabil Quart*. 1980;**3**:46–53.

Chapter 12

Oppositional defiant disorder and conduct disorder

Alison M. Cohn and Andrew Adesman

Introduction

Oppositional defiant disorder (ODD) and conduct disorder (CD) comprise the disruptive behavior disorders (DBDs) in the *Diagnostic and Statistical Manual of Mental Disorders* (DSM-5 [1]). ODD and CD, which are the most common conditions that are comorbid with ADHD, are the predominant juvenile disorders that are referred to mental health and community clinics. Features of DBDs can range from noncompliance and disobedience to more dangerous behavior, including aggressive hostility toward authorities or peers. These disorders cause noticeable impairment and pose immense complications in the lives of affected children and adolescents. When they are comorbid with ADHD, treatment of ADHD becomes more complicated and prognosis typically worsens. For example, ADHD is often effectively treated with medication alone, but ADHD with a comorbid diagnosis of ODD or CD requires a multimodal treatment approach, with a combination of medication and behavior therapy.

Beyond the disruptive and antisocial behavior in youth, DBDs can precede sociopathic behavior in adulthood. Developmental precursors and pathways to adult maladjustment can be seen even in children as young as 3 or 4 years old. Additionally, since ODD and CD frequently present with a variety of serious comorbid disorders, the lives of children and adolescents with these diagnoses can be even more turbulent and impaired. Since treatment of these disorders often requires multiple modalities – including a combination of pharmacological treatment, behavioral parent training (BPT), interpersonal skills training, and family therapy – early intervention may be the most critical step in preventing the progression of these disorders into more serious and stable problems [2]. Identifying

the key developmental precursors to DBDs and potential interventions to treat the behavioral disorders is crucial for attaining the optimal outcome in patients with these diagnoses and preventing further problems in their adult lives.

This chapter first presents an overview of the diagnostic criteria for and epidemiological features of ODD and CD individually, and then reviews the etiology, comorbid diagnoses, evaluation, and treatment for both DBDs.

Oppositional defiant disorder

Definition and diagnostic criteria

ODD is characterized by a pattern of negativistic, hostile, defiant, and disobedient behavior, often directed toward authority figures. Since many of these features are seen in children and adolescents who do not have the disorder, ODD can be diagnosed only when the behaviors are more frequent and severe than would normally be expected at the child's developmental level. The behaviors must also cause clinically significant functional impairment in order to reach the threshold for diagnosis. The complete DSM-5 criteria for ODD can be seen in Table 12.1. Some examples of DSM criteria include "often loses temper," "often argues with adults," and "often blames others for his or her mistakes or misbehavior" [1]. At least four out of eight symptoms must be present for at least 6 months. To differentially diagnose ODD, criteria cannot be met for CD. An individual cannot simultaneously be diagnosed with ODD and CD because a diagnosis of CD subsumes the ODD symptoms. Lastly, in individuals over the age of 18, criteria cannot be met for antisocial personality disorder (ASPD).

Attention-Deficit Hyperactivity Disorder in Adults and Children, ed. Lenard A. Adler, Thomas J. Spencer and Timothy E. Wilens.
Published by Cambridge University Press. © Cambridge University Press 2015.

Table 12.1. Diagnostic criteria for oppositional defiant disorder

A. *A pattern of negativistic, hostile, and defiant behavior lasting at least 6 months, during which four (or more) of the following are present:*
 (1) often loses temper
 (2) often argues with adults
 (3) often actively defies or refuses to comply with adults' requests or rules
 (4) often deliberately annoys people
 (5) often blames others for his or her mistakes or misbehavior
 (6) is often touchy or easily annoyed by others
 (7) is often angry and resentful
 (8) is often spiteful or vindictive.

Note: Consider a criterion met only if the behavior occurs more frequently than is typically observed in individuals of comparable age and developmental level.

B. The disturbance in behavior causes clinically significant impairment in social, academic, or occupational functioning.

C. The behaviors do not occur exclusively during the course of a Psychotic or Mood Disorder.

D. Criteria are not met for Conduct Disorder, and, if the individual is age 18 years or older, criteria are not met for Antisocial Personality Disorder.

Source: American Psychiatric Association [1]. Reprinted with permission from the *Diagnostic and Statistical Manual of Mental Disorders, Fifth Edition* (Copyright © 2013). American Psychiatric Association. All rights reserved.

Epidemiology

Prevalence estimates for ODD can vary depending on the population demographics, diagnostic criteria and assessment tools, informant, and whether point prevalence or lifetime prevalence is considered. In the general population, prevalence estimates range from 2% to 16% in children and adolescents [3]. The National Comorbidity Survey Replication, which used DSM-IV criteria, studied over 3000 adults to establish prevalence figures. In this retrospective study, prevalence was found to be 10.2% overall, and 11.2% and 9.2% for males and females respectively [4].

In terms of demographic factors, slightly more boys than girls meet diagnostic criteria for ODD in childhood, but the gap decreases in adolescence, leaving no noticeable gender difference after age 13 [5]. Additionally, ODD is more prevalent among children and adolescents from families of low socioeconomic status.

Conduct disorder

Definition and diagnostic criteria

CD is a disruptive behavior disorder that goes beyond some of the defiant behavior seen in individuals with

ODD, and is characterized by a repetitive and persistent pattern of behavior in which the basic rights of others or major age-appropriate societal norms or rules are violated [1]. Some of the behaviors can include aggression, vandalism, theft, deceitfulness, and running away from home.

The complete DSM-5 criteria for CD are shown in Table 12.2. The DSM-5 breaks the criteria into four categories – aggression to people and animals, destruction of property, deceitfulness or theft, and serious violations of rules – although the categories are not relevant for diagnostic purposes. The manual lists 15 criteria and specifies that at least three of them must be present for at least 12 months, with at least one of them present in the past 6 months. Just as with ODD, in individuals above the age of 18, CD can only be diagnosed if criteria are not met for ASPD.

The DSM-5 also specifies subtypes for CD based on age of onset (childhood-onset versus adolescent-onset) and severity (mild, moderate, or severe). If at least one criterion characteristic of CD is present prior to age 10, the individual is said to have the childhood-onset type, whereas the absence of any criteria prior to age 10 would classify the individual as having the adolescent-onset type. The subtypes for severity are based on the number of conduct problems present and the degree of harm that the problems cause others.

Epidemiology

The lifetime prevalence of CD also varies depending on the sample, but studies of community samples have estimated anywhere from 1% to 16%, with the most common estimate being around 5% [3]. Gender differences in CD are more pronounced than they are in ODD, with an estimated male-to-female ratio of 4:1 before adolescence, and dropping down to 2:1 in adolescence [5]. These gender differences may reflect social biases, though, rather than biological differences. The prevalence of DBDs in girls is likely underestimated, and some people have suggested modifying the criteria for girls for this reason. Whereas males are more likely to exhibit physical violence, females are more likely to use relational and indirect aggression, which is covert, manipulative behavior aimed at harming or depriving another individual. Boys have a greater tendency to be overtly aggressive toward others, which is more noticeable to adults in their lives, while girls, on the other hand, might ostracize or defame another person, which is harder to detect

Table 12.2. Diagnostic criteria for conduct disorder

A. *A repetitive and persistent pattern of behavior in which the basic rights of others or major age-appropriate societal norms or rules are violated as manifested by the presence of three (or more) of the following criteria in the past 12 months with at least one criterion present in the past 6 months.*

Aggression to people and animals

  (1) often bullies, threatens, or intimidates others.
  (2) often initiates physical fights.
  (3) has used a weapon that can cause serious physical harm to others.
  (4) has been physically cruel to people.
  (5) has been physically cruel to animals.
  (6) has stolen while confronting a victim.
  (7) has forced someone into sexual activity.

Destruction of property

  (8) has deliberately engaged in fire setting with the intention of causing serious damage.
  (9) has deliberately destroyed others' property.

Deceitfulness or theft

  (10) has broken into someone else's house, building or car.
  (11) often lies to obtain goods or favors or to avoid obligations.
  (12) has stolen items of nontrivial value without confronting a victim.

Serious violations of rules

  (13) often stays out at night despite parental prohibitions, beginning before age 13 years.
  (14) has run away from home overnight at least twice while living in parental or parental surrogate home.
  (15) is often truant from school, beginning before age 13 years.

B. The disturbance in behavior causes clinically significant impairment in social, academic, or occupational functioning.

C. If the individual is age 18 years or older, criteria are not met for Antisocial Personality Disorder.

Code based on age at onset:

Childhood-Onset Type: onset of at least one criterion characteristic of Conduct Disorder prior to age 10 years.

Adolescent-Onset Type: absence of any criteria characteristic of Conduct Disorder prior to age 10 years.

Unspecified Onset: age at onset is not known.

Specify severity:

Mild: few if any conduct problems in excess of those required to make the diagnosis and conduct problems cause only minor harm to others.

Moderate: number of conduct problems and effect on others intermediate between "mild" and "severe."

Severe: many conduct problems in excess of those required to make the diagnosis or conduct problems cause considerable harm to others.

Source: American Psychiatric Association [1]. Reprinted with permission from the *Diagnostic and Statistical Manual of Mental Disorders, Fifth Edition* (Copyright © 2013). American Psychiatric Association. All rights reserved.

when making a diagnosis. During adolescence, male teens with CD are more likely to exhibit fighting, stealing, and vandalism, whereas teenage girls with CD are more likely to exhibit lying, truancy, running away, substance use, and prostitution [1].

Just as ODD is more prevalent in families of low socioeconomic status, the same is true for CD. CD is also more prevalent in children and adolescents who come from neighborhoods with high crime rates and community disorganization.

Etiology of ODD and CD

Biological factors

The idea that ODD and CD stem from a reduction of autonomic responsiveness is one of the strongest biological arguments for the development of the disorders [6]. This can be characterized by low levels of salivary cortisol in children with ODD and CD, low levels of skin conductance in the presence of affectively arousing stimuli, and lower baseline levels of heart rate. Some studies have even found that lower cortisol levels correlate with being more symptomatic for CD [7]. Contrary to the lower baseline heart rate in these individuals, though, children with these disorders sometimes show greater increases in heart rate in response to frustration than children without ODD [8].

Neurological imaging has suggested that an atypical frontal lobe activation pattern may reflect a biological substrate of a negative affective style in children with these diagnoses [9]. Neurological abnormalities may also involve problems with several neurotransmitter systems. Specifically, problems associated with the regulation of serotonin and with dopaminergic and noradrenergic activity have been found in individuals with antisocial behavior [10, 11]. The exact origin of these abnormalities is still unclear.

Genetic studies on heritability are not conclusive, but they have begun to yield preliminary results. Some researchers believe that there may be a significant contribution from genetics to ODD in both boys and girls [12], but it seems very likely that the interaction between genetic factors and environmental factors is more important than simply genetics alone. Since there is a clear difference in the prevalence of CD among males and females, it might appear that there is stronger evidence to support the contribution of genetics to CD. However, since this gender difference might arise more from social constructs and attitudes than from biological differences, there is not yet enough clear support of this link.

Lastly, additional well-known biological risk factors for ODD and CD include low birth weight, antenatal and perinatal complications, and any brain injuries or brain disease. Maternal cigarette smoking during pregnancy is an important perinatal risk factor; children whose mothers smoked during pregnancy are not only at increased risk for CD, but they are also more likely to have an earlier onset of behavioral problems and delinquent behavior.

Psychological factors

Some of the well-known psychological risk factors for the development of ODD and CD include a below-average IQ, attentional problems, reading problems, language impairment, impulsivity, and hyperactivity. Youth with CD who have some of the neuropsychological deficits listed above (including dysfunction in the frontal and prefrontal lobe, as well as the left hemisphere) may already suffer from more learning disabilities, which may further compromise functioning. Individuals who use an aggressive coping style are also at greater risk for developing ODD and CD. Children with DBDs are more vigilant and hypersensitive to hostile cues from others and appear to be twice as likely to respond aggressively to a problem than children without these disorders [13]. Deficits in social cognition may lead to the misinterpretation of social cues, including a tendency to incorrectly perceive others as hostile.

In terms of personality traits, individuals with ODD and CD often lack impulse control, self-restraint, and a sense of responsibility. Furthermore, they may also be less sensitive to potential punishment when they are focused on the possibility of a reward [14]. It has been speculated that these children likely have trouble with tasks requiring response preservation and motivational inhibition. These deficits are likely related to problems with executive functions, which include not just impulse control, but also anticipation and planning, as well as abstract reasoning.

Lastly, difficult temperament (including irritability and restlessness), which can be observed in a child shortly after birth, might also be a developmental precursor to ODD and CD symptoms. General links between early temperament and ODD symptoms have been suggested; however, the evidence linking temperament early in life with later psychopathology has not been thoroughly developed, and specific aspects of temperament have not yet been confirmed as predictors of ODD, CD, or other disruptive behavioral problems [15]. As with biological factors, the interplay between environment and temperament is likely more influential in the etiology of ODD and CD than temperament alone.

Sociological factors

Compared to ADHD, environmental factors appear to play a greater role in the development of ODD and CD. Sociological factors that may contribute to the development of ODD and CD range from family-related factors to school, neighborhood, and other social factors. Some of the factors in the family include domestic violence, exposure to parental antisocial behavior or substance use, maltreatment or neglect, parent–child conflict, and excessive or insufficient parental supervision. When parents set inconsistent or excessively harsh limits, this has the potential to set the scene for oppositional behavior later in life. Additionally, parent–child interactions can be critical, especially in terms of parental reactions to oppositional behavior early on in the child's life.

Other social factors include poverty or low socioeconomic status, a family history of criminal activity, peer rejection or bullying, dysfunctional schools, living in a high-crime neighborhood, and associations with deviant peers. Low socioeconomic status is likely a risk factor because it is often accompanied by high stress levels among family members, which can lead to dysfunction in other areas.

In addition to living in a high-crime area, other neighborhood factors such as poor housing and community disorganization correlate with increased diagnoses of CD. Constant exposure to violence, including violence at home, in the neighborhood, or through the media (e.g., movies and video games), may also increase aggression in children and adolescents. However, it is important to note that social, economic, and cultural context must be considered prior to making a diagnosis. For example, if a child grows up in an environment in which it is necessary to acquire certain behaviors (that may ordinarily appear to be dangerous) in order to survive, a diagnosis of ODD or CD would not necessarily be warranted. In a threatening environment, patterns of behavior that would otherwise be viewed as unacceptable and undesirable may actually be protective.

As the number of biological, psychological, and sociological risk factors increases, the detrimental effects are additive, and the risk for ODD or CD increases with each additional factor. Additionally, the way in which children are affected by certain factors is mediated by their developmental age, their current state of behavior (or the disorder), and any factors that are already interacting together. For instance, a child who initially has more severe behavioral problems, who also struggles with parent–child conflict at home or inadequate resources at school, will likely be more impaired than a child with fewer of these risk factors. Risk factors become more significant as their number increases, particularly when multiple risk factors (such as exposure to domestic violence and harsh or inconsistent discipline) build upon each additional factor's negative effects. Remaining aware of the harmful effects and noticing these risk factors as early as possible has important implications for both the prevention and treatment of disruptive behavior disorders.

Prevention of ODD and CD

At each of the levels previously mentioned, there is potential to intervene in an effort to prevent the development of increased behavioral problems that could develop into ODD or CD. Due to the large degree of symptom overlap between DBDs and ADHD, many of the prevention strategies are similar. At the biological level, prevention can start with improving prenatal care, including educating mothers who smoke cigarettes and use other substances about the importance of quitting during pregnancy.

At the individual level, early intervention (before age 8) has the potential to reduce early behavior problems and prevent the problems from becoming worse [16]. Programs to improve speech, language, and reading development are also important interventions if the child struggles in these areas, or is at risk for struggling.

Prevention interventions at the family level are especially important at halting the development of a DBD because stress in the home – especially conflict between the parents and child – can exacerbate preexisting problems. One of the most important prevention resources (which can also be effective as a treatment for ODD or CD) is parent management training. Positive parenting skills (based on evidence-based parent-training programs that have been shown to promote

social and emotional competence) can decrease early behavioral problems in children. Bauer and Webster-Stratton [17] reviewed a variety of evidence-based parenting programs for children between the ages of 2 and 8 years old. Finding effective ways to positively parent a child and to use discipline strategies productively can have a large impact on the child's behavior. Bauer and Webster-Stratton encouraged pediatricians to incorporate some positive parenting principles into well-child visits, since the techniques are relatively easy to teach and are highly effective. Additional family interventions include programs to reduce domestic violence, treat substance abuse problems, and identify and treat any psychological disorders afflicting the parents if the family is struggling with these problems.

Programs to reduce bullying and school truancy, enhance the quality of schools, and increase law enforcement in high-crime neighborhoods are all possible portals of entry to prevent behavioral problems at the school and community level. Encouraging children to get involved with activities outside of school may also be a protective factor against the development of ODD or CD.

Prognosis and stability of the diagnoses of ODD and CD

Though behavioral problems can be identified as early as preschool, ODD is typically diagnosed between the ages of 6 and 10, since this is around the time when most children will have outgrown many oppositional behaviors that were previously normative and developmentally appropriate. Children who demonstrate more severe symptoms are more likely to carry those symptoms over time. Most children with ODD do not go on to develop CD, but they are at greater risk for developing it, and they are also at risk for continued behavior problems.

If the behavior begins to include things such as violating the rights of others and violating social rules, this may be a sign that CD is beginning to develop. Childhood-onset CD (which requires a diagnosis before age 10) can be present as early as 5 or 6 years old, and some children present with mild conduct problems as early as preschool. If symptoms present after age 10, the individual would receive a diagnosis of the adolescent-onset subtype. In children with ADHD and comorbid CD, the onset of CD is typically prior to adolescence. After the age of 16, the onset of CD is much rarer. Compared to ODD, which usually improves with age, CD is typically a more stable diagnosis and is actually considered the most stable form of all childhood and adolescent psychosocial disorders. In follow-up studies of clinical populations, 45–90% still meet the criteria for CD after 3 to 4 years. In normal populations, up to 43% of individuals could be rediagnosed up to 2.5 years later [18].

Stability of CD varies based on the age of onset. Individuals who are diagnosed with the childhood-onset subtype of CD are more likely to show aggressive behaviors in childhood and adolescence and are more likely to show antisocial and criminal behavior in adulthood, compared to those diagnosed with the adolescent-onset subtype. Individuals with the childhood-onset subtype show more severe, chronic, and aggressive behavior and are at greater risk for adjustment problems throughout development.

Approximately 30–50% of children who develop CD will go on to develop ASPD in adulthood. Individuals who first develop CD in adolescence are less likely to develop ASPD. Of those who do not develop ASPD, though, the risk of manifesting significant impairment in relationships and occupational functioning is still high.

Some researchers have proposed an additional distinction to differentiate within the preexisting subgroups of antisocial youth based on the presence or absence of callous-unemotional (CU) traits [19]. Examples of CU traits include "does not feel bad or guilty," "does not show emotions," and "is unconcerned about the feelings of others." Those who are higher in CU traits tend to exhibit more severe and violent conduct problems and, on average, tend to have earlier police contact compared to those who do not show high levels of CU traits. It has been suggested that these traits are associated with the early onset of antisocial behaviors, so it is likely that they designate a particularly severe group of individuals within the childhood-onset subtype. High CU traits may also lead to poorer treatment progress [19].

Comorbidities of ODD and CD

Since DBDs rarely occur on their own and comorbid conditions can result in greater impairment than having a DBD alone, it is important to consider the disorders that are often comorbid with ODD or CD.

ODD, CD, and ADHD, Combined Type have extremely high co-associations. In a meta-analysis of 21 community studies, Angold *et al.* reported a

median odds ratio of 10.7 (range 7.7 to 14.8) between ADHD and ODD/CD [20] – making these two disruptive behavior disorders the most likely comorbidity between ADHD and any other set of disorders [21]. In normal populations, the comorbidity of ADHD and a DBD is about 30%, but in clinical populations, it can be as high as 80–90%. Comorbidity varies by age, however; almost all younger children (under the age of 12) with ODD or CD will meet criteria for ADHD, while only about one-third of adolescents with CD will meet criteria for ADHD. In short, childhood-onset CD is most likely associated with ADHD whereas adolescent-onset CD is most likely not associated with ADHD.

Sometimes it can be difficult to distinguish between ADHD and ODD because children with ADHD are often disruptive and may appear to have a DBD. However, children with ADHD may be inattentive, forgetful, or impulsive, rather than intentionally defiant. While it is sometimes hard to determine whether ADHD preceded the DBD or vice versa, it is certainly clear that ADHD influences the development and severity of these disorders. Individuals with CD and comorbid ADHD tend to have an earlier age of onset of disruptive behavior compared to individuals with CD alone [5]. Additionally, since ADHD and learning disorders are also highly comorbid, many children with ODD or CD also have a comorbid learning disorder, which can further compromise the progress of these individuals.

While ODD and CD are known as externalizing disorders (i.e., they often cause noticeable problems, such as bullying, theft, and aggression), these disorders are often comorbid with anxiety and mood disorders, which are internalizing disorders that present with less noticeable problems, such as nervousness and depression. The interaction between CD and anxiety disorders is somewhat complex, though, because children with anxiety disorders who do not have CD appear to be at reduced risk for later conduct problems. However, youth who do develop CD seem to be at increased risk for a comorbid anxiety disorder. Specifically, separating shyness and inhibition from social setting may be important because some research has shown that inhibition may protect against delinquency, while withdrawal may increase the risk for CD, especially in boys [22].

Children and adolescents with ODD or CD are also at greater risk for mood disorders. For CD in particular, the high rate of comorbidity with depression can be problematic because the combination of these disorders increases the risk for additional dangerous conditions such as substance abuse. This serious risk makes it even more critical to understand the connection between CD and depression so that more harmful and threatening consequences can be prevented. Additionally, if bipolar disorder co-occurs with CD, this can also be a dangerous combination because of the possibility for increased commission and greater severity of crimes and other delinquent behavior during elated moods and manic episodes [5]. More research needs to be done in this area to determine the intricacies of this possible link.

Substance use is another common comorbidity, especially with CD. CD typically precedes substance use, but sometimes the problems arise at the same time. Substance use early on can predict later criminality, so it seems likely that regardless of the order of onset, having both conditions makes the expression of each individual disorder significantly worse than either one would be on its own.

Lastly, there has been some investigation of the comorbidity of CD and somatoform disorders. Somatoform disorders may be characterized by pain, stomach problems, or sexual problems. The presence of somatic problems is associated with an increased likelihood of CD symptoms, especially among adolescent girls. The link between these symptom groups has also been documented in studies of ASPD [23].

Clinical assessment

To assess the presence of ODD or CD, it is necessary to conduct an interview with both the child and the parent or guardian. In addition to asking about DBDs and other behavioral problems, careful attention should be paid to any possible comorbid disorders, given the large number of conditions that are highly comorbid with ODD and CD. To differentially diagnose a DBD, it is also helpful to determine the onset of each symptom, how frequently each problem occurs, and how severe the behavior is. Interviewing the parent and child separately is typically helpful in order to make the child more comfortable with the interview process, and to avoid conflict between the parent and child that may arise from having the child listen to all of the parental complaints about his or her behavior.

If a parent describes the child as disobedient and unable to listen to directions, the interviewer must ensure that the behavior is not due to a different type of problem, such as inattention, hearing loss, or a receptive language problem. One way to get around this challenge is to ask for a specific or recent example of a time when the defiant behavior occurred to get a full picture of the situation [3].

To distinguish between behavior that crosses the diagnostic threshold and normative behavior, the interviewer should collect a complete developmental, family, and social history. Obtaining reports from other informants, such as teachers or peers, is also important when establishing whether the behavior problems occur only in certain contexts with the parent present or in multiple contexts. However, unlike a diagnosis of ADHD, which requires that symptoms and impairment be present in two or more settings, a diagnosis of ODD or CD does not include this criterion.

Asking a child with a potential behavior disorder about his or her defiance may initially seem like an unreliable method of assessment, since you may not expect to receive truthful and accurate accounts of his or her own behavior. However, obtaining this information in an interview is not always as difficult as it seems because the child will often believe that the behavior is appropriate and justified. Developing rapport with the child is also an important step toward a positive and helpful interview with honest answers. In developing rapport, it is critical to use a non-judgmental tone and to avoid blaming or criticizing the child.

When interviewing the parent, gauging how the parent responds to various behaviors is a crucial step in determining whether the situations are being handled appropriately. If they are not, this can be a key intervention point for treatment and prevention of any further disruptive behavior. Another important area to assess is whether there is any suspected physical, sexual, or psychological abuse of the child, since the child's safety must be a priority, and abuse is a risk factor in these situations.

In addition to the interview, there are numerous rating scales to help diagnose oppositional and defiant behavior problems. Some of these include the Child Behavior Checklist [24] and the Teacher Report Form that goes with it, the Eyberg Child Behavior Inventory and the Sutter–Eyberg Student Behavior Inventory – Revised [25], and the Home and School Situations Questionnaires [26]. For CD specifically, there are scales designed to measure aggression and sociopathic traits. These include the Overt Aggression Scale [27], the Children's Aggression Scale [28], and the

Antisocial Process Screening Device [29]. A more extensive list of questionnaires and rating scales that can be used for diagnosis and/or follow-up is available [2].

A general physical exam should be conducted to check for any underlying medical problems or possible signs of abuse. If there is concern about academic functioning, educational testing and a psychometric assessment should be done to identify any academic problems that have not already been reliably assessed. Especially in the case of CD, additional health issues such as pregnancy, sexually transmitted diseases, and head trauma may be suspected and can be screened as well. It is not necessary to conduct any biochemical or radiological investigations, with the exception of urine drug screens in adolescents to detect any substance abuse.

Treatment

Treatment of ODD and CD will work best if a multidisciplinary approach is taken. This includes pharmacological treatment, BPT, interpersonal skills training, and family therapy. The most successful outcomes are achieved when these elements are combined.

Pharmacological treatments

There are no medications indicated for the treatment of ODD or CD. Nonetheless, treatment with medication is sometimes helpful in reducing aggression and other behaviors associated with ODD and/or CD. Moreover, since ODD and CD are often comorbid with other disorders or conditions – particularly ADHD, which is often successfully treated with medication – treatment of these concurrent disorders may also lead to improvement of some ODD and CD symptoms.

Stimulants

Since many patients with ODD or CD also have ADHD, psychostimulants such as methylphenidate and dexamphetamine are among the most common medications used in the treatment of concurrent ADHD and a DBD. Stimulants are typically effective at not only reducing the core ADHD symptoms but can help to reduce aggressive and antisocial behavior. Up to 75% of individuals with ADHD will respond to the first stimulant that is chosen, and 80–90% will respond if two different stimulants are tried consecutively [30]. Stimulants can effectively reduce inattention, hyperac-

tivity, impulsivity, and oppositional behavior, and they have been shown to be effective in controlling these symptoms at home and in social settings. These medications can improve aggression control and noncompliance, making them a practical choice in the treatment of comorbid ODD/CD and ADHD.

Non-stimulants

Atomoxetine is a specific norepinephrine (noradrenaline) transporter inhibitor that is a nonstimulant alternative for the treatment of ADHD symptoms. This medication has a long duration, which can help with behavioral and attentional problems in the early morning and late evening. Although atomoxetine is typically considered for the treatment of ADHD in patients with a comorbid tic or anxiety disorder, in a recent randomized, placebo-controlled trial of atomoxetine in children and adolescents with ADHD and comorbid ODD, improvement was noted in youth with ADHD and ODD when higher doses were used (1.8 mg/kg/day, compared to the typical 1.2 mg/kg/day). At these higher doses, medium-to-large effect sizes were noted with respect to oppositional symptoms in the ODD group [31]. Atomoxetine is sometimes used as an adjunct to stimulants therapy, not just as an alternative.

Alpha-2 agonists

The α_2 agonists, clonidine and guanfacine, have long been used as second-line medications to treat ADHD since they stimulate the neurotransmitter norepinephrine, which is important for concentration. New, extended-release formulations of guanfacine and clonidine are now US Food and Drug Administration (FDA) approved and available for once- and twice-daily dosing, respectively. Specific groups who may benefit from trials with these drugs include patients with ADHD and more severe ODD, patients with ADHD and CD, patients with ADHD and a tic disorder, and patients with ADHD and ODD who do not respond to stimulants or atomoxetine [30]. These medications are generally well tolerated; sedation is the most common side effect with initiation of therapy and typically diminishes with time. As with atomoxetine, these adrenergic agents are sometimes used as an adjunct to stimulant therapy, not just as an alternative. The combination of the extended-release preparations of α agonists with stimulants are FDA approved.

Antidepressants

Antidepressants with various mechanisms of action are occasionally used as a treatment for ADHD in the absence of a mood disorder, and improvement in aggressive symptoms has been shown in several open-label trials. Tricyclic antidepressants (TCAs) such as imipramine or desipramine can be considered, since they have been effective in treating ADHD. However, newer antidepressants such as selective serotonin reuptake inhibitors (SSRIs) may be beneficial to patients with associated anxiety or mood disorders. Their specific effects on the treatment of ODD symptoms have not yet been well established though [30]. Since there is a relationship between serotonin and aggression, serotonergic agents may be useful in treating individuals with aggressive and impulsive symptoms of CD [32]. It is important to use caution when prescribing antidepressants to children, however, since there is an increased risk of suicidality. Blood levels and EKG monitoring is generally recommended for patients treated with TCAs. Treatment with an antidepressant should be considered in patients with ODD or CD if there is a comorbid mood disorder.

Mood regulators

The most common mood regulators to treat aggression and mood dysregulation are carbamazepine and valproate semisodium, though lithium has also been shown to be effective with inpatient populations. Treatment of children and adolescents with bipolar disorder and ODD or CD must be closely monitored if stimulants are added to these other drugs, since this can sometimes provoke a manic or hypomanic episode [30]. In fact, whenever a stimulant medication is prescribed for ADHD and the medication significantly exacerbates a child's mood or behavior, the possibility of bipolar disorder must be considered as the primary diagnosis.

Antipsychotics

Antipsychotic medications can also be used to treat ODD and CD if other medications have been ineffective. Atypical or "second-generation" antipsychotics may be used to treat aggression and oppositional behavior in these cases, though this treatment is also "off-label" and has not been approved by the FDA for treating ODD/CD. The most commonly studied atypical antipsychotic is risperidone. While risperidone may be effective, it can have many adverse effects, including sedation, hypotension, extrapyramidal symptoms, and excessive weight gain or diabetes (due to metabolic syndrome). In children, the recommended starting dose is 0.02 mg/kg/day; the dose can be gradually increased up to 0.06 mg/kg/day [30]. Laboratory monitoring is recommended, especially if atypical antipsychotics are to be prescribed for an extended period. Newer atypical antipsychotic formulations are available (olanzapine, quetiapine, ziprasidone, aripiprazole, asenapine, and others); however, less data are available for the treatment of aggression and other symptoms associated with ODD and CD. Since children may be at increased risk for serious adverse events (extrapyramidal symptoms as well as endocrine or metabolic abnormalities), clinicians must always balance the potential risks and benefits associated with any medication trial.

Medication combinations

In addition to using the above medications alone, some medication combinations that have been shown to be effective are stimulants and clonidine (for aggressive ADHD patients), stimulants and antidepressants (for ADHD and comorbid depressive disorder), and stimulants and antipsychotics (for ODD or CD patients with sub-average IQ) [30, 32].

Psychotherapeutic treatments

Since ODD and CD are complex conditions with a variety of risk factors and potential problems, pharmacological treatments alone are often not enough [33]. One study that demonstrated this was the Multimodal Treatment of ADHD (MTA) study, conducted by the National Institute of Mental Health. The MTA study examined the effects of pharmacological and psychosocial treatment (alone and combined) on children with ADHD, many of whom had one or more comorbid psychiatric disorders [34]. In the study, 40% of patients with ADHD also had ODD, so the treatment effects provided useful information for patients with ODD symptoms. When patients had ADHD without a DBD, medication alone was just as effective at treating the core ADHD symptoms as medication and behavior therapy combined. However, when ODD was also present, children benefited more from combined therapy.

BPT is a common treatment for ADHD, ODD, and CD and can improve maladaptive parenting behavior that is exacerbating the effects of these disorders.

Techniques of BPT are based on social learning principles. Parents are taught how to attend to appropriate, compliant behavior and to ignore minor, inappropriate behavior. They are also taught how to identify antecedents to their child's behavior, as well as consequences of their behavior, to learn how to manipulate the outcomes. Parents learn to give appropriate commands and punishments, set effective limits, and give positive rewards (such as praise, as well as tangible rewards through a point system) when the child behaves properly and follows rules.

A variety of factors can influence the outcome of BPT, such as the specific type of BPT (e.g., format, maintenance, and setting), parental factors (e.g., maternal depression, parental ADHD, parental substance abuse, parental ASPD, marital problems, and father participation), and child factors (e.g., comorbid conditions and developmental considerations) [35].

Interpersonal skills training is a common treatment intervention for DBDs. Multisystemic therapy (MST) [36] and multidimensional treatment foster care (MTFC) [37] are two possible interventions for high-risk adolescents. MST is designed for youth and their families and incorporates a range of therapy, including BPT, family therapy, interpersonal skills training, and marital therapy. MTFC, which is generally a 6-month program, is targeted at individuals within the context of therapeutic foster homes. Two of the components of MTFC are family therapy and school interventions. An adolescent gets placed in special foster care under the supervision of foster parents who have been trained to properly discipline and supervise the child and positively reinforce good behavior. Adolescents are also taught problem-solving skills. When the treatment program is over, the individuals return home and continue to receive exposure to some of the skills training, including BPT (since their parents or guardians at home should be utilizing positive parenting skills) [35].

More recent analyses from the MTA study support the value of psychosocial treatment (which includes a parent-training component) when incorporated in a multimodal approach to treatment of children with ADHD, combined type. In short, medication alone may not be enough in some cases – especially if there is one or more comorbid diagnosis.

Overall, treatment programs should effectively integrate the proper skills training into an environment that is conducive to practicing and utilizing those skills.

Conclusion

ODD and CD are two of the most stable behavioral disorders in children and adolescents. Since they are highly comorbid with ADHD and can significantly complicate treatment and the individual's overall prognosis, it is important to identify these disorders as early as possible in order to intervene quickly and achieve the optimal outcome.

References

1. American Psychiatric Association: *Diagnostic and Statistical Manual of Mental Disorders*, 5th edn. (DSM-5). Arlington, VA: American Psychiatric Publishing; 2013.

2. Steiner H, Remsing L. Practice parameter for the assessment and treatment of children and adolescents with oppositional defiant disorder. *J Am Acad Child Adolesc Psychiatry*. 2007;**46**:126–41.

3. Thomas CR. Oppositional defiant disorder and conduct disorder. In: Dulcan MK, ed. *Dulcan's Textbook of Child and Adolescent Psychiatry*. Arlington, VA: American Psychiatric Publishing, Inc. 2010; 223–39.

4. Nock MK, Kazdin AE, Hirpi E, *et al.* Prevalence, subtypes, and correlates of DSM-IV conduct disorder in the National Comorbidity Survey Replication. *Psychol Med*. 2006;**36**:699–710.

5. Loeber R, Burke JD, Lahey B, *et al.* Oppositional defiant and conduct disorder: a review of the past 10 years, part I. *J Am Acad Child Adolesc Psychiatry*. 2000;**39**:1468–84.

6. Herpertz SC, Mueller B, Qunaibi M, *et al.* Response to emotional stimuli in boys with conduct disorder. *Am J Psychiatry*. 2005;**162**:1100–7.

7. Oosterlaan J, Geurts HM, Knol DL, *et al.* Low basal salivary cortisol is associated with teacher-reported symptoms of conduct disorder. *Psychiatry Res*. 2005;**134**:1–10.

8. van Goozen SHM, Matthys W, Kettenis PT, *et al.* Salivary cortisol and cardiovascular activity during stress in oppositional-defiant disorder boys and normal controls. *Biol Psychiatry*. 1998;**43**:531–9.

9. Baving L, Laucht M, Schmidt MH. Oppositional children differ from healthy children in frontal brain activation. *J Abnorm Child Psychol*. 2000;**28**:267–75.

10. Pliszka SR, Rogeness GA, Renner P, *et al.* Plasma neurochemistry in juvenile offenders. *J Am Acad Child Adolesc Psychiatry*. 1988;**27**:588–94.

11. Stadler C, Schmeck K, Nowraty I, *et al.* Platelet 5-HT uptake in boys with conduct disorder. *Neuropsychobiology*. 2004;**50**:244–51.

12. Hudziak JJ, Derks EM, Althoff RR. The genetic and environmental contributions to attention deficit hyperactivity disorder as measured by the Connors' Rating Scales-Revised. *Am J Psychiatry*. 2005;**162**: 1614–20.

13. Coy K, Speltz ML, DeKlyen M, *et al*. Social-cognitive processes in preschool boys with and without oppositional defiant disorder. *J Abnorm Child Psychol*. 2001;**29**:107–19.

14. van Goozen SH, Cohen-Kettenis PT, Snoek H, *et al*. Executive functioning in children: a comparison of hospitalized ODD and ODD/ADHD children and normal controls. *J Child Psychol Psychiatry*. 2004;**45**:284–92.

15. Loeber R, Burke J, Pardini DA. Perspectives on oppositional defiant disorder, conduct disorder, and psychopathic features. *J Child Psychol Psychiatry*. 2009;**50**:133–42.

16. Taylor TK, Biglan A. Behavioral family interventions for improving child-rearing: a review of the literature for clinicians and policy makers. *Clin Child Fam Psychol Rev*. 1998;**1**:41–60.

17. Bauer NS, Webster-Stratton C. Prevention of behavioral disorders in primary care. *Curr Opin Pediatr*. 2006;**18**:654–60.

18. Olsson M. DSM diagnosis of conduct disorder (CD) – a review. *Nord J Psychiatry*. 2009;**63**:102–12.

19. Frick PJ, Dickens C. Current perspectives on conduct disorder. *Curr Psychiatr Rep*. 2006;**8**:59–72.

20. Angold A, Costello EJ, Erkanli A. Comorbidity. *J Child Psychol Psychiatry*. 1999;**40**:57–87.

21. Barkley RA. *Attention-Deficit Hyperactivity Disorder*, 3rd edn. New York, NY: Guilford Press; 2006.

22. Kerr M, Tremblay R, Pagani L. *et al*. Boys' behavioral inhibition and the risk of later delinquency. *Arch Gen Psychiatry*. 1997;**54**:809–16.

23. Lilienfeld S. The association between antisocial personality and somatization disorders: a review and integration of theoretical models. *Clin Psychol Rev*. 1992;**12**:641–62.

24. Achenbach TM, Rescorla LA; for the ASEBA. *School-Age Forms and Profiles*. Burlington, VT: University of Vermont, Department of Psychiatry; 2000.

25. Eyberg SM, Pincus D. *Eyberg Child Behavior Inventory and Sutter-Eyberg Student Behavior Inventory – Revised, Professional Manual*. Odessa, FL: Psychological Assessment Resources; 1999.

26. Barkley RA. *A Clinician's Manual for Assessment and Parent Training*, 2nd edn. New York, NY: Guilford Press; 1997.

27. Yudofsky SC, Silber JM, Jackson W, *et al*. The Overt Aggression Scale for the objective rating of verbal and physical aggression. *Am J Psychiatry*. 1986;**143**:35–9.

28. Halperin JM, McKay KE, Newcorn JH. Development, reliability, and validity of the Children's Aggression Scale – Parent Version. *J Am Acad Child Adolesc Psychiatry*. 2002;**41**:425–52.

29. Frick PJ, Hare RD. *Antisocial Process Screening Device (APSD) Technical Manual*. North Tonawanda, NY: Multi-Health Systems, Inc.; 2001.

30. Turgay A. Psychopharmacological treatment of oppositional defiant disorder. *CNS Drugs*. 2009; **23**:1–17.

31. Newcorn J, Spencer T, Biederman J, *et al*. Atomoxetine treatment in children and adolescents with attention-deficit/hyperactivity disorder and comorbid oppositional defiant disorder. *J Am Acad Child Adolesc Psychiatry*. 2005;**44**:240–8.

32. Tcheremissine OV, Lieving LM. Pharmacological aspects of the treatment of conduct disorder in children and adolescents. *CNS Drugs*. 2006;**20**:549–65.

33. Kutcher S, Aman M, Brooks SJ, *et al*. International consensus statement on attention-deficit/hyperactivity disorder (ADHD) and disruptive behaviour disorders (DBDs): clinical implications and treatment practice suggestions. *Eur Neuropsychopharmacol*. 2004; **14**:11–28.

34. MTA Cooperative Group. Moderators and mediators of treatment response for children with attention-deficit/hyperactivity disorder. *Arch Gen Psychiatry*. 1995;**56**:1088–96.

35. Chronis AM, Chacko A, Fabiano GA, *et al*. Enhancements to the behavioral parent training paradigm for families of children with ADHD: review and future directions. *Clin Child Fam Psychol Rev*. 2004;**7**:1–27.

36. Henggeler SW, Cunningham PB, Pickrel SG, *et al*. Multisystemic therapy: an effective violence prevention approach for serious juvenile offenders. *J Adolesc*. 1996;**19**:47–61.

37. Fisher PA, Gunnar MR, Chamberlain P, *et al*. Preventive intervention for maltreated preschool children: impact on children's behavior, neuroendocrine activity, and foster parent functioning. *J Am Acad Child Adolesc Psychiatry*. 2000;**39**: 1356–64.

Chapter 13

Mimics of ADHD
Medical and neurological conditions

Phillip L. Pearl, Roy E. Weiss, and Mark A. Stein

Diagnostic process

The process of differential diagnosis involves distinguishing between the various disorders which may present with similar symptoms, and sorting out the different possible etiological factors that may lead to the same symptom [1]. Since many of the symptoms of attention-deficit hyperactivity disorder (ADHD) overlap with a wide range of psychiatric and medical disorders, the evaluation process should begin with a more general approach to identify potential medical mimics as well as comorbid disorders which will affect the diagnosis and treatment plan.

Although ADHD can be diagnosed at any age, the course is typically that of a developmental disorder with onset of symptoms during childhood. Suspicion of a medical mimic is increased, however, when symptoms occur acutely or there is a profound change or deterioration in function. In such cases, alternative explanations or "medical mimics" are more likely and should be more extensively pursued. Non-familial ADHD, or "ADHD-plus" syndromes where a patient is compromised by ADHD symptomatology plus other prominent deficits of cognitive processing or neurological functioning, should trigger a search for separate, more primary disorders which include ADHD symptoms as part of their typical presentation (e.g., neurofibromatosis, fetal alcohol syndrome, thyroid disorders including hyper- and hypothyroidism, intellectual deficiency, lead poisoning, obstructive sleep apnea, Tourette syndrome [TS]). In assessment of such patients one should be certain that the symptoms of ADHD are not associated with concomitant use of other medications, the side effects of which would have similar symptoms of inattentiveness and impaired cognitive function.

With the widespread recognition that ADHD is not limited to childhood, more and more adults are presenting for ADHD evaluation and, unlike children, are often self-referred. As a result, they may be less likely to have consistent medical care. Moreover, pediatricians who see children over time are most likely to identify medical mimics before pursuing ADHD diagnosis and treatment. The older adult who is a new patient and who presents for evaluation with current ADHD and neurocognitive symptoms but no prior history of ADHD represents a unique challenge to the clinician. As more older patients are now presenting for evaluation, the differential diagnosis should include deteriorating conditions, such as Alzheimer's disease, which may first present as problems with memory and attention. In such cases, neuropsychological testing (see Chapter 17) can be helpful in objectively quantifying the severity of the impairment and evaluating cognitive strengths and weaknesses.

This chapter addresses the medical and neurological conditions that may simulate or exacerbate ADHD. Primary care physicians as well as subspecialists who conduct ADHD evaluations should consider these conditions so that appropriate referral and evaluation procedures are instituted. Given the potential implications of misdiagnosing ADHD in the case of a primary medical disorder, as well as the frequent comorbidity of specific conditions which may affect treatment and course, all patients should receive a thorough medical examination that includes a physical examination and family medical and psychiatric history. Findings from the initial evaluation are then used to determine if additional diagnostic procedures, including laboratory tests, or consultation from other disciplines, such as neurology, genetics, cardiology, otolaryngology, or endocrinology, is warranted.

Attention-Deficit Hyperactivity Disorder in Adults and Children, ed. Lenard A. Adler, Thomas J. Spencer and Timothy E. Wilens.
Published by Cambridge University Press. © Cambridge University Press 2015.

Medical evaluation of ADHD

The medical evaluation of patients presenting with ADHD includes a complete medical, developmental, and family history, in addition to a physical examination. Evaluation procedures are well covered in standard texts of developmental pediatrics [2] as well as books and references concentrating in attention deficit disorder [3–5]. A logical way of viewing the myriad recommendations for a comprehensive neurodevelopmental history is to view brain development and insults in a temporal fashion, with somewhat arbitrary divisions into prenatal, perinatal, and postnatal lesions. Increasing understanding of fetal brain development, with an orderly progression of neural tube induction and development, cerebral lobar development, neuronal proliferation, migration, myelination, and synaptic organization, has led to a conceptualization of patterns of brain maldevelopment depending on the *timing* of the insult, whether etiologically teratogenic, ischemic, traumatic, infectious, or of other origin [6]. Thus, patients with heterotopias, i.e., misplaced nerve cell tissue, or bilateral perisylvian syndrome with polymicrogyria, have had insults occurring during gestational months 3–5 when neuronal migration is occurring. Fetal alcohol syndrome may result in congenital brain malformations ranging from primary microcephaly, affecting the stage of neuronal proliferation during months 2–4, to heterotopias during the somewhat later migrational period. If the general history and evaluation discloses the presence of failure to thrive, abnormal head size, unusual developmental patterns, facial or somatic dysmorphic features, or visceral anomalies, the most parsimonious diagnosis will take these findings into account.

Neurobehavioral effects of children exposed to drugs and toxins in utero are well described. These include alcohol [7], lead [8], and cocaine [9]. Fetal alcohol effects (FAE) serve as a diagnostic category for individuals whose history supports, either by known documentation or on the basis of epidemiological data for international orphans with very limited past information, the presence of alcohol exposure in utero who demonstrate sometimes striking symptoms of inattention, distractibility, hyperkinesis, and impulsivity along with cognitive impairments without the physical findings of growth deficiency, dysmorphic features, for example widened palpebral fissures, smooth philtrum, thin upper lip, and visceral anomalies, for example

palate and cardiac anomalies, generally reserved for a diagnosis of fetal alcohol syndrome (FAS).

The same principle holds true for perinatal lesions. A tenet in child neurology is that perinatal insults (e.g., birth asphyxia) do not cause developmental problems if there is not an associated newborn encephalopathy and deficit in motor function. Isolated ADHD without other stigmata of motor and cognitive handicaps has not been proven as secondary to perinatal distress. However, prematurity [10] and low birth weight [11, 12] are risk factors for ADHD and learning disorders. While an increased incidence of adverse maternal risk factors, including emotional distress and cigarette smoking [13], and perinatal complications during labor and delivery [14] have been reported in children with ADHD versus controls, the nature of the relationship of adverse maternal health during pregnancy and perinatal complications with ADHD is unclear.

Postnatal insults to the brain, again with a wide spectrum of causes, may lead to signs and symptoms of ADHD. A diagnosis of primary ADHD, in a child or adult, requires the presence of these symptoms during childhood and without the presence of a better *medical* explanation of etiology. Specific historical entities include past documentation of head injury with concussion or other complications, meningitis, encephalitis, or seizures. General pediatric disorders, ranging from plumbism to pinworms, can cause hyperactivity, inattention, and irritable behavior in children. Similarly, anemia and thyroid disorders are treatable conditions that may present with irritable, disruptive behavior. Specific endocrine considerations will be discussed later in this chapter. Anomalous developmental patterns, particularly with dysfunction in the areas of social relatedness, verbal and non-verbal communication, and aspects of play and interests are key clues in the identification of either specific learning disabilities or autism spectrum disorder (ASD) which are often confused with ADHD in children who are not intellectually impaired.

It cannot be overemphasized that the evaluation of adults presenting for an initial assessment includes active solicitation of any available documentation that a pattern of inattention, distractibility, impulsivity, and hyperactive behavior has been *long-standing, with evidence of dysfunction attributable to these factors during childhood*. Self-referred adults presenting to an ADHD program with cognitive dysfunction or a change in neurocognitive status require neurological evaluation with an emphasis on the time course and tempo of the disorder, as patients have been identified with a range of diagnoses varying from depression to HIV encephalopathy who have presented in this way [15]. Adults without a previous history of ADHD symptoms but with acute onset of psychiatric symptoms in late adolescence may also be suggestive of more serious forms of psychopathology that often begin in late adolescence, including schizophrenia, bipolar disorder, and substance use disorder.

The medical examination pays particular attention to primary sensory deficits of vision and hearing. Strabismus and amblyopia in particular require ophthalmological evaluation and follow-up, and hearing, especially in the presence of prior recurrent or chronic otitis media, should be tested. The presence of subtle or so-called soft neurological signs, such as cortical sensory processing affecting vestibular and proprioceptive functioning, or associative deficits affecting sensorimotor integration, may be assessed with more specific examinations out of the province of the primary care practitioner and of dubious relevance to diagnosis or treatment issues in ADHD.

The influence of medications that affect attention, including most psychotropic medications and anticonvulsants, antihistamines, benzodiazepines, beta-blockers, steroids, and theophylline, should be considered. Illicit substances, including alcohol, are particularly important in taking a history in adolescents and adults; in addition, medications that may partially target ADHD symptoms, such as caffeine and nicotine, should be inquired about and the patient questioned about frequency, effects, and comparative assessment of their functioning when these substances are not utilized.

Genetic disorders occupy an ever-increasing element in the differential diagnosis of ADHD, with an explosion of information on specific syndromes and greater availability of molecular diagnostic tests. Some particular syndromes merit concern, as they are not uncommon in patients presenting for an ADHD evaluation. Fragile X is the most common cause of inherited intellectual disability in boys and is typically associated with rather profound behavioral disturbance as well as altered facial features and body habitus. The disorder also affects girls, but more subtly, sometimes with attentional and cognitive difficulties that simulate attention deficit disorder (ADD) and learning disabilities [16]. A family history of intellectual disability, particularly in males, should trigger DNA testing

for the fragile X mutation. Other sex chromosome anomalies associated with ADHD include Klinefelter syndrome (XXY), Turner syndrome (45 XO), and extra-Y syndrome (47 XYY). Other dysmorphology syndromes that are recognizable clinically as ADHD-plus disorders, yet with their own unique characteristics, are the velo-cardio-facial syndrome (VCFS), previously known as the Catch-22 syndrome, and Williams syndrome, associated with elfin faces, small stature, and musical savant skills. These are verifiable in most cases with targeted DNA assays or genomic microarray studies.

Children may also present with common physiological manifestations such as elimination disorders and ultimately be identified as having ADHD. While nocturnal enuresis is common, affecting up to 10% of 7-year-old children, approximately 15% will have ADHD [17, 18]. Increased rates of ADHD are also reported in children with fecal incontinence [19].

Table 13.1 includes medical conditions to be ruled out in the evaluation of a child with suspected ADHD. Table 13.2 lists certain procedures which may be considered in this assessment depending on clinical considerations.

Specific neurological disorders

Seizure disorders

Epilepsy is a relatively common condition, having an incidence in the population of approximately 1%, with peak occurrences occurring in children and the elderly. Seizures are generally classified as generalized or focal based on whether their onset can be traced to a seizure focus. Focal, or partial seizures, are further subdivided into simple versus partial complex seizures, with the latter involving alteration of consciousness. Generalized seizures are classified as absence, clonic, tonic, tonic–clonic (grand mal), or myoclonic. The absence seizure, or petit mal, is of particular relevance with regard to the evaluation of children with ADHD.

Absence seizures have their own unique classification, with typical absence seizures being the prototypical epileptic "staring spell" during which the child may have associated symptomatology, including automatic behaviors, or "automatisms," or slight motor activity such as eyelid flutters or a retropulsive tonic body contraction [20]. The EEG has a stereotypical electrical signature manifest as generalized 3-cycle-per-second spike-and-wave paroxysms having abrupt onset and

Table 13.1. Medical conditions simulating ADHD

Autism spectrum disorder
Anemia
Congenital brain anomalies
Dementia (Lewy body dementia, see text)
Enterobius vermicularis (pinworms)
Epilepsy
Fetal alcohol effects/syndrome
Fragile X syndrome
Hearing loss
HIV encephalopathy
Lead poisoning
Learning disabilities
Medication effects
Mental retardation
Metabolic disorders, e.g., ALD
Narcolepsy
Neurofibromatosis I
PANDAS
Sex chromosome abnormalities
Sleep apnea
Sleep deprivation
Static encephalopathy
Sydenham's chorea
Thyroid disorder
Tourette syndrome
Vision loss

Abbreviations: ALD = adrenoleukodystrophy, PANDAS = pediatric autoimmune neuropsychiatric disorders associated with streptococcal infections.

Table 13.2. Laboratory evaluations to be considered based on differential diagnosis

Audiogram
CBC
DNA testing for microarray and fragile X
EEG (sleep-deprived)
Metabolic screening (may include long chain fatty acids)
MRI of brain
Neuropsychological evaluation
Polysomnography/MSLT (multiple sleep latency test), actigraphy
Ophthalmology exam
Thyroid function tests (thyrotrophin (TSH); free T4, free T3)

Abbreviations: CBC = complete blood count, TSH = thyroid-stimulating hormone, T4 = thyroxine, T3 = triiodothyronine.

offset and surrounded by otherwise normal background activity. In children, typical absence epilepsy is known as pyknolepsy, etymologically emanating from the Greek prefix *pyknos* for cluster [21]. These spells cluster into usually obvious discrete episodes of lapses of consciousness, associated with amnesia for events that transpired during the episode. These clinical features are very helpful in arriving at a suspected diagnosis of absence epilepsy. Hyperventilation for 3 minutes with good effort during the neurological examination is a very sensitive method at the bedside for the identification of absence seizures. The absence of absence seizures in an untreated and cooperative patient during this procedure, as judged by an experienced clinician, virtually rules out the presence of ongoing absence seizures. If the test is equivocal, a negative EEG under sleep-deprived conditions, which includes the hyperventilation and photic stimulation activating procedures, should be considered. Positive findings during hyperventilation, or EEG procedure, would mandate further neurological evaluation.

The more difficult, and not uncommon, scenario is when there are atypical features of either the ADHD presentation or the "spells" of concern and the classic scenario above does not apply. One straightforward example is that of adolescents. Juvenile absence epilepsy does not cluster into frequent, discrete episodes, but rather presents as sporadic, unpredictable events that sometimes last protracted periods, in the range of minutes to hours (versus <30 seconds, and on average approximately 10 seconds, in children) [22, 23]. There are also a multitude of clinical situations where absence seizures are atypical (i.e., having longer duration, less clear onset and offset, and associated with slower spike-and-wave EEG bursts, between 1.5 and 2.5 Hertz) in children with abnormal EEG backgrounds and abnormal cognition, oftentimes in the range of intellectual disability. Furthermore, any experienced clinician has seen cases of unexpected paroxysms of generalized spike-and-wave activity of variable duration in children with ADHD-plus syndromes, in whom treatment of the epileptiform activity with an anticonvulsant may or may not yield meaningful clinical improvement. Even in these cases, pharmacotherapy directed toward ADHD symptoms (with the important exception of bupropion, which can provoke seizures) can be helpful.

Suffice to say that there are multiple variations on the theme of epilepsy diagnoses in children with ADHD, and that the presence of discrete staring spells, or an atypical pattern of ADHD-plus symptomatology where either unusual physical or cognitive features are suspected, would be an indication to proceed with sleep-deprived EEG testing, to include a sleep recording, with subsequent neurological referral if needed.

Movement disorders

Movement disorders comprise the group of neurological disorders that present primarily with symptoms of either hyperactivity or hypoactivity. This has become an oversimplified approach, as the complex connections between the traditional localization of these disorders – the basal ganglia – and cortical, thalamic, subthalamic, and brainstem structures, as well as complex neurotransmitter systems comprising neural networks, have demonstrated that these disorders involve cerebral functioning well beyond the rate of movement. The term movement disorders, however, is retained in classical neurology as it preserves the important semiological distinctions between the different movements themselves: tics, myoclonus, chorea, athetosis, and ballismus.

TS, therefore, is recognized as a movement disorder that requires the presence of sufficiently chronic and disabling multiple motor and at least a single type of phonic tic and activity that the patient is impaired longer than 1 year and has no tic-free period longer than 3 months. Tics are often described as sudden, brief, involuntary or semi-voluntary movements or sounds that typically wax and wane in their presentation, can be temporarily suppressed, and usually first occur between ages 3 and 8 [24]. The comorbidities associated with TS include ADHD, learning disabilities, mood disorders, obsessive–compulsive disorder (OCD), phobias, anxiety disorders, and sleep disorders. Tics usually present with ocular or facial movements; repetitive eye blinking is the most common presenting tic. Tics typically follow a rostral–caudal pattern of evolution and will wax and wane in severity over time. Children with a history of both ADHD and TS typically have onset of the ADHD symptoms prior to the tic disorder [25]. This leads to the incorrect assumption that stimulant medications indicated to treat ADHD led to the TS manifestations. While stimulants rarely may cause self-limited, isolated simple motor tic activity, they do not lead to chronic tic activity or the plethora of characteristics

endogenous to TS as studies suggest no elevated risk of first-onset tics in children receiving stimulant medication [26]. Other psychiatric disorders specifically associated with TS have been OCD and phobias, whereby children with combined TS and ADHD have been identified as having more severe psychosocial dysfunction including disruptive behavior, mood disorders, anxiety disorders, and cognitive dysfunction [27]. The rate of comorbidity of ADHD with TS is between 30% and 50% [28, 29]. The presence of TS-associated symptomatology should be sought in patients presenting for evaluation of ADHD.

Sydenham's chorea describes a movement disorder in children which occurs as an autoimmune complication following streptococcal pharyngitis and is associated with rheumatic heart disease. It is manifest by chorea coupled with cognitive dysfunction, irritability, and mood lability. Chorea is a dance-like movement which in this disorder is most manifest in the distal upper extremities and is associated with inability to maintain hand grip. Patients may be extremely active motorically, but the purposeless movements of acute onset are distinguishable from the hyperkinesis of ADHD. Chorea minimi, representing a subtle form of chorea primarily manifest on outstretched arms (which also aggravates Sydenham's chorea), is considered one of the soft neurological signs, along with incoordination during rapid sequential movements and clumsiness, associated with ADHD.

PANDAS, or pediatric autoimmune neuropsychiatric disorders associated with streptococcal infections, refers to a post-infectious onset of OCD or tic disorder [30]. The clinical course is marked by a relapsing-remitting pattern with significant psychiatric comorbidity accompanying the exacerbations.

Sleep disorders

Sleep disturbances are common in children with ADHD [31, 32] and were previously part of the diagnostic criteria prior to DSM-IV. Impaired daytime functioning, manifest by irritable and hyperactive behavior in children with ADHD, may be at least partly attributable to impaired nocturnal sleep. The most common primary sleep disorders associated with ADHD symptoms are obstructive sleep apnea (OSA) and restless legs syndrome/periodic limb movement disorder (RLS/PLMD) [33]; however, any sleep disorder resulting in decreased quality and quantity of sleep may present clinically with ADHD-like symptoms. Clearly, sleep deprivation can mimic

ADHD in all ages, is highly prevalent in teenagers, and should be ruled out by obtaining a sleep history prior to beginning treatment. Children with ADHD are at increased risk of sleep-onset delays and difficulty settling, and stimulant treatment may exacerbate this [34, 35]. Increased latency to sleep onset and decreased sleep duration are strongly associated with stimulant use and are dose dependent [36, 37]. Consequently, individuals being evaluated for ADHD should be systematically screened for sleep symptoms (i.e., frequent snoring, restless sleep, daytime sleepiness) and risk factors (i.e., adenotonsillar hypertrophy, family history of RLS/PLMD) for primary sleep disorders. Overnight polysomnography should be strongly considered for children with symptoms or risk factors suggestive of the presence of OSA or RLS/PLMD.

Narcolepsy, an intrinsic primary sleep disorder, can also be missed in children and adolescents referred for ADHD. Patients with narcolepsy display excessive daytime somnolence related to a disorder involving abnormal intrusions of REM (rapid eye movement) sleep. Narcolepsy is estimated to affect 0.05% of the population, with half having onset in childhood or adolescence, yet latency from clinical onset to actual diagnosis of about 10 years is reported [38]. The classic tetrad of clinical features in narcolepsy, excessive sleepiness with sleep attacks, cataplexy, sleep paralysis, and hypnagogic hallucinations, do not necessarily appear in all patients with narcolepsy, particularly in children and adolescents. More common clinical features in children are weight gain, fragmented overnight sleep, and worsening in school performance. Substances to maintain alertness may be chosen by the patients. The disorder has no gender predilection and is linked to the HLA gene *DQB1*0602*. The pathophysiology has been associated with deficiency of the neurotransmitter hypocretin, and autoimmune destruction of hypocretin-producing hypothalamic neurons has been invoked. While the diagnostic criteria for narcolepsy include the presence of at least two sleep-onset REM episodes during daytime MSLT (multiple sleep latency test), not all children will demonstrate this, and the entire clinical picture must be considered. Testing for *DQB1*0602* gene typing or cerebrospinal fluid hypocretin levels may also be helpful for diagnosis. Narcolepsy treatment includes appropriate counseling and support, scheduled naps, and pharmacotherapy with a stimulant medication. Modafinil for alertness, venlafaxine for cataplexy, and sodium oxybate for all symptoms appear to be particularly useful, with lower rates of patient discontinuation [39]. Other sleep disorders to consider in adolescence as well in the differential diagnosis are delayed sleep phase syndrome, insufficient sleep time, sleep apnea, substance use, and less common neurological disorders such as the periodic hypersomnia of Klein Levin syndrome.

Restless legs syndrome (RLS), a syndrome of akathisias relieved with movement, is associated with periodic limb movement disorder of sleep, or PLMS. RLS/PLMS has long been associated with iron deficiency. There is increasing evidence that iron deficiency may be important as well in ADHD [40–42]. Iron supplementation (80 mg/day) was associated with improved ADHD symptoms in children with low serum ferritin levels (<30 ng/mL) [43]. Current research is focused on biomarkers (e.g., MRI relaxometry) to study brain iron levels, with evidence for lower thalamic iron levels in children with ADHD compared to healthy children [44].

Neurogenetic disorders

Neurogenetic disorders comprise a huge category of diseases which are viewed as genetically based neurological or multisystem disorders that frequently have a metabolic basis and sometimes a progressive, degenerative course. These may be lumped or split in many ways, but certain entities bear mention in this context because of having either a prominent ADHD component or initial features which closely simulate ADHD with only later development of more ominous features.

The phakomatoses, or neurocutaneous disorders, may prominently include ADHD-symptoms. These disorders include neurofibromatosis, tuberous sclerosis, and Sturge–Weber syndrome as well as many other less common entities. A careful skin examination is important in the medical assessment of children presenting for evaluation of ADHD. Neurofibromatosis type I, in particular, manifest as multiple café-au-lait skin maculae as well as peripheral neurofibromata, optic nerve gliomas, and cerebral hamartomas, characteristically have prominent features of both learning disabilities and ADHD. Myotonic dystrophy, a neuromuscular disorder associated with a trinucleotide repeat mutation involving chromosome 19, characteristically produces rather prominent features of learning disorders and ADHD in children otherwise having muscle weakness with similar, although sometimes very subtle and undiagnosed, problems in their mothers.

Adrenoleukodystrophy, known popularly as Lorenzo's disease following the movie named for the cooking oil discovered by Lorenzo's parents as a potential therapy for presymptomatic or early symptomatic cases, often presents in preschool- or kindergarten-age boys as ADHD. This is a metabolic disease based on impaired breakdown of very long chain fatty acids. Unlike ADHD, however, there is a progressive deterioration in this neurodegenerative white matter disease. Childhood-onset metachromatic leukodystrophy can also present with ADHD symptomatology, and children presenting with motor impairment, especially if suggestive of long-tract, upper motor neuron, pathology (spasticity, hyperreflexia, scanning/dysrhythmic speech, ataxia, and incoordination) should receive neurological evaluation for degenerative or metabolic nervous system disorders.

Dementia

As longevity increases with the aging of the population, the clinical question of ADHD in adults and even the elderly, both as an ongoing issue from a long-standing diagnosis, and as a new diagnosis that may become "uncovered" over time, looms as an expanding problem. Distinguishing ADHD from dementia requires a skillful history and sometimes neuropsychological evaluation. Recent evidence suggests that dementia with Lewy bodies, the second most prevalent dementia in the elderly after Alzheimer's, is linked to patients with ADHD [45]. Both dementia with Lewy bodies and ADHD are viewed as hypodopaminergic states. Dementia with Lewy bodies is clinically associated with Parkinson's disease, but is distinguishable because of the presence of recurrent visual hallucinations in patients with dementia with Lewy bodies [46]. Golimstok et al. determined that nearly half of patients with dementia with Lewy bodies had preceding ADHD symptoms, compared with 15% in the general population, and that patients diagnosed with dementia with Lewy bodies had a high prevalence of ADHD symptoms [45]. Any specific relationship between ADHD and dementia with Lewy bodies requires further study.

Endocrinopathies

Thyroid disorders

Thyroid hormone is responsible for normal growth and development as well as maintenance of metabolism in the adult. Perturbations in the hormonal milieu of the body can have profound and non-specific effects on behavior. The influence of thyroid hormone on the developing brain has been known for more than 100 years when cretinism and mental retardation were recognized in children with thyroid hormone deprivation. Thyroid hormone also influences behavior in the adult. Abnormalities in the concentration of serum thyroid hormone can result in behavior that is erratic and may resemble ADHD [47]. There are three conditions of the thyroid that have been reported to be associated with ADHD-like symptoms: hypothyroidism, hyperthyroidism, and the syndrome of resistance to thyroid hormone (RTH).

Hypothyroidism

Hypothyroidism is caused by insufficient production of thyroid hormone. This is usually due to a failure of the gland to produce thyroxine caused by an autoimmune process resulting in destruction of the gland (Hashimoto's thyroiditis), or less commonly due to a failure of the pituitary to appropriately stimulate the thyroid. Hypothyroidism may result in symptoms of lethargy and inattention. Thyroid hormone deprivation is usually accompanied by cold intolerance, weight gain, skin and hair changes, and constipation. Elevation of serum thyrotrophin (thyroid stimulating hormone [TSH]) and decreased levels of serum thyroxine (T4) and triiodothyronine (T3) define primary hypothyroidism (due to failure of the thyroid gland to synthesize or release thyroid hormone). In a recent study, Haddow et al. demonstrated that children of mothers who were hypothyroid during the pregnancy had a 4.1 ± 2.1 decrease in Full Scale IQ score (p = 0.06) and a 3 ± 2 point decrease in the Wechsler Intelligence Scale for Children (WISC)-III freedom-from-distractibility score (a measure of attention) (p = 0.08) [48]. Although these are subtle differences and the clinical significance in a larger population is unknown, it is suggestive that the thyroid status of the mother may influence the subsequent neurocognitive development of the child.

Treatment of hypothyroidism is usually easily achieved with T4 supplementation with the goal to normalize the serum TSH and T4 levels. In most instances hormone replacement results in return of behavior and psychological profiles to baseline. It has been suggested that subjective improvement of various behavioral parameters could be further improved with the addition of T3. Bunevicius et al. demonstrated in

33 patients with hypothyroidism, among 17 scores of mood, 6 were better or closer to normal after treatment with T4 plus T3 than with treatment with T4 only [49]. Although this was a rather small study, the results are provocative and warrant further investigation on the use of T3 along with T4 in the treatment of behavioral symptoms of hypothyroidism.

Hyperthyroidism

Hyperthyroidism is caused by an overproduction of thyroid hormone. This is usually due to an antibody directed to the TSH receptor on the thyrocyte, stimulating release of thyroid hormone in the absence of TSH. Less commonly hyperthyroidism can be the result of an autonomous production of thyroid hormone due to a nodule of the thyroid. Hyperthyroidism is usually associated with symptoms of tremors, palpitations with tachycardia, weight loss, fatigue, insomnia, hair and skin changes, heat intolerance, and frequent bowel movements. Commonly, these patients present with altered cognition, inability to concentrate, and inattentiveness. Elevated concentrations of serum T3 and T4 and suppression of serum TSH confirm the diagnosis of hyperthyroidism.

Treatment of hyperthyroidism is aimed at decreasing production of T4 and T3 by the thyroid gland by the use of antithyroid medication (such as propylthiouracil or methimazole), radioactive iodine ablation, or surgery. The latter two treatments usually result in hypothyroidism. Correction of the thyroid hormone concentration completely reverses the symptoms of hyperthyroidism.

Resistance to thyroid hormone

RTH is a rare thyroid hormone disorder that is characterized by reduced responsiveness to thyroid hormone [50]. It is usually due to a mutation in the thyroid hormone receptor beta gene such that the tissues are no longer able to respond to normal concentrations of thyroid hormone. Careful evaluation of subjects with RTH has shown that almost one-half have some degree of learning disability with or without ADHD [51]. About one-quarter of subjects have intellectual quotients (IQ) less than 85 but frank mental retardation (IQ < 60) has been found only in 3% of cases. IQ is on average lower in subjects with RTH with or without ADHD [52]. Although, the behavioral characteristics of children with ADHD and RTH are similar to those with ADHD only, the former have significantly weaker ability of perceptual organization and

lower school achievement, suggesting a more severe cognitive impairment [52]. Impaired mental function was found to be associated with impaired or delayed growth (<5th percentile) in 20% of subjects, though growth retardation alone is rare (4%) [51]. Despite the high prevalence of ADHD in patients with RTH, the occurrence of RTH in children with ADHD must be very rare, none having been detected in 412 such children studied [53]. Furthermore, current data do not support a genetic linkage of RTH with ADHD. Rather the association with low IQ scores may confer a higher likelihood for subjects with RTH to exhibit ADHD symptoms [54], a conclusion that has been recently contested [55]. The reason such a rare disorder is included in the list of thyroid diseases associated with ADHD, while other more common diseases are not, is that more than 40–60% of children with RTH have ADHD.

RTH is usually diagnosed by the presence of goiter along with elevated serum free T4 and T3 with nonsuppressed serum TSH. These children are usually brought to clinical attention because of the goiter, growth disturbance, hyperactive behavior, or tachycardia. Thyroid function tests are then obtained and the classic blood tests are obtained. Since most patients with RTH have compensated for their defect, in the absence of concurrent thyroid disease or previous antithyroid treatment, no treatment is necessary. Occasionally treatment with beta-adrenergic blockers can help with symptoms related to tachycardia. In a limited small study, it was suggested that T3 treatment may be beneficial for some of the inattentive symptoms in this group [56].

The link between ADHD and RTH has been further suggested by a mouse model of RTH which is reported to display some characteristics of ADHD, although methylphenidate seems to worsen the symptoms in this not well defined mouse model [57, 58].

Abnormality in the hypothalamic–pituitary–adrenal axis (HPA)

Cortisol, like thyroid hormone, is necessary for normal growth and development and is necessary for normal functioning of most biological systems within an organism from cognition to inflammation. The release of cortisol into the blood is exquisitely regulated by the pituitary and hypothalamus by control of adrenocorticotrophic hormone (ACTH) release by corticotrophin-releasing hormone (CRH), respectively. Conditions that result in over stimulation of the hypothalamus and pituitary would result in high levels of serum cortisol, while other conditions with inhibition of normal ACTH and CRH would result in lower amounts of circulating cortisol. There is a growing body of evidence to suggest that in ADHD there is a lower plasma cortisol level, possibly due to impaired hypothalamic pituitary simulation, for reasons that are not well known [59–61]. While there are no reports of hypoadrenalism presenting as ADHD, it is quite possible that in the subset of children with an underactive HPA axis or even mild adrenal insufficiency that replacement of glucocorticoid may affect the ADHD. Causes for low HPA activity may be due to an insult of the pituitary or hypothalamus secondary to radiation or surgery. In addition, children treated with pharmacological doses of glucocorticoids for inflammatory conditions such as asthma or rheumatoid arthritis would have suppression of the HPA upon withdrawal of the steroid and this should be considered when such a child presents with ADHD.

References

1. Weinberg WA, Emslie GJ. Attention deficit hyperactivity disorder: the differential diagnosis. *J Child Neurol.* 1991;**6**:S23–36.

2. Batshaw ML. *Children with Disabilities*, 6th edn. Baltimore, MD: Paul H. Brookes Pub. Co.; 2007.

3. Accardo PJ, Blondis TA, Whitman BY, Stein MA. *Attention Deficits and Hyperactivity in Children and Adults*. New York, NY: Marcel Dekker; 1999.

4. Goldman LS, Genel M, Bezman RJ, Slanetz PJ. Diagnosis and treatment of attention-deficit/hyperactivity disorder in children and adolescents. Council on Scientific Affairs, American Medical Association. *JAMA.* 1998;**279**:1100–7.

5. Lavenstein B. Neurological comorbidity patterns/differential diagnosis in adult attention deficit disorder. In: Nadeau KG, ed. *A Comprehensive Guide to Attention Deficit Disorder in Adults*. New York, NY: Brunnel/Mazel Pubs. 1995; 74–92.

6. Volpe JJ. *Neurology of the Newborn*, 5th edn. Philadelphia, PA: Elsevier Health Science; 2008.

7. Steinhausen HC, Willms J, Spohr HL. Long-term psychopathological and cognitive outcome of children with fetal alcohol syndrome. *J Am Acad Child Adolesc Psychiatry.* 1993;**32**:990–4.

8. Emory E, Ansari Z, Pattillo R, Archibold E, Chevalier J. Maternal blood lead effects on infant intelligence at age 7 months. *Am J Obstet Gynecol.* 2003;**188**:S26–32.

9. Chiriboga CA, Kuhn L, Wasserman GA. Prenatal cocaine exposures and dose-related cocaine effects on infant tone and behavior. *Neurotoxicol Teratol.* 2007;**29**:232–30.

10. Szatmari P, Saigal S, Rosenbaum P, Campbell D, King S. Psychiatric disorders at five years among children with birthweights <1000 g: a regional perspective. *Dev Med Child Neurol.* 1990;**32**:954–62.

11. Anderson PJ, De Luca CR, Hutchinson E, *et al.* Attention problems in a representative sample of extremely preterm/extremely low birth weight children. *Dev Neuropsychol.* 2011;**36**:57–73.

12. Hawdon JM, Hey E, Klovin L, *et al.* Born too small: is outcome still affected? *Dev Med Child Neurol.* 1990;**32**:943–53.

13. Motlagh MG, Katsovich L, Thompson N, *et al.* Severe psychological stress and heavy cigarette smoking during pregnancy: an examination of the pre- and perinatal risk factors associated with ADHD and Tourette syndrome. *Eur Child Adolesc Psychiatry.* 2010;**19**:755–64.

14. Sprich-Buckminster S, Biederman J, Milberger S, *et al.* Are perinatal complications relevant to the manifestations of ADD? Issues of comorbidity and familiarity. *J Am Acad Child Adolesc Psychiatry.* 1993;**32**:1032–7.

15. Stein MA, Rubinoff A, Pliskin N, Weiss RE. Adult ADHD and AIDS. *Am J Psychiatry.* 1995;**157**:1100.

16. Borghgraef M, Fryns JP, van den Berghe H. The female and the fragile X syndrome: data on clinical and psychological findings in 7 fra (x) carriers. *Clin Genet.* 1990;**37**:341–6.

17. Joinson C, Heron J, Emond A *et al.* Psychological problems in children with bedwetting and combined (day and night) wetting: A UK population-based study. *J Pediatr Psychol.* 2007;**32**:650.

18. Shreeram A, He JP, Kalaydjian A, *et al.* Prevalence of enuresis and its association with attention-deficit/hyperactivity disorder among U.S. children: results from a nationally representative study. *J Am Acad Child Adolesc Psychiatry.* 2009;**48**:35–41.

19. Joinson C, Heron J, Butler U, *et al.* Psychological differences between children with and without soiling problems. *Pediatrics.* 2006;**117**:1575–84.

20. Pearl PL, Holmes GL Absence seizures. In: Dodson WE, Pellock JM, eds. *Pediatric Epilepsy: Diagnosis and Treatment,* 2nd edn. New York, NY: Demos Publications. 1999.

21. Pearl PL, Holmes GL. Epilepsy syndromes and their prognosis. In: Wyler A, Hermann BP, eds. *The Surgical Management of Epilepsy*. New York, NY: Demos Publications. 1991.

22. Holmes GL, McKeever M, Adamson M. Absence seizures in children: clinical and electrographic features. *Ann Neurol.* 1987;**21**:268–73.

23. Alves-Leon SV, Cardoso MF, Pereira VC, Meira ID. Clinical and electroencephalographic characteristics of a cohort of patients with epilepsy and absence seizures. *Arq Neuropsiquiatr.* 2009;**67**:986–94.

24. Jankovic J. Tourette syndrome. *N Engl J Med.* 2001;**341**:1184–92.

25. Comings D, Comings B. Tourette's syndrome and attention deficit disorder. In: Cohen DJ, Bruun RD, Leckman JF, eds. *Tourette's Syndrome and Tic Disorders: Clinical Understanding and Treatment.* New York, NY: John Wiley & Sons. 1988; 119–35.

26. Roessner V, Robatzek M, Knapp G, Banascewski T, Rothenberger A. First-onset tics in patients with attention-deficit-hyperactivity disorder: impact of stimulants. *Dev Med Child Neurol.* 2006;**48**: 616–21.

27. Spencer T, Biederman J, Harding M, *et al.* Disentangling the overlap between Tourette's disorder and ADHD. *J Child Psychol Psychiatry.* 1998;**39**: 1037–44.

28. Chee KY, Sachdev P. The clinical features of Tourette's disorder: an Australian study using a structured interview schedule. *Aust N Z J Psychiatry.* 1994;**28**:313–18.

29. Gorman DA, Thompson N, Plessen KJ, *et al.* Psychosocial outcome and psychiatric comorbidity in older adolescents with Tourette syndrome: controlled study. *Br J Psychiatry.* 2010;**197**:36–44.

30. Swedo SE, Leonard HL, Garvey M, *et al.* Pediatric autoimmune neuropsychiatric disorders associated with streptococcal infections: clinical description of the first 50 cases. *Am J Psychiatry.* 1998;**155**: 264–71.

31. Konofal E, Lecendreux M, Cortese S. Sleep and ADHD. *Sleep Med.* 2010;**11**:652–8.

32. Owens JA. A clinical overview of sleep and attention-deficit/hyperactivity disorder in children and adolescents. *J Can Acad Child Adolesc Psychiatry.* 2009;**18**:92–102.

33. Cortese S, Konofal E, Lecendreux M, *et al.* Restless legs syndrome and attention-deficit/hyperactivity disorder: a review of the literature. *Sleep.* 2005;**28**:1007–13.

34. Corkum P, Moldofsky H, Hogg-Johnson S, Humphries T, Tannock R. Sleep problems in children with attention-deficit/hyperactivity disorder: impact of subtype, comorbidity, and stimulant medication. *J Am Acad Child Psychol.* 1999;**38**:1285–93.

35. Stein MA. Unraveling sleep problems in treated and untreated children with ADHD. *J Child Adolesc Psychopharmacol.* 1999;**9**:157–68.

36. Stein MA, Sarampote CS, Waldman ID, *et al.* A dose-response study of OROS methylphenidate in children and adolescents with ADHD. *Pediatrics.* 2003;**112**:e404.

37. Stein M, Weiss M, Hlavaty L. ADHD treatments, sleep, and sleep problems: complex associations. *Neurotherapeutics.* 2012;**9**:509–17.

38. Sullivan SS. Narcolepsy in adolescents. *Adolesc Med State Art Rev.* 2010;**21**:542–55.

39. Aran A, Einen M, Lin L, *et al.* Clinical and therapeutic aspects of childhood narcolepsy-cataplexy: a retrospective study of 51 children. *Sleep.* 2010;**33**: 1457–64.

40. Calarge C, Farmer C, DiSilvestro R, Arnold LE. Serum ferritin and amphetamine response in youth with attention-deficit/hyperactivity disorder. *J Child Adolesc Psychopharmacol.* 2010;**20**:495–502.

41. Konofal E, Lecendreux M, Arnulf I, Mouren MC. Iron deficiency in children with attention-deficit/ hyperactivity disorder. *Arch Pediatr Adolesc Med.* 2004;**158**:1113–15.

42. Konofal E, Cortese S, Marchand M, *et al.* Impact of restless legs syndrome and iron deficiency on attention deficit/hyperactivity disorder in children. *Sleep Med.* 2007;**8**:711–15.

43. Konofal E, Lecendreux M, Deron J, *et al.* Effects of iron supplementation on attention deficit hyperactivity disorder in children. *Pediatr Neurol.* 2008;**38**: 20–6.

44. Cortese S, Azoulay R, Castellanos F, *et al.* Brain iron levels in Attention-Deficit/Hyperactivity Disorder: a pilot MRI study. *World J Biol Psychiatry.* 2012;**13**: 223–31.

45. Golimstok A, Rojas JI, Romano M, *et al.* Previous adult attention-deficit and hyperactivity disorder symptoms and risk of dementia with Lewy bodies: a case-control study. *Eur J Neurol.* 2011;**18**: 78–84.

46. Weintraub D, Hurtig HI. Presentation and management of psychosis in Parkinson's disease and dementia with Lewy Bodies. *Am J Psychiatry.* 2007;**164**:1491–8.

47. Weiss RE, Stein MA. Thyroid function and attention deficit hyperactivity disorder. In: Accardo P, Blondis T, Whitman B, Stein M, eds. *Attention Deficits and Hyperactivity in Children and Adults*, New York, NY: Marcel Dekker. 1999; 419–30.

48. Haddow JE, Palomaki GE, Allan WC, *et al.* Maternal thyroid deficiency during pregnancy and subsequent neuropsychological development of the child. *N Engl J Med.* 1999;**341**:549–55.

49. Bunevicius R, Kazanavicius G, Zalinkevicius R, Prange AJ. Effects of thyroxine as compared with thyroxine

plus triiodothyronine in patients with hypothyroidism. *N Engl J Med*. 1999;**340**:424–9.

50. Refetoff S, Weiss RE. Resistance to thyroid hormone. In: Thakker TV, ed. *Molecular Genetics of Endocrine Disorders*. London: Chapman & Hill. 1997; 85–122.

51. Refetoff S, Weiss RE, Usala SJ. The syndromes of resistance to thyroid hormone. *Endocr Rev*. 1993;**14**:348–99.

52. Stein MA, Weiss RE, Refetoff S. Neurocognitive characteristics of individuals with resistance to thyroid hormone: comparisons to individuals with attention deficit hyperactivity disorder only. *J Dev Behav Pediatr*. 1995;**16**:406–11.

53. Spencer T, Biederman J, Wilens T, Guite J, Harding M. ADHD and thyroid abnormalities: a research note. *J Child Psychol Psychiatry*. 1995;**35**:878–85.

54. Weiss RE, Stein MA, Duck SC, *et al*. Low intelligence but not attention deficit hyperactivity disorder is associated with resistance to thyroid hormone caused by mutation R316H in the thyroid hormone receptor beta gene. *J Clin Endocrinol Metab*. 1994;**78**:1525–8.

55. Brucker-Davis F, Skarulis MC, Grace MB, *et al*. Genetic and clinical features of 42 kindreds with resistance to thyroid hormone. The National Institutes of Health Prospective Study. *Ann Intern Med*. 1995;**123**:572–83.

56. Weiss RE, Stein MA, Refetoff S. Behavior effects of liothyronine (L-T3) in children with attention deficit hyperactivity disorder in the presence of an absence of resistance to thyroid hormone. *Thyroid*. 1997;**7**: 389–93.

57. Siesser WB, Cheng S-Y, McDonald MP. Hyperactivity, impaired learning on a vigilance task, and a differential response to methylphenidate in the TRbetaPV knock-in mouse. *Psychopharmacology (Berl)*. 2005;**181**: 53–63.

58. Siesser WB, Zhao J, Miller L, Cheng S-Y, McDonald MP. Transgenic mice expressing a human mutant β1 thyroid receptor are hyperactive, impulsive, and inattentive. *Genes Brain Behav*. 2006;**5**:282–97.

59. Ma L, Chen Y-H, Chen H, Liu Y-Y, Wang Y-X. The function of hypothalamus-pituitary-adrenal axis in children with ADHD. *Brain Res*. 2010;**1368**: 159–62.

60. Stadler C, Kroeger A, Weyers P, *et al*. Cortisol reactivity in boys with attention-deficit/hyperactivity disorder and disruptive behavior problems: the impact of callous unemotional traits. *Psychiatry Res*. 2011;**187**(1–2):204–9.

61. Lee SH, Shin, DW, Stein M. Increased cortisol after stress is associated with variability in response time in ADHD children. *Yonsei Med J*. 2010;**51**(2):206–11.

Catecholamine influences on prefrontal cortex circuits and function

Amy F. T. Arnsten and Craig W. Berridge

Introduction

The symptoms of poor impulse control, impaired regulation of attention and locomotor hyperactivity in patients with attention-deficit hyperactivity disorder (ADHD) involve dysfunction of prefrontal cortical circuits. The prefrontal cortex (PFC) guides attention, actions, and emotions using representational knowledge, and is highly dependent on neurochemical state: moderate levels of dopamine (DA) D_1 and norepinephrine (NE) alpha-2A (α_{2A})-adrenoceptor stimulation are essential to strong prefrontal working memory function. ADHD is sometimes associated with genetic insults that dysregulate catecholamine signaling, for example reduced synthesis of NE is associated with poor sustained attention and impulse control. Approved treatments for ADHD (including stimulants, atomoxetine, and guanfacine) optimize catecholamine signaling in the PFC and strengthen PFC regulation of attention and impulse control. For example, low, therapeutic doses of methylphenidate increase levels of both NE and DA in the PFC in animals, enhance prefrontal physiology and cognitive function, and reduce locomotor hyperactivity in juvenile rats. These prefrontal actions likely contribute to methylphenidate's therapeutic effects in ADHD.

Deficits in PFC function underlie many of the symptoms of ADHD, including problems such as poor impulse control, weak sustained attention, heightened distractibility, and increased locomotor activity. The PFC in the right hemisphere is particularly important for inhibiting inappropriate responses [1], and both functional and structural imaging studies have shown weakness in this brain region in subjects with ADHD [2–5]. Basic research has shown that the PFC is especially sensitive to stimulation by the catecholamines NE and DA [6]. Importantly, all approved medications

for ADHD strengthen or mimic catecholamine transmission in the PFC, enhancing PFC function and ameliorating ADHD symptoms [7]. The following chapter briefly reviews the importance of catecholamines to PFC physiology and function, and their relevance to the etiology and treatment of ADHD.

The prefrontal association cortices regulate attention, behavior, and emotion

The primate PFC is topographically organized such that the dorsal and lateral surfaces monitor attention and action, while the ventral and medial regions monitor emotion [8]. These regions interconnect for the coordinated regulation of behavior.

The PFC regulates attention and thought through extensive projections back to the temporal and parietal association cortices, i.e., "top-down" attention [9–11]. The PFC provides the ability to inhibit distractions and gate sensory inputs based on internal goals [12]; it also facilitates sustained attention (especially over long delays) [13], and inhibits interference from irrelevant information [14]. Like patients with ADHD, those with PFC lesions are easily distracted, have poor concentration and organization, have difficulty dividing or focusing attention, and are more vulnerable to disruption from proactive interference [15].

The PFC is also essential for the inhibition of inappropriate behaviors; lesions in this region in monkeys and humans can induce locomotor hyperactivity and impulsive responses (e.g., on Go/No-Go tasks) [16, 17]. The PFC guides behavioral output via projections to the motor cortices, to basal ganglia structures (including the caudate and subthalamic nucleus), and to the cerebellum (by way of the

Attention-Deficit Hyperactivity Disorder in Adults and Children, ed. Lenard A. Adler, Thomas J. Spencer and Timothy E. Wilens. Published by Cambridge University Press. © Cambridge University Press 2015.

pons) [18]. In humans, the right inferior PFC is particularly important for behavioral inhibition [19, 20]; functional imaging studies reveal activity in the right inferior PFC when subjects successfully inhibit or stop movements [19]. Indeed, transmagnetic stimulation over the right inferior PFC can impair the ability to stop motor responses in healthy controls [21]. There are some PFC regions that project to the subthalamic nucleus (the "hyper-direct pathway") and are able to rapidly stop an ongoing movement, for example as in the Stop Signal task [22]. Emerging research suggests that this form of "emergency" behavioral inhibition may have different neurochemical needs than PFC circuits involved in inhibitory motor planning (e.g., the Go/No-Go task) [23].

The ventral (orbital) and medial PFC is extensively interconnected with structures involved with emotion, including the amygdala, hypothalamus, nucleus accumbens, and brainstem nuclei [24–26]. The PFC is positioned to activate or inhibit these structures, and studies in rats have shown that the PFC is essential for inhibition of the fear response [27, 28]. Studies in monkeys have shown the importance of the orbital PFC for the flexible regulation of emotional responses to reward and punishment [29, 30]. In humans, damage to this region produces unregulated emotional behavior, for example the famous case of Phineas Gage [31]. Importantly, damage to this area early in childhood can induce sociopathy, including reduced response to reward and punishment [32].

ADHD is associated with weaker PFC structure and function

Imaging studies of subjects with ADHD show reduced size and reduced functional activity of the PFC [33–35]. These differences are particularly prominent in the right hemisphere, consistent with the important role of the right PFC in the regulation of behavior and attention [20]. ADHD is also associated with alterations in structure/function in regions that receive PFC projections, such as the caudate and cerebellum [36]. Recent studies also have reported disorganized white matter tracks emanating from the PFC in subjects with ADHD, consistent with weaker functional connectivity [2, 4]. The PFC matures more slowly than less evolved brain regions, and there is evidence of slower PFC development in some subjects with ADHD [3]. However, for many patients, ADHD is a lifelong disorder, and imaging studies continue to show evidence

of weakened PFC function and reduced right PFC volume in adults with ADHD [4, 37]. Consistent with these imaging data, subjects with ADHD show deficits on tasks that depend on the PFC, including tests of executive function, working memory, attention regulation, and inhibitory control [20, 38, 39].

Many patients with ADHD have comorbid emotional dysregulation, for example, anxiety, oppositional defiant disorder (ODD), or conduct disorder. These affective symptoms have been related to abnormal activity in the orbital and/or ventral medial PFC [5]. Thus, global deficits in PFC function may result in impaired regulation of attention, behavior, and emotion.

Genetic insults in ADHD can involve changes to catecholamine signaling

ADHD is a highly heritable disorder, and many gene variants have been associated with increased risk of ADHD [40]. Although there are likely many genetic insults that can compromise the integrity of the PFC, and the contribution of any single gene to the development of ADHD symptoms appears to be small, it is of interest that several genes associated with ADHD involve catecholamines. These include genes encoding molecules involved in catecholamine signaling (e.g., NE and DA receptors) [41–46], DA and NE and DA transporters [41, 45, 46], and dopamine beta-hydroxylase (DBH), the enzyme required for NE synthesis [41, 43]. For example, genetic alterations in DBH are associated with weakened ability to regulate attention [47, 48], impaired executive functions [49], increased impulsivity [50], and the ADHD symptoms [51]. These genetic findings are consistent with basic research showing that the PFC is highly sensitive to catecholamine stimulation, and dysregulation of catecholamine actions can markedly impair PFC function.

The PFC requires optimal levels of NE and DA for proper function

NE and DA neurons arise from the brainstem and project across the entire cortical mantle, including the PFC [52]. NE acts at α_1, α_2, and beta (β) adrenoceptors, and has the highest affinity for α_2 adrenoceptors [53]. There are three subtypes of α_2 adrenoceptors: α_{2A}, α_{2B}, and α_{2C} [54]. The most prominent DA receptors in the PFC are the D_1 receptor family, which includes D_1 and D_5 receptors; these receptors are very similar, and there are currently no drugs that distinguish between them (thus, in this review, D_1 refers to both D_1 and D_5). A second DA receptor family, the D_2 receptor family, includes the D_2, D_3, and D_4 receptors. The D_4 receptor is actually a generalized catecholamine receptor, as both NE and DA have affinity for this receptor [55].

The PFC requires an optimal level of NE and DA for proper function: either too little (when we are fatigued) or too much (when we are stressed) markedly impairs PFC regulation of behavior, thought, and emotion. This dose–response relationship is often referred to as the "inverted-U" dose–response [56]. Studies in animals have found that NE and DA are so critical to PFC function that depleting them is as detrimental as ablating the cortex itself [57].

Receptor actions

Many of the beneficial effects of NE and DA on PFC-dependent behavior occur through actions at α_{2A} and D_1 receptors, respectively [56]. NE has its beneficial actions at α_{2A} receptors that reside on PFC neurons, postsynaptic to NE axons [58]. Although previous research has emphasized the important role of presynaptic α_2 receptors on NE neurons (which reduce NE cell firing and decrease NE release) [59], it is now appreciated that the majority of α_2 receptors in the brain are actually postsynaptic on non-NE neurons [60]. Within the PFC, these postsynaptic α_2 receptors facilitate PFC function [58]. Electron microscopic studies indicate that α_{2A} and D_1 receptors reside on separate dendritic spines on PFC pyramidal cells, near synaptic inputs from other PFC neurons [58, 61]. Stimulation of these receptors gates nearby synaptic inputs [62], with α_{2A} adrenoceptor stimulation strengthening behaviorally appropriate inputs ("signals") [58], and D_1 receptor stimulation weakening inappropriate inputs ("noise") [63]. These gating actions likely occur through cAMP opening of hyperpolarization-activated cyclic nucleotide-gated (HCN) channels on spines near α_{2A} or D_1 receptors, as illustrated in Figure 14.1A. Blockade of either the α_{2A} [64] or the D_1 [65] receptor markedly impairs PFC function, demonstrating the critical importance of these modulatory actions. This has been observed at the cellular level as well, where blockade of α_{2A} receptors in the PFC markedly reduces PFC neuronal firing in monkeys performing a working memory

task [58, 66], and produces a profile of deficits similar to ADHD: locomotor hyperactivity [67], poor impulse control [68], and weakened working memory needed to overcome distractors [64]. In contrast, α_{2A} receptor stimulation with guanfacine enhances PFC task-related firing [58], and improves dorsolateral [69], ventrolateral [70], and orbital [71] PFC functions (Figure 14.1B). Thus, α_{2A} receptor stimulation can enhance working memory and attention as well as behavioral inhibition. Similarly, moderate doses of D_1 agonists can enhance PFC function, especially in subjects with DA depletion [72–74].

However, excessive release of the catecholamines NE and DA (e.g., during exposure to uncontrollable stress) markedly impairs PFC function [75]. High levels of NE release engage lower affinity α_1 and β_1 receptors that are detrimental to PFC function, and suppress PFC neuronal firing [76]. Similarly, high levels of DA release during stress produce excessive D_1 receptor stimulation which suppresses PFC cell firing through excessive cAMP signaling [63]. These detrimental actions may be incurred with inappropriate doses of stimulant medications.

The pharmacology of attention-deficit hyperactivity disorder

Pharmacological treatments are currently the most effective form of treatment for ADHD. Several drug classes have been shown to be effective. These include the psychostimulants (primarily methylphenidate and amphetamine), selective NE reuptake blockers (desipramine, atomoxetine), and α_2 agonists, particularly α_{2A}-preferring, such as guanfacine. As reviewed below, most of these drugs share the ability to increase *both* NE and DA neurotransmission within the PFC, with the exception of α_2 agonists, which mimic NE neurotransmission at α_2 receptors.

Psychostimulants

Psychostimulants have been used in the treatment of ADHD since the 1930s. Across the different drug classes currently available for the treatment of ADHD, stimulants remain the most widely used. Extensive clinical studies demonstrate that these drugs are effective in treating the attentional and hyperactivity/impulsivity components of ADHD in children, adolescents, and adults [77, 78]. The therapeutic effects of low-dose stimulants are observed acutely

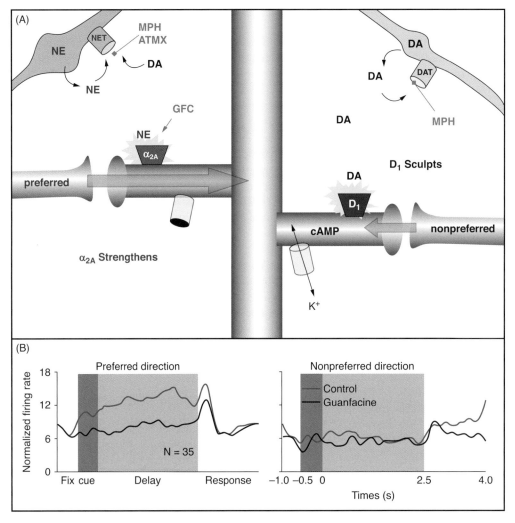

Figure 14.1. Catecholamine modulation of PFC networks. (A) NE and DA have complementary effects on PFC network inputs: NE α_{2A} strengthens preferred inputs, while DA D_1 weakens nonpreferred inputs. These actions occur through inhibition vs. activation of cAMP-HCN channel signaling, respectively. Both α_{2A} and D_1 receptors have been localized on spines in primate PFC near cAMP-HCN channel signaling proteins. See Arnsten *et al.* [62] for review.
(B) Iontophoretic application of guanfacine onto neurons in monkey dorsolateral PFC increases firing for the neurons' preferred direction, thus enhancing the spatially-tuned persistent firing during the delay period needed for working memory. Based on Wang *et al.* [58] and Vijayraghavan *et al.* [63]. ATMX = atomoxetine, DAT = dopamine transporter, GFC = guanfacine, MPH = methylphenidate, NET = norepinephrine transporter.

with neither pronounced tolerance nor sensitization observed with repeated treatment over many months [78]; however, see Swanson and Volkow [79].

At high doses, psychostimulants increase arousal, motor activity, and euphoria, while impairing PFC-dependent cognition [56, 80–84]. Historically, the behavioral/cognitive actions of low-dose stimulants were viewed as unique to ADHD (the so-called paradoxical actions of psychostimulants). A major advance

in our understanding of the pharmacology of ADHD was the discovery that low and clinically relevant doses improve PFC-dependent cognitive function and reduce impulsivity in *normal* human subjects [85–89]. Consistent with these findings, low-dose stimulants are commonly used as cognitive enhancers by individuals without ADHD [90]. Combined, these observations demonstrate that the cognition-enhancing and behavior-calming actions of stimulants occur only at low doses, and at these doses, psychostimulants exert similar cognition-enhancing effects in normal subjects and in subjects with ADHD.

Clinically, the therapeutic actions of methylphenidate occur with plasma concentrations in the range of 8 ng/mL to 40 ng/mL [79]. Recent studies demonstrate that doses of methylphenidate that result in similar plasma concentrations in monkeys and rodents suppress locomotor activity and exert an inverted-U shaped facilitation of PFC-dependent cognition similar to that seen in humans [7, 56, 80, 91–93].

Neurochemically, stimulants inhibit NE and DA reuptake and, depending on the drug and dose, serotonin reuptake. Within this drug class, amphetamine also actively stimulates the efflux of DA and, at high doses, NE [94]. Although amphetamine also blocks serotonin reuptake, this only occurs at high and clinically inappropriate doses [95]. In contrast to amphetamine, methylphenidate acts only as a reuptake blocker for NE and DA [96]. Combined, these observations indicate that the therapeutic/cognition-enhancing actions of low-dose stimulants involve inhibition of NE and/or DA reuptake and are not dependent on inhibition of serotonin reuptake or active stimulation of catecholamine efflux. A lack of involvement of serotonin in the therapeutic actions of stimulants is consistent with previous observations indicating that selective serotonin reuptake inhibitors are relatively ineffective in the treatment of ADHD [97].

When administered at relatively high doses associated with hyperactivity or stereotypy, stimulants elicit large increases in extracellular levels of brain NE and DA widely throughout the brain [95, 98, 99]. Stimulant-induced increases in accumbens DA and PFC α_1-signaling contribute to the locomotor-activating and reinforcing actions of the psychostimulants [100–103].

In contrast to behaviorally activating doses of stimulants, low and clinically relevant doses of these drugs produce a qualitatively different pattern of action on brain catecholamine systems. Specifically, at clinically relevant doses, methylphenidate produces a prominent increase in extracellular levels of NE and DA within the PFC while having substantially reduced actions in cortical (somatosensory cortex, hippocampus) and subcortical regions (accumbens, medial septum) outside the PFC (Figure 14.2) [7, 91, 104, 105]. This preferential sensitivity of PFC NE and DA to low-dose stimulants may involve low DA transporter levels within the PFC combined with an ability of the NE transporter to clear both NE and DA [106, 107].

Electrophysiological studies in rats indicate that at these low and cognition-enhancing doses, psychostimulants preferentially strengthen PFC neuronal responsiveness to afferent signals, while having only modest effects on spontaneous discharge of PFC neurons (Figure 14.3) [92]. In contrast, modestly higher doses that fail to improve PFC-dependent cognition no longer enhance the responsiveness of PFC neurons, while high and behaviorally activating doses profoundly suppress evoked discharge of PFC neurons (Figure 14.3) [92]. Consistent with the neurochemical observations described above, low-dose methylphenidate does not affect neuronal activity outside the PFC [92]. Thus, cognition-enhancing doses of psychostimulants act to increase catecholamine neurotransmission and signaling processing preferentially within the PFC. Evidence reviewed above suggests the hypothesis that the cognition-enhancing actions of low-dose stimulants involve preferential targeting of PFC catecholamine signaling at PFC α_{2A} and D_1 receptors. Consistent with this, the cognition-enhancing actions of low-dose methylphenidate in both rats and monkeys are prevented by systemic pretreatment with an α_2 antagonist or a D_1 antagonist, at doses that have no impact on baseline cognitive function [56, 80].

Non-stimulant medications: NET selective reuptake blockers

Low-dose methylphenidate and amphetamine act as NE and DA reuptake inhibitors. However, selective NE reuptake inhibitors are also effective in treating ADHD. These include the tricyclic antidepressants, desipramine and nortriptyline, as well as the non-tricyclic compound, atomoxetine (Strattera®). Among the tricyclics, the most intensively studied for the treatment of ADHD is desipramine [108]. For reasons that are poorly understood, desipramine appears effective in a subset of patients unresponsive to psychostimulants [108]. Atomoxetine (originally "tomoxetine") is a non-tricyclic selective NE reuptake blocker that has been approved by the US Food and Drug Administration (FDA) for treating ADHD [109–111]. Atomoxetine lacks the affinity for neurotransmitter receptors associated with the tricyclic antidepressants and, correspondingly, is largely devoid of tricyclic-like side effects [112, 113]. Atomoxetine, like stimulants, improves PFC cognitive function in

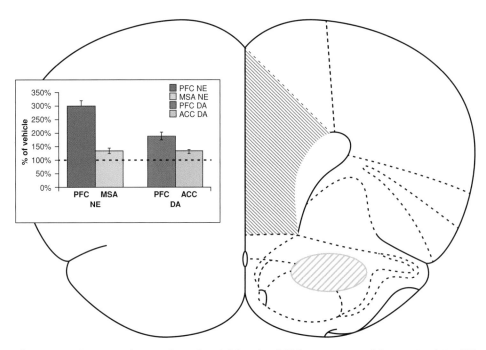

Figure 14.2. Cognition-enhancing doses of methylphenidate (MPH) increase extracellular norepinephrine (NE) and dopamine (DA) preferentially within the prefrontal cortex (PFC). Shown are the effects of a cognition-enhancing dose of MPH that produces clinically relevant peak plasma concentrations (0.5 mg/kg, intraperitoneally) on extracellular levels of NE and DA in the PFC, NE in the medial septal area (MSA), and DA in the nucleus accumbens core (ACC). Data are an average ($\pm$ SEM) of two 15-minute samples collected 15 to 45 minutes following drug treatment and are expressed as percent of vehicle treatment. At this dose, MPH produced only a modest ($\sim$30%) increase in NE and DA levels outside the PFC. In contrast, within the PFC, this dose of MPH produced a substantially larger increase in NE and DA levels. Moreover, the increase in PFC NE levels ($\sim$200%) was significantly larger than that seen for PFC DA ($\sim$85%). A similar pattern of effects was observed with oral administration of a cognition-enhancing dose (2.0 mg/kg) of MPH that produced plasma concentrations comparable to those seen with intraperitoneal administration of 0.5 mg/kg MPH. All groups differ significantly from vehicle treatment. For a given neurotransmitter, the cortical responses are significantly larger than the subcortical responses. Finally, the PFC NE response is significantly larger than the PFC DA response.

animals [56, 114], normal human subjects [115], and subjects with ADHD [116].

The neural circuitry underlying the therapeutic actions of selective NE reuptake inhibitors is not well understood. However, despite the selectivity of these compounds for the NE transporter, they nonetheless increase extracellular levels of both NE and DA in the PFC [106, 117]. Consistent with their primary pharmacological action (i.e., NE reuptake blockade), these drugs have minimal effects on DA levels outside the PFC, at least in regions largely devoid of NE fibers [106, 117]. Similar to that discussed with the psychostimulants, the ability of selective NE reuptake blockers to increase *both* NE and DA in the PFC is posited to result from the fact that the NE transporter displays a high affinity for DA [118, 119] and plays a prominent role in DA clearance in the PFC due to a limited density of DA transporters in this region.

Recent studies have shown that atomoxetine, like methylphenidate, produces an inverted-U dose response on working memory in monkeys [56], similar to the inverted-U shown in normal humans on tests of error monitoring [120]. Moreover, the cognition-enhancing effects of atomoxetine are blocked by either an α_2 or D_1 receptor antagonist [56]. Similarly, although the tricyclic compound mianserin also displays high selectivity for the NE transporter (relative to the other monoamine transporters), nonetheless, this compound is ineffective in the treatment of ADHD [121]. An important difference between mianserin and other tricyclics effective in treating ADHD is that mianserin displays a relatively high affinity for α_2 receptors, acting as an antagonist at these receptors [122]. Thus, the cognition-enhancing/therapeutic effects of selective NE reuptake blockers are similar to those seen with the stimulants [56, 80], and are dependent on α_2 as well as D_1 receptors.

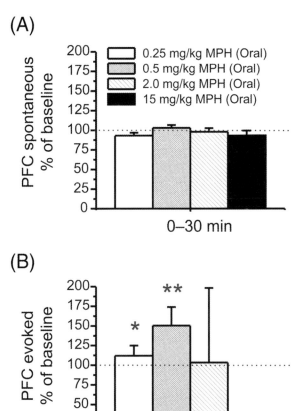

Figure 14.3. Cognition-enhancing doses of methylphenidate (MPH) preferentially increase the responsiveness of prefrontal cortex (PFC) neurons. Shown are the effects of varying doses of methylphenidate on spontaneous discharge and excitatory evoked responses (elicited by brief electrical stimulation of the hippocampus) of PFC neurons in the awake, freely moving rat. Doses examined included the cognition-enhancing dose of 0.5 mg/kg [92]. All data are expressed as the percent change from pre-drug conditions for the first 30 minutes following treatment (± SEM). (A) Spontaneous discharge of PFC neurons was minimally affected by low doses of methylphenidate. (B) Hippocampal stimulus-evoked excitatory discharge in PFC neurons exhibited a dose-dependent inverted-U facilitation/suppression. The maximal facilitation of PFC responses to hippocampal input was observed following the 0.5-mg/kg dose. A behaviorally activating dose of MPH (15.0 mg/kg) resulted in a suppression of stimulus-evoked activity well below baseline levels. *$p < 0.05$; **$p < 0.01$.

At the cellular level, iontophoresis of low doses of atomoxetine was observed to enhance spatially tuned, delay-related firing of PFC neurons by increasing delay-related firing for the neuron's preferred direction and/or decreasing delay-related firing for the neuron's nonpreferred directions [56]. These effects were mediated by α_2 and D_1 receptor actions, respectively [56]. In contrast, higher doses of atomoxetine suppressed PFC cell firing for all directions [56].

Non-stimulant medications: noradrenergic α_2-agonists

The nonselective α_2 agonist clonidine has long been used in the treatment of ADHD [123]. The ability of clonidine to decrease extracellular levels of NE is opposite to the effect observed with the stimulants, tricyclics, and atomoxetine. This difference between clonidine and other drug classes effective in treating ADHD was initially difficult to reconcile. A significant advance in our understanding of noradrenergic function was the identification of postsynaptic α_2 receptors within the PFC and the demonstration that these receptors promote PFC-dependent cognition (for reviews see Arnsten *et al.* [15] and Arnsten and Li [124]). Although it has been known for more than 30 years that most α_2 receptors in the brain are postsynaptic to NE terminals [60], this information has often not been appreciated. However, a variety of evidence suggests that the cognition-enhancing effects of α_{2A} agonists likely stem from the direct stimulation of postsynaptic α_{2A} receptors within the PFC [58].

Consistent with this hypothesis, the α_{2A}-preferring agonist guanfacine is effective in the treatment of ADHD while lacking the potent sedative actions of clonidine [125–127]. A limiting factor in the use of clonidine in ADHD is its sedative/hypotensive effects [123], which likely involve clonidine-induced suppression of NE release via stimulation of α_2 autoreceptors (for review see Berridge [128]) and stimulation of brainstem blood pressure-regulating imidazoline I1 receptors [129]. Guanfacine displays lower sedative/hypotensive effects presumably due to its lower affinity, relative to clonidine, for α_{2B}, α_{2C}, imidazoline I1, and presynaptic α_{2A} receptors [129–131]. In addition, guanfacine (along with the selective NE reuptake inhibitors) may be beneficial in patients who respond suboptimally to stimulants or for whom psychostimulants are contraindicated, for example due to tics [125] or ODD-like symptoms [132].

As is seen with the psychostimulants and atomoxetine, guanfacine improves PFC-dependent behavior in normal human and animal subjects [133, 134], although it is less effective in young, normal subjects than those with PFC deficits [133–135]. As discussed above (Figure 14.1), research in animals shows that guanfacine improves PFC working memory functions by strengthening the efficacy of PFC network connections [58]. Functional imaging studies in monkeys [136] and humans [137, 138] have shown increased PFC activity following systemic guanfacine administration, consistent with the physiological data.

Conclusion

The PFC plays a crucial role in regulating attention, behavior, and emotion. Deficits in PFC structure and function, including impaired regulation of subcortical structures, likely contribute to the etiology of ADHD symptoms. The PFC requires optimal levels of catecholamines to function properly – moderate levels of NE engaging postsynaptic α_{2A} adrenoceptors and DA stimulating a modest number of D_1 receptors. Approved treatments for ADHD increase or mimic catecholamine signaling in the PFC; both stimulants and atomoxetine exert their cognition-enhancing effects through indirect stimulation of NE α_2 and DA D_1 receptors, while guanfacine mimics NE actions at postsynaptic α_{2A} adrenoceptors on PFC neurons. Higher doses of stimulants and atomoxetine can impair PFC function through excessive catecholamine actions. Proper doses of ADHD medications may ameliorate symptoms by strengthening PFC regulation of behavior and attention.

Disclosures

Dr. Arnsten and Yale University have a license agreement with Shire Pharmaceuticals for the development of guanfacine (Intuniv™) for the treatment of attention-deficit hyperactivity disorder.

References

1. Robbins TW. Dissociating executive functions of the prefrontal cortex. *Philos Trans R Soc Lond B Biol Sci.* 1996;**351**:1463–71.

2. Casey BJ, Epstein JN, Buhle J, *et al.* Frontostriatal connectivity and its role in cognitive control in parent-child dyads with ADHD. *Am J Psychiatry.* 2007;**164**:1729–36.

3. Shaw P, Eckstrand K, Sharp W, *et al.* Attention-deficit/hyperactivity disorder is characterized by a delay in cortical maturation. *Proc Natl Acad Sci U S A.* 2007; **104**:19649–54.

4. Makris N, Buka SL, Biederman J, *et al.* Attention and executive systems abnormalities in adults with childhood ADHD: a DT-MRI study of connections. *Cereb Cortex.* 2008;**18**:1210–20.

5. Rubia K, Smith AB, Halari R, *et al.* Disorder-specific dissociation of orbitofrontal dysfunction in boys with pure conduct disorder during reward and ventrolateral prefrontal dysfunction in boys with pure ADHD during sustained attention. *Am J Psychiatry.* 2009; **166**:83–94.

6. Arnsten AF. Catecholamine and second messenger influences on prefrontal cortical networks of "representational knowledge": a rational bridge between genetics and the symptoms of mental illness. *Cereb Cortex.* 2007;**17**(Suppl 1):i6–15.

7. Berridge CW, Devilbiss DM, Andrzejewski ME, *et al.* Methylphenidate preferentially increases catecholamine neurotransmission within the prefrontal cortex at low doses that enhance cognitive function. *Biol Psychiatry.* 2006;**60**:1111–20.

8. Goldman-Rakic PS. Circuitry of the primate prefrontal cortex and the regulation of behavior by representational memory. In: Plum F, ed. *Handbook of Physiology, The Nervous System, Higher Functions of the Brain.* Bethesda: American Physiological Society. 1987; 373–417.

9. Chao LL, Knight RT. Human prefrontal lesions increase distractibility to irrelevant sensory inputs. *Neuroreport.* 1995;**6**:1605–10.

10. Moore T, Armstrong KM. Selective gating of visual signals by microstimulation of frontal cortex. *Nature.* 2003;**421**:370–3.

11. Gazzaley A, Rissman J, Cooney J, *et al.* Functional interactions between prefrontal and visual association cortex contribute to top-down modulation of visual processing. *Cereb Cortex.* 2007;**17**(Suppl 1):i125–35.

12. Buschman TJ, Miller EK. Top-down versus bottom-up control of attention in the prefrontal and posterior parietal cortices. *Science.* 2007;**315**:1860–2.

13. Wilkins AJ, Shallice T, McCarthy R. Frontal lesions and sustained attention. *Neuropsychologia.* 1987; **25**:359–65.

14. Bunge SA, Ochsner KN, Desmond JE, Glover GH, Gabrieli JD. Prefrontal regions involved in keeping information in and out of mind. *Brain.* 2001;**124**: 2074–86.

15. Arnsten AFT, Steere JC, Hunt RD. The contribution of alpha-2 noradrenergic mechanisms to prefrontal cortical cognitive function: potential significance to attention deficit hyperactivity disorder. *Arch Gen Psychiatry.* 1996;**53**:448–55.

16. French GM. Locomotor effects of regional ablation of frontal cortex in rhesus monkeys. *J Comp Physiol Psychol.* 1959;**52**:18–24.

17. Drewe EA. Go-no go learning after frontal lobe lesions in humans. *Cortex*. 1975;**11**:8–16.

18. Middleton FA, Strick PL. Basal ganglia and cerebellar loops: motor and cognitive circuits. *Brain Res Brain Res Rev*. 2000;**31**:236–50.

19. Aron AR, Robbins TW, Poldrack RA. Inhibition and the right inferior frontal cortex. *Trends Cogn Sci*. 2004;**8**:170–7.

20. Clark L, Blackwell AD, Aron AR, *et al.* Association between response inhibition and working memory in adult ADHD: a link to right frontal cortex pathology? *Biol Psychiatry*. 2007;**61**:1395–401.

21. Chambers CD, Bellgrove MA, Stokes MG, *et al.* Executive "brake failure" following deactivation of human frontal lobe. *J Cogn Neurosci*. 2006;**18**:444–55.

22. Aron AR, Behrens TE, Smith SD, Frank MJ, Poldrack RA. Triangulating a cognitive control network using diffusion-weighted magnetic resonance imaging (MRI) and functional MRI. *J Neurosci*. 2007;**27**: 3743–52.

23. Eagle DM, Davies KR, Towse BW, *et al.* Beta-adrenoceptor-mediated action of atomoxetine during behavioral inhibition on the stop-signal task in rats. *Soc Neurosci Abst*. 2010;**508**:510.

24. Price JL, Amaral DG. An autoradiographic study of the projections of the central nucleus of the monkey amygdala. *J Neurosci*. 1981;**1**:1242–59.

25. Ghashghaei HT, Barbas H. Pathways for emotion: interactions of prefrontal and anterior temporal pathways in the amygdala of the rhesus monkey. *Neuroscience*. 2002;**115**:1261–79.

26. Price JL. Definition of the orbital cortex in relation to specific connections with limbic and visceral structures and other cortical regions. *Ann N Y Acad Sci*. 2007;**1121**:54–71.

27. Morgan MA, Romanski LM, LeDoux JE. Extinction of emotional learning: contribution of medial prefrontal cortex. *Neurosci Lett*. 1993;**163**:109–13.

28. Quirk GJ, Mueller D. Neural mechanisms of extinction learning and retrieval. *Neuropsychopharmacology*. 2008;**33**:56–72.

29. Butter C, Snyder D, McDonald J. Effects of orbital frontal lesions on aversive and aggressive behaviors in Rhesus monkeys. *J Comp Physiol Psychol*. 1970;**72**: 132–44.

30. Iversen S, Mishkin M. Perseverative interference in monkeys following selective lesions of the inferior prefrontal convexity. *Exp Brain Res*. 1970;**11**:376–86.

31. Stuss DT, Gow CA, Hetherington CR. "No longer Gage": frontal lobe dysfunction and emotional changes. *J Consult Clin Psychol*. 1992;**60**:349–59.

32. Anderson SW, Bechara A, Damasio H, Tranel D, Damasio AR. Impairment of social and moral behavior related to early damage in human prefrontal cortex. *Nat Neurosci*. 1999;**2**:1032–7.

33. Rubia K, Overmeyer S, Taylor E, *et al.* Hypofrontality in attention deficit hyperactivity disorder during higher-order motor control: a study with functional MRI. *Am J Psychiatry*. 1999;**156**:891–6.

34. Bush G, Valera EM, Seidman LJ. Functional neuroimaging of attention-deficit/hyperactivity disorder: a review and suggested future directions. *Biol Psychiatry*. 2005;**57**:1273–84.

35. Sheridan MA, Hinshaw S, D'Esposito M. Efficiency of the prefrontal cortex during working memory in attention-deficit/hyperactivity disorder. *J Am Acad Child Adolesc Psychiatry*. 2007;**46**:1357–66.

36. Castellanos FX, Lee PP, Sharp W, *et al.* Developmental trajectories of brain volume abnormalities in children and adolescents with attention-deficit/hyperactivity disorder. *JAMA*. 2002;**288**:1740–8.

37. Seidman LJ, Valera EM, Makris N, *et al.* Dorsolateral prefrontal and anterior cingulate cortex volumetric abnormalities in adults with attention-deficit/hyperactivity disorder identified by magnetic resonance imaging. *Biol Psychiatry*. 2006;**60**:1071–80.

38. Barkley RA. *ADHD and the Nature of Self-Control*. New York, NY: Guilford Press; 1997.

39. Loo SK, Humphrey LA, Tapio T, *et al.* Executive functioning among Finnish adolescents with attention-deficit/hyperactivity disorder. *J Am Acad Child Adolesc Psychiatry*. 2007;**46**:1594–604.

40. Faraone SV, Perlis RH, Doyle AE, *et al.* Molecular genetics of attention-deficit/hyperactivity disorder. *Biol Psychiatry*. 2005;**57**:1313–23.

41. Daly G, Hawi Z, Fitzgerald M, Gill M. Mapping susceptibility loci in attention deficit hyperactivity disorder: preferential transmission of parental alleles at DAT1, DBH and DRD5 to affected children. *Mol Psychiatry*. 1999;**4**:192–6.

42. Tahir E, Yazgan Y, Cirakoglu B, *et al.* Association and linkage of DRD4 and DRD5 with attention deficit hyperactivity disorder (ADHD) in a sample of Turkish children. *Mol Psychiatry*. 2000;**5**:396–404.

43. Roman T, Schmitz M, Polanczyk GV, *et al.* Further evidence for the association between attention-deficit/hyperactivity disorder and the dopamine-beta-hydroxylase gene. *Am J Med Genet*. 2002;**114**:154–8.

44. Kustanovich V, Ishii J, Crawford L, *et al.* Transmission disequilibrium testing of dopamine-related candidate gene polymorphisms in ADHD: confirmation of association of ADHD with DRD4 and DRD5. *Mol Psychiatry*. 2004;**9**:711–17.

45. Bobb AJ, Addington AM, Sidransky E, *et al*. Support for association between ADHD and two candidate genes: NET1 and DRD1. *Am J Med Genet B Neuropsychiatr Genet*. 2005;**134**:67–72.

46. Mill J, Caspi A, Williams BS, *et al*. Prediction of heterogeneity in intelligence and adult prognosis by genetic polymorphisms in the dopamine system among children with attention-deficit/hyperactivity disorder: evidence from 2 birth cohorts. *Arch Gen Psychiatry*. 2006;**63**:462–9.

47. Bellgrove MA, Hawi Z, Gill M, Robertson IH. The cognitive genetics of attention deficit hyperactivity disorder (ADHD): sustained attention as a candidate phenotype. *Cortex*. 2006;**42**:838–45.

48. Greene CM, Bellgrove MA, Gill M, Robertson IH. Noradrenergic genotype predicts lapses in sustained attention. *Neuropsychologia*. 2009;**47**: 591–4.

49. Kieling C, Genro JP, Hutz MH, Rohde LA. The -1021 C/T DBH polymorphism is associated with neuropsychological performance among children and adolescents with ADHD. *Am J Med Genet B Neuropsychiatr Genet*. 2008;**147B**:485–90.

50. Hess C, Reif A, Strobel A, *et al*. A functional dopamine-beta-hydroxylase gene promoter polymorphism is associated with impulsive personality styles, but not with affective disorders. *J Neural Transm*. 2009;**116**:121–30.

51. Kopecková M, Paclt I, Goetz P. Polymorphisms of dopamine-beta-hydroxylase in ADHD children. *Folia Biol (Praha)*. 2006;**52**:194–210.

52. Lewis DA. The catecholamine innervation of primate cerebral cortex. In: Solanto MV, Arnsten AFT, Castellanos FX, eds. *Stimulant Drugs and ADHD: Basic and Clinical Neuroscience*. New York, NY: Oxford University Press. 2001; 77–103.

53. Arnsten AFT. Through the looking glass: differential noradrenergic modulation of prefrontal cortical function. *Neural Plast*. 2000;**7**:133–46.

54. Haapalinna A, Viitamaa T, MacDonald E, *et al*. Evaluation of the effects of a specific alpha 2-adrenoceptor antagonist, atipamezole, on alpha 1- and alpha 2-adrenoceptor subtype binding, brain neurochemistry and behaviour in comparison with yohimbine. *Naunyn Schmiedebergs Arch Pharmacol*. 1997;**356**:570–82.

55. Van Tol HHM, Bunzow JR, Guan H-C, *et al*. Cloning of the gene for a human dopamine D4 receptor with high affinity for the antipsychotic clozapine. *Nature*. 1991;**350**:610–14.

56. Gamo NJ, Wang M, Arnsten AFT. Methylphenidate and atomoxetine improve prefrontal cortical function via noradrenergic alpha-2 and dopaminergic D1 receptor stimulation. *J Am Acad Child Adolesc Psychiatry*. 2010;**49**:1011–23.

57. Brozoski T, Brown RM, Rosvold HE, Goldman PS. Cognitive deficit caused by regional depletion of dopamine in prefrontal cortex of rhesus monkey. *Science*. 1979;**205**:929–31.

58. Wang M, Ramos B, Paspalas C, *et al*. Alpha2A-adrenoceptor stimulation strengthens working memory networks by inhibiting cAMP-HCN channel signaling in prefrontal cortex. *Cell*. 2007;**129**: 397–410.

59. Cedarbaum JM, Aghajanian GK. Catecholamine receptors on locus coeruleus neurons: pharmacological characterization. *Eur J Pharmacol*. 1977;**44**:375–85.

60. U'Prichard DC, Bechtel WD, Rouot BM, Snyder SH. Multiple apparent alpha-noradrenergic receptor binding sites in rat brain: effect of 6-hydroxydopamine. *Mol Pharmacol*. 1979;**16**: 47–60.

61. Smiley JF, Williams SM, Szigeti K, Goldman-Rakic PS. Light and electron microscopic characterization of dopamine-immunoreactive processes in human cerebral cortex. *J Comp Neurol*. 1992;**321**: 325–35.

62. Arnsten AFT, Paspalas CD, Gamo NJ, Yang Y, Wang M. Dynamic network connectivity: a new form of neuroplasticity. *Trends Cogn Sci*. 2010;**14**: 365–75.

63. Vijayraghavan S, Wang M, Birnbaum SG, *et al*. Inverted-U dopamine D1 receptor actions on prefrontal neurons engaged in working memory. *Nat Neurosci*. 2007;**10**:376–84.

64. Li B-M, Mei Z-T. Delayed response deficit induced by local injection of the alpha-2 adrenergic antagonist yohimbine into the dorsolateral prefrontal cortex in young adult monkeys. *Behav Neural Biol*. 1994;**62**: 134–9.

65. Sawaguchi T, Goldman-Rakic PS. D1 dopamine receptors in prefrontal cortex: Involvement in working memory. *Science*. 1991;**251**:947–50.

66. Li B-M, Mao Z-M, Wang M, Mei Z-T. Alpha-2 adrenergic modulation of prefrontal cortical neuronal activity related to spatial working memory in monkeys. *Neuropsychopharmacology*. 1999;**21**: 601–10.

67. Ma C-L, Arnsten AFT, Li B-M. Locomotor hyperactivity induced by blockade of prefrontal cortical alpha-2-adrenoceptors in monkeys. *Biol Psychiatry*. 2005;**57**:192–5.

68. Ma C-L, Qi X-L, Peng J-Y, Li B-M. Selective deficit in no-go performance induced by blockade of prefrontal cortical alpha2-adrenoceptors in monkeys. *Neuroreport*. 2003;**14**:1013–16.

69. Mao Z-M, Arnsten AFT, Li B-M. Local infusion of alpha-1 adrenergic agonist into the prefrontal cortex impairs spatial working memory performance in monkeys. *Biol Psychiatry*. 1999;**46**:1259–65.

70. Wang M, Tang ZX, Li BM. Enhanced visuomotor associative learning following stimulation of alpha 2A-adrenoceptors in the ventral prefrontal cortex in monkeys. *Brain Res*. 2004;**1024**:176–82.

71. Steere JC, Arnsten AFT. The alpha-2A noradrenergic agonist, guanfacine, improves visual object discrimination reversal performance in rhesus monkeys. *Behav Neurosci*. 1997;**111**:1–9.

72. Arnsten AFT, Cai JX, Murphy BL, Goldman-Rakic PS. Dopamine D1 receptor mechanisms in the cognitive performance of young adult and aged monkeys. *Psychopharmacology*. 1994;**116**:143–51.

73. Cai JX, Arnsten AFT. Dose-dependent effects of the dopamine D1 receptor agonists A77636 or SKF81297 on spatial working memory in aged monkeys. *J Pharmacol Exp Ther*. 1997;**283**:183–9.

74. Granon S, Passetti F, Thomas KL, *et al.* Enhanced and impaired attentional performance after infusion of D1 dopaminergic receptor agents into rat prefrontal cortex. *J Neurosci*. 2000;**20**:1208–15.

75. Arnsten AFT. Stress signaling pathways that impair prefrontal cortex structure and function. *Nat Rev Neurosci*. 2009;**32**:267–87.

76. Birnbaum SB, Yuan P, Wang M, *et al.* Protein kinase C overactivity impairs prefrontal cortical regulation of working memory. *Science*. 2004;**306**:882–4.

77. Shenker A. The mechanism of action of drugs used to treat attention-deficit hyperactivity disorder: focus on catecholamine receptor pharmacology. *Adv Pediatr*. 1992;**39**:337–82.

78. Greenhill LL. Clinical effects of stimulant medication in ADHD. In: Solanto MV, Arnsten AFT, Castellanos FX, eds. *Stimulant Drugs and ADHD: Basic and Clinical Neuroscience*. New York, NY: Oxford University Press. 2001; 31–71.

79. Swanson J, Volkow N. *Pharmacokinetic and Pharmacodynamic Properties of Methylphenidate in Humans*. New York, NY: Oxford University Press; 2001.

80. Arnsten AFT, Dudley AG. Methylphenidate improves prefrontal cortical cognitive function through alpha2 adrenoceptor and dopamine D1 receptor actions: relevance to therapeutic effects in attention deficit hyperactivity disorder. *Behav Brain Funct*. 2005; **1**:2.

81. Berridge CW, Stalnaker TA. Relationship between low-dose amphetamine-induced arousal and extracellular norepinephrine and dopamine levels within prefrontal cortex. *Synapse*. 2002;**46**:140–9.

82. Rebec GV, Bashore TR. Critical issues in assessing the behavioral effects of amphetamine. *Neurosci Biobehav Rev*. 1984;**8**:153–9.

83. McGaughy J, Sarter M. Behavioral vigilance in rats: task validation and effects of age, amphetamine, and benzodiazepine receptor ligands. *Psychopharmacology (Berl)*. 1995;**117**:340–57.

84. Segal DS. Behavioral and neurochemical correlates of repeated d-amphetamine administration. *Adv Biochem Psychopharmacol*. 1975;**13**:247–62.

85. Rapoport JL, Buchsbaum MS, Weingartner H, *et al.* Dextroamphetamine – its cognitive and behavioral-effects in normal and hyperactive boys and normal men. *Arch Gen Psychiatry*. 1980;**37**:933–43.

86. Vaidya CJ, Austin G, Kirkorian G, *et al.* Selective effects of methylphenidate in attention deficit hyperactivity disorder: a functional magnetic resonance study. *Proc Natl Acad Sci U S A*. 1998;**95**: 14494–9.

87. Mehta MA, Owen AM, Sahakian BJ, *et al.* Methylphenidate enhances working memory by modulating discrete frontal and parietal lobe regions in the human brain. *J Neurosci*. 2000;**20**:RC651–6.

88. Mehta MA, Sahakian BJ, Robbins TW. Comparative psychopharmacology of methylphenidate and related drugs in human volunteers, patients with ADHD, and experimental animals. In: Solanto MV, Arnsten AFT, Castellanos FX, eds. *Stimulant Drugs and ADHD: Basic and Clinical Neuroscience*. New York, NY: Oxford University Press. 2001; 303–31.

89. Rapoport JL, Inoff-Germain G. Responses to methylphenidate in Attention-Deficit/Hyperactivity Disorder and normal children: update 2002. *J Atten Disord*. 2002;**6**:S57–60.

90. Maher B. Poll results: look who's doping. *Nature*. 2008;**452**:674–5.

91. Kuczenski R, Segal DS. Exposure of adolescent rats to oral methylphenidate: preferential effects on extracellular norepinephrine and absence of sensitization and cross-sensitization to methamphetamine. *J Neurosci*. 2002;**22**:7264–71.

92. Devilbiss DM, Berridge CW. Cognition-enhancing doses of methylphenidate preferentially increase prefrontal cortex neuronal responsiveness. *Biol Psychiatry*. 2008;**64**:626–35.

93. Zdrale A, Meier TB, Berridge CW, Populin LC. Effect of methylphenidate on monkey prefrontal cortex-mediated behavior. *Soc Neurosci Abst*. 2008;**388**:318.

94. Kuczenski R, Segal DS. Neurochemistry of amphetamine. In: Cho AK, Segal DS, eds. *Amphetamine and Its Analogues: Psychopharmacology, Toxicology and Abuse*. San Diego: Academic Press. 1994; 81–113.

95. Kuczenski R, Segal DS, Cho AK, Melega W. Hippocampus norepinephrine, caudate dopamine and serotonin, and behavioral responses to the stereoisomers of amphetamine and methamphetamine. *J Neurosci.* 1995;**15**:1308–17.

96. Kuczenski R, Segal DS. Effects of methylphenidate on extracellular dopamine, serotonin, and norepinephrine: comparison with amphetamine. *J Neurochem.* 1997;**68**:2032–7.

97. Green WH. Nonstimulant drugs in the treatment of attention-deficit hyperactivity disorder. *Child Adolesc Psychiatr Clin North Am.* 1992;**1**:449–65.

98. Kuczenski R, Segal DS. Regional norepinephrine response to amphetamine using dialysis: comparison with caudate dopamine. *Synapse.* 1992;**11**:164–9.

99. Moghaddam B, Berridge CW, Goldman-Rakic PS, Bunney BS, Roth RH. In vivo assessment of basal and drug-induced dopamine release in cortical and subcortical regions of the anesthetized primate. *Synapse.* 1993;**13**:215–22.

100. Kelly PH, Seviour PW, Iversen SD. Amphetamine and apomorphine responses in the rat following 6-OHDA lesions of the nucleus accumbens septi and corpus striatum. *Brain Res.* 1975;**94**:507–22.

101. Koob GF, Bloom FE. Cellular and molecular mechanisms of drug dependence. *Science.* 1988;**242**: 715–23.

102. Blanc G, Trovero F, Vezina P, *et al.* Blockade of prefronto-cortical alpha 1-adrenergic receptors prevents locomotor hyperactivity induced by subcortical D-amphetamine injection. *Eur J Neurosci.* 1994;**6**:293–8.

103. Drouin C, Darracq L, Trovero F, *et al.* Alpha1b-adrenergic receptors control locomotor and rewarding effects of psychostimulants and opiates. *J Neurosci.* 2002;**22**:2873–84.

104. Kuczenski R, Segal DS. Locomotor effects of acute and repeated threshold doses of amphetamine and methylphenidate: relative roles of dopamine and norepinephrine. *J Pharmacol Exp Ther.* 2001;**296**: 876–83.

105. Drouin C, Page M, Waterhouse B. Methylphenidate enhances noradrenergic transmission and suppresses mid- and long-latency sensory responses in the primary somatosensory cortex of awake rats. *J Neurophysiol.* 2006;**96**:622–32.

106. Carboni E, Tanda GL, Frau R, Di CG. Blockade of the noradrenaline carrier increases extracellular dopamine concentrations in the prefrontal cortex: evidence that dopamine is taken up in vivo by noradrenergic terminals. *J Neurochem.* 1990;**55**:1067–70.

107. Sesack SR, Hawrylak VA, Matus C, Guido MA, Levey AI. Dopamine axon varicosities in the prelimbic division of the rat prefrontal cortex exhibit sparse immunoreactivity for the dopamine transporter. *J Neurosci.* 1998;**18**:2697–708.

108. Biederman J, Baldessarini RJ, Wright V, Knee D, Harmatz JS. A double-blind placebo controlled study of desipramine in the treatment of ADD: I. Efficacy. *J Am Acad Child Adolesc Psychiatry.* 1989;**28**:777–84.

109. Spencer T, Biederman J, Wilens T, *et al.* Effectiveness and tolerability of tomoxetine in adults with attention deficit hyperactivity disorder. *Am J Psychiatry.* 1998; **155**:693–5.

110. Michelson D, Adler L, Spencer T, *et al.* Atomoxetine in adults with ADHD: two randomized, placebo-controlled studies. *Biol Psychiatry.* 2003;**53**:112–20.

111. Newcorn JH, Kratochvil CJ, Allen AJ, *et al.* Atomoxetine and osmotically released methylphenidate for the treatment of attention deficit hyperactivity disorder: acute comparison and differential response. *Am J Psychiatry.* 2008;**165**: 721–30.

112. Wong DT, Threlkeld PG, Best KL, Bymaster FP. A new inhibitor of norepinephrine uptake devoid of affinity for receptors in rat brain. *J Pharmacol Exp Ther.* 1982; **222**:61–5.

113. Zerbe RL, Rowe H, Enas GG, *et al.* Clinical pharmacology of atomoxetine, a potential antidepressant. *J Pharmacol Exp Ther.* 1985;**232**: 139–43.

114. Seu E, Lang A, Rivera RJ, Jentsch JD. Inhibition of the norepinephrine transporter improves behavioral flexibility in rats and monkeys. *Psychopharmacology (Berl).* 2009;**202**:505–19.

115. Chamberlain SR, Hampshire A, Müller U, *et al.* Atomoxetine modulates right inferior frontal activation during inhibitory control: a pharmacological functional magnetic resonance imaging study. *Biol Psychiatry.* 2009;**65**:550–5.

116. Chamberlain SR, Del Campo N, Dowson J, *et al.* Atomoxetine improved response inhibition in adults with attention deficit/hyperactivity disorder. *Biol Psychiatry.* 2007;**62**:977–84.

117. Bymaster FP, Katner JS, Nelson DL, *et al.* Atomoxetine increases extracellular levels of norepinephrine and dopamine in prefrontal cortex of rat: a potential mechanism for efficacy in attention deficit/ hyperactivity disorder. *Neuropsychopharmacology.* 2002;**27**:699–711.

118. Horn AS. Structure-activity relations for the inhibition of catecholamine uptake into synaptosomes from noradrenaline and dopaminergic neurones in rat brain homogenates. *Br J Pharmacol.* 1973;**47**:332–8.

119. Raiteri M, del Carmine R, Bertollini A, Levi G. Effect of sympathomimetic amines on the synaptosomal

transport of noradrenaline, dopamine and 5-hydroxytryptamine. *Eur J Pharmacol*. 1977;**41**: 133–43.

120. Graf H, Abler B, Freudenmann R, *et al*. Neural correlates of error monitoring modulated by atomoxetine in healthy volunteers. *Biol Psychiatry*. 2011;**69**:890–7.

121. Winsberg BG, Camp-Bruno JA, Vink J, Timmer CJ, Sverd J. Mianserin pharmacokinetics and behavior in hyperkinetic children. *J Clin Psychopharmacol*. 1987; **7**:143–7.

122. Baldessarini RJ. Antidepressant agents. In: *Chemotherapy in Psychiatry: Pharmacologic Basis of Treatments for Major Mental Illness*. Cambridge, MA: Harvard University Press. 1985; 130–234.

123. Hunt RD, Mindera RB, Cohen DJ. Clonidine benefits children with attention deficit disorder and hyperactivity: reports of a double-blind placebo-crossover therapeutic trial. *J Am Acad Child Psychiatry*. 1985;**24**:617–29.

124. Arnsten AFT, Li B-M. Neurobiology of executive functions: catecholamine influences on prefrontal cortical function. *Biol Psychiatry*. 2005;**57**:1377–84.

125. Scahill L, Chappell PB, Kim YS, *et al*. Guanfacine in the treatment of children with tic disorders and ADHD: A placebo-controlled study. *Am J Psychiatry*. 2001;**158**:1067–74.

126. Biederman J, Melmed RD, Patel A, *et al*. SPD503 Study Group. A randomized, double-blind, placebo-controlled study of guanfacine extended release in children and adolescents with attention-deficit/hyperactivity disorder. *Pediatrics*. 2008;**121**:e73–84.

127. Sallee FR, McGough JJ, Wigal T, *et al*. SPD503 Study Group. Guanfacine extended release in children and adolescents with attention-deficit/hyperactivity disorder: a placebo-controlled trial. *J Am Acad Child Adolesc Psychiatry*. 2009;**48**:155–65.

128. Berridge CW. Noradrenergic modulation of arousal. *Brain Res Rev*. 2008;**58**:1–17.

129. van Zwieten PA, Chalmers JP. Different types of centrally acting antihypertensives and their targets in the central nervous system. *Cardiovasc Drugs Ther*. 1994;**8**:787–99.

130. Engberg G, Eriksson E. Effects of alpha-2-adrenoceptor agonists on locus coeruleus firing rate and brain noradrenaline turnover in EEDQ-treated rats. *Naunyn-Schmiedebergs Arch Pharmacol*. 1991; **343**:472–7.

131. Uhlén S, Muceniece R, Rangel N, Tiger G, Wikberg JE. Comparison of the binding activities of some drugs on alpha 2A, alpha 2B and alpha 2C-adrenoceptors and non-adrenergic imidazoline sites in the guinea pig. *Pharmacol Toxicol*. 1995;**76**:353–64.

132. Connor DF, Findling RL, Kollins SH, *et al*. Effects of guanfacine extended release on oppositional symptoms in children aged 6–12 years with attention-deficit hyperactivity disorder and oppositional symptoms: a randomized, double-blind, placebo-controlled trial. *CNS Drugs*. 2010;**24**: 755–68.

133. Franowicz JCS, Arnsten AFT. The alpha-2A noradrenergic agonist, guanfacine, improves delayed response performance in young adult rhesus monkeys. *Psychopharmacology*. 1998;**136**:8–14.

134. Jakala P, Riekkinen M, Sirvio J, *et al*. Guanfacine, but not clonidine, improves planning and working memory performance in humans. *Neuropsychopharmacology*. 1999;**20**:460–70.

135. Muller U, Clark L, Lam ML, *et al*. Lack of effects of guanfacine on executive and memory functions in healthy male volunteers. *Psychopharmacology*. 2005;**182**:205–13.

136. Avery RA, Franowicz JS, Studholme C, van Dyck CH, Arnsten AFT. The alpha-2A-adenoceptor agonist, guanfacine, increases regional cerebral blood flow in dorsolateral prefrontal cortex of monkeys performing a spatial working memory task. *Neuropsychopharmacology*. 2000;**23**:240–9.

137. Swartz BE, Kovalik E, Thomas K, Torgersen D, Mandelkern MA. The effects of an alpha-2 adrenergic agonist, guanfacine, on rCBF in human cortex in normal controls and subjects with focal epilepsy. *Neuropsychopharmacology*. 2000;**23**:263–75.

138. Clerkin SM, Schulz KP, Halperin JM, *et al*. Guanfacine potentiates the activation of prefrontal cortex evoked by warning signals. *Biol Psychiatry*. 2009;**66**: 307–12.

Chapter 15

Molecular genetics of ADHD

Guy M. L. Perry and Stephen V. Faraone

Summary

Attention-deficit hyperactivity disorder (ADHD) is highly heritable ($h^2 \approx 0.76$), but its molecular genetic basis is unclear. ADHD candidate gene associations vary and genome-wide linkage and association studies have been unable to detect effects at significant thresholds. The identification of the genetic basis for ADHD is further complicated by the likely existence of both rare and common genetic risk variants, higher-order genetic interactions such as genotype-by-environment ($G \times E$) interaction, and parental imprinting of alleles which creates a diverse genetic architecture. Many candidate genes that have been studied are neurobiologically compelling but much of the data are inconsistent or contradictory, suggesting complex interactive or epigenetic modifiers, or of analytical and functional complexities in the expression of this disorder.

Introduction

ADHD is a common psychiatric disorder of childhood (8–12%) [1] which persists into adulthood in two-thirds of affected children [2]. ADHD risk among parents and siblings of children with ADHD was two- to eightfold higher than in those of unaffected children (see Faraone and Biederman [3]) with higher risk rates for the relatives of adults with ADHD [4]. Because many twin studies from the United States, Europe, and Australia show ADHD to be highly heritable [5, 6], molecular genetic studies have begun searching for genes that increase susceptibility to ADHD.

Genetic linkage studies

Linkage analysis – genotype–phenotype correlation based on recombinative distance between markers and traits – has been attempted in the search for genes responsible for ADHD. Genetic linkage studies have the advantage of screening the entire genome for potential susceptibility genes, which means they are not biased by prior neurobiological hypotheses. The main disadvantage of such studies is that they can only discover genes that have relatively large effects in causing a disease. Four genomic regions (5p12, 10q26, 12q23, 16p13) were suggestively linked to ADHD in 126 American affected sib-pairs (logarithm of the odds [LOD] scores >1.5) [7]: the 16p13 region was detected again (LOD = 4.0) in an expanded sample of 203 families [8]. Another peak (LOD = 3.5) was identified in a study of 164 Dutch affected sib-pairs at 15q15. Two other peaks were detected at 7p13 (LOD 3.0) and 9q33 (LOD = 2.1) [9]. A genome-wide scan from a genetically isolated community in Colombia implicated 4q13, 8q12, 8p23, 11q23, 12q23, and 17p11 [10]. A study of 155 sib-pairs from Germany reported linkage of ADHD to chromosomes 5p (LOD = 2.59) and suggestive linkage to 6q, 7p, 9q, 11q, 12q, and 17p [11].

A genome scan using 400 microsatellite markers in nine related affected and unaffected individuals found a non-significant heterogenetic LOD (HLOD) = 1.67 for 6p22 and HLOD = 2.13 for 18q21–22 [12], and HLOD = 2.0 for inattention alone at 6p22 [12]. A large multifamilial linkage analysis (1410 families) found a haplotype associated with ADHD embedded within the latrophilin 3 gene (*LPHN3*) (62.4–62.7 Mb, chromosome 4 (odds ratio [OR] = 1.23) [13]. Nonparametric linkage mapping in a Dutch family with ADHD and associated comorbidities found two markers with suggestive LOD for diagnosed ADHD on chromosomes 7 (7p15.1–q31.33; *D7S502*) and 14 (14q11.2–q22.3; *D14S275*) [14]. However, Faraone *et al.* found no linkage in a sib-pair analysis of 601 affected

Attention-Deficit Hyperactivity Disorder in Adults and Children, ed. Lenard A. Adler, Thomas J. Spencer and Timothy E. Wilens.
Published by Cambridge University Press. © Cambridge University Press 2015.

siblings in 217 full-sib families [15]. Interestingly, the 6p region, associated with ADHD in the study of Amin *et al.* [12], has also been linked to reading disability, which co-occurs with the former [16]. Some workers have restricted observational heterogeneity by filtering on comorbid traits: Joo *et al.* found a likelihood peak at 10p14 (LOD = 3.35) for inattention and 12q24 (LOD = 2.06) for total Wender Utah Rating Scale (WURS) score in 57 bipolar-afflicted families by excluding bipolarity [17].

Meta-analysis of linkage studies has been used to identify probable locations for ADHD genes: a pooled analysis found associations between variants at 5p13 and ADHD symptoms across several studies, possibly indicating a locus of general risk [8, 9, 18]. A meta-analysis by Zhou *et al.* found genome-wide significant linkage across seven linkage studies ($P_{SR} = 0.00034$, $P_{OR} = 0.04$) for a region on chromosome 16 between 64 Mb and 83 Mb ($\approx$16q22.1–24.1) [19].

Despite these intriguing findings, the main conclusion from genetic linkage studies is that no one gene has a very large effect on the manifestation of ADHD for most patients. Thus, researchers have gone on to consider two other possibilities: (1) that ADHD is caused by the cumulative effects of many common DNA variants and (2) that much of ADHD can be accounted for by rare DNA variants that occur in some, but not most, families.

The search for common variants: candidate gene studies

Genetic association studies are well suited for finding common variants that individually have small effects on disease expression. Correspondingly, there have been many genetic association studies of ADHD and most have focused on candidate genes, i.e., genes implicated in ADHD by what is known or hypothesized by the disorder's neurobiology.

The most compelling results from candidate gene studies have been summarized in meta-analyses. Meta-analysis of several individual studies has associated ADHD with the 7-repeat allele of a 48-bp VNTR at dopamine D_4 receptor (*DRD4*) [20, 21], a 148-bp microsatellite allele at dopamine D_5 receptor (*DRD5*) [20, 22], the 5′ taq1 A allele at dopamine beta-hydroxylase (*DBH*) [5], a T1065G single nucleotide polymorphism (SNP) at synaptosomal-associated protein 25 gene (*SNAP-25*), a 44-bp insertion/deletion in the promoter region of serotonin transporter

gene (*SLC6A4*) (*5HTTLPR*) [5], and the G861C SNP at serotonin 1B receptor gene (*HTR1B*) [5]. Other meta-analyses indicate weaker associations between ADHD and the 480-bp VNTR in the 3′ untranslated region (UTR) of the dopamine transporter gene (*SLC6A3*) [20, 23, 24], but not with association with the *Val108Met* polymorphism at catechol-O-methyltransferase gene (*COMT*) [25] despite associations between *COMT* and ADHD in other studies [26–31]. A recent meta-analysis by Neale *et al.* [32] found no associations between ADHD and SNPs collected by the International Multicenter ADHD Genetics (IMAGE) project (see below).

A meta-analytic review by Gizer *et al.* found significant associations between ADHD and *DAT1*, *DRD4*, *DRD5*, *5HTT*, *HTR1B*, and *SNAP-25* [33]; simultaneously, however, there was significant heterogeneity in the association of ADHD with *DAT1*, *DRD4*, *DRD5*, *DBH*, *ADRA2A*, *5HTT*, *TPH2*, *MAO-A*, and *SNAP-25*. *DAT1* may be associated with ADHD specifically in individuals without conduct disorder [34]. This strongly suggests that the effect of these genes is subject to modification by external or internal environment.

Other potential sources of heterogeneity also exist. Not all ratings scores of ADHD phenotype are analytically equal: maternal–teacher ratings of ADHD produced the strongest evidence for associations between ADHD symptoms and *DAT1* and *DRD4* SNPs in a proband of 99 children referred for problems in externalized behavior [35]. The genetics of ADHD may also be complicated by diversity in the nature of inheritance for the disorder. In the meta-analysis of Nikolas and Burt [36], dominant components of genetic variance were significantly greater for inattention, but additive genetic variance was greater for hyperactivity, suggesting critical differences in the etiology of ADHD. The assumption of common genetic structure in such disorders may be integral limitations on the repeatability of marker–ADHD correlations.

In the following, we discuss some of the individual studies that contributed to these meta-analyses.

Association studies of catecholaminergic genes

The dopamine D_4 receptor (*DRD4*)

Physiology strongly suggests the importance of *DRD4* in ADHD: dopamine is a potent agonist of this gene

[37]. Neuroimaging indicates that the D_4 receptor is prevalent in the frontal-subcortical networks implicated in the pathophysiology of ADHD [38].

The 7-repeat (7R) allele of an exon III *DRD4* VNTR is associated with poor response to dopamine [39, 40] and with ADHD [10] in case–control (OR = 1.45) and family-based (OR = 1.16) association tests [5]. Individuals inheriting the 7R allele were more likely (OR = 2.8) to develop a combined ADHD subtype [41]. A pooled OR of 1.34 (95% confidence interval [CI] 1.23–1.45) was obtained from a meta-analysis of 33 studies [20]. The association of the 7R allele appears to persist developmentally: 76% of 7R carriers with ADHD at the age of 25 had persistent ADHD in a sample of 539 probands and controls compared to 66% without it [42]. The 7R allele was also associated with persistent ADHD in a prospective study of 265 German boys [43] and a sample of 151 children interviewed in childhood and at adolescence [44].

Associations of *DRD4* appear to be slightly heterogeneous: both the 6- and 7-repeat alleles were linked to ADHD in 44 Indian trios (relative risk [RR] = 1, P = 0.03) [45]. There was no association of the 7-repeat with ADHD in the IMAGE project (p > 0.09) or in a small (36 families) trio study by Niederhofer *et al.* [46]. Kramer *et al.* found that 7R carriers without ADHD had, conversely, more accurate Go/No-Go performance than those carrying the 4R allele [47]. It is also possible that *DRD4* is a predisposing factor to ADHD: infants with regulatory problems were more likely to develop ADHD if they possessed the 7R genotype [48].

Alternatively, the effect of *DRD4* on ADHD may require multiple linked elements: a small (n = 26) case–control study found no main effect of the 7-repeat but did detect an interactive effect of the 7R allele with a 10-repeat *DAT1* VNTR allele [49]. Neither the 7-repeat *DRD4* allele nor the 10-repeat *DAT1* allele were independently associated with ADHD in a sample of 105 affected individuals and 84 controls, but homozygotes at both loci predicted membership in ADHD patients with associated comorbities [50]. A 5′ 120-bp repeat 1.2 kb upstream of the *DRD4* initiation codon has been variously associated with ADHD [51–56]. The effect of *DRD4* 7R may also vary over racial/ethnic background, being greatest in South Americans (OR = 2.4; p = 0.001), followed by Europeans (OR = 1.6; p < 0.00001) and Arabs (OR = 0.7; p = 0.014) [57].

The association of two promoter SNPs (rs747302, rs1800955) with ADHD was inconclusive [53, 58]; a third nearby *DRD4*, rs9195457, was nominally associated with the disorder [59]. Similarly, evidence for interaction between prenatal smoking and the 7-repeat allele is contradictory [60–62]. In 126 Korean ADHD trios, there were no 7-repeat probands, while the 5-repeat VNTR appeared protective for hyperactivity-impulsiveness compared to the 4-repeat [63]. The 4-repeat has also been associated with fewer commission errors in continuous performance tests (CPT) in a sample of Korean children [64].

DRD4 may be associated with specific symptoms of ADHD, although the evidence for this effect is also variable. Fathers of ADHD children with the 7R allele themselves had higher levels of inattention [65] and was associated with self-reported childhood inattention in women with seasonal affective disorder [66]. The presence of the rs747302-A allele at *DRD4* was correlated with deficits in sustained attention [67]. However, other evidence indicates better attention in 7R carriers [67–69] or no genotypic difference in attention at all [70]. Kim *et al.* found suggestive evidence that hyperactivity/impulsiveness was actually higher for Korean boys with the 5R *DRD4* exon III allele [63]. There was no association between the severity of ADHD symptoms and genotype at *DRD4* in 110 adults diagnosed for adult ADHD [71]. There was no association between the 7R allele and ADHD symptoms or subtypes in a pool of 2090 children studied by Todd *et al.* [72], or in 329 pairs of male English and Welsh twins [73]. A prospective longitudinal study (6, 11, and 15 years) found no association between ADHD symptoms and the 7R allele in care-deprived children from Romanian orphanages [74]. Loo *et al.* found associations of beta frequencies in electroencephalograms and ADHD (irrespective of subtype) with *DRD4* genotype in 132 ADHD families [75].

The effects of *DRD4* might act via modulation of environmental promoters of ADHD: Martel *et al.* found moderating effects of the 120-bp *DRD4* promoter on effects of inconsistent parenting care and marital conflict on vulnerability to ADHD in 548 ADHD and control children [76]. A few studies have suggested a *DRD4*–ADHD relationship based on comorbid or related traits, including autism [77], novelty seeking temperament [78], and eating behavior [79], the latter two via interaction with *COMT* (see below). Grady *et al.* found that ADHD children had four times the over-representation of rare *DRD4* variants compared to autistic children [77]. Lynn *et al.* found that the 7R allele predicted the incidence of

ADHD, but not novelty seeking despite the association of ADHD and novelty seeking behavior [78].

Catechol-*O*-methyltransferase (*COMT*)

COMT is a biallelic gene – one active, thermostable allele and one low-activity labile allele – involved with dopamine, norepinephrine, and epinephrine degradation [80]. Adult German MET homozygotes have higher ADHD symptom scores than other genotypes (26). DeYoung *et al.* found associations between the *Met* allele and ADHD symptoms in a sample of Russian delinquent adolescents [30]. The risk of ADHD was fivefold higher for *Met* carriers in 55 subjects with velo-cardio-facial syndrome and comorbid ADHD compared to unaffected individuals [27]. Palmason *et al.* found a significant association of *Met* with the incidence and severity of ADHD [31]. A *COMT* NlaIII VNTR was associated with ADHD symptoms in 160 Korean case–control individuals [29]. A haplotype analysis of SNPs tagging the common variants at *COMT* in 435 ADHD-affected adults and 383 controls found that the rs6269 SNP was associated with hyperactivity/impulsivity (p = 0.007) [81]. ADHD symptoms were weakly associated with *COMT* genotype in a set of 82 ADHD-affected subjects in a study of methylphenidate medication [28].

However, neither the IMAGE project SNP assay [82] nor meta-analysis by Cheuk *et al.* [25] found an association of ADHD with *COMT* in case–control or family studies (p > 0.5). The effect of this locus may be complicated by interaction: Nobile *et al.* found associations between socioeconomic status and ADHD [83], so that *Val* homozygotes with low socioeconomic status had higher scores for ADHD symptoms on the Child Behavior Check List 6/18 DSM oriented scales. In a sample of ADHD-affected Chinese males, Qian *et al.* found that full scale and performance IQ were associated with *MAO-A* × *COMT* interaction [84].

The dopamine D₅ receptor (*DRD5*)

The most widely studied polymorphism for *DRD5* is a 148-bp dinucleotide repeat 18.5 kb 5′ to the gene initiation site [85]. Transcript production for *DRD5* in the medial prefrontal cortex (mPFC) is associated with impulsiveness in rats [86]. Several meta-analyses support the effects of gene variants at *DRD5* on ADHD, including a meta-analysis of 14 family-based studies (OR = 1.2) by Lowe *et al.* [22], a meta-analysis of association studies to 2005 by Li *et al.* [20] (OR = 1.34), and

a meta-analysis of case–control [87–89] and transmission disequilibrium test (TDT) studies (p < 0.0027) [33]. Two- and three-marker haplotypes near *DRD5* support its association with ADHD (p = 0.0013) [85].

Meta-analyses of this gene have not produced consistent associations; ADHD was associated with *DRD5* in the IMAGE study [90], but not in a meta-analysis of TDT assays (OR = 1.17) [33]. A prospective study by Muller *et al.* [71] found no correlation of adult ADHD symptoms with genotype at the 148-bp marker, although the 148-bp allele was associated with the persistence of ADHD in children aged 6–12 years [44]. There is a suggestion of either transgressive segregation or epistasis at this gene: Mill *et al.* found that the 148-bp allele was significantly associated with lower scores for hyperactivity in 329 pairs of male English and Welsh twins [73].

The dopamine transporter gene (*DAT1*, *SLC6A3*)

Pharmacological evidence suggests the importance of *DAT* in ADHD: stimulants block dopamine [91]. *SLC6A3* knockout mice express hyperactivity and impulsiveness which may be ameliorated with stimulants [92, 93]. The *SLC6A3* locus is located near the 5p linkage peak for an ADHD gene [7, 18].

Several *DAT* alleles have been linked to ADHD. Cook *et al.* reported the first association between ADHD and the 10-repeat 3′ UTR VNTR at *DAT* [94]. Lee *et al.* found associations between the 10-repeat allele, hyperactivity, and impulsiveness [95]. Kopeckova *et al.* found that the risk of ADHD was higher in heterozygotes (OR = 1.6) and homozygotes (OR = 6.6) for the risk allele at *DAT1* [96]. A SNP at *DAT1*, rs11564750, was associated with ADHD (p = 0.02) in 450 ADHD probands by Doyle *et al.* [97]. However, no differences in the severity of symptoms were observed among *DAT1* genotypes in a sample of 110 adult sufferers of ADHD by Muller *et al.* [71]. A six-copy 30-bp VNTR allele was associated with ADHD symptoms in 94 affected and 481 control Brazilian adults [98]. The 9-repeat allele has also been associated with hyperactivity, impulsiveness, and oppositional defiant disorder. A meta-analysis of 29 studies by Kebir *et al.* [99] found four studies with conflicting results for the association of CPT tasks with *DAT1* genotype. Xu *et al.* found an association between the T allele at a promoter polymorphism (−67A > T) in 212 Taiwanese ADHD patients but not in 197 British patients, and over-transmission of this allele into ADHD patients in the combined samples (p = 0.003) [100].

As for *DRD5*, the association of this locus with ADHD has been variable: a meta-analysis of family-based studies by Li *et al.* found no association of the 10R allele with ADHD (OR = 1.04; 95% confidence interval [CI] = 0.99–1.14) [20]. There was significant heterogeneity in the odds ratio associated with the *DAT1* risk allele in six case–control studies, suggesting lability in effect [23].

Risk associated with the *DAT1* risk allele may be environmentally mediated: twins inheriting the *DAT1* 440-bp allele exposed to prenatal maternal smoking were more likely (OR = 2.6) to develop ADHD than unexposed twins without the risk allele. The 7-repeat allele at *DAT* has also been associated with increased risk in children prenatally exposed to maternal smoking [60, 101]. Stevens *et al.* found that the risk allele at *DAT1* moderated the development of ADHD symptoms in a sample of care-deprived institutionalized Romanian children [74]. Risk associated with the 10–6 *DAT* haplotype was only significantly greater for individuals with prenatal maternal alcohol exposure [90].

Alternatively, *DAT1* may be involved with ADHD through comorbidities: Sharp *et al.* indicate that *DAT1* is associated with ADHD in individuals without conduct disorder [34]. There was an association between ADHD symptoms and a 10R–6R haplotype in families from England and Taiwan in intron 8 including a significant interaction with maternal alcoholism [90]. The association of the 10–6 haplotype was replicated by Brookes *et al.* [59] (OR = 1.19) and Asherson *et al.* [102] (OR = 1.27) in 383 ADHD IMAGE probands, but not by Bakker *et al.* [88] in 198 Dutch probands (p = 0.2). Children homozygous for the 10–6 haplotype in an Irish sample of 50 affected and 65 controls had greater deficits in spatial inattention [103]. The 10–6 allele might be subject to longitudinal deactivation; Franke *et al.* found persistent ADHD was associated with the 9–9 and 9–6 haplotypes at *DAT1* in 1440 ADHD patients and 1769 controls [104].

Familial behavioral interactions appear to have an effect on genotypic risk for ADHD. Interaction between psychosocial adversity and the 3′ UTR 10-repeat allele, the 6-repeat intron 8 allele, and the 10–6 haplotype was associated with ADHD [105]. Conduct problems were only affected by positive maternal reinforcement for non-homozygotes for the 10R allele at *DAT1* in a sample of 728 males with combined-type ADHD [106].

Dopamine beta-hydroxylase (*DBH*)

DBH is the primary enzyme responsible for conversion of dopamine to norepinephrine, and appears to be involved with ADHD. Plasma DBH is higher in children with ADHD than unaffected individuals [107]. The *DBH*-A1 allele is associated with ADHD symptoms in children with Tourette's [108, 109] and in a sample of 105 Caucasian ADHD children and 68 controls (OR = 1.96; 95% CI 1.01–3.79) [110]. Over-transmission of the A2 allele in ADHD-affected children in conjunction with parental history has variably been observed [111, 112]. Paternal over-transmission of the G allele at rs2519152, also linked to DBH production, was observed in East Indian ADHD-affected children (p = 0.02) [113]. The TT homozygous genotype at *DBH* C-1021T genotype was associated with impulsiveness and aggression in a sample of 387 healthy individuals, 637 with personality disorder, 407 with ADHD, and 182 with affective disorder [114]. A prospective study of 200 individuals found that those with the T allele at C-1021T made more errors of commission in the Sustained Attention to Response Task [115]. Muller *et al.* detected no association between DBH and symptom severity at DBH in 110 ADHD adults [71].

Several studies disagree with the above: no effect of A2 was detected in case–control studies in Indian ADHD children [116] and case–control and family-based analyses of Canadian ADHD cases [117]. Neither the dinucleotide polymorphism nor a 5′ in/del marker (both of which were associated with serum DBH) were associated with ADHD in a study by Wigg *et al.* [112]. Two trio studies found no association between a G/T SNP in exon 5 of *DBH* and ADHD [85, 118]. None of the 33 *DBH* SNPs in the IMAGE study were associated with ADHD [59]. A 5′ –1021C>T polymorphism was associated with a major proportion of plasma DBH expression (>50%), and was also associated with ADHD in a Han Chinese sample [119], but not in Indian ADHD children [116]. Haplotype analysis in 100 ADHD children and 100 controls found a significantly increased risk of ADHD for an upstream +444A and +1603T haplotype (OR = 15) [96].

Monoamine oxidase A (*MAO-A*)

The MAO-A enzyme moderates norepinephrine, dopamine, and serotonin. *MAO-A* knockout mice exhibit marked disturbances in these neurotransmitters [120]. The 4R and 5R alleles of a 30-bp VNTR at

MAO-A were significantly associated with ADHD in 133 Israeli families [121] and suggestively associated with ADHD in 129 Israeli ADHD-affected individuals; this latter association was particularly strong in affected females (n = 19) [121]. Lawson *et al.* found no effect of *MAO-A*, in 171 British children [122]. Roohi *et al.* found that children with the 4R allele at the *MAO-A* VNTR had higher parent-rated inattention and impulsiveness than those with the 3R [123]. The risk genotype at *MAO-A* was strongly associated (OR = 1.94) with ADHD in a screen of 245 SNPs at gene-wide permutational thresholds in a sample of 182 Han Chinese ADHD children and 184 controls [124]. An intron 2 CA-repeat microsatellite was associated with ADHD by Jiang *et al.* in 82 Chinese [125], but this was not replicated in Caucasian samples by Payton *et al.* [118] or Domschke *et al.* [126]. Domschke *et al.* [126] and Xu *et al.* [127] found that the high activity G941T allele at the exon 8 SNP was associated with ADHD; furthermore, ADHD was associated with a G941T-3R-6R [CA] microsatellite haplotype [126], and with over-transmission of a haplotype containing G941T and the 3-repeat VNTR allele in 212 affected Taiwanese probands [127]. The IMAGE study identified five tagged SNPs (overlapping the 941G>T SNP) with significant associations with ADHD [59]. *MAO-A* may also be involved with the response to treatment: methylphenidate effectiveness was modulated by the 30-bp *MAO-A* allele during a 3-month treatment in 85 ADHD outpatient boys [128].

Monoamine oxidase B (*MAO-B*)

MAO-B was associated with adult ADHD (OR = 1.90, p = 0.0029) but not childhood ADHD in an association study of 188 ADHD-affected adults and 263 affected children and 400 controls [129]. A study of 84 ADHD-affected children and 64 controls found that platelet *MAO-B* activity was associated with hyperactive, inattentive, and combined ADHD [130].

The dopamine D_2 receptor (*DRD2*)

The *TaqIA1* allele at *DRD2* (rs1800497) was significantly associated with ADHD in a sample of 104 ADHD-affected individuals, most of which also suffered from Tourette's [131]. This finding was replicated by Comings *et al.* [108] and in ADHD-affected Czech boys by Sery *et al.* [132]. Carriers of the *TaqIA1* allele in a sample of 104 adolescents under psychiatric hos-

pitalization were more impulsive than other genotypes [133]. There was no association between ADHD and *TaqIA1* in a sample of Korean alcoholics [134]. A case–control study in 100 ADHD and 100 healthy children by Kopeckova *et al.* found significantly elevated risk for an allele at *DRD2* (OR = 7.5), which was particularly significant for homozygotes (OR = 54.8) [96]. This allele may affect ADHD via disregulation of dopamine efflux [135].

Family-based *DRD2* studies have not supported *DRD2*–ADHD associations. Transmission of the *Taq1A1* allele did not deviate from Mendelian ratios in 236 ADHD-affected children and siblings studied by Rowe *et al.* [136]. Huang *et al.* found no evidence of over-transmission of *Taq1A1* in 98 Taiwanese ADHD children and 154 parents [137]. Kirley *et al.* found only a marginally significant association between the *Ser311* polymorphism in 118 ADHD trios (p = 0.07) [138].

The dopamine D_3 receptor (*DRD3*)

Heterozygosity at an exon 1 *Ser9Gly* polymorphism was associated with greater impulsivity in 146 German patients with a history of violence [139], and the IMAGE study found nominal associations between 28 SNPs at *DRD3* [59]. However, *Ser9Gly* was not linked to ADHD in 100 Canadian nuclear families [140], 105 British nuclear families [118], or 39 families of ADHD adults [141]. Barr *et al.* [140] found no association of an intron 5 *Msp*I restriction site polymorphism with ADHD and Comings *et al.* [142] found no association of the *Ser9Gly* polymorphism with ADHD or Tourette's, although one *DRD3* variant was linked to autism spectrum disorder [143].

Noradrenergic receptors (*ADRA1A, A2A, 2C,* and *1C*)

The G-1291C SNP at the alpha-2A-adrenergic receptor (*ADRA2A*) has been associated with ADHD, oppositional defiant disorder, or conduct disorder, and the C-1291G with obsessive–compulsive disorder (OCD), panic, addictions, and schizophrenia [144]. The G-1291C allele was included in a significantly over-transmitted haplotype in 51 trios [145]. The *Msp*I G-1291C site was associated with symptoms of inattention in 128 ADHD Brazilian outpatients [146], inattention and hyperactivity in a sample of 96 Brazilian ADHD children and adolescents and their parents [147], and in 177 affected nuclear families from Michigan [145]. Deupree *et al.* found no linkage between *Msp*I, *Hha*I or *Dra*I *ADRA2A* polymorphisms and

ADHD in 93 ADHD probands and 50 siblings [148]. Several family-based studies have detected no association between ADHD and 1291 genotype [147–152]. Roman et al. detect an effect of MspI ADRA2A polymorphism on inattentive and combined ADHD (p < 0.04) [147]. In a sample of 177 families, the DraI polymorphism was associated with the combined ADHD subtype (p = 0.03), inattentive (p = 0.003) and hyperactive–impulsive (p = 0.015) traits [145]. A DraI C > T risk polymorphism [145] was nominally associated with ADHD diagnosis in a sample of 331 normal and 320 ADHD-affected boys [76]. Wang et al. found a trend toward lower ADHD symptom score in G-1291C homozygotes [152].

As in other gene candidates for ADHD, heterogeneity in presentation or expression among comorbid phenotypes may be partially responsible for variance in the detectable effect of candidate genes for ADHD. G-1291C (rs1800544) was associated with the inattentive subtype using case–control analysis, but not in family-based association analysis [150]. Xu et al. similarly found no association of G-1291C with ADHD using family-based analysis in ADHD probands in 94 nuclear families [149]. The association of ADRA2A with ADHD was also stronger in children having poor cognition [153]. Stevenson et al. found significant over-transmission of the G-1291C allele in children with reading disability, but not in their complete sample of 152 ADHD-affected boys in 110 parent–child trios and 42 parent–child duos [154]. De Cerqueira et al. found no association between ADHD and 403 affected adults and 232 controls, but did detect significant (p < 0.05) associations between a -1291 G-rs1800544/-262 G-rs1800545/1780 T-rs553668 haplotype, reduced harm avoidance, and greater novelty seeking [155]. It was suggested that some of the heterogeneity in ADRA2A-ADHD associations might be due to concomitant variability in temperament profile [155].

A 6-kb upstream dinucleotide repeat at alpha-2C-adrenergic receptor (ADRA2C) was nominally associated with ADHD by Comings et al. [156]. Guan et al., however, found an empirically significant association between ADRA2C (p < 0.05) and combined ADHD [124]. Other family-based analyses have not detected any association between ADRA2C and ADHD [157, 158]; the IMAGE study also detected no association between either ADRA2A or ADRA2C [59]. Elia et al. found, again, nominal associations of 7 of 27 candidate

genes with ADHD in 270 full-sib families (ADRA1A having the strongest association), but none were significant after multiple correction [159].

The norepinephrine transporter (NET; SLC6A2)

Drugs that block the norepinephrine transporter are efficacious in treating ADHD [160]. Genetic associations of SLC6A2 with ADHD have been variably successful. A SNP in SLC6A2 was associated with ADHD by Comings et al. [142], but not in a subsequent study of three SNPs (exon 9, intron 9, and intron 13) by Barr et al. in 122 ADHD families [161]. McEvoy et al. similarly found no association with SNPs in intron 7 or 9 [162]. Xu et al. reported nominal associations between the SNP rs3785157 and ADHD in an investigation of 21 SLC6A2 SNPs in 180 cases and 334 controls [163], which was replicated by Bobb et al. [89], who detected an additional SNP associated with ADHD (rs998424). In the IMAGE study, two SNPs at this locus (rs3785143 and rs11568324) were associated with ADHD [59]. An upstream promoter polymorphism at NET (−3081T) was associated with ADHD in 68 DSM-IV ADHD individuals [164]. A further test using 94 ADHD-diagnosed individuals and 60 controls found significantly (p = 0.008) higher frequency of the T allele in ADHD-affected individuals in a pattern suggesting dominance. The T allele may interact with the neural transcription repressors Slug and Scratch to repress SLC6A2 activity [165]. Interestingly, SLC6A2 may modulate the atomoxetine treatment of ADHD: SNPs across exons 4–9 were associated with response to treatment in two cohorts of ADHD-affected children [166].

Neurotrophin-3 (NTF3)

Cho et al. found a significantly higher T-score for errors of commission in commission performance tests (CPT) for individuals carrying an AA genotype at the SNP rs6332 than AG heterozygotes at NTF3 (p = 0.045) [167]. NTF3 is involved with the development and differentiation of mesolimbic dopaminergic neurons, noradrenergic locus ceruleus neurons, and hippocampal glutaminergic neurons [168].

Association studies of serotonergic genes

Serotonin receptors (HTR1B, HTR2A, HTR2C)

Although several studies of the serotonin HTR1B receptor found no association with ADHD [89,

169–171], Hawi *et al.* detected a significant association between ADHD and the G681C allele in a multi-site study [172]. Similarly, a pooled analysis by Smoller *et al.* found significant over-transmission of G681C (OR = 1.35 (1.13–1.62), p = 0.009), primarily paternal (p = 0.00005) rather than maternal transmission (p = 0.2) [170]. Li *et al.* found marginal evidence (p = 0.087) of over-transmission for G681C in a sample of inattentive ADHD subjects [173]. An *HTR1B* haplotype consisting of six SNPs (including G681C) was also linked to inattention by Smoller *et al.* [170]. Guimaraes *et al.* found over-transmission of the -261G/-161T/861G haplotype into affected children in a sample of 343 full-sib families (p = 0.014), but no over-transmission in a second set of 143 families with children having the inattentive subtype [174]. Heiser *et al.* did not detect an association between combined ADHD and the G681C allele [171]; the IMAGE project analysis similarly found no association with any tagged SNPs [59].

Ribases *et al.* detected an association between *5HT2A* and ADHD in 400 healthy control and 188 affected adults (OR = 1.63, p = 0.0036) and 263 children (OR = 1.49, p = 0.0084) [129]. The C102T allele at *HTR2A* has been associated with self-reported childhood ADHD symptoms in women with seasonal affective disorder [175] and the A1438G allele with functional remission from ADHD in Han Chinese adolescents [173]. ADHD was associated with a coding polymorphism (His452Tyr) in *HTR2A* by both Quist *et al.* [176] and Guimaraes *et al.* [177]. Several case–control and family-based studies, however, have detected no association between *HTR2A* SNPs and ADHD [71, 89, 171, 177–179]. Li *et al.* found significant over-transmission of the C-759T/G-697C *HTR2C* haplotype [180], but this association was not observed by Bobb *et al.* [89] or the IMAGE project [59]. Li *et al.* reported significant undertransmission of the C83097T/G83198A haplotype in the *HTR4* gene [181], but other serotonin receptor genes show no association with ADHD (*HTR5A*, *HTR6* [179]; HTR1D [182]; *HTR1E*, *HTR3B* [59]).

HTR2C has been linked to inattentive behavior: two *HTR2C* SNPs (rs2770296, rs927544) were associated with novelty seeking in samples of 366 and 355 healthy Caucasians [183]. Xu *et al.* detected over-transmission of the G allele at the G-697C polymorphism at *HTR2C* into ADHD affecteds in a sample of 180 British probands and their parents [184].

Serotonin transporter (*5HTT*, *SLC6A4*)

The 44-bp in/del promoter polymorphism (*5HTTLPR*) of *SLC6A4* has been associated with bipolar disorder, major depressive disorder, and suicidal behavior [185, 186]. A meta-review of gene effects including *5HTTLPR* found a pooled odds ratio of 1.31 for the long (L) allele [5]. The L allele was also linked to a composite index of ADHD by Curran *et al.* [187]. These associations have not been repeated in studies of 126 Korean [188], 197 British [189], 196 Taiwanese [189, 190], 56 Indian [191], 209 Canadian [192], and 102 German ADHD families [171] and a study of 279 Han Chinese ADHD families [193] actually found significant over-transmission of the S allele rather than the L allele. A case–control study by Kopeckova *et al.* found that the risk was significantly higher for heterozygotes (OR = 2.7) and homozygotes (OR = 6.7) for the risk allele at *5HTT* [96]. Other markers at this gene have been associated with ADHD. The 12–12 genotype at a 17-bp VNTR in intron 2 of *SLC6A4* has been variably over- or under-represented in ADHD cases [178, 191], although no differences in transmission were found by Heiser *et al.* [171], Xu *et al.* [189], or Kim *et al.* [188]. Li *et al.* found undertransmission of a *5HTTLPR*-L /17-bp intron 2-repeat haplotype in ADHD-affected individuals [193]. The IMAGE project found no association between ADHD and any *SLC6A4* SNPs [59]. Wigg *et al.* found no association of two functional *SLC6A4* polymorphisms (rs3813034 T-G and Ile425Val A-G) with ADHD [192]. Based on position relative to seed sequence for *SLC6A4*, Banerjee *et al.* determined that neither G689T nor G482T polymorphisms in the 3′ UTR were causally linked to ADHD [194]. The effects of *5HTT* may be subject to moderation by correlated traits; the *5HTT* in/del is associated with violent behavior [195] and positive maternal emotion moderated ADHD symptoms for non-I allele homozygotes at *5HTT* in a sample of 758 males with combined ADHD [106]. Nikolas *et al.* found significant interactions between *5HTTLPR* genotype and ratings of self-blame on the Child's Perception of Inter-Parental Conflict scale for symptoms of ADHD, and positive associations between self-blame and low- or high-serotonin genotypes at *5HTTLPR* [196].

Tryptophan hydroxylase (*TPH* and *TPH2*)

Li *et al.* found that a rare 218A/-6526G haplotype at *TPH* was transmitted at significantly lower frequency to probands of all ADHD subtypes (p = 0.034) [197]. A family-based study of *TPH* found no association with nearby genetic markers [198].

Walitza *et al.* found preferential transmission of the *TPH*-linked SNPs rs4570625 and rs11178997 into 225 affected children [199]. These SNPs were also associated with Go/No-Go continuous performance tests in 124 ADHD adults and 84 healthy controls [200]. Sheehan *et al.* found significant associations between the SNPs rs1843809-T (p = 0.0006) and rs1386497-A (p = 0.048) in 179 ADHD families [201], but these findings were not replicated in a sample of 63 ADHD trios [202].

In the IMAGE project [59], different alleles at rs1843809 and rs1386497 were significantly associated with ADHD at these SNPs. A SNP in linkage disequilibrium with rs1386497 (rs1007023) was associated with ADHD [59], but neither rs4570625 nor rs11178997 were linked to ADHD. Johansson *et al.* found no association between variants at *TPH1* or *TPH2* and ADHD in 1636 adult ADHD cases [203].

Dopa decarboxylase (*DDC*)

In a population association study involving 19 serotonergic genes in 188 adults and 263 children with ADHD, *DDC* was strongly associated with ADHD in both children (OR = 1.90) and adults (OR = 2.17).

Association studies of other candidate genes

Synaptosomal associated protein (25 kDa) (*SNAP-25*)

Coloboma mice, which have a hemizygous two-centimorgan chromosome 2q deletion encompassing *SNAP-25*, expresses hyperactivity, and deficits in motor development, hippocampal physiology, and Ca^{2+}-dependent dorsal striatum dopamine release [204]. Spontaneously hypertensive rats (SHR), an animal model of ADHD [205], have lower expression of *SNAP-25* compared to Wistar-Kyoto (WKY) controls [206].

Meta-analysis of four family-based studies of *SNAP-25* on two linked 3' SNPs (1069T>C and 1065T>G) [207–211] detected an association between T1065G (OR = 1.19; 95% CI 1.03–1.38). Feng *et al.* found significant over-transmission of four SNP alleles (rs66039806-C, rs362549-A, rs362987-A, and rs362998-C) in Canadian but not Californian ADHD families [212]. The IMAGE project found nominally statistically significant association with other 5' UTR markers and *SNAP-25* (rs363020 and rs362567)

[59]. Kim *et al.* examined the previously implicated SNPs and five additional SNPs (rs6077699, rs363006, rs362549, rs362987, rs362998) but found no evidence of association with ADHD in tests of individual markers or haplotypes [213]. A combined TDT analysis of pooled data was modestly significant for rs3746544-T (p = 0.048) and rs6077690-T (p = 0.031). Stratification by psychiatric comorbidities found stronger associations between ADHD and *SNAP-25* [213].

Acetylcholine receptors (*CHRNA4*, *CHRNA7*)

In a case–control study of Tourette syndrome (TS) children, Comings *et al.* linked the intron 1 dinucleotide repeat of *CHRNA4* to symptoms of ADHD [214]. A 3' exon 2 intronic G/A SNP was associated with ADHD by Todd *et al.* [215]. The IMAGE project found an association with a SNP in the 5' flanking region [59]. However, there was no association of a *Cfo1* restriction in exon 5 with ADHD [216], and no association of any of these markers with combined ADHD in two other studies [89, 217]. Lee *et al.* did detect over-transmission of two linked SNPs (rs2273505-G, rs3787141-T) in individuals having the combined ADHD subtype and hyperactivity–impulsivity [217]. A SNP at *CHRNA4* (rs1044396) was associated with visual attention. Also, at rs1044396 and carriers of the G allele at the *DBH*-linked SNP rs1108580 were associated with superior attentive working memory [218]. Kent *et al.* found no association of nicotinic acetylcholine receptor alpha-7 (*CHRNA7*) in 206 ADHD proband trios [219].

Glutamate receptors

GRIN2A encodes a subunit of the N-methyl D-aspartate (NMDA) receptor. Cognition in animals and humans has been linked to the NMDA receptor; notably, the *GRIN2A* gene is located in the region of the linkage peak at 16p13 [7, 8]. An exon 5 SNP (*Grin2a_5*) was associated with ADHD (p = 0.01) in 238 affected full-sib families [220], but Adams *et al.* found no such association in a group of 183 full-sib families (p = 0.74) [221].

Brain-derived neurotrophic factor (*BDNF*)

The association of *BDNF* with ADHD, as other genes, varies. A codon 66 *Val-Met* substitution at *BDNF* appears to downregulate its intracellular trafficking [222]. The *Val*66 allele was over-transmitted (p = 0.0005) in 341 Caucasians [223], but not in samples from either the UK or Taiwan [224]; contrarily, there was undertransmission of a haplotype containing the *Val*66 allele and the T allele at a 5′ intron 1 270C>T SNP in Taiwanese ADHD individuals [224]. There was also possible interaction of *BDNF* with the 3′ VNTR *DAT1* genotype (p = 0.02) [71]. *BNDF* was not associated with adult ADHD symptoms in a study of 110 affected adults [71]. The IMAGE project found no associations between 20 *BDNF* SNPs and ADHD [59]. The effects of *BDNF* on ADHD may be partially mediated by environment: a study of 10 SNPs around *BDNF* in 229 ADHD families found multiple genotype-by-socioeconomic status interactions for several haplotype blocks [225].

Nitric oxide synthase (*NOS1*)

A short repeat variant in a VNTR in exon 1 of the *NOS1* gene was associated with adult ADHD in a sample of 3272 individuals (383 of which had ADHD) and with lower transcription of the *NOS1* Ex1f promoter [226]. Altered transcription of *RGS4* and *GRIN1* and hypoactivation of the anterior cingulate cortex were also associated with this short repeat variant [226]. The effect of *NOS1* on impulsiveness was modified by the activity of platelet *MAO* in 637 males with self-reported impulsiveness [227].

Substance-preferring receptor (*Tacr1*)

Mice with the *Tacr1* gene knocked out are hyperactive [228]; this hyperactivity is prevented by treatment with *d*-amphetamine or methylphenidate [229]. Yan *et al.* subsequently found associations (p < 0.05) between four SNPs at *Tacr1* and ADHD in a sample of 450 ADHD patients and 600 controls [229].

The search for common variants: genome-wide association studies

Several searches have been made for genes responsible for ADHD using genome-wide association studies (GWAS). The IMAGE project identified families through ADHD patients at outpatient clinics, and 958 proband–parent trios were selected for the GWAS. Family members were Caucasians of European origin from Europe and Israel. Based on the Parental Account of Children's Symptoms (PACS), all probands met clinical criteria for ADHD according to the fourth edition of the American Psychiatric Association's diagnostic manual (DSM-IV). DNA had been extracted from blood samples. Genotyping was conducted at Perlegen Sciences using their genotyping platform of

600,000 SNPs. Lasky-Su *et al.* [230, 231] and Neale *et al.* [232] found several genes with nominal associations with ADHD, including *ADRB1*, *ADRB2*, *ARRB2*, *CHRNA4*, *DRD1*, *HTR2A*, *NFIL3*, *SLC6A3*, *SLC9A9*, and *SYT1*, although none with genome-wide significance (p > 10^{-7}). Six SNPs at *SLC9A9* were nominally associated with ADHD.

In a sample of 343 German ADHD in- and outpatients and 250 controls an unexpected array of genes associated with ADHD was found [233]. Genes found include *MOBP*, *REEP5*, *MAP1B*, *CTNNA2*, *ASTN2*, *CSMD2*, *CHD23*, and the cell adhesion gene *CDH13* which was also associated with ADHD by Lasky-Su *et al.* [230, 231]. CDH13 is found under the 16q peak for a quantitative trait locus (QTL) for ADHD.

An extension of the IMAGE project, called IMAGE 2, collected 903 ADHD cases from: (1) some of the original IMAGE sites; and (2) additional sites that had collected data that were assessed in a manner similar to IMAGE [234]. Based on the PACS interview, all probands met criteria for ADHD according to DSM-IV and were of Caucasian-European ethnicity. DNA had been extracted from blood samples. These were genotyped on the Affymetrix 5.0 platform at the SUNY Upstate Microarray Core Facility. The Affymetrix 5.0 platform was used due to cost considerations. The IMAGE 2 cases were genotypically matched to preexisting controls from the National Institute of Mental Health (NIMH) genetics repository which had been genotyped on the Affymetrix 6.0 platform. Genotypically matched controls were selected, adjusted for residual population stratification, and imputed Affymetrix 6.0 SNPs. No genome-wide significant associations were found. The most significant results implicated the following genes: *PRKG1*, *FLNC*, *TCERG1L*, *PPM1H*, *NXPH1*, *PPM1H*, *CDH13*, *HK1*, and *HKDC1*.

Another consortium (PUWMa) collected trio families at UCLA, Washington University, and the Massachusetts General Hospital [235]. Family members were Caucasian of European origin. Based on the Schedule for Affective Disorders and Schizophrenia for School Age Children (K-SADS), all probands met criteria for DSM-IV ADHD. DNA had been extracted from blood samples. Genotyping was completed at Genizon using the Illumina 1M platform. Their smallest p value did not reach the threshold for genome-wide statistical significance, but one of the most significant associations was for *SLC9A9*, a candidate gene for ADHD.

All the samples described above were subjected to uniform quality control procedures to create a dataset suitable for meta-analysis [32]. This sample also included data from the Children's Hospital of Philadelphia (CHOP). The CHOP ADHD trio families were recruited from pediatric and behavioral health clinics in the Philadelphia area. Inclusion criteria included families of European descent with an ADHD proband (age 6–18). Exclusionary criteria included prematurity (<36 weeks), mental retardation, major medical and neurological disorders, pervasive developmental disorder, psychoses, and major mood disorders. Diagnostic data were collected using the K-SADS interview. Samples were assayed on the Illumina HumanHap550. The final, clean sample comprised 2064 trios, 896 cases, and 2455 controls. The lambda statistic (1.025) for all SNPs showed no appreciable inflation of the test statistic. The lambdas for each individual study were 1.085 for IMAGE 2, 1.012 for IMAGE, 0.970 for PUWMa, and 1.047 for CHOP, which yields an expected lambda of 1.028 based on the average lambda, weighted by case size. No SNP achieved genome-wide significance but a joint analysis of candidate genes suggested they are involved in the disorder.

The search for common variants: genotype × environment interaction

Environmental effects on ADHD may be complex and occur along various dimensions from prenatal toxin exposure to perinatal stress to maternal emotionality [106, 236–239]. Waldman found evidence for interaction between DRD2 and maternal marital status in the development of ADHD [240]. Associations between DAT1 and DRD4 and ADHD may be affected by prenatal exposure to environmental factors such as nicotine and alcohol [241]. Significant interaction between smoking and DRD4 in the incidence of ADHD subtypes was detected by Neuman et al. [60], but not for parental ratings of ADHD symptoms in a study by Altink et al. [242]. However, a smaller study by Langley et al. found no effects of maternal use of alcohol, maternal smoking, DRD4 genotype, or interaction between these factors on ADHD [62]. ADHD in 229 families was affected by interaction between socioeconomic status for several BDNF haplotype blocks [225].

The number of such interactions may be substantial. Individual risk genes/alleles often explain ≤1% of the variance in ADHD phenotype, suggesting the influences of multiple characters and complex genotype–environmental interactions ([243, 244] but see Pennington et al. [245]). The resolution of such effects may require a more advanced, collaborative mapping effort, or the use of higher-order environmental×genotypic modeling to resolve such effects. Many individual surveys and meta-analytical tests indicate heterogeneity in ADHD among various effects, such as gender or comorbid disorders [246].

Despite these intriguing results, a meta-analysis of genotype-by-environment (G × E) interaction in 13 studies of inattention and 9 studies of hyperactivity found that G × E was insignificant [36].

The search for rare variants: parent-of-origin effects

Imprinting of genetic effects by parent or parental gender is another possible complication to statistical investigations of the molecular genetics of ADHD. Imprinting occurs when the DNA variant transmitted by one parent has a different effect than the DNA variant transmitted by the other parent. This occurs when the genome is modified by an epigenetic event such as methylation, which changes the degree to which the gene is expressed without changing the structure of the gene. A whole-genome survey found that more than 35,000 gene sites may be sensitive to methylation [247]; methylation affected 1.5% of SNP-labeled alleles in a study of 30 parent–child trios [247]. As for classical genetic effects on ADHD, the evidence for imprinting has varied. Hawi et al. found a joint paternal odds ratio of the transmission of ADHD-associated alleles of 2.0 at DRD4, DRD5, DAT1, TH, DDC, SNAP-25, 5HT1B, SERT, and TPH2 compared to 1.3 for affective alleles carried by the maternal parent in a sample of 179 ADHD-affected and 155 autism-affected Irish families [248]. In three new samples consisting of 108 nuclear Irish families, 107 nuclear English families, and 1033 nuclear families from the IMAGE study, Hawi et al. found both over-transmission of and strong evidence for imprinting effects at DAT1 associated with allele 6 in intron 8 and the 10-repeat allele [249]. However, Kim et al. found no evidence of parent-origin effects on ADHD associated with DAT1, BDNF, DRD5, SNAP-25, and HTR1B, in a sample of 291 trios [250]. Paternal over-transmission has been detected for several risk alleles for ADHD (i.e., rs2519152-G, DBH; G681C, HTR1B; Val66, BDNF) [113, 170, 223].

The search for rare variants: copy number variation and ADHD

Part of the difficulty in consistently identifying genes responsible for ADHD may be the existence of rare variants that cause the disorder. Some rare mutations have been documented to cause ADHD or ADHD-like symptoms: for example, a missense mutation of *FGD1* [251] and a familial translocation that disrupts the *DOCK3* and *SLC9A9* genes [252]. A SNP 3' from *SLC9A9* was significantly associated with hyperactive–impulsive DSM-IV scores, and another (rs2360867) with errors of commission in a study of ADHD-affected families by Markunas *et al.* [253]. Several studies have searched for rare copy number variants (CNVs) in ADHD patients. CNVs are insertions or deletions of DNA. They are of particular interest if they occur within a gene or a regulatory region as they are very likely to have an effect on the functioning of the gene.

Elia *et al.* found 222 inherited CNVs among 335 ADHD patients [254]. These inherited, rare CNVs were not detected in 2026 unrelated healthy individuals. Although, overall, no excess deletions or duplications were found in the ADHD cohort relative to controls, the genes harboring inherited rare CNVs were significantly enriched for genes reported as candidates in studies of autism, schizophrenia, and TS. The ADHD CNV gene set was also enriched for genes involved in learning, behavior, synaptic transmission, and central nervous system development.

Lesch and coworkers found several CNVs in 99 affected children and adolescents compared to 100 unscreened controls at several candidate genes, including acetylcholine-metabolizing butyrylcholinesterase (*BCHE*), pleckstrin domain-containing protein (*PLEKHB1*), NADH dehydrogenase 1A subcomplex assembly factor 2 (*NDUFAF2*), phosphodiesterase 4D isoform 6 (*PDE4D6*), and glucose transporter 3 (*SLC2A3*) [255]. CNVs were inherited from both affected and unaffected parents, and included two *de novo* CNVs.

A genome-wide analysis of CNVs in 366 British Caucasian ADHD children and 1047 unrelated controls found that the rate of large ($>$500 kb) rare ($f(a)$ $<$1%) CNVs in ADHD-affected children was twice that of controls [256]. ADHD children with intellectual disability (IQ $<$ 70) were 5.7 times as likely to carry such CNVs (p = $2.0{\times}10^{-6}$). There was a significant excess of large, rare duplication CNVs on chromosome 16p13.11 (p = 0.0008). An Icelandic sample of 825 ADHD patients and 35,243 controls also had a significant excess (p = 0.031) of duplications at this position [256].

Summary

The high heritability of ADHD, documented by numerous twin studies, is not in question. But, despite the high heritability of ADHD, the search for DNA variants that cause the disorder has been difficult. Perhaps the most progress has been made in the search for rare variants, where several groups have found insertions and deletions (CNVs) in the genome that appear to explain a small subset of ADHD cases. Future work is needed to see if most ADHD cases can be accounted for by such rare variants. If so, it is possible that the genetic causes of ADHD are extremely heterogeneous.

The variable association of the array of common genetic variants in several areas of neural functioning with the disorder signals an extraordinary complexity. Genome-wide and candidate analysis has been unable to detect consistent effects for common DNA variants if one requires a finding to achieve genome-wide significance. In part, this is due to the very stringent level of statistical significance required: i.e., p $<$ 0.00000005. Even genes that are compelling as candidate genes (*DBH*, *DAT1*, *MAO-A*) or have been implicated by meta-analysis (*DRD4*, *DRD5*, *SLC6A3*, *SNAP-25*, and *HTR1B*) have not achieved genome-wide levels of significance.

Attempts to improve the detection of common variants through gene-by-environment interaction studies or phenotypic refinement and the construction of discrete endophenotypes (see [257–260]) may help resolve this issue. But, unless subsets of patients carrying variants with very strong genetic effects can be created, it is likely that very large sample sizes will be needed: for example 10,000 cases and 10,000 controls. Such work will require more widespread collaboration and effective modeling of non-genetic variance sources, in addition to a more advanced appreciation of the basal genetic construction of each trait or the disorder as a whole.

More progress needs to be made before molecular genetic studies of ADHD can be translated into clinical practice. Currently, there is no genetic test for ADHD and genetic tests are not useful for predicting treatment response. The only exception to this is the documented ability of variants in the cytochrome P450 system to predict slow and fast drug metabolism, for example for atomoxetine. Yet, because standard practice is typically to titrate patients from low to high doses, genetic tests predictive of pharmacokinetic factors are typically not useful. From a clinical perspective, the most useful information from genetic studies is the fact that parents, siblings, and children of ADHD patients are at risk for ADHD. This should encourage clinicians to screen for the presence of ADHD in family members, especially when the relationship of the family member with the patient has implications for the patient's response to treatment.

References

1. Faraone SV, Sergeant J, Gillberg C, Biederman J. The worldwide prevalence of ADHD: is it an American condition? *World Psychiatry.* 2003;**2**(2):104–13.

2. Faraone S, Biederman J, Mick E. The age dependent decline of attention-deficit/hyperactivity disorder: a meta-analysis of follow-up studies. *Psychol Med.* 2006;**36**(2):159–65.

3. Faraone SV, Biederman J. Nature, nurture, and attention deficit hyperactivity disorder. *Dev Rev.* 2000;**20**:568–81.

4. Faraone SV, Biederman J, Spencer TJ, *et al.* Diagnosing adult attention deficit hyperactivity disorder: are late onset and subthreshold diagnoses valid? *Am J Psychiatry.* 2006;**163**(10):1720–9.

5. Faraone SV, Perlis RH, Doyle AE, *et al.* Molecular genetics of attention-deficit/hyperactivity disorder. *Biol Psychiatry.* 2005;**57**(11):1313–23.

6. Freitag C, Rohde L, Lempp T, Romanos M. Phenotypic and measurement influences on heritability estimates in childhood ADHD. *Eur Child Adolesc Psychiatry.* 2010;**19**:311–23.

7. Fisher SE, Francks C, McCracken JT, *et al.* A genomewide scan for loci involved in attention-deficit/hyperactivity disorder. *Am J Hum Genet.* 2002;**70**(5):1183–96.

8. Smalley SL, Kustanovich V, Minassian SL, *et al.* Genetic linkage of attention-deficit/hyperactivity disorder on chromosome 16p13, in a region implicated in autism. *Am J Hum Genet.* 2002;**71**(4):959–63.

9. Bakker S, van der Meulen E, Buitelaar J, *et al.* A whole-genome scan in 164 Dutch sib pairs with attention-deficit/hyperactivity disorder: suggestive evidence for linkage on chromosomes 7p and 15q. *Am J Hum Genet.* 2003;**72**(5):1251–60.

10. Arcos-Burgos M, Castellanos FX, Konecki D, *et al.* Pedigree disequilibrium test (PDT) replicates association and linkage between DRD4 and ADHD in multigenerational and extended pedigrees from a genetic isolate. *Mol Psychiatry.* 2004;**9**(3):252–9.

11. Hebebrand J, Dempfle A, Saar K, *et al.* A genome-wide scan for attention-deficit/hyperactivity disorder in 155 German sib-pairs. *Mol Psychiatry.* 2006;**11**(2):196–205.

12. Amin N, Aulchenko Y, Dekker M, *et al.* Suggestive linkage of ADHD to chromosome 18q22 in a young genetically isolated Dutch population. *Eur J Hum Genet.* 2009;**17**:958–66.

13. Arcos-Burgos M, Jain M, Acosta M, *et al.* A common variant of the latrophilin 3 gene, LPHN3, confers susceptibility to ADHD and predicts effectiveness of stimulant medication. *Mol Psychiatry.* 2010;**15**(1):1053–66.

14. Vegt R, Bertoli-Avella A, Tulen J, *et al.* Genome-wide linkage analysis in a Dutch multigenerational family with attention deficit hyperactivity disorder. *Eur J Hum Genet.* 2010;**18**(2):206–11.

15. Faraone SV, Doyle AE, Lasky-Su J, *et al.* Linkage analysis of attention deficit hyperactivity disorder. *Am J Med Genet B Neuropsychiatr Genet.* 2008;**147B**(8):1387–91.

16. Couto JM, Gomez L, Wigg K, *et al.* Association of attention-deficit/hyperactivity disorder with a candidate region for reading disabilities on chromosome 6p. *Biol Psychiatry.* 2009;**66**(4):368–75.

17. Joo E, Greenwood T, Schork N, *et al.* Suggestive evidence for linkage of ADHD features in bipolar disorder to chromosome 10p14. *Am J Med Genet B Neuropsychiatr Genet.* 2010;**153**(1):260–8.

18. Ogdie MN, Bakker SC, Fisher SE, *et al.* Pooled genome-wide linkage data on 424 ADHD ASPs suggests genetic heterogeneity and a common risk locus at 5p13. *Mol Psychiatry.* 2006;**11**(1):5–8.

19. Zhou K, Dempfle A, Arcos-Burgos M, *et al.* Meta-analysis of genome-wide linkage scans of attention deficit hyperactivity disorder. *Am J Med Genet B Neuropsychiatr Genet.* 2008;**147B**(8):1392–8.

20. Li D, Sham PC, Owen MJ, He L. Meta-analysis shows significant association between dopamine system genes and attention deficit hyperactivity disorder (ADHD). *Hum Mol Genet.* 2006;**15**(14):2276–84.

21. Faraone SV, Doyle AE, Mick E, Biederman J. Meta-analysis of the association between the 7-repeat allele of the dopamine d(4) receptor gene and attention deficit hyperactivity disorder. *Am J Psychiatry.* 2001;**158**(7):1052–7.

22. Lowe N, Kirley A, Hawi Z, *et al.* Joint analysis of DRD5 marker concludes association with ADHD confined to the predominantly inattentive and combined subtypes. *Am J Hum Genet.* 2004;**74**(2):348–56.

23. Yang B, Chan RC, Jing J, *et al.* A meta-analysis of association studies between the 10-repeat allele of a VNTR polymorphism in the 3′-UTR of dopamine transporter gene and attention deficit hyperactivity disorder. *Am J Med Genet B Neuropsychiatr Genet.* 2007;**144B**(4):541–50.

24. Purper-Ouakil D, Wohl M, Mouren MC, *et al.* Meta-analysis of family-based association studies between the dopamine transporter gene and attention deficit hyperactivity disorder. *Psychiatr Genet.* 2005; **15**(1):53–9.

25. Cheuk DK, Wong V. Meta-analysis of association between a catechol-O-methyltransferase gene polymorphism and attention deficit hyperactivity disorder. *Behav Genet.* 2006;**36**(5):651–9.

26. Reuter M, Kirsch P, Hennig J. Inferring candidate genes for attention deficit hyperactivity disorder (ADHD) assessed by the World Health Organization Adult ADHD Self-Report Scale (ASRS). *J Neural Transm.* 2006;**113**(7):929–38.

27. Gothelf D, Michaelovsky E, Frisch A, *et al.* Association of the low-activity COMT 158 Met allele with ADHD and OCD in subjects with velocardiofacial syndrome. *Int J Neuropsychopharmacol.* 2007;**10**(3):301–8.

28. McGough JJ, McCracken JT, Loo SK, *et al.* A candidate gene analysis of methylphenidate response in attention-deficit/hyperactivity disorder. *J Am Acad Child Adolesc Psychiatry.* 2009;**48**(12):1155–64.

29. Song EY, Paik KC, Kim HW, Lim MH. Association between catechol-O-methyltransferase gene polymorphism and attention-deficit hyperactivity disorder in Korean population. *Genet Test Mol Biomarkers.* 2009;**13**(2):233–6.

30. DeYoung CG, Getchell M, Koposov RA, *et al.* Variation in the catechol-O-methyltransferase Val 158 Met polymorphism associated with conduct disorder and ADHD symptoms, among adolescent male delinquents. *Psychiatr Genet.* 2010;**20**(1):20–4.

31. Palmason H, Moser D, Sigmund J, *et al.* Attention-deficit/hyperactivity disorder phenotype is influenced by a functional catechol-O-methyltransferase variant. *J Neural Transm.* 2010;**117**(2):259–67.

32. Neale BM, Medland SE, Ripke S, *et al.* Meta-analysis of genome-wide association studies of attention-deficit/ hyperactivity disorder. *J Am Acad Child Adolesc Psychiatry.* 2010;**49**(9):884–97.

33. Gizer IR, Ficks C, Waldman ID. Candidate gene studies of ADHD: a meta-analytic review. *Hum Genet.* 2009;**126**(1):51–90.

34. Sharp SI, McQuillin A, Gurling HM. Genetics of attention-deficit hyperactivity disorder (ADHD). *Neuropharmacology.* 2009;**57**(7–8):590–600.

35. Gizer I, Waldman I, Abramowitz A, *et al.* Relations between multi-informant assessments of ADHD symptoms, DAT1, and DRD4. *J Abnorm Psychol.* 2008;**117**(4):869–80.

36. Nikolas M, Burt S. Genetic and environmental influences on ADHD symptom dimensions of inattention and hyperactivity: a meta-analysis. *J Abnorm Psychol.* 2010;**119**:1–17.

37. Lanau F, Zenner M, Civelli O, Hartman D. Epinephrine and norepinephrine act as potent agonists at the recombinant human dopamine D4 receptor. *J Neurochem.* 1997;**68**(2):804–12.

38. Faraone SV, Biederman J. Neurobiology of attention-deficit hyperactivity disorder. *Biol Psychiatry.* 1998;**44**(10):951–8.

39. Van Tol HH, Wu CM, Guan HC, *et al.* Multiple dopamine D4 receptor variants in the human population. *Nature.* 1992;**358**(6382):149–52.

40. Asghari V, Sanyal S, Buchwaldt S, *et al.* Modulation of intracellular cyclic AMP levels by different human dopamine D4 receptor variants. *J Neurochem.* 1995;**65**(3):1157–65.

41. Pluess M, Belsky J, Neuman RJ. Prenatal smoking and attention-deficit/hyperactivity disorder: DRD4–7R as a plasticity gene. *Biol Psychiatry.* 2009;**66**(4):e5–6.

42. Biederman J, Petty C, Ten Haagen K, *et al.* Effect of candidate gene polymorphisms on the course of attention deficit hyperactivity disorder. *Psychiatry Res.* 2009;**170**:199–203.

43. El-Faddagh M, Laucht M, Maras A, Vohringer L, Schmidt MH. Association of dopamine D4 receptor (DRD4) gene with attention-deficit/hyperactivity disorder (ADHD) in a high-risk community sample: a longitudinal study from birth to 11 years of age. *J Neural Transm.* 2004;**111**(7):883–9.

44. Langley K, Fowler TA, Grady DL, *et al.* Molecular genetic contribution to the developmental course of attention-deficit hyperactivity disorder. *Eur Child Adolesc Psychiatry.* 2009;**18**(1):26–32.

45. Bhaduri N, Sinha S, Chattopadhyay A, *et al.* Analysis of polymorphisms in the dopamine beta hydroxylase gene: association with attention deficit hyperactivity disorder in Indian children. *Indian Pediatr.* 2005;**42**(2):123–9.

46. Niederhofer H, Menzel F, Gobel K, *et al.* A preliminary report of the dopamine receptor D(4) and the dopamine transporter 1 gene polymorphism and its association with attention deficit hyperactivity disorder. *Neuropsychiatr Dis Treat.* 2008;**4**(4): 701–5.

47. Kramer UM, Rojo N, Schule R, *et al.* ADHD candidate gene (DRD4 exon III) affects inhibitory control in a healthy sample. *BMC Neurosci.* 2009;**10**:150.

48. Becker K, Blomeyer D, El-Faddagh M, *et al*. From regulatory problems in infancy to attention-deficit/hyperactivity disorder in childhood: a moderating role for the dopamine D4 receptor gene? *J Pediatr*. 2010;**156**(5):798–803, 803.e1–e2.

49. Carrasco X, Rothhammer P, Moraga M, *et al*. Genotypic interaction between DRD4 and DAT1 loci is a high risk factor for attention-deficit/hyperactivity disorder in Chilean families. *Am J Med Genet B Neuropsychiatr Genet*. 2006;**141**(1):51–4.

50. Gabriela ML, John DG, Magdalena BV, *et al*. Genetic interaction analysis for DRD4 and DAT1 genes in a group of Mexican ADHD patients. *Neurosci Lett*. 2009;**451**(3):257–60.

51. McCracken JT, Smalley SL, McGough JJ, *et al*. Evidence for linkage of a tandem duplication polymorphism upstream of the dopamine D4 receptor gene (DRD4) with attention deficit hyperactivity disorder (ADHD). *Mol Psychiatry*. 2000;**5**(5):531–6.

52. Kustanovich V, Ishii J, Crawford L, *et al*. Transmission disequilibrium testing of dopamine-related candidate gene polymorphisms in ADHD: confirmation of association of ADHD with DRD4 and DRD5. *Mol Psychiatry*. 2004;**9**(7):711–17.

53. Barr CL, Feng Y, Wigg KG, *et al*. 5′-untranslated region of the dopamine D4 receptor gene and attention- deficit hyperactivity disorder. *Am J Med Genet*. 2001;**105**(1):84–90.

54. Todd RD, Neuman RJ, Lobos EA, *et al*. Lack of association of dopamine D4 receptor gene polymorphisms with ADHD subtypes in a population sample of twins. *Am J Med Genet*. 2001;**105**(5):432–8.

55. Brookes KJ, Xu X, Chen CK, *et al*. No evidence for the association of DRD4 with ADHD in a Taiwanese population within-family study. *BMC Med Genet*. 2005;**6**:31.

56. Bhaduri N, Das M, Sinha S, *et al*. Association of dopamine D4 receptor (DRD4) polymorphisms with attention deficit hyperactivity disorder in Indian population. *Am J Med Genet B Neuropsychiatr Genet*. 2006;**141B**(1):61–6.

57. Nikolaidis A, Gray J. ADHD and the DRD4 exon III 7-repeat polymorphism: an international meta-analysis. *Soc Cogn Affect Neurosci*. 2010;**5**(2–3): 188–93.

58. Lowe N, Kirley A, Mullins C, *et al*. Multiple marker analysis at the promoter region of the DRD4 gene and ADHD: evidence of linkage and association with the SNP-616. *Am J Med Genet B Neuropsychiatr Genet*. 2004;**131B**(1):33–7.

59. Brookes K, Xu X, Chen W, *et al*. The analysis of 51 genes in DSM-IV combined type attention deficit hyperactivity disorder: association signals in DRD4,

60. Neuman RJ, Lobos E, Reich W, *et al*. Prenatal smoking exposure and dopaminergic genotypes interact to cause a severe ADHD subtype. *Biol Psychiatry*. 2007;**61**(12):1320–8.

61. Altink M, Arias-Vasquez A, Franke B, *et al*. The dopamine receptor D4 7-repeat allele and prenatal smoking in ADHD-affected children and their unaffected siblings: no gene–environment interaction. *J Child Psychol Psychiatry*. 2008;**49**:1053–60.

62. Langley K, Turic D, Rice F, *et al*. Testing for gene × environment interaction effects in attention deficit hyperactivity disorder and associated antisocial behavior. *Am J Med Genet B Neuropsychiatr Genet*. 2008;**147B**:49–53.

63. Kim YS, Leventhal BL, Kim SJ, *et al*. Family-based association study of DAT1 and DRD4 polymorphism in Korean children with ADHD. *Neurosci Lett*. 2005;**390**(3):176–81.

64. Kim B, Koo MS, Jun JY, *et al*. Association between dopamine D4 receptor gene polymorphism and scores on a continuous performance test in Korean children with attention deficit hyperactivity disorder. *Psychiatry Investig*. 2009;**6**(3):216–21.

65. Rowe DC, Stever C, Chase D, *et al*. Two dopamine genes related to reports of childhood retrospective inattention and conduct disorder symptoms. *Mol Psychiatry*. 2001;**6**(4):429–33.

66. Levitan RD, Masellis M, Lam RW, *et al*. Childhood inattention and dysphoria and adult obesity associated with the dopamine D4 receptor gene in overeating women with seasonal affective disorder. *Neuropsychopharmacology*. 2004;**29**(1):179–86.

67. Bellgrove MA, Hawi Z, Lowe N, *et al*. DRD4 gene variants and sustained attention in attention deficit hyperactivity disorder (ADHD): effects of associated alleles at the VNTR and -521 SNP. *Am J Med Genet B Neuropsychiatr Genet*. 2005;**136**(1):81–6.

68. Swanson J, Oosterlaan J, Murias M, *et al*. Attention deficit/hyperactivity disorder children with a 7-repeat allele of the dopamine receptor D4 gene have extreme behavior but normal performance on critical neuropsychological tests of attention. *Proc Natl Acad Sci U S A*. 2000;**97**(9):4754–9.

69. Manor I, Tyano S, Eisenberg J, *et al*. The short DRD4 repeats confer risk to attention deficit hyperactivity disorder in a family-based design and impair performance on a continuous performance test (TOVA). *Mol Psychiatry*. 2002;**7**(7):790–4.

70. Langley K, Marshall L, van den Bree M, *et al*. Association of the dopamine D4 receptor gene 7-repeat allele with neuropsychological test

performance of children with ADHD. *Am J Psychiatry.* 2004;**161**(1):133–8.

71. Muller DJ, Chiesa A, Mandelli L, *et al.* Correlation of a set of gene variants, life events and personality features on adult ADHD severity. *J Psychiatr Res.* 2010;**44**(9): 598–604.

72. Todd RD, Huang H, Smalley SL, *et al.* Collaborative analysis of DRD4 and DAT genotypes in population-defined ADHD subtypes. *J Child Psychol Psychiatry.* 2005;**46**(10):1067–73.

73. Mill J, Xu X, Ronald A, *et al.* Quantitative trait locus analysis of candidate gene alleles associated with attention deficit hyperactivity disorder (ADHD) in five genes: DRD4, DAT1, DRD5, SNAP-25, and 5HT1B. *Am J Med Genet B Neuropsychiatr Genet.* 2005;**133B** (1):68–73.

74. Stevens SE, Kumsta R, Kreppner JM, *et al.* Dopamine transporter gene polymorphism moderates the effects of severe deprivation on ADHD symptoms: developmental continuities in gene-environment interplay. *Am J Med Genet B Neuropsychiatr Genet.* 2009;**150B**(6):753–61.

75. Loo SK, Hale ST, Hanada G, *et al.* Familial clustering and DRD4 effects on electroencephalogram measures in multiplex families with attention deficit/ hyperactivity disorder. *J Am Acad Child Adolesc Psychiatry.* 2010;**49**(4):368–77.

76. Martel M, Nikolas M, Jernigan K, Friderici K, Nigg J. Personality mediation of genetic effects on attention-deficit/hyperactivity disorder. *J Abnorm Child Psychol.* 2010;**38**(5):633–43.

77. Grady DL, Harxhi A, Smith M, *et al.* Sequence variants of the DRD4 gene in autism: further evidence that rare DRD4 7R haplotypes are ADHD specific. *Am J Med Genet B Neuropsychiatr Genet.* 2005;**136**(1):33–5.

78. Lynn DE, Lubke G, Yang M, *et al.* Temperament and character profiles and the dopamine D4 receptor gene in ADHD. *Am J Psychiatry.* 2005;**162**(5):906–13.

79. Hersrud SL, Stoltenberg SF. Epistatic interaction between COMT and DAT1 genes on eating behavior: a pilot study. *Eat Behav.* 2009;**10**(2):131–3.

80. Syvanen AC, Tilgmann C, Rinne J, Ulmanen I. Genetic polymorphism of catechol-O-methyltransferase (COMT): correlation of genotype with individual variation of S-COMT activity and comparison of the allele frequencies in the normal population and parkinsonian patients in Finland. *Pharmacogenetics.* 1997;**7**(1):65–71.

81. Halleland H, Lundervold AJ, Halmoy A, Haavik J, Johansson S. Association between catechol O-methyltransferase (COMT) haplotypes and severity of hyperactivity symptoms in adults. *Am J Med Genet B Neuropsychiatr Genet.* 2009;**150B**(3):403–10.

82. Brookes KJ, Knight J, Xu X, Asherson P. DNA pooling analysis of ADHD and genes regulating vesicle release of neurotransmitters. *Am J Med Genet B Neuropsychiatr Genet.* 2005;**139B**(1):33–7.

83. Nobile M, Rusconi M, Bellina M, *et al.* COMT Val158Met polymorphism and socioeconomic status interact to predict attention deficit/hyperactivity problems in children aged 10–14. *Eur Child Adolesc Psychiatry.* 2010;**19**(7):549–57.

84. Qian QJ, Yang L, Wang YF, *et al.* Gene-gene interaction between COMT and MAOA potentially predicts the intelligence of attention-deficit hyperactivity disorder boys in China. *Behav Genet.* 2010;**40**(3):357–65.

85. Hawi Z, Lowe N, Kirley A, *et al.* Linkage disequilibrium mapping at DAT1, DRD5 and DBH narrows the search for ADHD susceptibility alleles at these loci. *Mol Psychiatry.* 2003;**8**(3):299–308.

86. Loos M, Pattij T, Janssen MC, *et al.* Dopamine receptor D1/D5 gene expression in the medial prefrontal cortex predicts impulsive choice in rats. *Cereb Cortex.* 2010;**20**(5):1064–70.

87. Mill J, Curran S, Richards S, Taylor E, Asherson P. Polymorphisms in the dopamine D5 receptor (DRD5) gene and ADHD. *Am J Med Genet B Neuropsychiatr Genet.* 2004;**125B**(1):38–42.

88. Bakker SC, van der Meulen EM, Oteman N, *et al.* DAT1, DRD4, and DRD5 polymorphisms are not associated with ADHD in Dutch families. *Am J Med Genet B Neuropsychiatr Genet.* 2005;**132**(1):50–2.

89. Bobb AJ, Addington AM, Sidransky E, *et al.* Support for association between ADHD and two candidate genes: NET1 and DRD1. *Am J Med Genet B Neuropsychiatr Genet.* 2005;**134B**(1):67–72.

90. Brookes KJ, Mill J, Guindalini C, *et al.* A common haplotype of the dopamine transporter gene associated with attention-deficit/hyperactivity disorder and interacting with maternal use of alcohol during pregnancy. *Arch Gen Psychiatry.* 2006;**63**(1):74–81.

91. Spencer T, Biederman J, Wilens T. Pharmacotherapy of attention deficit hyperactivity disorder. *Child Adolesc Psychiatr Clin North Am.* 2000;**9**(1): 77–97.

92. Giros B, Jaber M, Jones SR, Wightman RM, Caron MG. Hyperlocomotion and indifference to cocaine and amphetamine in mice lacking the dopamine transporter. *Nature.* 1996;**379**(6566):606–12.

93. Gainetdinov RR, Wetsel WC, Jones SR, *et al.* Role of serotonin in the paradoxical calming effect of psychostimulants on hyperactivity. *Science.* 1999;**283**:397–402.

94. Cook EH, Stein MA, Krasowski MD, *et al.* Association of attention deficit disorder and the dopamine transporter gene. *Am J Hum Genet.* 1995;**56**:993–8.

95. Lee S, Lahey B, Waldman I, *et al.* Association of dopamine transporter genotype with disruptive behavior disorders in an eight-year longitudinal study of children and adolescents. *Am J Med Genet B Neuropsychiatr Genet.* 2007;**144B**:310–17.

96. Kopeckova M, Paclt I, Petrasek J, *et al.* Some ADHD polymorphisms (in genes DAT1, DRD2, DRD3, DBH, 5-HTT) in case-control study of 100 subjects 6–10 age. *Neuro Endocrinol Lett.* 2008;**29**(2):246–51.

97. Doyle C, Brookes K, Simpson J, *et al.* Replication of an association of a promoter polymorphism of the dopamine transporter gene and Attention Deficit Hyperactivity Disorder. *Neurosci Lett.* 2009;**462**(2): 179–81.

98. Silva MA, Cordeiro Q, Louza M, Vallada H. Association between a SLC6A3 intron 8 VNTR functional polymorphism and ADHD in a Brazilian sample of adult patients. *Rev Bras Psiquiatr.* 2009;**31**(4):387–95.

99. Kebir O, Tabbane K, Sengupta S, Joober R. Candidate genes and neuropsychological phenotypes in children with ADHD: review of association studies. *J Psychiatry Neurosci.* 2009;**34**(2):88–101.

100. Xu X, Mill J, Sun B, *et al.* Association study of promoter polymorphisms at the dopamine transporter gene in attention deficit hyperactivity disorder. *BMC Psychiatry.* 2009;**9**:3.

101. Todd RD. Neural development is regulated by classical neurotransmitters: dopamine D2 receptor stimulation enhances neurite outgrowth. *Biol Psychiatry.* 1992;**31**:794–807.

102. Asherson P, Brookes K, Franke B, *et al.* Confirmation that a specific haplotype of the dopamine transporter gene is associated with combined-type ADHD. *Am J Psychiatry.* 2007;**164**(4):674–7.

103. Bellgrove MA, Johnson KA, Barry E, *et al.* Dopaminergic haplotype as a predictor of spatial inattention in children with attention-deficit/ hyperactivity disorder. *Arch Gen Psychiatry.* 2009;**66**(10):1135–42.

104. Franke B, Vasquez AA, Johansson S, *et al.* Multicenter analysis of the SLC6A3/DAT1 VNTR haplotype in persistent ADHD suggests differential involvement of the gene in childhood and persistent ADHD. *Neuropsychopharmacology.* 2010;**35**(3):656–64.

105. Laucht M, Skowronek MH, Becker K, *et al.* Interacting effects of the dopamine transporter gene and psychosocial adversity on attention-deficit/ hyperactivity disorder symptoms among 15-year-olds from a high-risk community sample. *Arch Gen Psychiatry.* 2007;**64**(5):585–90.

106. Sonuga-Barke EJ, Oades RD, Psychogiou L, *et al.* Dopamine and serotonin transporter genotypes moderate sensitivity to maternal expressed emotion: the case of conduct and emotional problems in attention deficit/hyperactivity disorder. *J Child Psychol Psychiatry.* 2009;**50**(9):1052–63.

107. Paclt I, Koudelova J, Pacltova D, Kopeckova M. Dopamine beta hydroxylase (DBH) plasma activity in childhood mental disorders. *Neuro Endocrinol Lett.* 2009;**30**(5):604–9.

108. Comings DE, Muhleman D, Gysin R. Dopamine D2 receptors (DRD2) gene and susceptibility to posttraumatic stress disorder: a study and replication. *Soc Biol Psychiatry.* 1996;**40**:368–72.

109. Comings DE, Wu H, Chiu C, *et al.* Polygenic inheritance of Tourette syndrome, stuttering, attention deficit hyperactivity, conduct and oppositional defiant disorder: the additive and subtractive effect of the three dopaminergic genes – DRD2, DβH and DAT1. *Am J Med Genet.* 1996;**67**:264–88.

110. Smith KM, Daly M, Fischer M, *et al.* Association of the dopamine beta hydroxylase gene with attention deficit hyperactivity disorder: genetic analysis of the Milwaukee longitudinal study. *Am J Med Genet B Neuropsychiatr Genet.* 2003;**119B**(1):77–85.

111. Roman T, Schmitz M, Polanczyk GV, *et al.* Further evidence for the association between attention-deficit/hyperactivity disorder and the dopamine-beta-hydroxylase gene. *Am J Med Genet.* 2002;**114**(2): 154–8.

112. Wigg K, Zai G, Schachar R, *et al.* Attention deficit hyperactivity disorder and the gene for dopamine beta-hydroxylase. *Am J Psychiatry.* 2002;**159**(6): 1046–8.

113. Bhaduri N, Sarkar K, Sinha S, Chattopadhyay A, Mukhopadhyay K. Study on DBH genetic polymorphisms and plasma activity in attention deficit hyperactivity disorder patients from Eastern India. *Cell Mol Neurobiol.* 2010;**30**(2):265–74.

114. Hess C, Reif A, Strobel A, *et al.* A functional dopamine-beta-hydroxylase gene promoter polymorphism is associated with impulsive personality styles, but not with affective disorders. *J Neural Transm.* 2009;**116**(2):121–30.

115. Greene CM, Bellgrove MA, Gill M, Robertson IH. Noradrenergic genotype predicts lapses in sustained attention. *Neuropsychologia.* 2009;**47**(2):591–4.

116. Bhaduri N, Mukhopadhyay K. Lack of significant association between -1021C–>T polymorphism in the dopamine beta hydroxylase gene and attention deficit hyperactivity disorder. *Neurosci Lett.* 2006;**402**(1–2): 12–16.

117. Inkster B, Muglia P, Jain U, Kennedy JL. Linkage disequilibrium analysis of the dopamine beta-hydroxylase gene in persistent attention deficit

hyperactivity disorder. *Psychiatr Genet*. 2004;**14**(2): 117–20.

118. Payton A, Holmes J, Barrett JH, *et al*. Examining for association between candidate gene polymorphisms in the dopamine pathway and attention-deficit hyperactivity disorder: a family-based study. *Am J Med Genet*. 2001;**105**(5):464–70.

119. Zhang HB, Wang YF, Li J, Wang B, Yang L. [Association between dopamine beta hydroxylase gene and attention deficit hyperactivity disorder complicated with disruptive behavior disorder]. *Zhonghua Er Ke Za Zhi*. 2005;**43**(1):26–30.

120. Cases O, Lebrand C, Giros B, *et al*. Plasma membrane transporters of serotonin, dopamine, and norepinephrine mediate serotonin accumulation in atypical locations in the developing brain of monoamine oxidase A knock-outs. *J Neurosci*. 1998;**18**(17):6914–27.

121. Manor I, Tyano S, Mel E, *et al*. Family-based and association studies of monoamine oxidase A and attention deficit hyperactivity disorder (ADHD): preferential transmission of the long promoter-region repeat and its association with impaired performance on a continuous performance test (TOVA). *Mol Psychiatry*. 2002;**7**(6):626–32.

122. Lawson DC, Turic D, Langley K, *et al*. Association analysis of monoamine oxidase A and attention deficit hyperactivity disorder. *Am J Med Genet B Neuropsychiatr Genet*. 2003;**116B**(1):84–9.

123. Roohi J, DeVincent CJ, Hatchwell E, Gadow KD. Association of a monoamine oxidase-a gene promoter polymorphism with ADHD and anxiety in boys with autism spectrum disorder. *J Autism Dev Disord*. 2009;**39**(1):67–74.

124. Guan L, Wang B, Chen Y, *et al*. A high-density single-nucleotide polymorphism screen of 23 candidate genes in attention deficit hyperactivity disorder: suggesting multiple susceptibility genes among Chinese Han population. *Mol Psychiatry*. 2009;**14**(5):546–54.

125. Jiang S, Xin R, Lin S, *et al*. Linkage studies between attention-deficit hyperactivity disorder and the monoamine oxidase genes. *Am J Med Genet*. 2001;**105**(8):783–8.

126. Domschke K, Sheehan K, Lowe N, *et al*. Association analysis of the monoamine oxidase A and B genes with attention deficit hyperactivity disorder (ADHD) in an Irish sample: preferential transmission of the MAO-A 941G allele to affected children. *Am J Med Genet B Neuropsychiatr Genet*. 2005;**134B**(1): 110–14.

127. Xu X, Brookes K, Chen CK, *et al*. Association study between the monoamine oxidase A gene and attention

deficit hyperactivity disorder in Taiwanese samples. *BMC Psychiatry*. 2007;**7**(1):10.

128. Guimaraes AP, Zeni C, Polanczyk G, *et al*. MAOA is associated with methylphenidate improvement of oppositional symptoms in boys with attention deficit hyperactivity disorder. *Int J Neuropsychopharmacol*. 2009;**12**(5):709–14.

129. Ribases M, Ramos-Quiroga JA, Hervas A, *et al*. Exploration of 19 serotoninergic candidate genes in adults and children with attention-deficit/hyperactivity disorder identifies association for 5HT2A, DDC and MAOB. *Mol Psychiatry*. 2009;**14**(1):71–85.

130. Nedic G, Pivac N, Hercigonja D-K, *et al*. Platelet monoamine oxidase activity in children with attention-deficit hyperactivity disorder. *Psychiatry Res*. 2010;**175**:252–5.

131. Comings DE, Comings BG, Muhleman D, *et al*. The dopamine D2 receptor locus as a modifying gene in neuropsychiatric disorders. *J Am Med Assoc*. 1991; **266**(13):1793–800.

132. Sery O, Drtilkova I, Theiner P, *et al*. Polymorphism of DRD2 gene and ADHD. *Neuro Endocrinol Lett*. 2006;**27**(1–2):236–40.

133. Esposito-Smythers C, Spirito A, Rizzo C, McGeary JE, Knopik VS. Associations of the DRD2 TaqIA polymorphism with impulsivity and substance use: preliminary results from a clinical sample of adolescents. *Pharmacol Biochem Behav*. 2009;**93**(3): 306–12.

134. Kim JW, Park CS, Hwang JW, *et al*. Clinical and genetic characteristics of Korean male alcoholics with and without attention deficit hyperactivity disorder. *Alcohol Alcohol*. 2006;**41**(4):407–11.

135. Bowton E, Saunders C, Erreger K, *et al*. Dysregulation of dopamine transporters via dopamine D2 autoreceptors triggers anomalous dopamine efflux associated with attention-deficit/hyperactivity disorder. *J Neurosci*. 2010;**30**(17):6048–57.

136. Rowe DC, den Oord EJ, Stever C, *et al*. The DRD2 TaqI polymorphism and symptoms of attention deficit hyperactivity disorder. *Mol Psychiatry*. 1999;**4**(6): 580–6.

137. Huang YS, Lin SK, Wu YY, Chao CC, Chen CK. A family-based association study of attention-deficit hyperactivity disorder and dopamine D2 receptor TaqI A alleles. *Chang Gung Med J*. 2003;**26**(12): 897–903.

138. Kirley A, Hawi Z, Daly G, *et al*. Dopaminergic system genes in ADHD: toward a biological hypothesis. *Neuropsychopharmacology*. 2002;**27**(4):607–19.

139. Retz W, Rosler M, Supprian T, Retz-Junginger P, Thome J. Dopamine D3 receptor gene polymorphism

and violent behavior: relation to impulsiveness and ADHD-related psychopathology. *J Neural Transm.* 2003;**110**(5):561–72.

140. Barr CL, Wigg KG, Wu J, *et al.* Linkage study of two polymorphisms at the dopamine D3 receptor gene and attention-deficit hyperactivity disorder. *Am J Med Genet.* 2000;**96**(1):114–17.

141. Muglia P, Jain U, Kennedy JL. A transmission disequilibrium test of the Ser9/Gly dopamine D3 receptor gene polymorphism in adult attention-deficit hyperactivity disorder. *Behav Brain Res.* 2002;**130** (1–2):91–5.

142. Comings DE, Gade-Andavolu R, Gonzalez N, *et al.* Comparison of the role of dopamine, serotonin, and noradrenaline genes in ADHD, ODD and conduct disorder: multivariate regression analysis of 20 genes. *Clin Genet.* 2000;**57**(3):178–96.

143. de Krom M, Staal WG, Ophoff RA, *et al.* A common variant in DRD3 receptor is associated with autism spectrum disorder. *Biol Psychiatry.* 2009;**65**(7): 625–30.

144. Comings DE, Gonzalez NS, Cheng Li SC, MacMurray J. A "line item" approach to the identification of genes involved in polygenic behavioral disorders: the adrenergic alpha2A (ADRA2A) gene. *Am J Med Genet B Neuropsychiatr Genet.* 2003;**118B**(1):110–14.

145. Park L, Nigg JT, Waldman ID, Nummy KA, *et al.* Association and linkage of alpha-2A adrenergic receptor gene polymorphisms with childhood ADHD. *Mol Psychiatry.* 2005;**10**(6):572–80.

146. Roman T, Polanczyk GV, Zeni C, *et al.* Further evidence of the involvement of alpha-2A-adrenergic receptor gene (ADRA2A) in inattentive dimensional scores of attention-deficit/hyperactivity disorder. *Mol Psychiatry.* 2006;**11**(1):8–10.

147. Roman T, Schmitz M, Polanczyk GV, *et al.* Is the alpha-2A adrenergic receptor gene (ADRA2A) associated with attention-deficit/hyperactivity disorder? *Am J Med Genet B Neuropsychiatr Genet.* 2003;**120B**(1):116–20.

148. Deupree JD, Smith SD, Kratochvil CJ, *et al.* Possible involvement of alpha-2A adrenergic receptors in attention deficit hyperactivity disorder: radioligand binding and polymorphism studies. *Am J Med Genet B Neuropsychiatr Genet.* 2006;**141**(8):877–84.

149. Xu C, Schachar R, Tannock R, *et al.* Linkage study of the alpha2A adrenergic receptor in attention-deficit hyperactivity disorder families. *Am J Med Genet.* 2001;**105**(2):159–62.

150. Schmitz M, Denardin D, Silva TL, *et al.* Association between alpha-2a-adrenergic receptor gene and ADHD inattentive type. *Biol Psychiatry.* 2006;**60**(10): 1028–33.

151. Stevenson J, Asherson P, Hay D, *et al.* Characterizing the ADHD phenotype for genetic studies. *Dev Sci.* 2005;**8**(2):115–21.

152. Wang B, Wang Y, Zhou R, *et al.* Possible association of the alpha-2A adrenergic receptor gene (ADRA2A) with symptoms of attention-deficit/hyperactivity disorder. *Am J Med Genet B Neuropsychiatr Genet.* 2006;**141B**(2):130–4.

153. Waldman ID, Nigg JT, Gizer IR, *et al.* The adrenergic receptor alpha-2A gene (ADRA2A) and neuropsychological executive functions as putative endophenotypes for childhood ADHD. *Cogn Affect Behav Neurosci.* 2006;**6**(1):18–30.

154. Stevenson J, Langley K, Pay H, *et al.* Attention deficit disorder with reading disabilities: preliminary findings on the involvement of the *ADRA2A* gene. *J Child Psychol Psychiatry.* 2005;**46**:1081–8.

155. de Cerqueira C, Polina E, Contini V, *et al.* ADRA2A polymorphisms and ADHD in adults: possible mediating effect of personality. *Psychiatry Res.* 2010;**186**(2–3):345–50.

156. Comings D, Gade-Andavolu R, Gonzalez N, Blake H, MacMurray J. Additive effect of three noradenergic genes (ADRA2A, ADRA2C, DBH) on attention-deficit hyperactivity disorder and learning disabilities in Tourette syndrome subjects. *Clin Genet.* 1999;**55**(3): 160–72.

157. Barr CL, Wigg K, Zai G, *et al.* Attention-deficit hyperactivity disorder and the adrenergic receptors alpha1C and alpha2C. *Mol Psychiatry.* 2001;**6**(3): 334–7.

158. De Luca V, Muglia P, Vincent JB, *et al.* Adrenergic alpha 2C receptor genomic organization: association study in adult ADHD. *Am J Med Genet B Neuropsychiatr Genet.* 2004;**127B**(1):65–7.

159. Elia J, Capasso M, Zaheer Z, *et al.* Candidate gene analysis in an on-going genome-wide association study of attention-deficit hyperactivity disorder: suggestive association signals in ADRA1A. *Psychiatr Genet.* 2009;**19**(3):134–41.

160. Biederman J, Spencer T. Non-stimulant treatments for ADHD. *Eur Child Adolesc Psychiatry.* 2000;**9** (Suppl 1):I51–9.

161. Barr CL, Kroft J, Feng Y, *et al.* The norepinephrine transporter gene and attention-deficit hyperactivity disorder. *Am J Med Genet.* 2002;**114**(3):255–9.

162. McEvoy B, Hawi Z, Fitzgerald M, Gill M. No evidence of linkage or association between the norepinephrine transporter (NET) gene polymorphisms and ADHD in the Irish population. *Am J Med Genet.* 2002;**114**(6): 665–6.

163. Xu X, Knight J, Brookes K, *et al.* DNA pooling analysis of 21 norepinephrine transporter gene SNPs with

attention deficit hyperactivity disorder: no evidence for association. *Am J Med Genet B Neuropsychiatr Genet.* 2005;**134B**(1):115–18.

164. Kim CH, Hahn MK, Joung Y, *et al.* A polymorphism in the norepinephrine transporter gene alters promoter activity and is associated with attention-deficit hyperactivity disorder. *Proc Natl Acad Sci U S A.* 2006;**103**(50):19164–9.

165. Kim C, Waldman I, Blakely R, Kim K. Functional gene variation in the human norepinephrine transporter: association with attention deficit hyperactivity disorder. *Ann N Y Acad Sci.* 2008;**1129**:256–60.

166. Ramoz N, Boni C, Downing AM, *et al.* A haplotype of the norepinephrine transporter (Net) gene Slc6a2 is associated with clinical response to atomoxetine in attention-deficit hyperactivity disorder (ADHD). *Neuropsychopharmacology.* 2009;**34**(9):2135–42.

167. Cho SC, Kim HW, Kim BN, *et al.* Neurotrophin-3 gene, intelligence, and selective attention deficit in a Korean sample with attention-deficit/hyperactivity disorder. *Prog Neuropsychopharmacol Biol Psychiatry.* 2010;**34**(6):1065–9.

168. Maness LM, Kastin AJ, Weber JT, *et al.* The neurotrophins and their receptors: structure, function, and neuropathology. *Neurosci Biobehav Rev.* 1994;**18**:143–59.

169. Quist JF, Barr CL, Schachar R, *et al.* The serotonin 5-HT1B receptor gene and attention deficit hyperactivity disorder. *Mol Psychiatry.* 2003;**8**(1): 98–102.

170. Smoller JW, Biederman J, Arbeitman L, *et al.* Association between the 5HT1B receptor gene (HTR1B) and the inattentive subtype of ADHD. *Biol Psychiatry.* 2006;**59**(5):460–7.

171. Heiser P, Dempfle A, Friedel S, *et al.* Family-based association study of serotonergic candidate genes and attention-deficit/hyperactivity disorder in a German sample. *J Neural Transm.* 2007;**114**(4):513–21.

172. Hawi Z, Dring M, Kirley A, *et al.* Serotonergic system and attention deficit hyperactivity disorder (ADHD): a potential susceptibility locus at the 5-HT(1B) receptor gene in 273 nuclear families from a multi-centre sample. *Mol Psychiatry.* 2002;**7**(7):718–25.

173. Li J, Kang C, Wang Y, *et al.* Contribution of 5-HT2A receptor gene -1438A>G polymorphism to outcome of attention-deficit/hyperactivity disorder in adolescents. *Am J Med Genet B Neuropsychiatr Genet.* 2006;**141B**(5):473–6.

174. Guimaraes A, Schmitz M, Polanczyk G, *et al.* Further evidence for the association between attention deficit/hyperactivity disorder and the serotonin receptor 1B gene. *J Neural Transm.* 2009;**116**: 1675–80.

175. Levitan R, Masellis M, Basile V, *et al.* Polymorphism of the serotonin-2A receptor gene (HTR2A) associated with childhood attention deficit hyperactivity disorder (ADHD) in adult women with seasonal affective disorder. *J Affect Disord.* 2002;**71**(1–3):229–33.

176. Quist JF, Barr CL, Schachar R, *et al.* Evidence for the serotonin HTR2A receptor gene as a susceptibility factor in attention deficit hyperactivity disorder (ADHD). *Mol Psychiatry.* 2000;**5**(5):537–41.

177. Guimaraes AP, Zeni C, Polanczyk GV, *et al.* Serotonin genes and attention deficit/hyperactivity disorder in a Brazilian sample: Preferential transmission of the HTR2A 452His allele to affected boys. *Am J Med Genet B Neuropsychiatr Genet.* 2007;**144**(1):69–73.

178. Zoroglu SS, Erdal ME, Alasehirli B, *et al.* Significance of serotonin transporter gene 5-HTTLPR and variable number of tandem repeat polymorphism in attention deficit hyperactivity disorder. *Neuropsychobiology.* 2002;**45**(4):176–81.

179. Li J, Wang Y, Zhou R, *et al.* No association of attention-deficit/hyperactivity disorder with genes of the serotonergic pathway in Han Chinese subjects. *Neurosci Lett.* 2006;**403**(1–2):172–5.

180. Li J, Wang Y, Zhou R, *et al.* Association between polymorphisms in serotonin 2C receptor gene and attention-deficit/hyperactivity disorder in Han Chinese subjects. *Neurosci Lett.* 2006;**407**(2):107–11.

181. Li J, Wang Y, Zhou R, *et al.* Association of attention-deficit/hyperactivity disorder with serotonin 4 receptor gene polymorphisms in Han Chinese subjects. *Neurosci Lett.* 2006;**401**(1–2):6–9.

182. Li J, Zhang X, Wang Y, *et al.* The serotonin 5-HT1D receptor gene and attention-deficit hyperactivity disorder in Chinese Han subjects. *Am J Med Genet B Neuropsychiatr Genet.* 2006;**141B**(8):874–6.

183. Heck A, Lieb R, Ellgas A, *et al.* Investigation of 17 candidate genes for personality traits confirms effects of the HTR2A gene on novelty seeking. *Genes Brain Behav.* 2009;**8**(4):464–72.

184. Xu X, Brookes K, Sun B, Ilott N, Asherson P. Investigation of the serotonin 2C receptor gene in attention deficit hyperactivity disorder in UK samples. *BMC Res Notes.* 2009;**2**:71.

185. Anguelova M, Benkelfat C, Turecki G. A systematic review of association studies investigating genes coding for serotonin receptors and the serotonin transporter: I. Affective disorders. *Mol Psychiatry.* 2003;**8**(6):574–91.

186. Anguelova M, Benkelfat C, Turecki G. A systematic review of association studies investigating genes coding for serotonin receptors and the serotonin transporter: II. Suicidal behavior. *Mol Psychiatry.* 2003;**8**(7):646–53.

187. Curran S, Purcell S, Craig I, Asherson P, Sham P. The serotonin transporter gene as a QTL for ADHD. *Am J Med Genet B Neuropsychiatr Genet*. 2005;**134B**(1): 42–7.

188. Kim SJ, Badner J, Cheon KA, *et al.* Family-based association study of the serotonin transporter gene polymorphisms in Korean ADHD trios. *Am J Med Genet B Neuropsychiatr Genet*. 2005;**139**(1):14–18.

189. Xu X, Mill J, Chen CK, *et al.* Family-based association study of serotonin transporter gene polymorphisms in attention deficit hyperactivity disorder: no evidence for association in UK and Taiwanese samples. *Am J Med Genet B Neuropsychiatr Genet*. 2005;**139**(1):11–13.

190. Xu M, Hu XT, Cooper DC, *et al.* Elimination of cocaine-induced hyperactivity and dopamine-mediated neurophysiological effects in dopamine D1 receptor mutant mice [see comments]. *Cell*. 1994; **79**(6):945–55.

191. Banerjee E, Sinha S, Chatterjee A, *et al.* A family-based study of Indian subjects from Kolkata reveals allelic association of the serotonin transporter intron-2 (STin2) polymorphism and attention-deficit-hyperactivity disorder (ADHD). *Am J Med Genet B Neuropsychiatr Genet*. 2006;**141**(4):361–6.

192. Wigg KG, Takhar A, Ickowicz A, *et al.* Gene for the serotonin transporter and ADHD: no association with two functional polymorphisms. *Am J Med Genet B Neuropsychiatr Genet*. 2006;**141B**(6):566–70.

193. Li J, Wang Y, Zhou R, *et al.* Association between polymorphisms in serotonin transporter gene and attention deficit hyperactivity disorder in Chinese Han subjects. *Am J Med Genet B Neuropsychiatr Genet*. 2007;**144**(1):14–19.

194. Banerjee E, Sinha S, Chatterjee A, Nandagopal K. No causal role for the G482T and G689T polymorphisms in translation regulation of serotonin transporter (SLC6A4) or association with attention-deficit-hyperactivity disorder (ADHD). *Neurosci Lett*. 2009;**454**(3):244–8.

195. Retz W, Rosler M. The relation of ADHD and violent aggression: what can we learn from epidemiological and genetic studies? *Int J Law Psychiatry*. 2009; **32**(4):235–43.

196. Nikolas M, Friderici K, Waldman I, Jernigan K, Nigg JT. Gene x environment interactions for ADHD: synergistic effect of 5HTTLPR genotype and youth appraisals of inter-parental conflict. *Behav Brain Funct*. 2010;**6**:23.

197. Li J, Wang Y, Zhou R, *et al.* Association between tryptophan hydroxylase gene polymorphisms and attention deficit hyperactivity disorder in Chinese Han population. *Am J Med Genet B Neuropsychiatr Genet*. 2006;**141B**:126–9.

198. Tang G, Ren D, Xin R, *et al.* Lack of association between the tryptophan hydroxylase gene A218C polymorphism and attention-deficit hyperactivity disorder in Chinese Han population. *Am J Med Genet*. 2001;**105**(6):485–8.

199. Walitza S, Renner TJ, Dempfle A, *et al.* Transmission disequilibrium of polymorphic variants in the tryptophan hydroxylase-2 gene in attention-deficit/hyperactivity disorder. *Mol Psychiatry*. 2005;**10**(12):1126–32.

200. Baehne CG, Ehlis AC, Plichta MM, *et al.* Tph2 gene variants modulate response control processes in adult ADHD patients and healthy individuals. *Mol Psychiatry*. 2009;**14**(11):1032–9.

201. Sheehan K, Lowe N, Kirley A, *et al.* Tryptophan hydroxylase 2 (TPH2) gene variants associated with ADHD. *Mol Psychiatry*. 2005;**10**(10):944–9.

202. Sheehan K, Hawi Z, Gill M, Kent L. No association between TPH2 gene polymorphisms and ADHD in a UK sample. *Neurosci Lett*. 2007;**412**(2):105–7.

203. Johansson S, Halmoy A, Mavroconstanti T, *et al.* Common variants in the TPH1 and TPH2 regions are not associated with persistent ADHD in a combined sample of 1,636 adult cases and 1,923 controls from four European populations. *Am J Med Genet B Neuropsychiatr Genet*. 2010;**153B**:1008–15.

204. Wilson MC. Coloboma mouse mutant as an animal model of hyperkinesis and attention deficit hyperactivity disorder. *Neurosci Biobehav Rev*. 2000;**24**(1):51–7.

205. Sagvolden T, Johansen E, Woien G, *et al.* The spontaneously hypertensive rat model of ADHD – the importance of selecting the appropriate reference strain. *Neuropharmacology*. 2009;**57**(7–8):619–26.

206. Li Q, Wong JH, Lu G, *et al.* Gene expression of synaptosomal-associated protein 25 (SNAP-25) in the prefrontal cortex of the spontaneously hypertensive rat (SHR). *Biochim Biophys Acta*. 2009;**1792**(8): 766–76.

207. Barr CL, Feng Y, Wigg K, *et al.* Identification of DNA variants in the SNAP-25 gene and linkage study of these polymorphisms and attention-deficit hyperactivity disorder. *Mol Psychiatry*. 2000;**5**(4): 405–9.

208. Brophy K, Hawi Z, Kirley A, Fitzgerald M, Gill M. Synaptosomal-associated protein 25 (SNAP-25) and attention deficit hyperactivity disorder (ADHD): evidence of linkage and association in the Irish population. *Mol Psychiatry*. 2002;**7**(8):913–17.

209. Kustanovich V, Merriman B, McGough J, *et al.* Biased paternal transmission of SNAP-25 risk alleles in attention-deficit hyperactivity disorder. *Mol Psychiatry*. 2003;**8**(3):309–15.

210. Mill J, Curran S, Kent L, *et al.* Association study of a SNAP-25 microsatellite and attention deficit hyperactivity disorder. *Am J Med Genet.* 2002;**114**(3): 269–71.

211. Mill J, Richards S, Knight J, *et al.* Haplotype analysis of SNAP-25 suggests a role in the aetiology of ADHD. *Mol Psychiatry.* 2004;**9**(8):801–10.

212. Feng Y, Crosbie J, Wigg K, *et al.* The SNAP25 gene as a susceptibility gene contributing to attention-deficit hyperactivity disorder. *Mol Psychiatry.* 2005;**10**(11): 998–1005, 973.

213. Kim JW, Biederman J, Arbeitman L, *et al.* Investigation of variation in SNAP-25 and ADHD and relationship to co-morbid major depressive disorder. *Am J Med Genet B Neuropsychiatr Genet.* 2007;**144B**(6): 781–90.

214. Comings DE, Gade-Andavolu R, Gonzalez N, *et al.* Multivariate analysis of associations of 42 genes in ADHD, ODD and conduct disorder. *Clin Genet.* 2000;**58**(1):31–40.

215. Todd RD, Lobos EA, Sun LW, Neuman RJ. Mutational analysis of the nicotinic acetylcholine receptor alpha 4 subunit gene in attention deficit/hyperactivity disorder: evidence for association of an intronic polymorphism with attention problems. *Mol Psychiatry.* 2003;**8**(1):103–8.

216. Kent L, Middle F, Hawi Z, *et al.* Nicotinic acetylcholine receptor alpha4 subunit gene polymorphism and attention deficit hyperactivity disorder. *Psychiatr Genet.* 2001;**11**(1):37–40.

217. Lee J, Laurin N, Crosbie J, *et al.* Association study of the nicotinic acetylcholine receptor alpha4 subunit gene, CHRNA4, in attention-deficit hyperactivity disorder. *Genes Brain Behav.* 2007;**7**(1):53–60.

218. Greenwood PM, Sundararajan R, Lin MK, *et al.* Both a nicotinic single nucleotide polymorphism (SNP) and a noradrenergic SNP modulate working memory performance when attention is manipulated. *J Cogn Neurosci.* 2009;**21**(11):2139–53.

219. Kent L, Green E, Holmes J, *et al.* No association between CHRNA7 microsatellite markers and attention-deficit hyperactivity disorder. *Am J Med Genet.* 2001;**105**(8):686–9.

220. Turic D, Langley K, Mills S, *et al.* Follow-up of genetic linkage findings on chromosome 16p13: evidence of association of N-methyl-D aspartate glutamate receptor 2A gene polymorphism with ADHD. *Mol Psychiatry.* 2004;**9**(2):169–73.

221. Adams J, Crosbie J, Wigg K, *et al.* Glutamate receptor, ionotropic, N-methyl D-aspartate 2A (GRIN2A) gene as a positional candidate for attention-deficit/hyperactivity disorder in the 16p13 region. *Mol Psychiatry.* 2004;**9**(5):494–9.

222. Egan MF, Kojima M, Callicott JH, *et al.* The BDNF val66met polymorphism affects activity-dependent secretion of BDNF and human memory and hippocampal function. *Cell.* 2003;**112**(2):257–69.

223. Kent L, Green E, Hawi Z, *et al.* Association of the paternally transmitted copy of common Valine allele of the Val66Met polymorphism of the brain-derived neurotrophic factor (BDNF) gene with susceptibility to ADHD. *Mol Psychiatry.* 2005;**10**(10): 939–43.

224. Xu X, Mill J, Zhou K, *et al.* Family-based association study between brain-derived neurotrophic factor gene polymorphisms and attention deficit hyperactivity disorder in UK and Taiwanese samples. *Am J Med Genet B Neuropsychiatr Genet.* 2007;**144**(1):83–6.

225. Lasky-Su J, Faraone SV, Lange C, *et al.* A study of how socioeconomic status moderates the relationship between SNPs encompassing BDNF and ADHD symptom counts in ADHD families. *Behav Genet.* 2007;**37**:487–97.

226. Reif A, Jacob CP, Rujescu D, *et al.* Influence of functional variant of neuronal nitric oxide synthase on impulsive behaviors in humans. *Arch Gen Psychiatry.* 2009;**66**(1):41–50.

227. Laas K, Reif A, Herterich S, *et al.* The effect of a functional NOS1 promoter polymorphism on impulsivity is moderated by platelet MAO activity. *Psychopharmacology (Berl).* 2010;**209**(3):255–61.

228. Fisher A, Stewart R, Yan T, Hunt S, Stanford S. Disruption of noradrenergic transmission and the behavioural response to a novel environment in NK1R -/- mice. *Eur J Neurosci.* 2007;**25**:1195–204.

229. Yan T, McQuillin A, Thapar A, *et al.* NK1 (TACR1) receptor gene 'knockout' mouse phenotype predicts genetic aassociation with ADHD. *J Psychopharmacol.* 2010;**24**(1):27–38.

230. Lasky-Su J, Anney RJ, Neale BM, *et al.* Genome-wide association scan of the time to onset of attention deficit hyperactivity disorder. *Am J Med Genet B Neuropsychiatr Genet.* 2008;**147B**(8):1355–8.

231. Lasky-Su J, Neale BM, Franke B, *et al.* Genome-wide association scan of quantitative traits for attention deficit hyperactivity disorder identifies novel associations and confirms candidate gene associations. *Am J Med Genet B Neuropsychiatr Genet.* 2008;**147B** (8):1345–54.

232. Neale BM, Lasky-Su J, Anney R, *et al.* Genome-wide association scan of attention deficit hyperactivity disorder. *Am J Med Genet B Neuropsychiatr Genet.* 2008;**147B**(8):1337–44.

233. Lesch KP, Timmesfeld N, Renner TJ, *et al.* Molecular genetics of adult ADHD: converging evidence from genome-wide association and extended pedigree

linkage studies. *J Neural Transm.* 2008;**115**(11): 1573–85.

234. Neale BM, Medland S, Ripke S, *et al.* Case-control genome-wide association study of attention-deficit/ hyperactivity disorder. *J Am Acad Child Adolesc Psychiatry.* 2010;**49**(9):906–20.

235. Mick E, Todorov A, Smalley S, *et al.* Family-based genome-wide association scan of attention-deficit/ hyperactivity disorder. *J Am Acad Child Adolesc Psychiatry.* 2010;**49**(9):898–905.e3.

236. Banerjee TD, Middleton F, Faraone SV. Environmental risk factors for attention-deficit hyperactivity disorder. *Acta Paediatr.* 2007;**96**(9): 1269–74.

237. Kim H, Cho S, Kim B, *et al.* Perinatal and familial risk factors are associated with full syndrome and subthreshold attention-deficit hyperactivity disorder in a Korean community sample. *Psychiatry Investig.* 2009;**6**(4):278–85.

238. Frisell T, Lichtenstein P, Rahman Q, Langstrom N. Psychiatric morbidity associated with same-sex sexual behaviour: influence of minority stress and familial factors. *Psychol Med.* 2010;**40**:315–24.

239. Wermter AK, Laucht M, Schimmelmann BG, *et al.* From nature versus nurture, via nature and nurture, to gene x environment interaction in mental disorders. *Eur Child Adolesc Psychiatry.* 2010;**19**(3):199–210.

240. Waldman ID. Gene-environment interactions reexamined: does mother's marital stability interact with the dopamine receptor D2 gene in the etiology of childhood attention-deficit/hyperactivity disorder? *Dev Psychopathol.* 2007;**19**(4):1117–28.

241. Ficks C, Waldman I. Gene-environment interactions in attention-deficit/hyperactivity disorder. *Curr Psychiatry Rep.* 2009;**11**:387–92.

242. Altink M, Arias-Vasquez A, Franke B, *et al.* The dopamine receptor D4 7-repeat allele and prenatal smoking in ADHD-affected children and their unaffected siblings: no gene-environment interaction. *J Child Psychol Psychiatry.* 2008;**49**:1053–60.

243. Plomp E, Van Engeland H, Durston S. Understanding genes, environment and their interaction in attention-deficit hyperactivity disorder: is there a role for neuroimaging? *Neuroscience.* 2009;**164**(1): 230–40.

244. Smith AK, Mick E, Faraone SV. Advances in genetic studies of attention-deficit/hyperactivity disorder. *Curr Psychiatry Rep.* 2009;**11**(2):143–8.

245. Pennington BF, McGrath LM, Rosenberg J, *et al.* Gene x environment interactions in reading disability and attention-deficit/hyperactivity disorder. *Dev Psychol.* 2009;**45**(1):77–89.

246. Steinhausen HC. The heterogeneity of causes and courses of attention-deficit/hyperactivity disorder. *Acta Psychiatr Scand.* 2009;**120**(5):392–9.

247. Schalkwyk L, Meaburn E, Smith R, *et al.* Allelic skewing of DNA methylation is widespread across the genome. *Am J Hum Genet.* 2010;**86**: 196–212.

248. Hawi Z, Segurado R, Conroy J, *et al.* Preferential transmission of paternal alleles at risk genes in attention-deficit/hyperactivity disorder. *Am J Hum Genet.* 2005;**77**(6):958–65.

249. Hawi Z, Kent L, Hill M, *et al.* ADHD and DAT1: Further evidence of paternal over-transmission of risk alleles and haplotype. *Am J Med Genet B Neuropsychiatr Genet.* 2010;**153**:97–102.

250. Kim JW, Waldman ID, Faraone SV, *et al.* Investigation of parent-of-origin effects in ADHD candidate genes. *Am J Med Genet B Neuropsychiatr Genet.* 2007;**144**(6): 776–80.

251. Orrico A, Galli L, Buoni S, *et al.* Attention-deficit/ hyperactivity disorder (ADHD) and variable clinical expression of Aarskog-Scott syndrome due to a novel FGD1 gene mutation (R408Q). *Am J Med Genet A.* 2005;**135**(1):99–102.

252. de Silva MG, Elliott K, Dahl HH, *et al.* Disruption of a novel member of a sodium/hydrogen exchanger family and DOCK3 is associated with an attention deficit hyperactivity disorder-like phenotype. *J Med Genet.* 2003;**40**(10):733–40.

253. Markunas CA, Quinn KS, Collins AL, *et al.* Genetic variants in SLC9A9 are associated with measures of attention-deficit/hyperactivity disorder symptoms in families. *Psychiatr Genet.* 2010;**20**(2):73–81.

254. Elia J, Glessner JT, Wang K, *et al.* Genome-wide copy number variation study associates metabotropic glutamate receptor gene networks with attention deficit hyperactivity disorder. *Nat Genet.* 2011;**44**(1): 78–84.

255. Lesch K-P, Selch S, Renner T, *et al.* Genome-wide copy number variation analysis in attention-deficit/ hyperactivity disorder: association with neuropeptide Y gene dosage in an extended pedigree. *Mol Psychiatry.* 2011;**16**(5):491–503.

256. Williams N, Zaharieva I, Martin A, *et al.* Rare chromosomal deletions and duplications in attention-deficit hyperactivity disorder: a genome-wide analysis. *Lancet.* 2010;**376**(9750): 1401–8.

257. Doyle AE, Willcutt EG, Seidman LJ, *et al.* Attention-deficit/hyperactivity disorder endophenotypes. *Biol Psychiatry.* 2005;**57**(11): 1324–35.

258. Rommelse NN, Arias-Vasquez A, Altink ME, *et al.* Neuropsychological endophenotype approach to genome-wide linkage analysis identifies susceptibility loci for ADHD on 2q21.1 and 13q12.11. *Am J Hum Genet.* 2008;**83**(1):99–105.

259. Wood AC, Neale MC. Twin studies and their implications for molecular genetic studies: endophenotypes integrate quantitative and molecular genetics in ADHD research. *J Am Acad Child Adolesc Psychiatry.* 2010;**49**(9):874–83.

260. Wood AC, Asherson P, van der Meere JJ, Kuntsi J. Separation of genetic influences on attention deficit hyperactivity disorder symptoms and reaction time performance from those on IQ. *Psychol Med.* 2010;**40**(6):1027–37.

Neuroimaging of ADHD

Jesse M. Jun and F. Xavier Castellanos

Introduction

Neuroimaging of attention-deficit hyperactivity disorder (ADHD) involves the application of increasingly sophisticated approaches to an intermittently moving target. The first imaging studies, which are reviewed elsewhere [1], used computed-axial tomography even before the diagnosis of attention deficit disorders with or without hyperactivity had been formulated in 1980 and did not detect differences when applied quantitatively [2]. The second generation of imaging studies harnessing positron emission tomography methods first detected substantial differences between individuals with ADHD and healthy controls [3], but the use of injected radioligands meant that this approach was mostly limited to studies of adults [1] with rare exceptions [4].

The widespread availability of high-resolution three-dimensional magnetic resonance imaging (MRI) by the early 1990s revolutionized ADHD structural imaging, as the technique could be applied to children and adolescents without entailing risks greater than those encountered in daily life. The designation as a minimal risk procedure was particularly important for the inclusion of healthy children as comparison subjects and for the conduct of longitudinal studies. The resulting profusion of investigations has become too voluminous to even enumerate. For example a PubMed search on March 16, 2013 with the abbreviated search terms MRI and ADHD returned 846 results.

Fortunately, much of the ADHD neuroimaging literature has been condensed through systematic meta-analyses [5–11]. These abbreviate the process of evaluating the growing literature, and also can provide deeper insights than may be available when individual findings are considered in isolation. After all,

quantitative spatial meta-analyses are optimized for neuroimaging. Valid findings are most likely to emerge repeatedly in similar locations in standardized brain space, whereas spurious or false-positive results are less likely to converge [12]. Accordingly, we will focus on the major meta-analyses that have recently examined brain imaging studies related to ADHD. We begin with structural studies, whether focusing on gray or white matter, followed by syntheses of task-based functional MRI (fMRI) investigations. We also briefly review resting-state imaging using fMRI (R-fMRI), as this approach is rapidly gaining adherents among investigators who are developing novel methods of pursuing open science approaches that will likely advance the field in the coming decade.

Structural MRI studies of ADHD

Volumetric (morphometric) studies

Although MRI data are always acquired slice-by-slice, the improvements in spatial resolution afforded by the refinement of scanning at 1.5 Tesla, and subsequently at 3.0 Tesla, made it possible to obtain sufficiently thin slices that could be convincingly concatenated into three-dimensional virtual structures *in silico*. Once acquired digitally, the same high-resolution T1-weighted structural image data can be used as the raw material for studies. Importantly, there is no upper limit on how many times imaging data can be queried with scientifically distinct questions.

Typical MRI images quantify a physical property referred to as T1 relaxation, and are described as T1-weighted. T1-weighted images depict cerebrospinal fluid (CSF) as black, white matter as nearly white, and gray matter in various shades of gray. The most straightforward manner of quantifying T1 images is to

Attention-Deficit Hyperactivity Disorder in Adults and Children, ed. Lenard A. Adler, Thomas J. Spencer and Timothy E. Wilens.
Published by Cambridge University Press. © Cambridge University Press 2015.

draw boundaries around the margins of a structure of interest on a slice-by-slice basis. Software then calculates the area inside the perimeter, which is multiplied by the thickness of the slice (generally about 1 mm). Then the value for each bounded figure within the structure is added to equal an estimate of the total volume. Such hand-tracing of brain structures has been performed since the early days of the field, and is still performed, particularly for structures with complex geometries, such as the hippocampus or amygdala. Hand-tracing by a trained anatomist represents the gold standard in anatomical volumetric quantification, but maintaining reliability of hand-traced measurements, both intra-rater and inter-rater, is always a challenge. This is because humans cannot be prevented from learning. As raters become increasingly proficient, they become more sensitive, increasingly contributing a-priori knowledge of the latent geometry of the structure, to the information displayed on the screen. While this arguably results in even more valid results, the implicitly changing criteria are problematic.

Rater-drift effects can be handled by counter-balancing groups and blinding raters in cross-sectional studies. In longitudinal studies, rater drift is particularly pernicious, as all images must be re-measured contemporaneously, and counter-balanced not only by group but also by study phase. New measurements of previously collected data are rarely identical to previously published values, which raises questions investigators would prefer to ignore. One alternative is to adopt fully algorithmic procedures which have theoretically perfect intra-rater reliability [13]. In other words, the same image will yield exactly the same values when processed by the same algorithm. The trade-off is in validity. Computer algorithms can be prevented from learning, and they will apply the programmed rules no matter the consequences. Sometimes this results in grossly abnormal or impossible values, which requires that investigators view the derived images, to ascertain that such errors are excluded from further analyses.

Meta-analyses of structural imaging in ADHD

Region-of-interest quantification

The first meta-analysis of anatomical findings in ADHD grappled with the diversity of approaches manifest in the extant literature at the time [6]. Valera

and colleagues cataloged 21 reports of structural results published by 15 groups of investigators. They computed standardized mean differences (SMD) between ADHD and healthy controls and found significant differences in several regions. The largest differences were observed in the posterior inferior cerebellar vermis, i.e., lobules VIII–X (SMD = 0.77), cerebellar vermis in general (SMD = 0.67), splenium of the corpus callosum (SMD = 0.59), total cerebral volume (SMD = 0.50), cerebellum (SMD ∼ 0.45), and right caudate nucleus (SMD = 0.34). Comparable results for caudate volume were obtained by Frodl and Skokauskas [9] who reported 8% smaller right caudate (SMD = 0.57) and 7% smaller left caudate volume (SMD = 0.50) in seven studies including 218 children with ADHD and 228 controls that largely overlapped with those summarized earlier by Valera et al. [6]. The proportion of patients in a given study who had been treated with stimulants was associated with decreasing between-group differences in both right and left caudate volumes, suggesting normalization with treatment, at least in terms of caudate volumes [9].

Besides the corpus callosum mid-sagittal area, the caudate is the easiest cerebral structure to trace manually. When cortical regions are quantified, Valera et al. noted the difficulty in combining values from studies with vastly different approaches to volumetric quantification, as some used anatomical boundaries and others adopted arbitrary planes to segment the cortex [6]. This difficulty has been circumvented by the subsequent adoption of fully automated and unbiased voxel-based morphometry.

Voxel-based morphometry

Total cerebral volume

Nakao et al. conducted a meta-analysis of voxel-based morphometry (VBM) studies of ADHD across both children and adults [7]. They first examined seven datasets comprising 191 patients with ADHD and 179 healthy controls. Patients with ADHD (mostly children, as only one study was of adults) were found to have significantly smaller global gray matter volumes than controls (SMD = 0.28). An earlier meta-analysis (published in Spanish) of eight studies reporting total cerebral volume included 250 patients with ADHD and 253 controls [14]. Castellanos and Acosta found SMD = 0.42 for total cerebral volume or its equivalent, which corresponded to an average volumetric reduction of 2.7% [14]. Castellanos and Acosta noted that such a small-to-medium between-group effect size would be expected to reach statistical significance only in substantially sized samples. For example, attaining 80% power for a two-tailed alpha level of 0.05 and a SMD = 0.42 requires samples containing at least 85 individuals per group [15]. Nevertheless, global differences in brain volume are consistently noted in volumetric studies of ADHD and they may represent an important clue pointing to factors that affect overall brain development [16, 17].

Regional differences in gray matter volumes

Nakao *et al.* identified 14 independent datasets reporting unbiased VBM results, based on 270 patients with ADHD and 378 controls [7]. In contrast to region-of-interest studies, which necessarily determine the locations to be quantified, VBM studies do not constrain the location of potential between-group differences. This unbiased property is a requirement for quantitative meta-analysis [12]. Nakao *et al.* found that patients with ADHD had significantly smaller gray matter volumes in a large cluster centered in the right lentiform nucleus (which comprises the putamen and globus pallidus) extending into the caudate nucleus and also into the thalamus and claustrum, all on the right [7]. Significantly larger gray matter volumes were found in a relatively small cluster in the left posterior cingulate cortex/precuneus. Additionally, these investigators examined the effects of age and stimulant medication on gray matter volume: age was significantly correlated with gray matter volume in the right putamen, while percentage of patients on stimulant medication was correlated with gray matter volume in the right caudate. These authors concluded that the accumulating evidence highlighted decreased volumes in the right basal ganglia, with a suggestion of increased volume in the posterior cingulate cortex/precuneus. The age and medication effects were interpreted as evidence for normalization with increased age in the putamen; they suggested that medication treatment may normalize right caudate volumes [12]. The authors acknowledged that these hypotheses can only be truly tested in longitudinal within-subject investigations. These are essentially impossible in humans, as they would require randomly assigning children to treatment or placebo for extensive periods. It is instructive that a carefully conducted study of chronic methylphenidate dosing in young non-human primates failed to find any evidence of toxic or enduring effects [18].

In another meta-analysis of VBM studies published at about the same time with largely overlapping studies, Frodl and Skokauskas examined 11 studies which included 320 patients with ADHD and 288 controls. Four of the studies focused on adults; the remainder on children [9]. Results differed by age. Children with ADHD had significantly decreased volumes in the right putamen and the right globus pallidus. When the proportion of treated individuals was used as a covariate of interest, significant differences were also found in the right anterior cingulate cortex (ACC), as untreated children were more likely to demonstrate abnormal ACC gray matter volumes. We presume the abnormality was a decrease in volume, although the authors did not specify the direction of the difference. Additionally, the proportion of treated children with ADHD was inversely associated with volumes of the left amygdala/uncus. Age and sex did not interact with group differences [9].

In the four studies limited to adults with ADHD, gray matter volumes were decreased in the left and right ACC. Despite the small number of studies, the proportion of treated patients once again was associated with differential effects. Between-group differences in both left and right ACC were larger in studies with greater proportions of medication-naïve patients. Also unspecified were the directions of age and sex effects, which were reported to be significantly associated with changes in both left and right ACC [9].

Diffusion-weighted imaging

While standard T1-weighted methods can be used to differentiate gray from white matter, they do not lend themselves well to regional quantification of white matter. The emergence of diffusion-based methods has produced a rich profusion of methods which provide insights into white matter ultrastructure. The most commonly used approach, diffusion-tensor imaging (DTI), quantifies the net distances traveled by water molecules undergoing Brownian motion during brief intervals. The diffusion of water molecules is unconstrained in CSF, so the path of potential diffusion is termed isotropic, i.e., equal in all directions. Deviations from isotropy are termed anisotropies. Water molecules diffusing within well-myelinated white matter tracts diffuse most easily along the long axis of the tract, and their potential trajectories describe an elongated ellipsoid with its long axis parallel to that of the tract. The theoretical maximum of such an ellipsoid would describe a linear path, and would have a maximal value of fractional anisotropy (FA) of 1.0. FA in CSF can be as low as 0; most white matter regions in brain have FA values exceeding 0.2.

FA values have been examined across the lifespan and in a range of neuropsychiatric conditions. Based on the expectation that myelination is a process that increases with age over the first decades of life, increased FA with increasing age has been interpreted as evidence of greater "white matter integrity" [19]. However, such interpretation is grossly incorrect, as there are many reasons why FA can vary in various brain regions, including most commonly when white matter fiber tracts cross, which is common [19]. Further, because diffusion-weighted data can be represented spatially in terms of differentially oriented ellipsoids, investigators can construct images that appear to recapitulate white matter fiber tracts, described as "tractography." Tractography images can be compelling, as they appear to precisely parallel the results of post-mortem dissections of major white matter tracts. At the same time, current generation DTI datasets are wholly inadequate to provide spatially accurate representations of white matter tracts for many reasons, including the still inadequate spatial resolution of even the best DTI data acquisition sequences [19]. Thus tractography is best considered a suggestive, quasi-quantitative process.

Despite these caveats, DTI and other diffusion-based methods represent an important advance over standard T1-weighted anatomical imaging. To address their shortcomings, investigators are increasingly limiting their examinations of FA to the central skeleton of major white matter tracts by using tract-based spatial statistics (TBSS) [20]. This approach removes from consideration all voxels except those lying on the predetermined network of linear tracts which has been incorporated into the Oxford Centre for Functional Magnetic Resonance Imaging of the Brain (FMRIB) Software Library (FSL), thus obviating difficulties inherent in determining the breadth or width of particular white matter tracts. Once co-located on the same linear structure, the FA values for groups of individuals can be easily submitted to statistical inferential testing, with correction for multiple comparisons, thus yielding regions of reliable between-group differences. This is the approach that has become most widely used in DTI studies of ADHD.

Meta-analysis of diffusion-tensor imaging studies

Van Ewijk *et al.* conducted the first meta-analysis of DTI studies in ADHD [10], while also summarizing region-of-interest and voxel-based whole-brain analyses. Their review culminated with an activation-likelihood estimation (ALE) meta-analysis of nine voxel-based analyses, which included 173 patients with ADHD and 169 healthy controls [10]. In ALE, significant peak coordinates from specific studies are converted into three-dimensional Gaussian probability distributions which are then overlaid on brain standard space. The likelihood that the convergence of significant foci across multiple studies exceeds what would be expected by chance is computed through permutation analysis [8]. In ADHD, ALE analysis revealed five significant clusters in the right forceps minor, right anterior corona radiata, left and right internal capsule, and left cerebellum [10]. However, only four of nine studies contributed to these findings, based on 69 children or adolescents with ADHD and 81 controls. Confusingly, the ALE abnormalities associated with ADHD were mixed; some clusters exhibited increased FA and others decreased FA, although the authors of the meta-analysis did not provide details. Examination of the original papers shows that increases [21, 22] and decreases [23, 24] in FA were reported by two papers each. These four studies had small to moderate sample sizes, ranging from 14 to 26 per group. The most reasonable conclusion is that no firm conclusions can be reached at this time, as a surfeit of underpowered studies predicts that most published findings will fail to replicate once tested in sufficiently powered designs [25]. Fortunately, many groups of investigators are actively collecting diffusion-weighted imaging data in ADHD, and this situation should resolve in time.

Task-based functional MRI studies of ADHD

In contrast to structural studies, which can provide high-resolution information regarding gray and white matter structure, fMRI studies open a window into brain functioning, typically through fluctuations in blood oxygen level-dependent (BOLD) signals which are quantified at approximately two-second intervals throughout the brain. The BOLD technique depends on the differences in magnetic properties of hemoglobin, depending on whether it is fully oxygenated (and thus magnetically inert) or partially deoxygenated, as in venous blood, and thus magnetically disruptive. Remarkably, modern MRI scanners using echo-planar imaging (EPI) approaches can detect the infinitesimal differences in BOLD signal reflecting the interplay between hemoglobin flowing through the brain and the magnetic fields induced by the scanner. The trade-off for obtaining so much information is a reduction in spatial resolution. While typical T1-weighted high-resolution structural images provide data on voxels in the range of 1 mm^3 (1 mm $\times$ 1 mm $\times$ 1 mm), most fMRI studies use voxels that are 3 mm $\times$ 3 mm $\times$ 3 mm (i.e., 27 mm^3) every 2 or 2.5 seconds. Beyond the dramatic loss of spatial resolution, EPI is also particularly susceptible to spatial distortions at interfaces between air and brain tissues, such as near the sinuses. This susceptibility artifact makes it difficult to image some of the most psychiatrically interesting brain regions, such as orbitofrontal cortex, medial temporal lobes or temporal poles.

Despite these limitations, fMRI is a remarkably informative technique, particularly for advancing cognitive neuroscience [26]. Sophisticated task designs can be used to examine differences in BOLD patterns between two conditions, which are designed to only differ by the factor of interest. Statistically significant differences in BOLD signal are interpreted as evidence that the implicated region is differentially involved more or less in one of the task conditions. Studies using fMRI designs with patients tend to be briefer than those focusing on cognitive neuroscience questions targeting only healthy volunteers. In ADHD, the preponderance of fMRI studies has examined various aspects of inhibition, although tasks addressing attention/vigilance, and working memory have also been studied.

Meta-analyses of functional imaging in ADHD

The first ALE meta-analysis of fMRI studies in ADHD, conducted in 2006 [5], was based on 16 neuroimaging studies that provided activation results for ADHD and control samples separately. Despite relatively primitive methodology, this meta-analysis detected widespread evidence of frontal hypoactivation in ADHD, extending across the anterior cingulate cortex, dorsolateral prefrontal cortex, inferior prefrontal and orbitofrontal cortex, as well as parietal cortex and basal ganglia [5].

Towards systems neuroscience of ADHD

An updated search was conducted by Cortese *et al.* covering from 2005 through June 30, 2011. They identified 55 fMRI studies (16 in adults, 39 in children), based on 741 subjects with ADHD and 801 controls [8]. An updated version of ALE known as GingerALE (version 2.1.1, www.brainmap.org/ale/) was used to examine between-group differences in activation across a wide range of tasks, in children and adults separately, and in a combined, omnibus meta-analysis. Beyond diagnostic group differences, Cortese *et al.* also probed the effects of stimulant medication, psychiatric comorbidities, and various task types in secondary meta-analyses.

In children with ADHD compared to controls, significant hypoactivation was found in frontal regions and putamen bilaterally and in right parietal and right temporal regions. Significant hyperactivation was found in the right angular gyrus, middle occipital gyrus, posterior cingulate cortex, and midcingulate cortex.

In adults with ADHD compared to controls, significant hypoactivation was found in the right central sulcus, precentral gyrus, and middle frontal gyrus. Significant hyperactivation was found in the right angular and middle occipital gyri.

In a secondary analysis which contrasted only stimulant-naïve ADHD subjects compared to controls, significant hypoactivation was observed in several frontal regions bilaterally, the right superior temporal gyrus, right posterior cingulate cortex, right postcentral gyrus, putamen bilaterally, and right thalamus. Significant hyperactivation was observed in only one cluster, in the right superior longitudinal fasciculus underlying the insula.

In a meta-analysis limited to studies of comorbidity-free ADHD subjects compared to controls, significant hypoactivation was observed in frontal regions and putamen bilaterally, right superior temporal gyrus, and right occipital pole. Significant hyperactivation was observed in the left inferior frontal gyrus, left Heschl's gyrus, and several right posterior regions.

Separate GingerALE meta-analyses were conducted for three task modalities: inhibition, working memory, and vigilance/attention. In the meta-analysis of inhibition tasks, significant hypoactivation was observed in several frontal regions bilaterally as well as in the right superior temporal gyrus, left inferior occipital gyrus, right thalamus, and midbrain;

significant hyperactivation was observed in deep right parieto-occipital cortex and right intermediate frontal sulcus. In working memory tasks, significant hypoactivation was observed in the left inferior frontal gyrus and anterior insula and in the right middle frontal gyrus. In vigilance/attention tasks, significant hypoactivation was observed in the right paracingulate gyrus.

Rather than simply enumerating the implicated regions, Cortese et al. [8] related their findings to seven reference neuronal networks defined robustly on the basis of data-driven analyses of 1000 participants undergoing R-fMRI studies [27]. The seven networks were visual, somatomotor, dorsal attention, ventral attention, limbic, frontoparietal, and default [27].

The default network has become a focus of interest across many psychiatric diagnoses, including ADHD. Specifically, based on repeated observations of inconsistent performance across both clinical and neuropsychological contexts, Castellanos and Tannock highlighted increased intra-subject variability as a potential endophenotype in ADHD [28]. Increased intra-subject variability [29] was hypothesized to reflect lapses of attention that are produced by dysregulated interactions between the default network and top-down control networks, particularly the dorsal attention network and the frontoparietal network [30, 31].

In the Cortese et al. meta-analysis limited to studies of children, significant ADHD-related hypoactivation was predominantly observed in the ventral attention (44%) and frontoparietal (39%) networks, while hyperactivation was predominantly observed in default (37%), ventral attention (23%), and somatomotor (22%) networks. In adults, significant ADHD-related hypoactivation was almost exclusively observed in the frontoparietal network (97%), while hyperactivation was observed in visual (41%), dorsal attention (33%), and default (26%) networks.

In the meta-analysis limited to patients with non-comorbid ADHD, similar results emerged, with significant ADHD-related hypoactivations in the ventral attention (30%), frontoparietal (29%), and default (21%) networks, while most hyperactivation was found in the default (44%) and somatomotor (26%) networks. The presence of the default network among both hypoactivated and hyperactivated regions was noted, although default network hyperactivations prevailed overall.

In the meta-analysis limited to patients who were medication-naïve, significant ADHD-related hypoactivations were mostly located in the frontoparietal (27%), default (24%), and ventral attention (18%) networks, while few voxels exhibited hyperactivation, all in the somatomotor network. This meta-analysis also implicated thalamic hypoactivation, and the authors noted that the thalamus has generally been overlooked in models of ADHD, despite its central location in cortico-striato-thalamic-cortical circuits.

In summary, Cortese et al. quantitatively synthesized 55 fMRI studies and reported both evidence of hypoactivation in frontoparietal and ventral attention networks as well as hyperactivation in the default network, ventral attention and somatomotor networks [8]. These data indirectly support the default network interference hypothesis of ADHD [30] and lay the groundwork for targeted future investigations of the interplay of large-scale neural systems in ADHD [31].

Meta-analysis of fMRI studies of inhibition and attention

An alternative meta-analytic approach using effect size signed differential mapping (www.sdmproject.com/) was conducted by Hart et al. to probe differences between patients with ADHD and controls on tasks of inhibition and attention [11]. In their meta-analysis of inhibition studies, 21 independent datasets (7 of adults, 14 pediatric studies) were included with 287 patients with ADHD, and 320 controls. When all inhibition tasks were considered together, patients with ADHD versus controls were found to have significantly decreased activation in the right inferior frontal cortex (IFC) extending into the insula, in a cluster comprising the supplementary motor area (SMA) and the cognitive division of the ACC, in the left caudate head extending into the putamen and insula, and in the right thalamus [11].

In the meta-analysis limited to motor response inhibition tasks, patients with ADHD (n = 187) versus controls (n = 206) showed significantly decreased activation in the right IFC and insula, right SMA and ACC, right thalamus, left caudate, and right occipital lobe. In the meta-analysis limited to interference inhibition tasks, patients with ADHD (n = 100) versus controls (n = 114) showed significantly decreased activation in the left cognitive division of the ACC, in the right IFC and insula, in the right caudate head, and in the left posterior insula extending to the parietal lobe [11].

In the Hart et al. meta-analysis of attention studies, 13 independent datasets (2 in adults, 11 pediatric) were included, with 171 patients with ADHD and 178 controls. Patients with ADHD versus controls were found to have decreased activation in right dorsolateral prefrontal cortex, left putamen and globus pallidus, right posterior thalamus (pulvinar), and caudate tail extending into the posterior insula, and right inferior parietal lobe, precuneus, and superior temporal lobe. Significantly increased activation was found in right cerebellum and left cuneus.

In the inhibition task meta-analysis by Hart *et al.*, medication status did not reveal a significant effect across groups. However, in the attention meta-analysis, the percentage of patients on long-term stimulant medications correlated significantly with increasing activation in the right caudate tail, such that medication-naïve patients had significantly reduced activation while patients medicated long term were indistinguishable from healthy controls.

Meta-analysis of age effects was only conducted by Hart *et al.* for inhibition tasks due to an insufficient number of attention studies, but did not reveal any significant effects. However, when categorically analyzed separately for adult and pediatric groups, significant effects emerged. Children with ADHD versus controls had decreased activation in the left putamen and right caudate, SMA, and ACC, while adults with ADHD versus controls had decreased activation in the right IFC and right thalamus.

Comparisons between two meta-analytical approaches

Cortese *et al.* [8] and Hart *et al.* [11] both addressed the fMRI literature on ADHD but with different meta-analytical approaches and with mostly, but not completely, overlapping included studies. The meta-analysis by Hart *et al.* focused exclusively on studies of inhibition or attention, while Cortese *et al.* were more inclusive, but did perform secondary meta-analyses limited to inhibition tasks or to attention/vigilance tasks. With respect to inhibition tasks, the two meta-analyses overlapped on 16 of the 21 studies included by Hart *et al.* (76%), whereas for attention/vigilance the meta-analyses overlapped for 10 of the 13 studies included by Hart *et al.* (77%).

When the two sets of partially overlapping meta-analyses with differing approaches are considered for studies of inhibition, the regions identified as being hypoactivated in ADHD by both meta-analyses include the ACC, SMA, IFC, and thalamus. None of the other findings from either of the attention meta-analyses (ADHD > controls or controls > ADHD) or

from inhibition (ADHD > controls) overlapped across the two meta-analyses. Given the substantial overlap in starting points, this degree of discrepancy raises questions regarding the validity of meta-analyses with modest samples, as most still are. Doubts regarding the value of meta-analyses are not new in the medical literature [32]. An alternative that is becoming a practical reality is to combine the raw data directly, as we discuss in the next section.

Resting-state functional MRI studies of ADHD

Despite the extraordinary utility of task-based fMRI for cognitive neuroscience when applied to healthy young adult volunteers, this approach has been much less fruitful when applied to patients with psychiatric disorders, or to children or the elderly [26]. Functional imaging without an explicit task, known for historical reasons, as resting state fMRI (R-fMRI), has moved into the breech, becoming the fastest growing type of human imaging in the past decade [33, 34].

R-fMRI is a misnomer which raises needless controversy regarding whether rest can be adequately defined. R-fMRI approaches focus on spontaneous fluctuations of BOLD signals which can be appreciated in mammalian brain except during brain death. Thus R-fMRI can be obtained while participants are awake (the most common condition), with eyes open or closed, during sleep, or even during anesthesia [34]. All of these factors matter, as does time of day, whether preceding or following effortful tasks [35]. Still, R-fMRI data can be obtained in neonates, infants, sleeping toddlers, school-age children, adolescents, young adults, or the elderly. The lack of explicit cognitive task facilitates data collection with groups characterized by variable cognitive ability or by dementia. With all these advantages, R-fMRI approaches have one major weakness – vulnerability to even extremely small degrees of head movement [36–41]. The central problem is that even movements of 0.1 mm or 0.2 mm produce effects which are indistinguishable from correlations of nearby voxels, since movements occur with roughly the same frequencies as BOLD signal fluctuations. The best solution is to collect movement-free data, but this is certainly not possible with young children, and particularly not with young children who have ADHD. Thus the first generation of R-fMRI studies in ADHD [24, 42–52] need to be interpreted with caution until their results are confirmed to not be ascribable to between-group or between-individual differences in head micromovements.

Now that the field has been sensitized to the issue of movement, a number of approaches have been proposed for addressing it [36–41]. While consensus on a single method has yet to develop, a multimodal approach includes minimizing motion during acquisition (which is best accomplished by assuring participant comfort and providing snug placement in the scanner), monitoring movement indices, monitoring physiological parameters such as heart rate and respiration, and covarying individual motion parameters in group statistical analyses [41, 53].

Besides attending to in-scanner head motion, the field needs to take statistical power seriously. Fortunately, R-fMRI data are amenable to aggregation across multiple sites, despite differences in data acquisition parameters or in populations from which samples are drawn [34, 54–57]. In ADHD, this led to the creation of the ADHD-200 sample.

The ADHD-200 sample and global competition

Following the creation of the 1000 Functional Connectomes Project [57], which established an open science repository of 1093 structural and R-fMRI datasets collected from 24 labs across the world, a number of ADHD neuroimaging investigators decided to create a comparable resource for the scientific community. The ADHD-200 sample, which was collected from eight labs, was released on March 1, 2011 via Neuroimaging Informatics Tools and Resources Clearinghouse (NITRC.org) at http://fcon_1000.projects.nitrc.org/indi/adhd200/. The initial release of 776 R-fMRI and structural scans included 491 scans from typically developing individuals and 285 scans from children and adolescents with ADHD, all aged from 7 to 21 years [58]. To publicize the availability of the ADHD-200 sample, the ADHD-200 Consortium declared a global competition to develop novel strategies for predicting diagnosis based on R-fMRI and structural scan data, and to identify novel features of brain structure or function with the potential to yield ADHD biomarkers [58]. The global competition involved analyzing an additional 197 datasets that were released on July 1, 2011 without diagnostic labels. Fifty teams indicated their intent to participate and 21 teams competed. Competitors were invited to publish their approaches and results in a special

issue of an on-line open access journal [59–70]. Many of these approaches are highly technical, and many were submitted primarily by statisticians and applied mathematicians, whose participation was made possible by the provision of preprocessed data. Other investigators bypassed the competition and simply published their novel results based on these open access data in standard peer-reviewed outlets [71]. Interestingly, given the unbalanced demographic data of the various subsamples (male preponderance and lower IQ in patients, for example), one group obtained the highest classification accuracy by using only demographic data (site of data collection, age, sex, handedness, and IQ scores) and ignoring brain imaging data [60]. This result showed that neuroimaging results are far from being sufficient or necessary for diagnoses.

Distinct neural signatures detected for combined vs. inattentive ADHD

Nevertheless, the availability of the ADHD-200 sample also allowed a novel type of collaborative science to be conducted [67]. Fair *et al.* took on the problem of head micromovement by applying 10 different motion correction procedures. They showed variable efficacy for a number of options, and concluded that including an individual measure of micromovement as a nuisance covariate in group analyses is necessary regardless of what other methods are applied [67]. After including various methods of motion correction, including censoring data (also known as "scrubbing" [36, 37]), they limited subsequent analyses to three sets of 52 participants each who were either typical controls, children or adolescents with combined type ADHD, or children or adolescents with inattentive type ADHD. Thus analyses contrasting ADHD subtypes were limited to 20% of the starting sample, so as to arrive at groups that exhibited limited extents of micromovements and that did not differ significantly among each other [67].

With this refined subsample, Fair *et al.* applied a network based approach [72, 73] to examine differences in node strength in whole brain among controls and individuals with combined type or inattentive type ADHD. As shown in Figure 16.1, regional differences in functional networks emerge across all three pair-wise comparisons. All of these results represent hypotheses which invite replication and further extension.

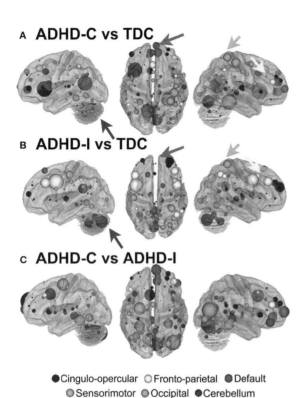

A ADHD-C vs TDC

B ADHD-I vs TDC

C ADHD-C vs ADHD-I

● Cingulo-opercular ○ Fronto-parietal ● Default
◐ Sensorimotor ◉ Occipital ● Cerebellum

Figure 16.1. Pair-wise comparisons based on features found to predict ADHD vs. typically developing controls (TDC) after applying one of 10 motion correction procedures by Fair *et al.* [67]. Differences in node strength are depicted by the sizes of the corresponding circles which are centered over the corresponding nodal coordinates. The colors of the circles indicate their membership in one of six functional networks defined by a prior study [73]. (A). Node strength for combined type ADHD (ADHD-C) vs. TDC differs particularly for anterior and posterior nodes of the default network. Also shown are prominent between-group differences in sensorimotor and occipital networks. (B). Contrast between inattentive type ADHD (ADHD-I) and TDC highlights between-group differences in frontoparietal and cerebellar networks. (C). Head-to-head contrast between the two subtypes of ADHD highlights between-group differences in the anterior nodes of the default network, occipital, and sensorimotor networks.

Reproduced from Fair *et al.* [67] copyright © 2013 by Fair, Nigg, Iyer, Bathula, Mills, Dosenbach, Schlaggar, Mennes, Gutman, Bangaru, Buitelaar, Dickstein, Di Martino, Kennedy, Luna, Schweitzer, Velanova, Want, Mostofsky, Castellanos, and Milham based on Creative Commons Attribution License which permits reproduction provided the original authors and source are credited. This figure can be found in full color at the following link (figure 7): http://www.frontiersin.org/Systems_Neuroscience/10.3389/fnsys.2012.00080/abstract

Conclusions

ADHD neuroimaging has advanced dramatically in slightly over two decades, yet there is still much work to be done. Recent work has been focusing on large-scale networks which are at least heuristically useful

and which may also be revealing fundamental aspects of neurobiology [31]. We note the repeated emergence of the default network in ADHD, particularly in combined type ADHD, from distinct types of imaging approaches, as well as the implication of top-down executive control networks such as the frontoparietal network. However, we also observe that sensorimotor and visual networks appear to be implicated in brain imaging studies of ADHD, which should motivate targeted investigations of the associated modalities. Finally, we expect that the encouragement by funding agencies for investigators to openly share data and the availability of computational tools designed for Big Data [74, 75] will likely transform our perspectives on ADHD and related disorders over the next decade.

References

1. Castellanos FX. Neuroimaging of attention-deficit hyperactivity disorder. *Child Adolesc Psychiatr Clin N Am.* 1997;**6**:383–411.

2. Shaywitz BA, Shaywitz SE, Byrne T, Cohen DJ, Rothman S. Attention deficit disorder: quantitative analysis of CT. *Neurology.* 1983;**33**:1500–3.

3. Zametkin AJ, Nordahl TE, Gross M, *et al.* Cerebral glucose metabolism in adults with hyperactivity of childhood onset. *N Engl J Med.* 1990;**323**:1361–6.

4. Zametkin AJ, Liebenauer LL, Fitzgerald GA, *et al.* Brain metabolism in teenagers with attention-deficit hyperactivity disorder. *Arch Gen Psychiatry.* 1993;**50**: 333–40.

5. Dickstein SG, Bannon K, Castellanos FX, Milham MP. The neural correlates of attention deficit hyperactivity disorder: an ALE meta-analysis. *J Child Psychol Psychiatry.* 2006;**47**:1051–62.

6. Valera EM, Faraone SV, Murray KE, Seidman LJ. Meta-analysis of structural imaging findings in attention-deficit/hyperactivity disorder. *Biol Psychiatry.* 2007;**61**:1361–9.

7. Nakao T, Radua J, Rubia K, Mataix-Cols D. Gray matter volume abnormalities in ADHD: voxel-based meta-analysis exploring the effects of age and stimulant medication. *Am J Psychiatry.* 2011;**168**: 1154–63.

8. Cortese S, Kelly C, Chabernaud C, *et al.* Towards systems neuroscience of ADHD: a meta-analysis of 55 fMRI studies. *Am J Psychiatry.* 2012;**169**:1038–55.

9. Frodl T, Skokauskas N. Meta-analysis of structural MRI studies in children and adults with attention deficit hyperactivity disorder indicates treatment effects. *Acta Psychiatr Scand.* 2012;**125**:114–26.

10. van Ewijk H, Heslenfeld DJ, Zwiers MP, Buitelaar JK, Oosterlaan J. Diffusion tensor imaging in attention deficit/hyperactivity disorder: a systematic review and meta-analysis. *Neurosci Biobehav Rev*. 2012;**36**: 1093–106.

11. Hart H, Radua J, Nakao T, Mataix-Cols D, Rubia K. Meta-analysis of functional magnetic resonance imaging studies of inhibition and attention in attention-deficit/hyperactivity disorder: exploring task-specific, stimulant medication, and age effects. *JAMA Psychiatry*. 2013;**70**:185–98.

12. Radua J, Mataix-Cols D. Meta-analytic methods for neuroimaging data explained. *Biol Mood Anxiety Disord*. 2012;**2**:6.

13. Collins DL, Holmes CJ, Peters TM, Evans AC. Automatic 3-D model-based neuroanatomical segmentation. *Hum Brain Mapp*. 1995;**3**:190–208.

14. Castellanos FX, Acosta MT. [The neuroanatomy of attention deficit/hyperactivity disorder]. *Rev Neurol*. 2004;**38**(Suppl 1):131–6.

15. Bartko JJ, Pulver AE, Carpenter WT, Jr. The power of analysis: statistical perspectives. Part 2. *Psychiatry Res*. 1988;**23**:301–9.

16. Gilmore JH, Schmitt JE, Knickmeyer RC, *et al*. Genetic and environmental contributions to neonatal brain structure: a twin study. *Hum Brain Mapp*. 2010;**31**:1174–82.

17. Peper JS, Brouwer RM, Boomsma DI, Kahn RS, Hulshoff Pol HE. Genetic influences on human brain structure: a review of brain imaging studies in twins. *Hum Brain Mapp*. 2007;**28**:464–73.

18. Gill KE, Pierre PJ, Daunais J, *et al*. Chronic treatment with extended release methylphenidate does not alter dopamine systems or increase vulnerability for cocaine self-administration: a study in nonhuman primates. *Neuropsychopharmacology*. 2012;**37**:2555–65.

19. Jones DK, Knosche TR, Turner R. White matter integrity, fiber count, and other fallacies: the do's and don'ts of diffusion MRI. *Neuroimage*. 2013;**73**: 239–54.

20. Smith SM, Jenkinson M, Johansen-Berg H, *et al*. Tract-based spatial statistics: voxelwise analysis of multi-subject diffusion data. *Neuroimage*. 2006;**31**:1487–505.

21. Davenport ND, Karatekin C, White T, Lim KO. Differential fractional anisotropy abnormalities in adolescents with ADHD or schizophrenia. *Psychiatry Res*. 2010;**181**:193–8.

22. Li Q, Sun J, Guo L, *et al*. Increased fractional anisotropy in white matter of the right frontal region in children with attention-deficit/hyperactivity disorder: a diffusion tensor imaging study. *Neuro Endocrinol Lett*. 2010;**31**:747–53.

23. Nagel BJ, Bathula D, Herting M, *et al*. Altered white matter microstructure in children with attention-deficit/hyperactivity disorder. *J Am Acad Child Adolesc Psychiatry*. 2011;**50**:283–92.

24. Qiu MG, Ye Z, Li QY, *et al*. Changes of brain structure and function in ADHD children. *Brain Topogr*. 2011;**24**:243–52.

25. Rossi JS. Statistical power of psychological research: what have we gained in 20 years? *J Consult Clin Psychol*. 1990;**58**:646–56.

26. Raichle ME, Mintun MA. Brain work and brain imaging. *Annu Rev Neurosci*. 2006;**29**:449–76.

27. Yeo BT, Krienen FM, Sepulcre J, *et al*. The organization of the human cerebral cortex estimated by functional connectivity. *J Neurophysiol*. 2011;**106**:1125–65.

28. Castellanos FX, Tannock R. Neuroscience of attention-deficit hyperactivity disorder: the search for endophenotypes. *Nat Rev Neurosci*. 2002;**3**:617–28.

29. Castellanos FX, Sonuga-Barke EJS, Scheres A, *et al*. Varieties of attention-deficit/hyperactivity disorder-related intra-individual variability. *Biol Psychiatry*. 2005;**57**:1416–23.

30. Sonuga-Barke EJ, Castellanos FX. Spontaneous attentional fluctuations in impaired states and pathological conditions: a neurobiological hypothesis. *Neurosci Biobehav Rev*. 2007;**31**:977–86.

31. Castellanos FX, Proal E. Large-scale brain systems in ADHD: beyond the prefrontal-striatal model. *Trends Cogn Sci*. 2012;**16**:17–26.

32. Feinstein AR. Meta-analysis: statistical alchemy for the 21st century. *J Clin Epidemiol*. 1995;**48**:71–9.

33. Snyder AZ, Raichle ME. A brief history of the resting state: the Washington University perspective. *Neuroimage*. 2012;**62**:902–10.

34. Kelly C, Biswal BB, Craddock RC, Castellanos FX, Milham MP. Characterizing variation in the functional connectome: promise and pitfalls. *Trends Cogn Sci*. 2012;**16**:181–8.

35. Barnes A, Bullmore ET, Suckling J. Endogenous human brain dynamics recover slowly following cognitive effort. *PLoS One*. 2009;**4**:e6626.

36. Power JD, Barnes KA, Snyder AZ, Schlaggar BL, Petersen SE. Spurious but systematic correlations in functional connectivity MRI networks arise from subject motion. *Neuroimage*. 2012;**59**:2142–54.

37. Power JD, Barnes KA, Snyder AZ, Schlaggar BL, Petersen SE. Steps toward optimizing motion artifact removal in functional connectivity MRI; a reply to Carp. *Neuroimage*. 2013;**76**:439–41.

38. Satterthwaite TD, Wolf DH, Loughead J, *et al*. Impact of in-scanner head motion on multiple measures of functional connectivity: relevance for studies of

neurodevelopment in youth. *Neuroimage*. 2012;**60**: 623–32.

39. Satterthwaite TD, Elliott MA, Gerraty RT, *et al*. An improved framework for confound regression and filtering for control of motion artifact in the preprocessing of resting-state functional connectivity data. *Neuroimage*. 2013;**64**:240–56.

40. Van Dijk KR, Sabuncu MR, Buckner RL. The influence of head motion on intrinsic functional connectivity MRI. *Neuroimage*. 2012;**59**:431–8.

41. Yan CG, Cheung B, Kelly C, *et al*. A comprehensive assessment of regional variation in the impact of micromovement head motion on functional connectomics. *Neuroimage*. 2013;**76**:183–201.

42. Cao Q, Zang Y, Sun L, *et al*. Abnormal neural activity in children with attention deficit hyperactivity disorder: a resting-state functional magnetic resonance imaging study. *Neuroreport*. 2006;**17**:1033–6.

43. Tian L, Jiang T, Wang Y, *et al*. Altered resting-state functional connectivity patterns of anterior cingulate cortex in adolescents with attention deficit hyperactivity disorder. *Neurosci Lett*. 2006;**400**: 39–43.

44. Zang YF, Yong H, Chao-Zhe Z, *et al*. Altered baseline brain activity in children with ADHD revealed by resting-state functional MRI. *Brain Dev*. 2007;**29**: 83–91.

45. Castellanos FX, Margulies DS, Kelly AMC, *et al*. Cingulate-precuneus interactions: a new locus of dysfunction in adult attention-deficit/hyperactivity disorder. *Biol Psychiatry*. 2008;**63**:332–7.

46. Tian L, Jiang T, Liang M, *et al*. Enhanced resting-state brain activities in ADHD patients: a fMRI study. *Brain Dev*. 2008;**30**:342–8.

47. Uddin LQ, Kelly AMC, Biswal BB, *et al*. Network homogeneity reveals decreased integrity of default-mode network in ADHD. *J Neurosci Methods*. 2008; **169**:249–54.

48. Cao X, Cao Q, Long X, *et al*. Abnormal resting-state functional connectivity patterns of the putamen in medication-naive children with attention deficit hyperactivity disorder. *Brain Res*. 2009;**1303**:195–206.

49. Wang L, Zhu C, He Y, *et al*. Altered small-world brain functional networks in children with attention-deficit/hyperactivity disorder. *Hum Brain Mapp*. 2009;**30**: 638–49.

50. Fair DA, Posner J, Nagel BJ, *et al*. Atypical default network connectivity in youth with attention-deficit/hyperactivity disorder. *Biol Psychiatry*. 2010;**68**: 1084–91.

51. Wilson TW, Franzen JD, Heinrichs-Graham E, *et al*. Broadband neurophysiological abnormalities in the medial prefrontal region of the default-mode network

in adults with ADHD. *Hum Brain Mapp*. 2013;**34**: 566–74.

52. Yang H, Wu QZ, Guo LT, *et al*. Abnormal spontaneous brain activity in medication-naive ADHD children: a resting state fMRI study. *Neurosci Lett*. 2011;**502**: 89–93.

53. Craddock RC, Jbabdi S, Yan CG, *et al*. Imaging human connectomes at the macroscale. *Nat Method*. 2013;**10**: 524–39.

54. Mennes M, Biswal B, Castellanos FX, Milham MP. Making data sharing work: the FCP/INDI experience. *Neuroimage*. 2013;**82**:683–91.

55. Milham MP. Open neuroscience solutions for the connectome-wide association era. *Neuron*. 2012;**73**: 214–18.

56. Nooner KB, Colcombe SJ, Tobe RH, *et al*. The NKI-Rockland Sample: a model for accelerating the pace of discovery science in psychiatry. *Front Neurosci*. 2012;**6**:152.

57. Biswal BB, Mennes M, Zuo XN, *et al*. Toward discovery science of human brain function. *Proc Natl Acad Sci U S A*. 2010;**107**:4734–9.

58. ADHD Consortium. The ADHD-200 Consortium: a model to advance the translational potential of neuroimaging in clinical neuroscience. *Front Syst Neurosci*. 2012;**6**:62.

59. Bohland JW, Saperstein S, Pereira F, Rapin J, Grady L. Network, anatomical, and non-imaging measures for the prediction of ADHD diagnosis in individual subjects. *Front Syst Neurosci*. 2012;**6**:78.

60. Brown MR, Sidhu GS, Greiner R, *et al*. ADHD-200 Global Competition: diagnosing ADHD using personal characteristic data can outperform resting state fMRI measurements. *Front Syst Neurosci*. 2012;**6**:69.

61. Chang CW, Ho CC, Chen JH. ADHD classification by a texture analysis of anatomical brain MRI data. *Front Syst Neurosci*. 2012;**6**:66.

62. Cheng W, Ji X, Zhang J, Feng J. Individual classification of ADHD patients by integrating multiscale neuroimaging markers and advanced pattern recognition techniques. *Front Syst Neurosci*. 2012;**6**:58.

63. Colby JB, Rudie JD, Brown JA, *et al*. Insights into multimodal imaging classification of ADHD. *Front Syst Neurosci*. 2012;**6**:59.

64. Dai D, Wang J, Hua J, He H. Classification of ADHD children through multimodal magnetic resonance imaging. *Front Syst Neurosci*. 2012;**6**:63.

65. Dey S, Rao AR, Shah M. Exploiting the brain's network structure in identifying ADHD subjects. *Front Syst Neurosci*. 2012;**6**:75.

66. Eloyan A, Muschelli J, Nebel MB, *et al.* Automated diagnoses of attention deficit hyperactive disorder using magnetic resonance imaging. *Front Syst Neurosci.* 2012;**6**:61.

67. Fair DA, Nigg JT, Iyer S, *et al.* Distinct neural signatures detected for ADHD subtypes after controlling for micro-movements in resting state functional connectivity MRI data. *Front Syst Neurosci.* 2012;**6**:80.

68. Olivetti E, Greiner S, Avesani P. ADHD diagnosis from multiple data sources with batch effects. *Front Syst Neurosci.* 2012;**6**:70.

69. Sato JR, Hoexter MQ, Fujita A, Rohde LA. Evaluation of pattern recognition and feature extraction methods in ADHD prediction. *Front Syst Neurosci.* 2012;**6**:68.

70. Sidhu GS, Asgarian N, Greiner R, Brown MR. Kernel Principal Component Analysis for dimensionality reduction in fMRI-based diagnosis of ADHD. *Front Syst Neurosci.* 2012;**6**:74.

71. Tomasi D, Volkow ND. Abnormal functional connectivity in children with attention-deficit/hyperactivity disorder. *Biol Psychiatry.* 2012;**71**: 443–50.

72. Dosenbach NU, Fair DA, Miezin FM, *et al.* Distinct brain networks for adaptive and stable task control in humans. *Proc Natl Acad Sci U S A.* 2007;**104**:11073–8.

73. Dosenbach NU, Nardos B, Cohen AL, *et al.* Prediction of individual brain maturity using fMRI. *Science.* 2010;**329**:1358–61.

74. Conger K. B!G DATA. What it means for our health and the future of medical research. *Stanford Medicine* 2012;Summer:1.

75. Raddick MJ, Szalay AS. The universe online. *Science.* 2010;**329**:1028–9.

Neuropsychological testing

Joel E. Morgan, Kira E. Armstrong, and Lisa G. Hahn

Introduction

Neuropsychology is the study of brain behavior relationships, the scientific underpinnings of cognition, emotion, and behavior as these human functions relate to the integrity of the central nervous system [1, 2]. Clinical neuropsychology specializes in the assessment and treatment of known or suspected abnormalities of brain function as they manifest themselves in cognition, emotion, and/or behavior. Often, neuropsychological evaluations are helpful in cases where diagnostic uncertainty is present (e.g., does my child have a learning disability; or, does mom have Alzheimer's?). Likewise, neuropsychological assessment is indicated in cases where, although the diagnosis is already identified, specific patterns of cognitive strengths and weaknesses are unclear and a patient's functional limitations may be unknown. For example, treating physicians may be interested in knowing the effects of a left hemisphere stroke on speech/language functions, or if a patient's right parietal neoplasm has disrupted visual-spatial processes or memory.

Readers of this volume will know that attention-deficit hyperactivity disorder (ADHD) is often diagnosed by history and observation, particularly in uncomplicated cases (i.e., absent comorbidities). Nonetheless, neuropsychological testing contributes to patient care by providing specifics about cognition that may help direct treatment and interventions, as well as educational and employment planning. Neuropsychological assessment is particularly informative for differential diagnoses and providing guidance for intervention in those cases of more complicated ADHD, where comorbidities are known or suspected (e.g., learning disabilities and/or psychiatric disorders such as anxiety or depression) [3]. This point becomes all the more salient when recognizing that it is "more

common to find a child with ADHD and a comorbidity than it is to find a child with ADHD alone" [4]. Indeed 58–87% of children with ADHD have at least one comorbid disorder and up to 20% have three or more comorbid disorders.

In this chapter we present a primer on neuropsychological assessment with particular relevance to ADHD. We will discuss the neuropsychological assessment process as well as the various areas of cognition (i.e., the traditional mental functions) that are assessed in typical neuropsychological examinations. In conjunction with the discussion of cognitive functions, we will present the cerebral systems underlying (subserving) these functions (i.e., *behavioral geography*, [1]), followed by a brief review of some of the many typical assessment instruments utilized in neuropsychological testing. Considerable heterogeneity of cognitive functions is observed among ADHD patients [5], examples of which are presented throughout the discussion. We hope the reader will come to appreciate the contribution that neuropsychological evaluations may play in the overall assessment and treatment of patients with known or suspected ADHD.

Neuropsychology, cognition and the brain: a primer

A neuropsychologist's primary role is to assess and interpret the intricacies of a patient's cognition or the details of mental abilities, in the context of his or her psychosocial history, behavioral presentation, and presenting complaints. This integrative process allows neuropsychologists to effectively assist with complicated differential diagnoses and to provide strong recommendations for clinical management. Thus, while the remainder of this chapter focuses primarily on the

Attention-Deficit Hyperactivity Disorder in Adults and Children, ed. Lenard A. Adler, Thomas J. Spencer and Timothy E. Wilens. Published by Cambridge University Press. © Cambridge University Press 2015.

testing process, it is critical to emphasize that a neuropsychological *assessment* also entails comprehensive diagnostic interviews with the patient and informants. The data derived from both processes allow the clinician to interpret test findings in a contextually meaningful (i.e., *accurate*) manner.

Within this context, abnormalities of brain structure and/or brain function may, and often do, adversely affect cognition. For example, readers of this volume will appreciate that abnormalities of frontal lobe structure and function have clearly been implicated in ADHD [6–10]. More recent literature has also begun to implicate the cerebellum's role in executive functioning and possibly even ADHD [11, 12]. Similarly, in addition to abnormal attention, some children and adults with ADHD have abnormalities of other areas of cognition related to frontal systems (e.g., executive functions), while still other patients with ADHD do not. The great heterogeneity of cognition among ADHD patients makes it challenging to offer a pathognomonic neuropsychological profile. Nonetheless, each patient's cognitive strengths and weaknesses can be useful in clarifying the accuracy of an ADHD diagnosis, and delineating its impact on a patient's day-to-day functioning.

Cognitive functions are broadly grouped into a number of areas, including: language and verbal skills; general intellectual skills; perceptual and visual-spatial skills; learning and memory; sensorimotor skills; and emotional adjustment/regulation. Executive functions are also considered a primary cognitive skill although they include a wide range of specific domains including: attention; organization and planning; abstract reasoning and problem solving; and inhibitory and higher cortical functions, among others.

These categories or classes of cognitive, neurological, and emotional functions are somewhat arbitrary and some neuropsychologists may use a slightly different grouping. For example, some may categorize abstract reasoning and higher cortical functions along with executive skills [13, 14] while others may not. It is also important to note that these various functions are not particularly discrete, that almost all of these different domains or skills require some degree of input from other functions. This is especially true of attention and other executive functions. Think of learning and memory for example and their relationship to attention. As attention is a fundamental function that largely underlies most of the various aspects of cognition, if one has impaired attention, information may not be adequately registered in order to be remembered. It stands to reason that, depending on the severity and nature of extant attentional deficits, many other higher-level cognitive skills may also be negatively affected. Similarly, if a patient is prone to cognitive impulsivity (i.e., if he/she frequently makes errors due to an impulsive response style) he/she may perform poorly on tasks that are more vulnerable to this characteristic (e.g., multiple choice tests) regardless of how knowledgeable he/she may otherwise be. That is, his/her score on a neurocognitive or academic test may *suggest* cognitive deficits in a discrete domain or lack of adequate knowledge when his/her problems are really more accurately recognized as being secondary to impulsivity.

Lateralization of cognition within the brain

For the vast majority of persons, the brain is functionally organized such that the left cerebral hemisphere subserves verbal and language skills (known as the dominant hemisphere, i.e., dominant for language) and the right cerebral hemisphere (the non-dominant hemisphere) subserves perceptual and spatial skills, i.e., non-verbal functions [1]. This functional organization pervades all cognitive functions; "materially specific" organization is broadly divided into verbal and non-verbal information processing, largely relative to the integrity of the left and right cerebral hemispheres, respectively. Other functional neuroanatomy pertinent to neuropsychology is integrated below in the discussions relating to specific cognitive domains.

General intellectual skills

The general public thinks of intelligence as a unitary concept encompassing all cognitive activity; this is sometimes referred to as *g*, representing a general unitary cognitive factor [15, 16]. However, neuropsychologists tend to view cognition not as a general or unitary factor embodied in the concept of a Full Scale Intelligence Quotient (FSIQ or "IQ"). Rather neuropsychology recognizes cognition as being made up of many discrete functions and abilities, all subserved by various brain regions [1, 2]. So unlike language skills (typically associated with the dominant hemisphere), or executive functions (mediated by the frontal/subcortical and cerebellar regions), intelligence may simplistically be thought of as a process or activity related to the entire brain. In other words, a patient's FSIQ is a composite of many discrete functions, subserved by many different brain regions. This is especially important to emphasize when attempting to document the IQ of a patient with ADHD, as their executive dysfunction will very often impact and even limit their overall performance across many if not all cognitive domains.

The FSIQ score from most neuropsychological measures represents a derived score, a composite of the various discrete functions assessed by an individually administered full scale intelligence test. In some cases, this composite may be an amalgamation of as many as 10 or more subtests, each tapping different cognitive skill sets. For this reason, the concept of "IQ" (at least in isolation) often has limited applicability since the focus of neuropsychological assessment is on the pattern of numerous discrete functions. Indeed, most commonly used intelligence tests assess a number of distinct abilities that largely fall within the verbal/non-verbal distinction, although several measures also incorporate subtests designed to assess working memory and processing speed. Summarizing one's performance across all of these domains with a single score can often be misleading if not altogether inaccurate. On the other hand, an analysis of the subtests of intelligence measures can provide insight into the nature of various cognitive functions of an examinee. It is also worth acknowledging that the American educational system typically relies on standardized, individually administered IQ tests (e.g., Wechsler Scales of Intelligence, Stanford–Binet, etc.) for the determination of whether or not a student may be eligible for special educational services. Thus, despite the issue of FSIQ scores being misleading, they are often utilized to provide a baseline of the individual's functioning, particularly in academic settings.

Regardless of whether an examinee's IQ score is an accurate summary of his/her full range of cognitive abilities, intellectual assessment with standardized tests of intelligence are considered an integral component of many neuropsychological assessments (depending on the diagnostic question being posed). The insights about cognition provided through a review of the various subtests and index scores are often useful not only for diagnostic purposes but also to help examiners determine what clinical interventions may be appropriate. In the case of assessment for ADHD and related cognitive disorders, for example, it would not be uncommon to see lower scores in some areas on certain Wechsler Index Scores (e.g., Processing Speed, Working Memory). Even the

Perceptual Reasoning Index subtests can be vulnerable to the effects of executive dysfunction as one's performance on each subtest can be significantly impacted by inattention to detail (e.g., on the Block Design subtest where a patient may rotate a single block without attending to his/her error), or impulsivity (e.g., on the Matrix Reasoning subtest where a patient may select the first close response without first determining whether there is a more accurate option).

One common lay misconception about ADHD is that individuals with ADHD are of low or limited intelligence. Nothing could be further from the truth, as children and adult patients with ADHD present with a full range of intelligence. Similarly, research indicates that high intelligence is not "protective" of ADHD. In fact, high-IQ individuals diagnosed with ADHD typically have greater problems in numerous domains of life relative to their non-ADHD-high-IQ peers, including in social, academic, vocational, and leisure pursuits, reflecting reduced achievement, success, and personal satisfaction [17, 18].

Executive and higher cortical functions

This group of mental skills refers to the highest level of cognition, those behaviors and abilities that separate humans from most all other animals. These cognitive skills manifest themselves in everyday living through tasks requiring fundamental reasoning skills, "judgment," planning, and organizing. Abstraction and reasoning abilities are crucial for solving problems of all kinds and there is an obvious difference between problems of a verbal nature and those that are visual/non-verbal, reflecting primarily left or right hemispheric processing, respectively. But integral to all problem solving is reasoning, logical analysis, and abstraction. Such functions employ the *executive system;* this cognitive system is responsible for organization, planning, sequencing, judging, etc., and provides the means by which problems are solved and how reasoning is effectuated [19]. Executive functions also may be said to be the components of abstract reasoning.

These higher skills, sometimes referred to as "higher cortical functions," are largely subserved by the vast frontal lobes, but clearly other brain systems play a role. And of course they are not just "cortical," since cognition is dependent on cortical and subcortical brain systems and their vast interconnections (or neural networks). For this reason neuropsychology can be used to clearly demonstrate how subcortical lesions can affect "cortical" functions. Finally, although the cerebellum was previously felt to be exclusively related to motor control, research is increasingly documenting many clear roles in higher cognitive skills and executive functions to the cerebellum [20, 21].

In addition to higher skills, the prefrontal region is significantly involved in attention, working memory, and the ability to sustain mental effort over time, as are other brain regions. As such it should come as no surprise that attention functions are often impaired with frontal lesions [1]. Children and adults with ADHD also frequently demonstrate developmental abnormalities of frontal structures [22–24] that may manifest themselves in neuropsychological testing, particularly relative to attention tests and executive functions [25].

There are three major frontal subsystems implicated in aspects of cognition and behavior: the orbital frontal prefrontal region, the dorsolateral region, and the medial/anterior cingulum system. These three systems concern the regulation of impulse control and inhibitory processes (orbital); integration of cognitive functions (dorsolateral); and the dampening of drive, emotional, and social behavior (medial/anterior cingulam) [26].

Language skills

Verbal skills encompass the totality of language functioning including naming (object recognition), fluency (word retrieval), expressive/receptive language, reading, writing, verbal reasoning, and others. While most people process verbal information in the left hemisphere (known as the dominant hemisphere, i.e., dominant for language), a minority of others process verbal information in the right hemisphere or in both, bilateral representation [27]. When the latter two occur developmentally (i.e., not due to an acquired brain injury), these individuals are primarily left-handed, though such right dominant or mixed dominant brain organization may occur "anomalously" in right-handed people. Furthermore, the majority of left-handed people have the same brain organization as right-handers. That is, they also tend to be left dominant for language, and right dominant for non-verbal, perceptual functions [28].

Patients who have ADHD do not intrinsically have language-based disorders as part of their etiology. However, because ADHD is associated with executive dysfunction it is not uncommon for these patients to struggle (at least qualitatively if not enough to suggest comorbid processes) with organized verbal tasks. For example, they may report a history of word finding difficulties and/or their verbal output may be tangential, disorganized, and verbose. Although reading skills are not directly limited by ADHD, many patients do complain of difficulties with reading that are secondary to inattention; people with ADHD frequently read entire paragraphs or pages only to lament, "Wait, what did I just read?" Additionally, the organizational deficits seen in many patients with ADHD can also contribute to very significant difficulties in organized written output.

Perceptual, visual-spatial skills

These non-verbal functions are largely subserved by the non-dominant hemisphere, usually the right. Among such skills are visual perception, perceptual judgment, visual analysis/discrimination, visual-motor integration, and non-verbal abstract reasoning and problem solving. Since research evidence is mounting that ADHD is predominantly a right-frontal disorder, some difficulties with this domain are not unexpected in ADHD patients [29–32]. Of course as has been discussed, there is great heterogeneity among patients with ADHD and many may not have difficulties in this area. Additionally, many examinees with ADHD exhibit non-verbal/visual-spatial impairments on neuropsychological testing that are related more to their executive dysfunction (e.g., inattention, cognitive impulsivity and/or organization) than true visual-spatial deficits. This distinction is important, as interpreting testing results correctly will guide the determination for appropriate interventions. In contrast, assuming poor scores on visual-spatial tasks are reflective of actual functional deficits may lead one to inaccurate diagnostic decisions and associated ineffective, if not altogether inappropriate, interventions. Clearly, competent neuropsychological practice requires far more than simple score interpretation at face value.

Nonetheless, some ADHD patients may have comorbid serious problems in the realm of non-verbal abilities that extend into multiple areas of perceptual skills that include social perception (e.g., non-verbal learning disabilities [NVLD] and Asperger's disorder, among others) [33, 34]. Similarly, some patients with ADHD may manifest serious difficulties with emotional regulation that go well beyond what are typically observed among most cases of ADHD. Depending on the presenting emotional symptoms, some of these patients may be more accurately identified as having a comorbid anxiety disorder. Or, in the case of more serious psychiatric presentations, they may actually be presenting with a comorbid bipolar disorder [35]. Research evidence suggests that anomalies of executive functions and non-verbal skills among some of these patients may be consistent with right-frontal dysfunction [36] and that bipolar disorder may be a right-frontal phenomenon, as is ADHD. While it is unlikely that these disorders differentiate themselves to any meaningful extent on the basis of neuropsychological test performance alone, the cognitive concomitants of these disorders would be important to recognize in patient assessments, so as to offer meaningful recommendations for clinical management. Additionally, a neuropsychological *assessment* can be an effective tool for differential diagnosis. That is, by interpreting a patient's test results in context of his psychosocial history and behavioral presentation a neuropsychologist can often provide accurate diagnostic conclusions.

Learning and memory

It is not unusual for patients with ADHD to have *functional* difficulties with their memory, particularly if severely inattentive. But not all patients with ADHD have memory problems, and most of those who do are experiencing their difficulties secondary to executive dysfunction rather than true memory impairments (i.e., their ability to learn [encode] and recall is not limited from a neurological perspective). The major brain systems involved in the learning and retention of new information (referred to as anterograde memory) encompass three main cerebral areas: mesial temporal structures, particularly the hippocampus, amygdala, and mammillary bodies; the frontal region; and the diencephalon and frontal subcortical structures including the thalamus and surrounding gray matter, and basal forebrain (i.e., nucleus basalis of Meynert). Retention of new verbal material appears largely based on the integrity of the dominant, left hemisphere while memory for non-verbal material is mediated by the non-dominant, right cerebral hemisphere [37]. Thus, memory functions follow the same basic hemispheric material specificity as broad-based intellectual functions.

A memory disorder in a child or adult may be entirely independent of whether or not the patient has ADHD. Conversely, as noted, if attentional functioning is grossly deficient in severe cases of ADHD, learning and therefore memory may be secondarily compromised; one cannot learn something without actually *attending* to it in the first place. Notably, the presence of a learning/memory *disorder* is not the same as a "learning *disability*." As noted in Chapter 11 of this volume, a *learning disability* is a legal term referring to a specific difficulty in acquiring academic knowledge and skills, and therefore makes one eligible for special education services. This difficulty may be due to any variety of causes, among which may or may not be an extant memory disorder [38].

One relatively common disorder of children that may disrupt both attention and memory is epilepsy. Many seizure disorders are often associated with abnormalities of mesial temporal structures such as hippocampal sclerosis or frontal structures, among others. Individuals with generalized, tonic–clonic seizures are more prone to have both attention and memory problems than patients with partial seizures [39]. We mention epilepsy in particular within this context, as it is not uncommon for many children to present with comorbid diagnoses of epilepsy and ADHD [40, 41]. In these cases, the distinction of what etiology is causing which symptoms is not necessarily important, at least in terms of directing decisions about medication for attentional difficulties; in these cases it is important to treat the seizure disorder *and* the ADHD symptoms regardless of the potential etiology underlying the latter disorder. However, it is critical to recognize that these comorbidities may exacerbate the presentation of symptoms. Additionally, even with successful treatment of a seizure disorder, patients with comorbid ADHD may still experience attentionally driven memory challenges.

The human memory system is vast, as noted above, and therefore extremely vulnerable to a variety of disorders of structural, and physiological abnormalities. Assessment of learning and memory is a crucial aspect of neuropsychological assessment that provides invaluable information about the basic functional abilities of the patient, clearly necessary for everyday living.

Sensorimotor skills

Sensory functions are broadly subserved by bilateral parietal (tactile) and occipital (visual) lobe structures. For the purposes of most common neuropsychological exams, sensory functions are confined to testing of bilateral tactile sensations, though some neuropsychologists test visual, auditory (temporal lobe), and olfactory functions (piriform cortex/entorhinal cortex), as well [42]. The area of the postcentral gyrus of the bilateral parietal lobes primarily subserves tactile sensory functions, with contralateral representation.

The frontal region and particularly the precentral gyrus of the frontal lobes largely subserve motor skills, bilaterally. Similar to the goals of a neurological examination, the assessment of these functions as part of a neuropsychological examination provides for a comparison of skills on both sides of the body and the brain structures subserving those senses. Significant disparity of functions relative to one or the other side of the body, in the context of similarly localizing neurocognitive data, may assist the neuropsychologist in the overall case formulation of the patient and provide for a complete assessment of skills. This may be beneficial in questions of cerebral functional integrity involving diagnosis, treatment planning, intervention, and functional status.

Neuropsychological tests

As is apparent to the reader, neuropsychologists administer, score, and interpret a vast array of tests of cognition and emotional status. In this section, we present some examples of the numerous tests available to the practicing neuropsychologist.

IQ

The Wechsler intelligence tests are considered the gold standard of individually administered intelligence tests that assess general cognition. The Wechsler scales contain a number of subtests assessing such knowledge and skills as vocabulary, general information, verbal and non-verbal reasoning, psychomotor speed, visual scanning, etc., which taken together form the FSIQ. As noted above, these subtests make special demands on particular, sometimes discrete, mental processes and brain systems. So the FSIQ is a composite, representing a kind of "shorthand" summary of one's overall general abilities. Certainly, where persons have wide deviations or discrepancies in one or more areas, referred to as "scatter," this variability is not captured by the FSIQ. For this reason, in these cases the FSIQ is an inadequate, sometimes misleading, representation of the person's abilities [43]. The Wechsler scales come in versions for preschool-age children, school-age children, and adults [43–45]. Other full scale tests assessing

general intelligence include the Stanford–Binet [46] and Kaufman intelligence tests [47, 48]. There are also briefer intelligence tests that have fewer subtests such as the Wechsler Abbreviated Scale of Intelligence – Second Edition (WASI-II) [49].

Executive, attention, and "frontal" tests

Commonly used tests of attention include the continuous performance tests (CPTs), which are computer-assisted tests of attention and impulse control. Among these is the popular Conners' Continuous Performance Test that assesses sustained attention (the test lasts some 14 minutes), visual attention, and motor response inhibition [50]. Other, similar CPTs include the Test of Variables of Attention (TOVA) [51] and the Gordon Diagnostic System [52]. These tests all operate under the premise that individuals with attention deficits will have difficulty in one or more areas of sustaining attention over time, multitasking, inhibiting inappropriate responses, attending to visual stimuli, and differentiating targets from foils [53]. However, these measures cannot and should never be used in isolation to confirm or rule out or diagnose a patient with ADHD [54].

Because the executive system is multidimensional, there are many different functions within this cognitive domain that are assessed in a typical neuropsychological exam. For example, measures of verbal fluency help to assess an aspect of what might be thought of as "initiation," or the ability to get started at a task, in this case verbal initiation. It can also document a patient's ability to sustain mental effort long enough to complete a task (or in this case until the time limit has expired). Research indicates that rapid retrieval of words beginning with specific first letters (phonemic retrieval, e.g., the letter "s") places greater demand on frontal systems (involving an active "search" and associated organizational strategies), while retrieval of words in a specific category (semantic/category retrieval, e.g., "different animals") taxes temporo-parietal systems to a greater extent [55, 56].

Trail Making Tests (Parts A and B) assess rapid graphomotor attention in a seemingly simplistic format of connecting letters in sequence (Part A), then alternating numbers and letters sequentially while switching between them (Part B) [57]. Part B obviously places greater demand on multitasking than Part A, requiring visual attention, scanning, working memory, alternating one's attention, and sequential thinking.

Inhibitory control, assessed in part by CPTs (motor response inhibition), is also assessed by Stroop-type tests. The Stroop Color and Word Test has a long history in psychology [58, 59], assessing an examinee's ability to refrain from responding to an over-learned (or "prepotent") response. In this case, one must inhibit the strong tendency to read a word and instead "merely" state the color of the ink in which the word is printed. This seemingly simple test is actually quite challenging to almost everyone, as it places demand on self-control mechanisms, inhibitory functions, subserved by the frontal executive system. One might say the task represents a type of cognitive conflict (called an interference, or Stroop effect), as for most individuals, reading is automatic. Therefore to actively suppress it, inhibit it, in favor of color naming is effortful and cognitively taxing.

Abstract reasoning and problem solving, sometimes referred to as the concept of "higher cortical functions," are assessed by many different tests, among which is the popular Wisconsin Card Sorting Test (WCST). In this task the examinee has little information about how to sort a deck of cards and must discover the unrevealed rules for sorting via trial and error [60]. Perseverative errors, categories completed, and failure to maintain sets are important variables in the analysis of performance. Somewhat similar to the WCST is the Category test, requiring the examinee to discern a principle or rule related to a spatial relationship [61]. Finally, the "Tower" tests integrate problem solving with planning, spatial reasoning, and cognitive flexibility by requiring examinees to move colored balls or discs from one peg to another, placing the discs in a specific pattern/array, while following specific rules. The Tower of London [62] and Tower of Hanoi are two such tests [63].

Some neuropsychologists use the original, free-standing versions of the executive function tests described above, while others may use the Delis–Kaplan Executive Function System (D-KEFS) [64], or the NEPSY – Second Edition (NEPSY-II) [65]; recently normed collections of similar tests purchased as a set.

Language

The assessment of verbal and language skills employs numerous tests of vocabulary, word reasoning, general fund of information, and expressive and receptive speech, among others. Several of these are included in the Wechsler tests (e.g., the Vocabulary and Similarities subtests). However, once again qualitative

observations can be critical; some patients can earn high *scores* on these measures despite very clear problems with verbal formulation. For example, a patient with ADHD may be noticeably verbose, circumlocutious and even somewhat imprecise in their verbal output, but still earn full or partial credit for his responses. In these instances a high score will fail to reflect some of the functional challenges they may be facing in their daily lives. Other tasks assess more precise skills. For example, verbal fluency (noted above in the discussion of executive functions) and naming are usually assessed with tests such as the Controlled Oral Word Association (COWA) Test [66] and the Boston Naming Test-2 (BNT-2) [67], among others.

Visual, spatial, and perceptual functions

The Wechsler tests of intelligence, include subtests that assess primarily visually based abilities (e.g., Block Design, Visual Puzzles, and Matrix Reasoning). The children's version of this measure (the WISC-IV) also includes the Picture Concepts subtest in the Perceptual Reasoning Index, which ostensibly measures non-verbal reasoning, although it can also be mediated by verbal reasoning skills. Since data are emerging supporting a primary right hemisphere focus of ADHD [29–32], deficient processing in this area would not be surprising. However, as noted above, some individuals with ADHD perform poorly on these tasks due to their executive dysfunction rather than true visual-spatial weaknesses or impairments. Consequently, qualitative assessment of the patient's performance can be as important as reviewing his or her scores. Given this caveat, the Block Design subtest assesses the ability to arrange colored blocks to match a sample geometric pattern. It requires spatial reasoning and part/whole analytic skills, and the task does not easily lend itself to verbal mediation. Non-verbal reasoning can also be measured with the Visual Puzzle and Matrix Reasoning subtests, both of which depend on normal visual perceptual skills and spatial analysis, although they are also vulnerable to inattention, impulsivity, and difficulties with sustained mental effort.

Other tests of visual processing not found within the Wechsler scales include some of the tests from the Benton Laboratory [68], including Judgment of Line Orientation (perceptual judgment) and Facial Recognition, assessing perception of facial characteristics, among others. Similar subtests as well as other visual-based tasks can be found in the NEPSY-II [65].

Still other tests of non-verbal skills include tests of drawing (visual-motor integration) that involve an array of skills involving executive input, organization, and motor planning. These include the Rey–Osterreith Complex Figure (RCOF) and Beery Tests of Developmental Visual-motor Integration, among others [1, 69, 70].

Learning and memory

No neuropsychological examination is complete without the assessment of learning and memory. Anterograde memory processes (new learning) are particularly vulnerable to a host of neurological, psychiatric, and medical conditions [71, 72], not to mention their obvious reliance on intact attention. Memory testing follows three formats: spontaneous free recall/retrieval of the learned information, cued recall, and recognition. In free recall, the examinee must spontaneously recall the previously learned information. In cued recall trials (which are not present on all memory tests) the examinee is given a semantic cue to help support/organize recall. In the recognition format, the patient must choose the correct item from among alternatives, often called foils.

Within this context, material-specific memory functions, verbal and visual, are assessed with a variety of standardized tests. Tests of verbal memory generally take two formats, both of which are auditory (i.e., the examiner reads material to the examinee): learning and retrieval of word lists and/or learning and retrieval of story material, i.e., prose. The former is generally thought to represent rote memorization primarily, though some word-list memory tests (e.g., the California Verbal Learning Test-II [CVLT-II]) [73] include inherent categorical relationships among the words (e.g., fruits, animals, etc.) and therefore provide organization that can potentially aid memory if the patient recognizes and applies this strategy. In story memory tasks, the examiner reads a paragraph length story to the examinee. Both of these formats typically require the examinee to recall material immediately after hearing it and then after a delay. They also often include recognition formats.

Non-verbal memory tests assess visual learning and recall. The typical paradigm for assessing visual memory is that the examiner shows the patient a picture(s), designs, or other visual array, which is followed by immediate and delayed recall tests. Some visual memory tests also include a recognition format.

Numerous standardized tests of memory are available to the neuropsychologist, including the CVLT-II, which comes in child and adult versions [73], Children's Memory Scale (CMS) [74], Wide Range Assessment of Memory of Learning – Second Edition (WRAML2) [75], Wechsler Memory Scale – Fourth Edition (WMS-IV) [76], and the memory trials of the ROCF, a test used for several purposes, including memory, drawing/visual-motor integration, and the executive system aspects of organization and motor planning [69, 70]. There are many others available.

As is not surprising, memory functions are often abnormal in individuals with ADHD, most likely attributable to poor initial registration (encoding) of information. Sometimes, however, disorders of memory are present that may be independent of deficient attentional processes, which may suggest an alternative or comorbid diagnosis. Regardless of the underlying etiology, it stands to reason that impaired memory has deleterious consequences for functional living.

Motor skills

Fine motor dexterity is often associated with developmental disabilities such as ADHD and Learning Disabilities, among others, likely reflecting greater involvement and dysfunction of frontal subcortical motor systems and/or the cerebellum [77, 78]. Tests assessing fine motor dexterity include the Grooved Pegboard Test [79] and Perdue Pegboard Test [80]. More generally, neuropsychologists are also interested in knowing how one side of the body relates to the other, referred to as lateralizing signs. In assessment of abilities and in diagnostic assessment, knowledge of these matters may make a significant difference, especially when the rest of the neuropsychological profile implicates a lateralizing profile. In these instances, ADHD may not ultimately be the primary diagnosis, or it may reflect a comorbid diagnostic picture.

Sensory functions

The assessment of sensory functions can also assist in overall case formulation. While some neuropsychologists prefer to leave sensory assessment to neurologists, others perform tasks of tactile, auditory, and/or visual discrimination, assessment essentially based on a neurological examination.

Emotional functioning

Emotional functioning can be assessed through clinical means (e.g., through an informal or semi-structured interview process such as the Schedule for Affective Disorders and Schizophrenia [SADS] or Kiddie-SADS [K-SADS]) [81, 82], as well as through standardized clinical measures. Questionnaires can be completed by patients, teachers, parents, and significant others (depending on the measure), and can encompass a broad range of emotional and behavioral characteristics. There are comprehensive questionnaires that attempt to sample all clinical areas including depression, anxiety, emotional regulation, aggression, psychosis, attention, and impulsivity. Common examples include the Conners' Rating Scale, 3rd Edition (Conners 3) [83], Behavior Assessment Scale for Children – Second Edition (BASC-2) [84], and the Minnesota Multiphasic Personality Inventory – 2nd Edition and Adolescent version (MMPI-2; MMPI-A) [85, 86]. Other measures are more circumspect, choosing to focus specifically on single domains such as anxiety (e.g., the Multidimensional Anxiety Scale for Children, Second Edition, MASC 2 [87]; Beck Anxiety Inventory, BAI [88]) or depression (e.g., the Children's Depression Inventory, CDI [89] or Beck Depression Inventory – Second Edition, BDI-II [90]).

One potential drawback of these measures is their strong face validity, which allows patients to easily deny or exaggerate symptoms depending on how they wish to present themselves. They can also be lengthy (some with more than 550 questions), which means that patients with waning attention may struggle to consistently focus on and accurately respond to the items. Some tests, such as the MMPI and the MASC 2, incorporate specific validity measures to evaluate how consistently a patient may be responding to the test and/or to determine whether they may be exaggerating their symptoms in a "cry for help" or to emphasize what they see as important clinical symptomatology (this latter index is found in the MMPI but not the MASC 2). On the other hand, some patients find they are more comfortable acknowledging symptoms through inventories than discussing them directly with a clinician.

Occasionally, examinees may present themselves in an exaggerated fashion in order to achieve what is referred to as "secondary gain." Secondary gain is contrasted with primary gain, wherein patients present themselves in forthright fashion with the motivation to find out what is wrong with them and to get better. Examinees in secondary gain contexts may be motivated not to get better, but to achieve some external favor, such as accommodations for extra time in standardized academic testing (i.e., SAT, GRE, MCAT, LSAT, etc.) or for medications, drugs of abuse (i.e., stimulants). Neuropsychologists in such cases may employ a host of assessment techniques addressing the validity of an examinee's presentation and symptom reports. Research unfortunately indicates that exaggerated or frankly malingered presentations are not uncommon [91].

Academic testing

Neuropsychologists who assess school-aged children and young adults attending colleges or graduate schools often administer academic achievement tests, as well as more cognitively based measures. Technically speaking, tests assessing academic achievement are not *neuropsychological* measures in the true sense of the word, as brain-based functions are not directly assessed with these tests. However, when administered and interpreted by neuropsychologists, they often reveal more information than a simple summary of academic achievement. For example, a child who scores below the average range on measures of math fluency and/or math computation may have a Mathematic Disorder/Disability (as would be supported by a review of the child's scores). Alternatively, he may actually have ADHD, which is contributing to frequent inattentive calculation errors. This distinction will lead to strikingly different recommendations for clinical management and educational planning. The Woodcock–Johnson Tests of Academic Achievement (now in its third edition, WJ-III) and the Wechsler Individual Achievement Test, also in its third edition (WIAT-III), represent the gold standard of such instruments [92, 93]. These are large battery tests that are designed to assess all academic areas. However, other gold standard measures that are specific to reading include the Gray Oral Reading Test (GORT-5) [94], now in its fifth edition, and the Test of Word Reading Efficiency (TOWRE), recently updated to a second edition [95].

Some case examples

Case 1: Comorbid ADHD and LD

Johnny was 8 years old and struggling in school despite having received informal academic supports. He had been previously diagnosed with ADHD by a competent and well-respected psychiatrist and appropriately medicated. Despite clear improvement in attention and reduced hyperactivity and impulsivity, reading remained significantly problematic, as did other subjects. Neuropsychological assessment when tested with his stimulant medication documented relatively intact working memory and attentional skills. However, even with the support of this intervention, his ability to decode words and to read fluently was significantly impaired. Although his academic problems had previously been felt to be related to his ADHD, testing helped to document that he also had a reading disorder (or dyslexia) that was contributing to a learning disability. Adjustments to Johnny's Individualized Education Plan (IEP) including specialized reading interventions were ultimately very helpful.

Case 2: ADHD or not?

Sarah seemed like a typical undiagnosed ADHD patient in many respects: she was disorganized, forgot her assignments and homework, could not find things, left a "wake" behind her of disorganization and clutter, and seemed impulsive if not outright flighty. Neuropsychological testing surprisingly revealed all attention tests within normal limits, including challenging tests of auditory and visual attention. The Working Memory and Processing Speed indices of the Wechsler tests, often (but not always) abnormal in ADHD, were also normal. But Sarah performed abnormally on Trail Making Part B, showing marked difficulty in sequential thinking and alternating. Her Wisconsin Card Sort showed a high number of perseverations, as well, and she had some difficulty with inhibition on the Stroop. Sarah had executive dysfunction, with normal attention, not ADHD. She required particular interventions as well as a trial of stimulant medication.

Case 3: ADHD and bipolar disorder of childhood

Mark was 8 years old and displaying tantrums at home after school. In school he was well behaved, though teachers noted occasional inattention and off-task behaviors. When completing homework, his parents reported that he very quickly had a meltdown and displayed uncontrollable anger and tantrums, sometimes with hitting of his mother or older brother. Neuropsychological assessment revealed many areas of impairment, with significant dysfunction of frontal systems as demonstrated by impairment on most all executive tests and tests of attention. Mark,

nonetheless, was very bright, with a Wechsler FSIQ of 134, he displayed very superior verbal ability, but had disproportionately low working memory (Standard Score 92) and Processing Speed (96), constituting serious intracognitive discrepancies. A more thorough review of his psychosocial history indicated that Mark had a history of difficulties with emotional regulation; Mark had periods of extremely happy, impulsive, and hyperactive behaviors followed quickly by either irritable or quiet and reserved activity. At times he also exhibited grandiose thought patterns and a reduced need for sleep. Mark was appropriately treated medically, had a comprehensive IEP, and within a semester began to show improvement.

Case 4: ADHD and NOT dyslexia

Jimmy was 11 years old and had been diagnosed with dyslexia by a learning specialist. He had just started attending a specialized private school setting developed for children with language-based learning disabilities. While most of his classmates thrived in this school (after having struggled for years in their public school), he was having a great deal of difficulty with the repetitive nature of the reading intervention program. He found it boring, redundant, and was not developing any improvement in reading comprehension, which had always been his primary challenge. Furthermore, teachers were raising concerns about his "negative attitude" in response to his inability to persist during reading tutorials. A neuropsychological assessment documented intact decoding (i.e., reading) ability as well as a relatively strong and efficient reading fluency both for real words and "nonwords" (a measure especially sensitive to reading-based disorders). However, consistent with his parents' and own report, Jimmy had marked difficulties responding to reading comprehension measures. In evaluating this further, and in the context of his overall neuropsychological profile and developmental history, it became apparent that Jimmy's problems were *attentionally* based rather than reflecting actual problems with reading. That is, he could read just fine, he just had difficulties attending to the text as he read it. This was the source of his reading comprehension difficulties (as you cannot comprehend something that you never process in the first place). His ADHD was also exacerbating his sense of boredom during the repetitive drills in his reading tutorials. Jimmy was placed on a stimulant medication, with positive effect. His reading support was modified; it no longer emphasized decoding skills, but included specific instruction in identifying key words and phrases to better support comprehension and learning. He transferred back to his public school system and began to excel academically.

Case 5: ADHD and anxiety

Charlie was an 8-year-old boy who had previously been diagnosed with oppositional defiant disorder (ODD). He had a seeming disregard for classroom rules that became disruptive for him and his peers. For example, he had a habit of touching or poking other children when he walked by them, and he insisted on touching the classroom pets despite frequent admonishments to keep his hands to himself. Additionally, when he felt wronged by another child, his first instinct was to use physical force, such as pushing or hitting. He would rush to be first in line, pushing children out of his way, and argued with his teachers if they attempted to correct his behavior. At times, he also fell apart emotionally and engaged in tantrums both at home and at school. While many of his behaviors did *appear* to be defiant, a closer look at his history, and his neuropsychological profile helped to provide a better description of the source of his difficulties. Charlie had ADHD, which led him to *impulsively* poke his classmates, even though he knew he was not supposed to. He also had an anxiety disorder characterized by an exquisite sensitivity to perceived criticism and judgment, which in combination with his ADHD, led him to react quickly and with force whenever he felt "wronged." Charlie often felt bad about his inappropriate behaviors, but he was so overwhelmed by his anxiety that he was often unable to express his remorse, leading adults in his life to incorrectly assume he did not care. When his interventions were changed from that of a punishment model (i.e., you did this incorrect behavior so we will remove something you like) to one that emphasized positive reinforcement, praise, and support, Charlie began to feel more confident at school and some of his negative behaviors reduced. This success was further supported with a stimulant medication, which helped Charlie to become an active, positive student in his classroom.

Final comment

This chapter provided a short primer on neuropsychological testing and its role in the assessment and treatment of ADHD. We hope the reader will come to appreciate some of the benefits that neuropsychology can provide to patients and their families by revealing what may be very important aspects of cognition and behavior that may not be particularly obvious at first glance, yet may be crucial to the welfare and successful treatment of the patient.

References

1. Lezak MD, Howieson DB, Loring DW. *Neuropsychological Assessment*, 4th edn. New York, NY: Oxford University Press; 2004.

2. Morgan JE, Ricker JH, eds. *Textbook of Clinical Neuropsychology*. New York, NY: Psychology Press: 2008.

3. Stefanatos GA, Baron IS. Attention deficit hyperactivity disorder: a neuropsychological perspective towards DSM-V. *Neuropsychol Rev.* 2007; **17**:5–38.

4. Brassett-Harknett A, Butler N. Attention-deficit/ hyperactivity disorder: an overview of the etiology and a review of the literature relating to the correlates and life course outcomes for men and women. *Clin Psychol Rev.* 2007;**27**:188–210.

5. Halperin JM, Marks DJ, Schultz KP. Neuropsychological perspectives on ADHD. In: Morgan JE, Ricker JH, eds. *Textbook of Clinical Neuropsychology*. New York, NY: Psychology Press. 2008; 333–45.

6. Chelune GJ, Ferguson W, Koon R, Dickey TO. Frontal lobe disinhibition in attention deficit disorder. *Child Psychiatry Hum Dev.* 1986;**16**:221–32.

7. Posner MI, Petersen SE. The attention system of the human brain. *Annu Rev Neurosci.* 1990;**13**:25–42.

8. Barkley RA, Grodzinsky G, DuPaul GJ. Frontal lobe functions in attention deficit disorder with and without hyperactivity: a review and research report. *J Abnorm Child Psychol.* 1992;**16**:511–25.

9. Devinsky O, D'Esposito MD. *Neurology of Cognitive and Behavioral Disorders*. New York, NY: Oxford University Press; 2004.

10. Nigg JT. Neuropsychological theory and findings in ADHD: the state of the field and salient challenges for the coming decade. *Biol Psychiatry.* 2005;**57**:1424–35.

11. Diamond A. Close interrelation of motor development and cognitive development and of the cerebellum and prefrontal cortex. *Child Dev.* 2000;**71**:44–56.

12. Krain AL, Castellanos FX. Brain development and ADHD. *Clin Psychol Rev.* 2006;**26**:433–44.

13. Strauss E, Sherman EMS, Spreen O. *A Compendium of Neuropsychological Tests: Administration, Norms, and Commentary*, 3rd edn. New York, NY: Oxford University Press; 2006.

14. Tranel D. Higher brain functions. In: Conn MP, ed. *Neuroscience in Medicine*, 2nd edn. New York, NY: Human Press, Inc.; 2003.

15. Neisser U, Boodoo G, Bouchard TJ, *et al.* Intelligence: knowns and unknowns. *Am Psychol*. 1996;**51**:77–101.

16. Sattler JM. *Assessment of Children: Cognitive Foundations*. San Diego, CA: Jerome Sattler, Publisher, Inc.; 2008.

17. Antshel KM, Faraone SV, Maglione K, *et al.* Executive functioning in high-IQ adults with ADHD. *Psychol Med*. 2010;**40**:1909–18.

18. Antshel KM, Faraone SV, Maglione K, *et al.* Is adult attention deficit hyperactivity disorder a valid diagnosis in the presence of high IQ? *Psychol Med*. 2009;**39**:1325–35.

19. Welsh MC, Pennington BF, Groisser DB. A normative-developmental study of executive function: a window on prefrontal function in children. *Dev Neuropsychol*. 1991;**7**:131–49.

20. Rivia D, Giorgi C. The cerebellum contributes to higher functions during development: evidence from a series of children surgically treated for posterior fossa tumors. *Brain*. 2000;**123**:1051–61.

21. Schmahmann JD. Disorders of the cerebellum: ataxia, dysmetria of thought, and the cerebellar cognitive affective syndrome. *J Neuropsychiatry Clin Neurosci*. 2004;**16**:367–78.

22. Makris N, Pandya DN. The extreme capsule in humans and rethinking of the language circuitry. *Brain Struct Funct*. 2009;**213**:343–58.

23. Sowell ER, Peterson BS, Thompson PM, *et al.* Mapping cortical change across the human life span. *Nat Neurosci*. 2003;**6**:309–15.

24. Mostofsky SH, Lasker AG, Singer HS, Denckla MB, Zee DS. Oculomotor abnormalities in boys with Tourette Syndrome with and without ADHD. *J Am Acad Child Adolesc Psychiatry*. 2001;**40**(12):1464–72.

25. Biederman J, Petty C, Fried R, *et al.* Stability of executive function deficits into young adult years: A prospective longitudinal follow-up study of grown up males with ADHD. *Acta Psychiatr Scand*. 2007;**116**:129–36.

26. Stuss DT, Levine B. Adult clinical neuropsychology: lessons from studies of the frontal lobes. *Annu Rev Psychol*. 2002;**53**:401–33.

27. Knecht S, Drager B, Deppe M, *et al.* Handedness and hemispheric language dominance in healthy humans. *Brain*. 2000;**123**:2512–18.

28. Warrington EK, Pratt RTC. Language laterality in left-handers assessed by unilateral E.C.T. *Neuropsychologia*. 1973;**11**:423–8.

29. Booth JR, Burman DD, Meyer JR, *et al.* Larger deficits in brain networks for response inhibition than for visual selective attention in attention deficit hyperactivity disorder (ADHD). *J Child Psychol Psychiatry*. 2005;**46**:94–111.

30. Carter CS, Krener P, Chaderjian M, Northcutt C, Wolfe V. Asymmetrical visual-spatial attentional performance in ADHD: evidence for a right hemispheric deficit. *Biol Psychiatry*. 1995;**37**:789–97.

31. Clark L, Blackwell AD, Aron AR, *et al.* Association between response inhibition and working memory in adult ADHD: a link to right frontal cortex pathology? *Biol Psychiatry*. 2006;**61**:1395–401.

32. Yeo RA, Hill DE, Campbell RA, *et al.* Proton magnetic resonance spectroscopy investigation of the right frontal lobe in children with attention-deficit hyperactivity disorder. *J Am Acad Child Adolesc Psychiatry*. 2003;**42**:303–10.

33. Brown TE. *Attention-Deficit Hyperactivity Disorders and Comorbidities in Children, Adolescents, and Adults*. Arlington, VA: American Psychiatric Publishing, Inc.; 2000.

34. Fine JG, Semrud-Clikeman M, Butcher B, Wallowiak J. Brief report: attention effect on a measure of social perception. *J Autism Dev Disord*. 2008;**38**:1797–802.

35. Wilens TE, Biederman J, Spencer TJ. Attention deficit hyperactivity disorder across the lifespan. *Annu Rev Med*. 2002;**53**:113–31.

36. Lyoo IK, Kim MJ, Stoll AL, *et al.* Frontal lobe gray matter density decreases in bipolar I disorder. *Biol Psychiatry*. 2004;**55**:648–51.

37. Golby AJ, Poldrack RA, Brewer JB, *et al.* Material-specific lateralization in the medial temporal lobe and prefrontal cortex during memory encoding. *Brain*. 2001;**124**:1841–54.

38. Miller E. On the nature of the memory disorder in presenile dementia. *Neuropsychologia*. 1971;**9**:75–81.

39. Dodrill C. Correlates of generalized tonic-clonic seizures with intellectual, neuropsychological, emotional, and social function in patients with epilepsy. *Epilepsia*. 1986;**27**:399–411.

40. Hermann B, Jones J, Dabbs K, *et al.* The frequency, complications, and aetiology of ADHD in new onset paediatric epilepsy. *Brain*. 2007;**130**:3135–48.

41. Kauffman R, Goldberg-Stern H, Shuper A. Attention-deficit disorders and epilepsy in childhood: incidence, causative relations and treatment possibilities. *J Child Neurol*. 2009;**24**:727–33.

42. Sweet JJ, Meyer DG, Nelson NW, Moberg PJ. The TCN/AACN 2010 "salary survey": professional practices, beliefs, and incomes of U.S. neuropsychologists. *Clin Neuropsychol*. 2011;**25**:12–61.

43. Wechsler D. *Manual for the Wechsler Intelligence Scale for Children – Fourth Edition*. New York, NY: Psychological Corporation; 2008.

44. Wechsler D. *Manual for the Wechsler Preschool and Primary Scale of Intelligence – Third Edition*. New York, NY: Psychological Corporation; 2002.

45. Wechsler D. *Manual for the Wechsler Adult Intelligence Scale – Fourth Edition*. New York, NY: Psychological Corporation; 2003.

46. Thorndike RL, Hagen EP, Sattler JM. *The Stanford-Binet Intelligence Scale, Fourth Edition: Guide for Administering and Score*. Chicago, IL: Riverside Publishing Company; 1986.

47. Kaufman AS. *Kaufman Brief Intelligence Test: KBIT*. Circle Pines, MN: American Guidance Service; 1990.

48. Kaufman AS. *Kaufman Adolescent and Adult Intelligence Test (KAIT)*. Circle Pines, MN: American Guidance Service; 1993.

49. Wechsler D. *Wechsler Abbreviated Scale of Intelligence*. New York, NY: Psychological Corporation; 1999.

50. Conners CK, MHS Staff. *Conners' Continuous Performance Test II CPT II Computer Program for Windows Technical Guide and Software Manual*. North Tonawanda, NY: Multi-Health Systems Inc.; 2000.

51. Greenberg L, Leark RA, Dupuy TR, Corman C, Kindschi CL. *Test of Variables of Attention, Version 8 (TOVA 8) Professional Manual*. Los Alamitos, CA: The TOVA Company; 2012.

52. Gordon M. *The Gordon Diagnostic Systems*. DeWitt, NY: Gordon Systems; 1983.

53. Epstein JN, Erkanli A, Conners CK, *et al.* Relations between continuous performance test performance measures and ADHD behaviors. *J Abnorm Child Psychol*. 2003;**31**:543–54.

54. Doyle AE, Biederman J, Seidman LJ, Weber W, Faraone SV. Diagnostic efficiency of neuropsychological test scores for discriminating boys with and without attention deficit–hyperactivity disorder. *J Consult Clin Psychol*. 2000;**68**:477–88.

55. Stuss DT, Alexander MP, Hamer L, *et al.* The effects of focal anterior and posterior brain lesions on verbal fluency. *J Int Neuropsychol Soc*. 1998;**4**:265–78.

56. Rascovsky K, Salmon DP, Hansen LA, Thal LJ, Galasko D. Disparate letter and semantic category fluency deficits in autopsy confirmed frontotemporal dementia and Alzheimer's disease. *Neuropsychology*. 2007;**21**:20–30.

57. Reitan RM. Validity of the Trail Making test as an indicator of organic brain damage. *Percept Mot Skills*. 1958;**8**:271–6.

58. Golden CJ, Freshwater SM. *Stroop Color and Word Test: Revised Examiner's Manual*. Wood Dale, IL: Stoelting Co.; 2002.

59. Golden CJ, Freshwater SM, Golden Z. *Stroop Color and Word Test Children's Version for Ages 5–14*. Wood Dale, IL: Stoelting Co.; 2003.

60. Heaton RK, Chelune GJ, Talley JL, Kay GG, Curtis G. *Wisconsin Card Sorting Test (WCST) manual, revised and expanded*. Odessa, FL: Psychological Assessment Resources; 1993.

61. DeFilippis NA, McCampbell E. *Manual for the Booklet Category Test*. Odessa, FL: Psychological Assessment Resources; 1997.

62. Shallice T. Specific impairments of planning. *Philos Trans R Soc Lond B Biol Sci*. 1982;**298**:199–209.

63. Glosser G, Goodglass H. Disorders in executive control functions among aphasic and other rain-damaged subjects. *J Clin Exp Neuropsychol*. 1990;**12**:485–501.

64. Delis DC, Kaplan E, Kramer JH. *Delis-Kaplan Executive Function System*. San Antonio, TX: The Psychological Corporation; 2001.

65. Korkman M, Kirk U, Kemp S. *NEPSY–Second Edition (NEPSY II)*. San Antonio, TX: The Psychological Corporation; 2007.

66. Benton AL, Hamsher K deS, Sivan AB. *Multilingual Aphasia Examination*, 3rd edn. San Antonio, TX: Psychological Corporation; 1994.

67. Kaplan EF, Goodglass H, Weintraub S. *The Boston Naming Test*, 2nd edn. Philadelphia, PA: Lippincott Williams & Wilkins; 2001.

68. Benton AL, Sivan AB, Hamsher K deS, Varney NR, Spreen O. *Contributions to Neuropsychological Assessment*, 2nd edn. Orlando, FL: Psychological Assessment Resources; 1994.

69. Rey A. "L'examen psychologique dans les cas d'encephalopathie traumatique. (Les Problems)." *Arch Psychol*. 1941;**28**:215–85.

70. Osterrieth PA. Le test de copie d'une figure complexe. *Arch Psychol*. 1944;**30**:206–356.

71. Fama R, Marsh L, Sullivan E. Dissociation of remote and anterograde memory impairment and neural correlates in alcoholic Korsakoff syndrome. *J Int Neuropsychol Soc*. 2004;**10**:427–41.

72. Speedie L, Heilman K. Anterograde memory deficits for visuospatial material after infarction of the right thalamus. *Arch Neurol*. 1983;**40**:183–6.

73. Delis DC, Kramer JH, Kaplan E, Ober BA. *California Verbal Learning Test – Second Edition, Adult Version*. San Antonio, TX: The Psychological Corporation; 2000.

74. Cohen MJ. *Children's Memory Scale*. San Antonio, TX: The Psychological Corporation; 1997.

75. Sheslow D, Adams W. *Wide Range Assessment of Memory and Learning, Second Edition administration and technical manual*. Wilmington, DE: Wide Range; 2003.

76. Wechsler D. *Wechsler Memory Scale – Fourth Edition*. San Antonio, TX: Pearson; 2009.

77. Bradshaw JL, Sheppard DM. The neurodevelopmental frontostriatal disorders: evolutionary adaptiveness and anomalous lateralization. *Brain Lang*. 2000;**73**(2): 297–320.

78. Harvey WJ, Reid G. Attention-deficit/hyperactivity disorder: a review of research on movement skill performance and physical fitness. *Adapt Phys Activ Q*. 2003;**20**:1–25.

79. Heaton RK, Grant I, Matthews C. *Comprehensive Norms for an Expanded Halstead-Reitan Neuropsychological Battery: Demographic Corrections, Research Findings, and Clinical Applications*. Odessa, FL: Psychological Assessment Resources, Inc.; 1991.

80. Tiffin J. *Purdue Pegboard: Examiner Manual*. Chicago: Science Research Associates; 1968.

81. Endicott J, Spitzer RL. A diagnostic interview: the schedule for affective disorders and schizophrenia. *Arch Gen Psychiatry*. 1978;**35**:837–44.

82. Puig-Antich J, Chambers W. *The Schedule for Affective Disorders and Schizophrenia for School-Age Children (Kiddie-SADS)*. New York, NY: New York State Psychiatric Institute; 1978.

83. Conners CK. *Conners 3rd Edition (Conners 3)*. North Tonawanda, NY: Multi-Health Systems, Inc.; 2008.

84. Reynolds CR, Kamphaus RW. *Behavior Assessment System for Children*, 2nd edn. Circle Pines, MN: American Guidance Service; 2004.

85. Butcher JN, Dahlstrom WG, Graham JR, Tellegen A, Kraemmer B. *The Minnesota Multiphasic Personality Inventory – 2 (MMPI-2): Manual for Administration and Scoring*. Minneapolis, MN: University of Minnesota Press; 1989.

86. Butcher JN, Williams CL, Graham JR, *et al*. *The Minnesota Multiphasic Personality Inventory – Adolescent Version (MMPI-A): Manual for Administration and Scoring*. Minneapolis, MN: University of Minnesota Press; 1992.

87. March J. *MASC 2: Multidimensional Anxiety Scale for Children, Second Edition*. North Tonawanda, NY: Multi-Health Systems Inc.; 2012.

88. Beck AT, Steer RA. *Beck Anxiety Inventory*. San Antonio, TX: The Psychological Corporation; 1993.

89. Kovacs M. *Children's Depression Inventory Manual*. North Tonawanda, NY: Multi-Health Systems, Inc.; 1992.

90. Beck AT, Steer RA, Brown GK. *Beck Depression Inventory*, 2nd edn. San Antonio, TX: The Psychological Corporation; 1996.

91. Morgan JE, Sweet JJ, eds. *Neuropsychology of Malingering Casebook*. New York, NY: Psychology Press/AACN; 2009.

92. Woodcock RW, McGrew KS, Mather N. *Woodcock-Johnson-III Tests of Achievement*. Itasca, IL: Riverside Publishing; 2001.

93. Wechsler D. *Wechsler Individual Achievement Test – Third Edition*. San Antonio, TX: NCS Pearson; 2009.

94. Wiederholt JL, Bryant BR. *Gray Oral Reading Test (5th edition)*. Austin, TX: PRO-ED; 2012.

95. Torgeson JK, Wagner RK, Rashotte CA. *Test of Word Reading Efficiency, 2nd Edition*. Austin, TX: Pro-Ed, Inc.; 2012.

Chapter 18

ADHD diagnostic and symptom assessment scales for adults

Lenard A. Adler, David M. Shaw, and Samuel Alperin

Although the diagnostic criteria for attention-deficit hyperactivity disorder (ADHD) were originally intended for children [1, 2], the criteria are the same for adults and can be reliably used to diagnose individuals who are currently experiencing symptoms of the disorder and have a history of these symptoms since early childhood [3, 4]. It is also necessary to document impairment in professional, academic, and personal settings and that the symptoms are due primarily to ADHD and not to another psychiatric condition or other environmental or personal circumstances. Rating scales can be quite helpful for documenting symptoms (ADHD symptom scales) or for more structured evaluations which can be used in fully establishing the diagnosis. A further utility of ADHD adult symptom scales can be in monitoring the response to treatment.

There are several diagnostic interviews and symptom rating scales that can be used in the clinical evaluation of adults for ADHD (Tables 18.1 and 18.2), which are generally economical and effective in obtaining a large amount of data quickly, including symptom severity and response to treatment. Many of these measures include adult-specific prompts and probes designed to assess the impact and severity of ADHD symptoms using a semi-structured interview, which is particularly advantageous for clinicians who have limited experience in working with adult ADHD patients. There are also measures that assess ADHD-related impairments in executive function (EF), emotional regulation (ER), occupational, and quality-of-life domains.

Adult ADHD diagnostic scales

A number of available scales can be used to assist in the diagnosis of adult ADHD.

The Conners' Adult ADHD Diagnostic Interview for DSM-IV (CAADID) is a semi-structured interview that assesses ADHD in adults using the *Diagnostic and Statistical Manual of Mental Disorders,* fourth edition (DSM-IV) criteria [5]. The CAADID is administered in two parts. Part I collects comprehensive information about the patient's demographic history, developmental course, risk factors for ADHD symptoms, and comorbid psychopathology [5]. Part I consists of questions that are primarily in a yes/no format and can be completed by either the patient or clinician. Part II is administered by a trained clinician and is designed to determine if the patient meets DSM-IV Criteria A–D for ADHD [5]. Part II is divided into three sections. The first two sections evaluate the presence, age of onset, and pervasiveness of all 18 DSM-IV symptoms of inattention and hyperactivity–impulsivity, respectively. Each symptom is accompanied by specific examples of typical behaviors related to the manifestation of that symptom in order to increase diagnostic reliability. The third section assesses the impairment caused by the symptoms endorsed in the first two sections. Clinicians are also provided with a checklist and space at the end of the interview for recording behaviors observed during the interview that are either consistent or inconsistent with ADHD. DSM-IV Criterion E regarding differential diagnosis of ADHD is assessed using information gathered in Part I, which can be supplemented with a separate clinical interview, such as the Structured Clinical Interview for DSM-IV-TR Axis I Disorders (SCID-I) [6]. The CAADID has been shown to have good test–retest reliability and concurrent validity [7] and has been used in a number of clinical trials of adult ADHD [8–13].

The Adult ADHD Clinician Diagnostic Scale version 1.2 (ACDS v1.2) is a semi-structured clinician-administered interview that is designed to assess

Attention-Deficit Hyperactivity Disorder in Adults and Children, ed. Lenard A. Adler, Thomas J. Spencer and Timothy E. Wilens. Published by Cambridge University Press. © Cambridge University Press 2015.

Table 18.1. Adult ADHD diagnostic rating scales

Scale	Description	Source
Conners' Adult ADHD Diagnostic Interview for DSM-IV (CAADID) [5]	Clinician-administered, semi-structured interview designed to assess ADHD in adults using the DSM-IV criteria. Assesses the presence, age of onset, pervasiveness, and impairment of all 18 DSM-IV symptoms of ADHD, as well as demographic history, developmental course, ADHD risk factors, and comorbid psychopathology	Multi-Health Systems, Inc.; www.mhs.com
Adult ADHD Clinician Diagnostic Scale (ACDS v1.2) [3]	Clinician-administered interview designed to retrospectively assess ADHD symptoms in childhood and adult symptoms in the past 6 months. Suggested prompts are paired with each symptom domain in the adult section that are designed to ensure adequate probing of the impact and severity of the symptoms in an adult-specific context	New York University School of Medicine; adultADHD@nyumc.org
Barkley Adult ADHD Rating Scale-IV (BAARS-IV) [19]	Assesses 18 items that correspond to the DSM-IV ADHD symptom domains. Available in four versions: DSM-IV ADHD symptom domains: Self-Report Current Symptoms, Self-Report Childhood Symptoms, Other Report Current Symptoms, and Other Report Childhood Symptoms. The Current Symptom versions include 9 additional items that assess symptoms of sluggish cognitive tempo. Childhood versions retrospectively assess childhood symptoms from ages 5 to 12. Scores from the Self-Report versions can be compared to normative data	The Guilford Press; http://www.guilford.com/
Adult ADHD Symptoms Scale [20]	Earlier version of the BAARS-IV. Assesses 18 items that correspond to the DSM-IV ADHD symptom domains and functional impairment in 10 life domains. Informant-report version available and can be used to retrospectively assess childhood symptoms from ages 5 to 12	In *Attention Deficit Hyperactivity Disorder: A Handbook for Diagnosis and Treatment*, 3rd edn.; The Guilford Press; http://www.guilford.com/
Brown ADD Scale Diagnostic Form [21]	Comprehensive assessment that collects information about the DSM-IV ADHD symptoms as well as the individual's clinical history, psychiatric comorbidities, family history, physical health, drug use, sleep habits, and functional and social impairments. The information is combined with the results from the Brown ADD Rating Scale	The Psychological Corporation; http://www.pearsonclinical.com/education/products/100000456/brown-attention-deficit-disorder-scales-brownaddscales.html?Pid=015-8029-240
ADHD module of the Kiddie Schedule for Affective Disorders and Schizophrenia (K-SADS) [23]	Includes prompts that can be used to assess adult ADHD according to DSM-IV criteria; utility in adults is limited because questions often refer to childhood-specific situations	University of Pittsburgh, Department of Psychiatry; http://www.psychiatry.pitt.edu/research/tools-research/ksads-pl
Diagnostic Interview for ADHD in Adults (DIVA) [24]	Clinician-administered structured interview designed to assess ADHD in adults using the DSM-IV criteria. Includes sections for 18 symptoms, age-of-onset, and five areas of impairment affected by ADHD. Includes examples (both childhood and adulthood) for each of the symptoms as well as areas of impairment. Available in English and Dutch online for free for clinicians and non-commercial researchers	DIVA Foundation; http://www.divacenter.eu/

and document childhood and adult ADHD symptoms. The interview begins with a retrospective childhood assessment of ADHD using the module adapted from the Kiddie Schedule for Affective Disorders and Schizophrenia (K-SADS) followed by an assessment of the 18 DSM-IV ADHD symptoms in the past 6 months. Each symptom domain in the adult assessment includes suggested prompts for clinicians that are intended to probe for the impact and severity of these symptoms in an adult-specific context. The prompts were developed for use in adult ADHD assessment and treatment research [3] but have been validated in the re-examination of the prevalence of adult ADHD in the National Comorbidity Survey Replication (NCS-R) [14] and a variety of treatment trials [15–17]. Consistent with DSM-IV, the ACDS v1.2 also requires

Table 18.2. ADHD symptom assessment, quality of life and functional impairment scales

Scale	Description
SYMPTOM SCALES	
Brown ADD Scale for Adults (BADDS) [21]	Developed before the DSM-IV. Assesses the frequency (0 = never, 1 = once a week, 2 = twice a week, or 3 = almost daily) of 40 items across these five symptom domains: organizing work, inattention, sustaining alertness and energy, managing frustration and other affective interference, and using working memory. This scale has been normed, standardized, and validated via clinician and patient rating and can yield a subset of scores, including executive function [48]*
Conners' Adult ADHD Rating Scales (CAARS) [49]	Include a self-report and observer-rated scale that have been developed into long, short, and screening versions. Measures DSM-IV criteria symptoms as well as specific manifestations of ADHD, such as mood lability. Both versions of this scale have been validated and normed [36]. The CAARS-Investigator (CAARS-INV) is clinician administered and contains 30 items that assesses the 18 DSM-IV criteria symptoms, as well as specific manifestations of ADHD, on a 4-point Likert scale (0 = not at all, never; 1 = just a little, once in a while; 2 = pretty much, often; and 3 = very much, very frequently) that combines frequency and severity [8]†
Wender–Reimherr Adult Attention Deficit Disorder Scale (WRAADDS) [9, 38]	This 28-item scale is based on the Utah Criteria [37] for adult ADHD. It assesses the severity of seven symptom domains: difficulties sustaining attention, disorganization, hyperactivity and restlessness, impulsivity, temper, mood lability, and emotional overreactivity. The individual items are rated on a scale from 0 to 2 (0 = not present, 1 = mild, 2 = clearly present), and the seven categories are summarized on a scale from 0 to 4 (0 = none, 4 = very much)‡
ADHD Rating Scale-IV (ADHD-RS-IV) [28]	This 18-item scale is derived from the DSM-IV criteria symptoms. It uses a 4-point, Likert severity scale (0 = none, 3 = severe). Can be divided into two subscales to measure either inattentive or hyperactive/impulsive symptoms. This scale was developed and standardized for use with children, but clinicians can be trained to use it with adults. It can be paired with the prompts from the adult component of the ACDS [3], which has been shown to be sensitive to drug effects in clinical trials of adults [15–17]
Adult ADHD Investigator Symptom Rating Scale (AISRS) [29]	This 18-item rating scale integrates symptom frequency, severity, and pervasiveness to assess each DSM-IV criterion on a 4-point Likert scale (0 = none, 3 = severe). The AISRS items are paired with prompts from the adult component of the ACDS and improve on aspects of the ADHD-RS. The AISRS uses adult-specific stem questions that aid clinicians in providing a context basis to the core symptom domains. For example, the symptom "difficulty waiting" in the ADHD-RS becomes "difficulty waiting your turn in situations when turn taking is required" in the AISRS. Also, "double-barreled" questions in the ADHD-RS that assess two symptom domains are replaced in the AISRS by questions that assess only one domain. For example, "difficulty playing quietly or engaging in leisure activities quietly" has been replaced by "difficulty unwinding or relaxing when you have time to yourself." The AISRS has been shown sensitive to drug effects in clinical trials of adults [50, 51]
Adult ADHD Self-Report Scale (ASRS) v1.1 Symptom Checklist [39, 52]	This 18-item, self-report scale derived from the DSM-IV criteria for ADHD is used to screen and identify adults using modified language to reflect the adult presentation of ADHD and to provide a context basis for the symptoms. The scale was developed by an adult ADHD workgroup for the World Health Organization. Respondents rate the frequency of each symptom on a scale of 0 (none) to 4 (very often)§
Adult Self-Report Scale (ASRS) Screener [39, 41]	This screening version of the 18-item ASRS Symptom Checklist is a self-administered scale consisting of the six symptoms of ADHD psychometrically determined to be most predictive of the disorder [39]. The ASRS Screener has shown good sensitivity and specificity and has a positive predictive value between 57% and 93% [39, 41]. In order for respondents to screen positively, they must rate at least four of the six symptoms as occurring significantly. The ASRS Screener should be used first to identify individuals who may be at risk for ADHD and then the ASRS Symptom Checklist should be used as a follow-up measure. The ASRS Screener can be found on the WHO website or at http://psych.med.nyu.edu/adhd-self-assessment-tools-and-information
QUALITY OF LIFE AND FUNCTIONAL IMPAIRMENT	
Adult ADHD Quality of Life (AAQoL) scale [42]	Consists of 29 items that assess the following quality-of-life domains on a 5-point scale (from "not at all" to "extremely"): life productivity, psychological health, relationships, and life outlook. The AAQoL was validated in a retrospective study of 989 adults [42]
ADHD Impact Module for Adults (AIM-A) [44]	Consists of five multi-item domains scored on a 5-point scale, along with questions on quality of life, and economic impact. The AIM-A has shown high correlation with the ADHD-RS, high validity, and also an ability to discriminate amongst the ADHD population based on severity, subtype, medication history, and sensitivity to change

Table 18.2. *(cont.)*

Scale	Description
Barkley Functional Impairment Scales (BFIS) [45]	Consists of Long-Form (LF) and Quick-Form (QF), both with self-report and other-reports. The LF consists of 15 domains of impairment while the QF only has 6, all of which are rated on a 0–9 scale (or 99 for "Does not apply"). BFIS includes normative data, has been validated with 1249 adults, and has a high reliability
Weiss Functional Impairment Rating Scale Self-Report (WFIRS-S) [46, 47]	Frequency/severity based scale ("0" – "never or not at all," "1" – "sometimes or somewhat," "2" – "often or much," "3" – "very often or very much," and "n/a" – "not applicable"), with domains in family, work, school, life skills, social and self-concept and risk, with 8 to 14 questions in each domain. Items which rate "2" or "3" are considered to denote significant impairment. Impairment for each of the domains noted above is characterized by two items rating "2" or "3" or one item scoring a "3" in the domain in question

* The Wechsler Adult Intelligence Scale can be used with the Brown Scale to aid in establishing an ADHD diagnosis.
† The CAARS total ADHD symptom score with adult ADHD prompts (the 18 DSM-IV symptoms of ADHD from the CAARS-INV) and ADHD symptom subscale scores (the nine inattentive and nine hyperactive/impulsive symptoms) have been shown to successfully assess the treatment response to atomoxetine in adult ADHD clinical trials [8, 53].
‡ A recent clinical trial of atomoxetine showed the WRAADDS to be sensitive to drug effects in the improvement of mood lability and dysregulation in adults with ADHD [9].
§ A recent study of 60 adults with ADHD found the ASRS to have high internal consistency and concurrent validity with the clinician-administered ADHD-RS [52]. The ASRS can be found at http://psych.med.nyu.edu/adhd-self-assessment-tools-and-information.

respondents to have at least some symptoms of ADHD before the age of 7, some impairment in at least two domains of functioning in the past 6 months due to the ADHD symptoms, and clinically significant impairment in at least one domain of functioning in the same period linked to the ADHD symptoms. Finally, a clinician evaluation or structured clinical interview, such as the SCID-I [18], should be used to rule out other psychiatric conditions that may account for the symptoms. The ACDS v1.2 has also been updated to allow assessment via DSM-IV and DSM-5 criteria.

The Barkley Adult ADHD Rating Scale-IV (BAARS-IV) assesses 18 items that correspond to the DSM-IV ADHD symptom domains as well as 9 additional items that assess symptoms of sluggish cognitive tempo (SCT) [19]. Symptoms of SCT include being prone to daydreaming, trouble staying awake and alert, being easily confused or bored, lethargy, and trouble processing information quickly [19]. Each item is rated for the past 6 months on a 4-point scale (1 = never or rarely; 2 = sometimes; 3 = often; 4 = very often) and information on age of onset and impairment domains is also collected. A total current ADHD symptom score is calculated as well as four subscale scores – Inattention, Hyperactivity, Impulsivity, and SCT – which can then be compared with normative data for the respondent's age group to obtain a percentile score [19]. The BAARS-IV is available in four versions: Self-Report Current Symptoms, Self-Report Childhood Symptoms, Other Report Current Symptoms, and Other Report Childhood Symptoms. The Childhood versions of the BAARS-IV

retrospectively assess the 18 DSM-IV symptoms of ADHD from ages 5 to 12 and do not contain the additional SCT symptoms. The BAARS-IV Other Report Forms allow clinicians to obtain ratings from an adult who knows the respondent well. Normative Data is not available for the Other Report Forms [19].

The earlier version of the BAARS-IV, the Adult ADHD Symptoms Scale, assessed 18 items that correspond to the DSM-IV ADHD symptom domains using a similar 4-point Likert scale [20]. However, the Adult ADHD Symptoms Scale contained a separate section that asked respondents to rate the degree of impairment they experienced from any ADHD symptoms in 10 life domains including school, relationships, work, and home life. The Adult ADHD Symptoms Scale also included informant-report versions and could be completed for a retrospective assessment of childhood ADHD symptoms from ages 5 to 12 [20]. These scales, along with assessments of developmental history, employment, medical health, social history, and driving behaviors can be combined in performing a structured diagnostic ADHD assessment in adults [20].

The Brown ADD Diagnostic Form is a comprehensive assessment that gathers information about the DSM-IV ADHD symptoms as well as clinical and family history, psychopathology, comorbidities, physical health, drug use, sleep habits, IQ, and impairments with work, school, leisure, peer interactions, and self-image [21]. Other assessments can be used to assess deficits in cognitive EF. A diagnosis is established by evaluating all of these data together with the results from the 40-item Brown ADD Rating Scale [21, 22].

The K-SADS module on ADHD includes extensive prompts that clinicians can use to assess for ADHD in adults according to the DSM-IV criteria. However, its use with adults is limited as the questions were developed for use with pediatric patients as they use childhood-based language [3, 23].

The Diagnostic Interview for ADHD in Adults (DIVA) is based on the 18 items for an ADHD diagnosis in the DSM-IV and is the first structured Dutch interview for ADHD in adults [24]. The DIVA includes three sections: (1) Criteria for Attention Deficits, (2) Criteria for Hyperactivity–Impulsivity, and (3) Age-of-Onset and Impairments due to the ADHD. Each of the 18 items provides a list of examples for both current and childhood to help the patient further understand the item and compare themselves to others. The impairments section also provides examples (for both adulthood and childhood) of how ADHD can affect the five major areas of work/education, relationships and family life, social contacts, free time and hobbies, and self-confidence/self-image.

Adult ADHD symptom assessment scales

Current-symptom surveys can be divided into clinician-administered and self-report forms. A number of the self-reported scales are normed and can provide population comparisons. Self-report scales are an effective way to capture the symptoms of adults with ADHD, as symptoms such as internalized restlessness, feeling disorganized, and distraction may be more readily apparent to the patient than to observers [25]. Semi-structured scales are also useful when assessing new patients who may be less aware about their symptoms as they allow the use of an extensive list of example prompts to establish a comprehensive baseline for impairment. Some scales adhere more strictly to the DSM-IV-TR symptom domains, whereas others expand the adult ADHD symptomatology to include assessment of mood regulation and EF [3].

The ADHD Rating Scale IV, Investigator Administered and Scored (ADHD-RS-IV), is a clinician-administered scale that is designed to assess current symptomatology. The ADHD-RS-IV consists of 18 items that directly correspond to the DSM-IV symptoms of ADHD and each item is scored on a 4-point

Likert scale ranging from 0 (none) to 3 (severe) using a combined rating of frequency and severity [26]. The ADHD-RS-IV was originally standardized for use in children [26, 27] but has been shown to be sensitive to drug effects in adults with ADHD [15, 16]. The prompts from the adult module of the ACDS v1.2 can be paired with each item of the ADHD-RS-IV to enable raters to probe for the impact and severity of ADHD symptomatology in an adult-specific context [28]. The ADHD-RS-IV with prompts has been shown to be a valid and reliable measure to assess ADHD in adults [17].

The Adult ADHD Investigator Symptom Rating Scale (AISRS) is another clinician-administered scale that assesses each DSM-IV symptom domain of ADHD. Similar to the ADHD-RS-IV, the AISRS consists of 18 items that are scored on a 4-point Likert scale (0 = none; 1 = mild; 2 = moderate; and 3 = severe) with a maximum total score of 54 and maximum scores of 27 for both the inattentive and hyperactive–impulsive subscales [29]. In addition to using the adult ADHD prompts from the ACDS v1.2, the AISRS stem questions are designed to better capture symptoms of the disorder presented in adulthood. The AISRS has been found to be a valid measure of medication response in adults with ADHD [29–31].

The Brown Attention-Deficit Disorder Scale (BADDS) for adults is a validated, normed 40-item self-report scale administered by a clinician (clinician-recorded responses). Each item is measured on a frequency-based scale (0 = never, 1 = once a week or less, 2 = twice a week, or 3 = almost daily) and can be grouped into five clusters of related ADHD symptoms: organizing and activating work; sustaining attention and concentration; sustaining energy and effort; managing affective interference; and utilizing working memory and accessing recall [21]. The BADDS can be used to assess ADHD-related EF, and has been previously used to evaluate EF in children and adults with ADHD [32–35].

The screening version of the Conners' Adult ADHD Rating Scale (CAARS) is a 30-item frequency scale with items such as "has difficulty organizing tasks and activities" and "is 'on the go' or acts as if 'driven by a motor.'" Symptoms are assessed on a combination of frequency and severity. Patients respond on a 4-point Likert-type scale (0 = not at all, never; 1 = just a little, once in a while; 2 = pretty much, often; and 3 = very much, very frequently). All 18 items from the DSM-IV can be extrapolated from the CAARS. There are also observer and self-report versions of the CAARS. Both the clinician-administered and self-rated versions of this scale have been validated. The self-rated version of the CAARS has been normed [36].

The Wender–Reimherr Adult Attention Deficit Disorder Scale (WRAADDS) is a clinician-administered scale based on the Utah Criteria [37] for adult ADHD. It assesses the severity of the seven ADHD symptom domains of the Utah Criteria using 27 individual items: attention difficulties, hyperactivity, affective lability, disorganization, temper, emotional overreactivity, and impulsivity. The individual items are rated on a scale from 0 to 2 (0 = not present, 1 = mild, 2 = clearly present), and the seven categories are summarized on a scale from 0 (none) to 4 (very much) [9, 38].

The Adult ADHD Self-Report Scales (ASRS) consist of a 6-item screening tool for general use and an 18-item symptom checklist for patients who might be at risk. These scales were developed by the workgroup on adult ADHD and are copyrighted by the World Health Organization. The ASRS has been translated into 24 languages. The ASRS is free and available on the NYU (http://psych.med.nyu.edu/adhd-self-assessment-tools-and-information) and Harvard School of Public Health (http://www.hcp.med.harvard.edu/ncs/asrs.php) websites. The ASRS symptom checklist asks patients about the 18 symptom domains identified in the DSM-IV, modified to reflect the adult presentation of ADHD symptoms, with a context basis of symptoms provided. Symptoms are rated on a frequency basis, ranging from 0 (none) to 4 (very often) [39]. There is also an expanded version of the ASRS v1.1 symptom checklist, which includes 14 additional ADHD-related symptoms of EF and emotional control which have been validated versus the ACDS v1.2 [40]. The 6-item screening version, the ASRS v1.1 screener (extracted from the full 18-item symptom assessment scale), is available for assessing patients in the community to establish whether they are at increased risk for ADHD and is designed to be used before the symptom checklist [39]. The six items in the ASRS Screener were selected based on psychometric factor analyses of the diagnostic interviews of patients with and without ADHD in the NCS-R [39, 41].

Neither the 6-item ASRS v1.1 screener nor the full ASRS 18-item symptom assessment version is meant to be a stand-alone diagnostic tool. The diagnosis of ADHD remains predicated on assessment of current symptoms, impairment, and childhood onset of symptoms. The ASRS symptom checklist and other symptom assessment tools are designed to assess the breadth of ADHD symptoms in fulfilling the first criteria. The ASRS Screener has shown good sensitivity and specificity and has a positive predictive value between 57% and 93% [39, 41].

The BAARS-IV and earlier scales assess ADHD symptoms, but have been described above in the section on diagnostic assessments as they can be used as part of a structured diagnostic assessment of adult ADHD [20].

Quality of life and functional impairment assessments

Assessments of impairment are part of the core DSM-IV and DSM-5 related diagnostic criteria. Additionally, assessment of quality of life can assist the clinician in establishing the impact and consequences of adult ADHD. There are two major scales in each of these categories of assessments.

The Adult ADHD Quality of Life (AAQoL) scale, which is in development, is a current-symptom psychometric scale that identifies and assesses five ADHD-related quality-of-life domains: daily activities, work, psychological well-being, physical well-being, and relationships [42]. The AAQoL consists of 29 self-rated items encompassing these five domains. Respondents rate each item on a 5-point scale, from "not at all" to "extremely." The AAQoL assists clinicians in determining the impact of ADHD symptomatology and of treatment on quality of life [42]. The AAQoL has been used to assess changes in quality of life in a number of adult ADHD treatment trials [43].

The ADHD Impact Module for Adults (AIM-A) is another current-symptom psychometric scale which includes five multi-item domains to assess the impact of ADHD [44]. The five domains include Living with ADHD, General Well-Being, Performance and Daily-Life (for home, work, and school), Relationships and Communication, and Impact of Symptoms (both emotional, including bothersome and concern, and daily interference), and within which each item is scored on a 5-point scale. The AIM-A also includes four questions assessing the limitations ADHD has put on the individual's life goals and achievements. Lastly, the scale includes questions on the economic impact (e.g., days of missed work, number of motor vehicle accidents), demographics (e.g., marital status, age), and medical questions (e.g., comorbidities, medication history). The AIM-A has been shown to have a moderate correlation with the ADHD-RS (>0.34), high validity, and sensitivity to change [44].

The Barkley Functional Impairment Scale (BFIS) is available to aid identifying functional impairments resulting from mental disorders [45]. BFIS consists of both a Long-Form (LF, which includes a Self- and Other-report), and a Quick-Form (QF, also Self- and Other-reports). The LF includes 15 major-life activity domains, while the QF only includes six (i.e., self-care routines, home-chores, home-family, social-friends, education, and work). Furthermore, once the BFIS is completed, the clinician can follow up with the BFIS Impairment Interview, and discover reasons for the specific impairments that were rated greater than moderate. The BFIS has the benefit of over 16 years of work and a lot of normative data for adults from 18 to 96 years of age (n = 1249). Each of the domains on the BFIS is rated from 0 to 9 (0 = not at all, 1–2 = somewhat, 3–4 = mild, 5–7 = moderate, 8–9 = severe) or 99 for "Does not apply." Data are also provided (in the appendix to the BFIS forms) to allow the clinician to rate each impairment domain as well as total impairment score and Percent Domain Impairment score at a clinically significant level (judged to be at the 93rd–95th percentile, or above). The BFIS (both LF and QF) has high test–retest reliability, internal consistency, and validity and can be used both in clinical and research settings [45].

The Weiss Functional Impairment Rating Scale Self-Report (WFIRS-S) is another self-rating scale of functional impairment [46]. The WFIRS-S is a frequency/severity-based scale ("0" – "never or not at all," "1" – "sometimes or somewhat," "2" – "often or much," "3" – "very often or very much," and "n/a" – "not applicable"), with domains in family, work, school, life skills, social and self-concept and risk, with 8 to 14 questions in each domain. A mean overall impairment score can be assessed via the average score in endorsed items (excluding "n/a'). Items which rate "2" or "3" are considered to denote significant impairment, as compared to two to three standard deviations above the normative sample. Impairment for each of the domains noted above is characterized by two items rating "2" or "3" or one item scoring a "3" in the domain in question. The WFIRS-S has high internal consistency, is noted to have reasonable sensitivity to change and has mild to moderate correlations against an ADHD symptoms rating scale (the ADHD-RS-IV) [47].

Summary

Although some areas of understanding of adult ADHD remain limited, there is a strong sense of how to proceed with diagnosis, using current DSM-IV-TR criteria as a guide. A thorough clinical interview, aided by the use of rating scales for current symptoms, collateral information about childhood from parents or siblings, and the use of a clinical evaluation to determine cross-situationality, onset, impairment, and comorbidity, forms the backbone of the diagnostic assessment. The poor psychosocial outcomes of patients with ADHD, often a consequence of unrecognized, untreated disorder manifestation, can also serve as a diagnostic indicator. Accordingly, adult ADHD remains a valid clinical diagnosis, and the clinician-administered interview that adheres to the cardinal DSM-IV-TR or DSM-5 criteria for making the diagnosis remains the cornerstone of the diagnostic evaluation.

References

1. Lahey BB, Applegate B, McBurnett K, *et al*. DSM-IV field trials for attention deficit hyperactivity disorder in children and adolescents. *Am J Psychiatry*. 1994;**151**(11):1673–85.

2. Spitzer RL, Davies M, Barkley RA. The DSM-III-R field trial of disruptive behavior disorders. *J Am Acad Child Adolesc Psychiatry*. 1990;**29**(5):690–7.

3. Adler L, Cohen J. Diagnosis and evaluation of adults with attention-deficit/hyperactivity disorder. *Psychiatr Clin North Am*. 2004;**27**(2):187–201.

4. Faraone SV. The scientific foundation for understanding attention-deficit/hyperactivity disorder as a valid psychiatric disorder. *Eur Child Adolesc Psychiatry*. 2005;**14**(1):1–10.

5. Epstein JN, Johnson DE, Conners CK. *Conners' Adult ADHD Diagnostic Interview for DSM-IV*. North Tonawanda, NY: Multi-Health Systems, Inc.; 2001.

6. First MB, Gibbons M, Williams JBW, Spitzer RL. *SCID Screen Patient Questionnaire-Extended Version*. North Tonawanda, NY: Multi-Health Systems, Inc.; 1997.

7. Epstein JN, Kollins SH. Psychometric properties of an adult ADHD diagnostic interview. *J Atten Disord*. 2006;**9**(3):504–14.

8. Michelson D, Adler L, Spencer T, *et al*. Atomoxetine in adults with ADHD: two randomized, placebo-controlled studies. *Biol Psychiatry*. 2003;**53**(2):112–20.

9. Reimherr FW, Marchant BK, Strong RE, *et al.* Emotional dysregulation in adult ADHD and response to atomoxetine. *Biol Psychiatry.* 2005;**58**(2): 125–31.

10. Adler LA, Sutton VK, Moore RJ, *et al.* Quality of life assessment in adult patients with attention-deficit/hyperactivity disorder treated with atomoxetine. *J Clin Psychopharmacol.* 2006;**26**(6):648–52.

11. Adler LA, Liebowitz M, Kronenberger W, *et al.* Atomoxetine treatment in adults with attention-deficit/hyperactivity disorder and comorbid social anxiety disorder. *Depress Anxiety.* 2009;**26**(3):212–21.

12. Durell T, Adler L, Wilens T, Paczkowski M, Schuh K. Atomoxetine treatment for ADHD: younger adults compared with older adults. *J Atten Disord.* 2010;**13**(4):401–6.

13. Solanto MV, Marks DJ, Wasserstein J, *et al.* Efficacy of meta-cognitive therapy for adult ADHD. *Am J Psychiatry.* 2010;**167**(8):958–68.

14. Kessler RC, Adler L, Barkley R, *et al.* The prevalence and correlates of adult ADHD in the United States: results from the National Comorbidity Survey Replication. *Am J Psychiatry.* 2006;**163**(4): 716–23.

15. Wilens TE, Haight BR, Horrigan JP, *et al.* Bupropion XL in adults with attention-deficit/hyperactivity disorder: a randomized, placebo-controlled study. *Biol Psychiatry.* 2005;**57**(7):793–801.

16. Spencer TJ, Adler LA, Weisler RH, Youcha SH. Triple-bead mixed amphetamine salts (SPD465), a novel, enhanced extended-release amphetamine formulation for the treatment of adults with ADHD: a randomized, double-blind, multicenter, placebo-controlled study. *J Clin Psychiatr.* 2008;**69**(9):1437–48.

17. Adler LA, Spencer TJ, Biederman J, *et al.* The internal consistency and validity of the Attention-Deficit/Hyperactivity Disorder Rating Scale (ADHD-RS) with adult ADHD prompts as assessed during a clinical treatment trial. *J ADHD Relat Disord.* 2009;**1**(1): 14–24.

18. First MB, Spitzer RL, Gibbon M, Williams J. *Structured Clinical Interview for DSM-IV-TR Axis I Disorders-Patient Edition (SCID-I/P).* New York, NY: Biometrics Research Department, New York State Psychiatric Institute; 2002.

19. Barkley RA. *Barkley Adult ADHD Rating Scale-IV (BAARS-IV).* New York, NY: Guilford Press; 2011.

20. Barkley RA. *Attention-Deficit Hyperactivity Disorder: A Handbook for Diagnosis and Treatment*, 3rd edn. New York, NY: Guilford Press; 2005.

21. Brown TE. *Brown Attention-Deficit Disorder Scales for Adolescents and Adults.* San Antonio, TX: The Psychological Corporation; 1996.

22. Rösler M, Retz W, Thome J, *et al.* Psychopathological rating scales for diagnostic use in adults with attention-deficit/hyperactivity disorder (ADHD). *Eur Arch Psychiatry Clin Neurosci.* 2006;**256** (Suppl 1):i3–11.

23. Kaufman J, Birmaher B, Brent D, *et al.* Schedule for Affective Disorders and Schizophrenia for School-Age Children-Present and Lifetime Version (K-SADS-PL): initial reliability and validity data. *J Am Acad Child Adolesc Psychiatry.* 1997;**36**(7):980–8.

24. Kooij JJS. *Adult ADHD. Diagnostic Assessment and Treatment*, 3rd edn. New York, NY: Springer; 2012

25. O'Donnell JP, McCann KK, Pluth S. Assessing adult ADHD using a self-report symptom checklist. *Psychol Rep.* 2001;**88**(3 Pt 1):871–81.

26. DuPaul GJ, George J, Power TJ, Anastopoulos AD. *ADHD Rating Scale–IV: Checklists, Norms, and Clinical Interpretation.* New York, NY: Guilford Press; 1998.

27. Faries DE, Yalcin I, Harder D, Heiligenstein JH. Validation of the ADHD Rating Scale as a clinician administered and scored instrument. *J Atten Disord.* 2001;**5**(2):107–15.

28. Adler LA, Spencer T, Faraone SV, *et al.* Training raters to assess adult ADHD: reliability of ratings. *J Atten Disord.* 2005;**8**(3):121–6.

29. Spencer TJ, Adler LA, Qiao M, *et al.* Validation of the adult investigator symptom rating scale (AISRS). *J Atten Disord.* 2010;**14**(1):57–68.

30. Biederman J, Mick E, Spencer T, *et al.* An open-label trial of OROS methylphenidate in adults with late-onset ADHD. *CNS Spectr.* 2006;**11**(5):390–6.

31. Adler LA, Spencer T, Brown TE, *et al.* Once-daily atomoxetine for adult attention-deficit/hyperactivity disorder: a 6-month, double-blind trial. *J Clin Psychopharmacol.* 2009;**29**(1):44–50.

32. Hervey AS, Epstein JN, Curry JF. Neuropsychology of adults with attention-deficit/hyperactivity disorder: a meta-analytic review. *Neuropsychology.* 2004;**18**(3):485–503.

33. Brown TE, Landgraf JM. Improvements in executive function correlate with enhanced performance and functioning and health-related quality of life: evidence from 2 large, double-blind, randomized, placebo-controlled trials in ADHD. *Postgrad Med.* 2010;**122**(5):42–51.

34. Brown TE, Brams M, Gasior M, *et al.* Clinical utility of ADHD symptom thresholds to assess normalization of executive function with lisdexamfetamine dimesylate treatment in adults. *Curr Med Res Opin.* 2011;**27** (Suppl 2):23–33.

35. Brown TE, Holdnack J, Saylor K, *et al*. Effect of atomoxetine on executive function impairments in adults with ADHD. *J Atten Disord*. 2011;**15**(2): 130–8.

36. Van Voorhees EE, Hardy KK, Kollins SH. Reliability and validity of self- and other-ratings of symptoms of ADHD in adults. *J Atten Disord*. 2011;**15**(3):224–34.

37. Wender PH, Reimherr FW, Wood DR. Attention deficit disorder ('minimal brain dysfunction') in adults. A replication study of diagnosis and drug treatment. *Arch Gen Psychiatry*. 1981;**38**(4):449–56.

38. Wender PH. *Attention-Deficit Hyperactivity Disorder in Adults*. New York, NY: Oxford University Press; 1995.

39. Kessler RC, Adler L, Ames M, *et al*. The World Health Organization Adult ADHD Self-Report Scale (ASRS): a short screening scale for use in the general population. *Psychol Med*. 2005;**35**(2):245–56.

40. Kessler RC, Green JG, Adler LA, *et al*. Structure and diagnosis of adult attention-deficit/hyperactivity disorder: analysis of expanded symptom criteria from the Adult ADHD Clinical Diagnostic Scale. *Arch Gen Psychiatry*. 2010;**67**(11):1168–78.

41. Kessler RC, Adler LA, Gruber MJ, *et al*. Validity of the World Health Organization Adult ADHD Self-Report Scale (ASRS) Screener in a representative sample of health plan members. *Int J Methods Psychiatr Res*. 2007;**16**(2):52–65.

42. Brod M, Johnston J, Able S, Swindle R. Validation of the adult attention-deficit/hyperactivity disorder quality-of-life scale (AAQoL): a disease-specific quality-of-life measure. *Qual Life Res*. 2006;**15**(1): 117–29.

43. Matza LS, Johnston JA, Faries DE, Malley KG, Brod M. Responsiveness of the Adult Attention-Deficit/ Hyperactivity Disorder Quality of Life Scale (AAQoL). *Qual Life Res*. 2007;**16**(9):1511–20.

44. Langraf J. Monitoring quality of life in adults with ADHD : reliability and validity of a new measure.

J Atten Disord. 2007;**11**:351 originally published online May 9, 2007, DOI: 10.1177/1087054707299400.

45. Barkley R. *Barkley Functional Impairment Scale (BFIS for Adults)*. New York, NY: Guilford Press; 2011.

46. The Canadian Attention Deficit Hyperactivity Disorder Resource Alliance (CADDRA). Weiss Functional Impairment Rating Scale Self-Report (WFIRS-S). http://www.caddra.ca/cms4/pdfs/ caddraGuidelines2011WFIRS_S.pdf.

47. The Canadian Attention Deficit Hyperactivity Disorder Resource Alliance (CADDRA). Weiss Functional Impairment Rating Scale Self-Report (WFIRS-S) instructions. http://naceonline.com/ AdultADHDtoolkit/assessmenttools/wfirs.pdf.

48. Murphy KR, Adler LA. Assessing attention-deficit/ hyperactivity disorder in adults: focus on rating scales. *J Clin Psychiatry*. 2004;**65**(Suppl 3):12–17.

49. Conners CK, Erhardt D, Sparrow E. *Conners' Adult ADHD Rating Scales*. North Tonawanda, NY: Multi-Health Systems, Inc.; 1999.

50. Spencer T, Biederman J, Wilens T, *et al*. A large, double-blind, randomized clinical trial of methylphenidate in the treatment of adults with attention-deficit/hyperactivity disorder. *Biol Psychiatry*. 2005;**57**(5):456–63.

51. Biederman J, Mick E, Surman C, *et al*. A randomized, placebo-controlled trial of OROS methylphenidate in adults with attention-deficit/hyperactivity disorder. *Biol Psychiatry*. 2006;**59**(9):829–35.

52. Adler LA, Spencer T, Faraone SV, *et al*. Validity of pilot adult ADHD self-report scale (ASRS) to rate adult ADHD symptoms. *Ann Clin Psychiatry*. 2006;**18**(3):145–8.

53. Adler LA, Spencer TJ, Williams DW, Moore RJ, Michelson D. Long-term, open-label safety and efficacy of atomoxetine in adults with ADHD: final report of a 4-year study. *J Atten Disord*. 2008;**12**(3):248–53.

Chapter 19

Assessment of ADHD in children and adolescents

Mark A. Stein, Laura Hans, and Sonali Nanayakkara

Introduction

The diagnosis of attention-deficit hyperactivity disorder (ADHD) is not based upon a single scale, score, biomarker, or laboratory test. Despite dramatic advances in our understanding through neuroimaging and molecular genetic studies [1], ADHD is a clinical diagnosis, made by a clinician who weighs and evaluates the available data before making a determination that diagnostic criteria (i.e., *Diagnostic and Statistical Manual of Mental Disorders* [DSM]-IV, soon to be DSM-5 [2]) are fulfilled. In this chapter, we will review the diagnostic process and describe common measures, such as rating scales and interviews, which help clinicians diagnose ADHD and monitor treatment response.

Diagnostic process

The diagnostic process and purpose of assessment goes well beyond determining whether ADHD is present or absent. The diagnostic evaluation sets the stage for the development and implementation of a successful treatment plan. In addition to providing baseline information for the diagnostician and treatment team, it is also an opportunity to educate the family and school about the unique needs of the patient and course of the disorder, to establish appropriate expectations for treatment and measures of response, and to motivate the patient and family to participate in and adhere to treatment recommendations. Following the recommendations of Cantwell and Baker [3], the diagnostic evaluation should address the following questions [4].

1. Are ADHD symptoms present? Are they disparate from developmental norms or developmentally inappropriate?
2. Is there significant impairment?

3. Are the symptoms better accounted for by another psychiatric disorder (e.g., depression, intellectual disability, mental retardation), medical condition (e.g., see Chapter 13, hypothyroidism, obstructive sleep disorder, oral steroid) [5] or social mimics (inappropriate academic expectations for a preschooler, chaotic home or school environment) that can cause, exacerbate, or obscure the clinical presentation of ADHD?
4. What other comorbid disorders or associated problems are also present (e.g., oppositional defiant disorder [ODD], articulation disorders, enuresis, developmental coordination disorder)?
5. Are there potential etiological or risk factors present (e.g., marital dysfunction, parental psychopathology, ADHD in parents)?
6. What are the child's strengths and protective factors (e.g., perceptual skills, peer relationships, empathy)?

To gather the information necessary to answer these questions, a variety of procedures, including diagnostic interviews with the patient and their parents, physical exam, psychological and laboratory tests, and parent and teacher rating scales, are utilized [6]. In this chapter, we will focus specifically on rating scales and diagnostic interviews.

Rating scales: history and function

The history of ADHD and dimensional ratings of behavior are closely intertwined. Noteworthy is the pioneering work of C. Keith Conners, who developed a rating scale in 1969 that could be used to select patients for study and to evaluate stimulant effects [7]. Subsequently, numerous dimensional rating scales have been developed and they have had a dramatic impact

Attention-Deficit Hyperactivity Disorder in Adults and Children, ed. Lenard A. Adler, Thomas J. Spencer and Timothy E. Wilens.
Published by Cambridge University Press. © Cambridge University Press 2015.

on ADHD research and clinical practice. Indeed, the wide use of behavior rating scales has been associated with increased precision in making and informing categorical (i.e., DSM-5) definitions of the disorder in the past and currently [8–12].

Description and use of rating scales

Common practice guidelines for ADHD recommend the use of behavior rating scales [13–17]. Presently, there are numerous rating scales available to assess ADHD. As described by Hinshaw and Nigg [18], rating scales have numerous advantages, including: ease of use, ability to capture or describe behaviors that may not be observable in the clinic or office setting such as school behavior or attention, generally good to excellent test–retest stability, and strong internal consistency. Rating scales provide a quantifiable measure of frequency, duration, or severity that can be used for screening, to evaluate prevalence in different cultures [19], and to track treatment outcome or course [20–22].

As pointed out by Achenbach [23], the meaning of scores obtained from multi-informant ratings depends on comparisons with norms for the child's age and gender, the informant, and the context for assessment. For treatment outcome, it is best to utilize the same rater or informant who initially provided information about the child, so as not to introduce additional sources of variance.

When parents disagree on the severity of ADHD symptoms, it is useful to have ratings obtained from each parent and then determine potential reasons for the discrepancy in perception. It should be noted, for example, that maternal depression is associated with more severe parent ratings of childhood behavior [24–26]. Other factors to be considered when interpreting discrepant ratings from the same setting include different expectations for childhood behavior as well as differing frames of reference.

Administering both a parent and a teacher rating scale are recommended for diagnostic purposes, because parents and teachers have different expectation, frames of reference, and samples of children's behavior. Furthermore, utilizing multiple informants who see the child in different settings (i.e., home, school) addresses the DSM-5 requirement that the symptoms be present in more than one more setting [27]. Although adding to the complexity of the diagnostic process over use of a single scale or informant, it is important to survey and understand the context in which ratings are made, especially rater, setting, and perception differences. Indeed, utilizing information from multiple sources is a key component of evidence-based practice [28]. Although most rating scales of ADHD symptoms demonstrate moderate correlations between informants that see the child in the same setting, informant discrepancies are common [29].

A prototypical broadband scale is the parent-completed Child Behavior Checklist (CBCL), which, along with the Teacher Report Form (TRF), is a component of the Achenbach System of Empirically Based Assessment (ASEBA). The CBCL has a long history of use, especially in clinic-based studies of ADHD [30]. In addition to providing Internalizing, Externalizing, and Total scores, the CBCL has an empirically derived "attention problems" factor as well as a DSM-5 based ADHD factor score. Examples of other broadband scales are the Behavior Assessment System for Children, second edition [31], and the Conners' Comprehensive Behavior Rating Scales. Examples of frequently used narrowband scales include the ADHD-RS-IV [11, 32], ADHD Symptom Checklist, Conners 3, Swanson, Nolan, and Pelham IV Teacher and Parent Rating Scales (SNAP-IV), and Vanderbilt ADHD Diagnostic Parent/Teacher Rating Scales [33]. Each of these scales has detailed manuals describing their psychometric characteristics, age- and gender-based norms, and versions for different informants or settings. Several excellent reviews are available for more detailed descriptions of rating scales used to assess ADHD and their psychometric characteristics [16, 34, 35].

In a seminal review of ADHD assessment measures, Pelham *et al.* summarize the reliability and validity of DSM-IV-based (e.g., ADHD-RS, Vanderbilt), empirically based (Conners, CBCL), and rationally developed (Brown Attention-Deficit Disorder Scale [BADDS]) scales. Generally, these measures demonstrate strong agreement with each other and with other diagnostic measures [36]. Furthermore, for treatment planning and studies on the nature of ADHD, information on the context (i.e., antecedents, consequences, setting of symptoms, and impact on day-to-day functioning) should be obtained. Presently there are numerous rating scales available to assess ADHD (see Table 19.1).

For diagnostic and research purposes, a broader item pool is desirable as investigators have questioned

Table 19.1. Rating scales

Assessment scales	Parent(P)/teacher(T)/self-report(S)? Ages assessed?	Description
ADHD Rating Scale IV [64, 65]	P, T forms available for ages 5–18	This scale is based on DSM criteria; it has 18 items, and scores are compared to norms by age and gender. May be less well normed for older ages and Spanish version
ADHD symptom checklist 4 (ADHD-SC4) [66] Early Childhood Inventory 4R (FCI-4R) [67, 68] Youth Inventory (YI-4R) [69] for self-report	ADHD-SC4: ages 3–18; YI-4R: ages 12 and up; ECI-4R: ages 3–5	This is a 50-item assessment, which is used to screen for ADHD and ODD. It is useful for following response to treatment. This assessment also has a scale of medication side effects, and a Peer Conflict scale
Behavioral Assessment Scale for Children, 2nd edn. (BASC 2) [70]	P, T, S; ages 2–25	This is a broad-spectrum assessment tool, which includes questions addressing anxiety, depression, ADHD, social skills, learning problems, etc. Of interest, it includes both positive and negative trait evaluations
Behavioral Rating Inventory of Executive Functioning (BRIEF) and Behavioral Rating Inventory of Executive Functioning for Preschoolers (BRIEF-P) [71, 72]	P, T forms available for ages 2–5 for BRIEF-P; 5–18 for BRIEF	Children from urban, rural, and suburban homes, with mixed clinical diagnoses as well as non-referred. Factor analysis of symptoms puts the focus on behavior and executive functioning, rather than DSM criteria. Validity testing compared to BASC, CBCL, and ADHD-IV-P
Brown Attention-Deficit Disorder Scales for Children and Adults (Brown ADD scales) [63]	Ages 3–18 P, T for ages 3–7 P, T, S for ages 8–12 P, S for ages 13–18	Based on factor analysis rather than DSM per se; also emphasized executive functioning concept over ADHD
Conners' Early Childhood (Conners' EC) and Conners' Early Childhood – Behavior (EC BEH) [73]	P, T for ages 2–6	This is a broad-range assessment if used in its entirety (Conners' EC); the shorter scale, focused on behavior (EC BEH) has 17 items and screens for ADHD, ODD
Conners' 3rd edn. long and short forms [74]	P, T forms for ages 6–18; self-assessment for ages 8–18	This is the third edition of the classic Conners' assessment tool, normed on 7000 rating responses. The short form focuses on ADHD, while the long form also screens for other conditions, including ODD and anxiety
Conners' Comprehensive Behavior Rating Scales (CBRS) and Clinical Index (CI) [74, 75]	P, T forms for ages 6–18; S for ages 8–18	As indicated, this is a comprehensive survey of symptoms of multiple disorders, including ADHD, Asperger's, and symptom areas, such as violence and disturbing thoughts. The tool is meant to assist not only with diagnosis, but also with forming treatment plans and following the results; it is based on DSM-IV-TR criteria. The Conners' Clinical Index (CI) is shorter, and may be used for screening. Many of the scales are administered and/or scored online
Pediatric Attention Disorders Diagnostic Screener (PADDS), with a Rating Scale adopted from Swanson, Nolan, and Pelham (SNAP-IV) [76]	For ages 6–12	This assessment tool relies on accumulation of evidence from multiple sources and testing devices. The parent–teacher rating scales are only part of the evidence collected
Vanderbilt ADHD Diagnostic Parent Rating Scale and Teacher Rating Scale [77]	P, T for ages 6–12	Normed on 6591 children from grades 1 to 4 in urban, rural, and suburban Tennessee settings. It is freely available at http://www.brightfutures.org/mentalhealth/pdf/professionals/bridges/adhd.pdf. ODD, anxiety/depression, and academic problems are also addressed

whether the current item pool of DSM-5-based scales is too restricted, especially for a wider age range. For example, it has been advocated that sleep behaviors, sluggish cognitive tempo [37, 38], and emotional dysregulation [39, 40] are salient associated behaviors that may define important subgroups or developmental features of ADHD. Narrowband scales are best suited for screening for ADHD symptoms and monitoring treatment response, due to their brevity and limited burden on the rater. However, these scales are limited in their ability to detect changes in other domains which may be clinically significant, such as emotional reactivity, an emerging mood disorder, or improvement in self-esteem [40].

Choosing a rating scale

In choosing a rating scale, it is important to first consider the *purpose of the evaluation*. For diagnostic purposes, a longer instrument with broader content validity may be recommended so that ADHD symptoms as well as associated problems are identified. It may also be desirable to utilize a rating scale system that can be administered to different informants and tap information from different settings. However, for screening purposes or to use as an outcome measure that is repeated frequently, a shorter, "narrowband" scale of ADHD symptoms should be utilized.

The next step in choosing an instrument is to consider the *psychometric characteristics*, namely reliability and validity. These are heterogeneous constructs, as there are multiple types of reliability and validity. Internal consistency means that the construct being measured is internally consistent. Also, estimates of reliability and validity are highly dependent on the population studied. Most empirically developed rating scales have strong internal consistency. Of greater concern to clinicians, however, is the test–retest reliability or stability over time of the measure and the inter-rater reliability. Normative data on the measure should also be available, ideally for both typically developing and clinical samples. This information should be contained in previous articles or they should be reported in a manual.

The third step in selecting a diagnostic instrument, after reliability and validity, is considering *clinical utility*. Will the instrument perform the function that it is intended for in the specific setting where it is to be used? Aspects of clinical utility include cost (i.e., some scales are free and available on the internet), burden on the informant in terms of time and complexity, convenience in administering and scoring, and sensitivity to treatment effects. Clinical utility is enhanced further when rating scales can provide additional information relevant for treatment. For example, Langberg *et al.* recently reported that the Vanderbilt questionnaire, in combination with an interview, was helpful in screening for the presence of a comorbid learning disability [42]. This is quite an advantage as learning disabilities are common in youth with ADHD, and typically require psychometric testing to pinpoint the learning disorder.

Importantly, when evaluating treatment response, raters who evaluate the child before treatment and can observe the child in a similar situation or time period after treatment should be utilized. For example, in studies of stimulants whose duration of action is limited to school hours, teachers would be the ideal raters for efficacy. With the advent of long-acting stimulants, parents' ratings appear to be quite sensitive and similar in most cases to teacher reports [43]. Child self-report of ADHD symptoms in general is less reliable and generally has less correspondence with parent and teacher reports of disruptive behavior [44]. However, in a 2006 study, adolescent self-report, especially for older adolescents, was valid and sensitive to treatment effects [45].

Rating scales for specific purposes: impairment

Impaired functioning is typically the reason for referral, is predictive of long-term outcome, and leads directly to identification of appropriate treatment targets [31, 36]. Moreover, impairment is a requirement for diagnosing ADHD. However, as noted by Gordon *et al.* [46], and Buitelaar *et al.* [47] there is only a modest relationship between ADHD symptoms and impairment. Although a 30% reduction of symptoms is sometimes used as a categorical definition of response in short-term studies, further work is needed in longer-term studies that also examine functional impairment since symptom improvement does not automatically result in functional improvement. The main point is that it is crucial to measure impairment as well as symptoms.

In addition to assessing symptoms of ADHD and associated behavioral and emotional symptoms, rating scales are also useful for assessing impairment. During the diagnostic phase it is important to identify impairments to distinguish treatment of a psychiatric disorder from performance enhancement in cases of mild symptoms without corresponding impairment. This is a crucial point, as providing accommodations or pharmacological treatment to individuals who are not displaying impairment raises several ethical concerns, especially for children. Thus, impairment as well as ADHD symptoms should be routinely assessed.

Several behavior rating scales described above have specific items related to impairment. For example, the CBCL and Vanderbilt scales have the informant rate impairment in several areas (e.g., academic or social functioning, extracurricular activities). However, these scales have limited content validity and are seldom utilized as treatment outcome measures.

There are two main types of measures developed specifically to assess impairment, those that assess global impairment, such as the Clinical Global Impression-Severity (CGI-S) and Children's Global Assessment of Functioning [48], and those that assess more specific domains and are assessed with either a semi-structured interview or rating scale.

The global scales are quick, simple to utilize, and sensitive to treatment effects. Moreover, clinicians are familiar with these scales as they are used for a variety of disorders besides ADHD. Clinician-rated impairment is related not just to severity of ADHD symptoms per se, but also to comorbid externalizing and internalizing psychopathology, peer relationship difficulties, and family health problems [48]. For example, the CGI-S has the clinician rate the patient on the question "Considering your total clinical experience with this particular population, how mentally ill is the subject at this time?" from "1 = normal" to "7 = among the most extremely ill." The main limitation of these ratings is that they are quite subjective and depend on the frame of reference of the clinician and their previous experience. Also, unlike the more detailed impairment measures (described below) they do not have normative data and do not identify specific targets for treatment.

The Swanson, Kotkin, Agler, Mylnn, and Pelham Rating Scale (SKAMP) [49], is a 15-item scale that assesses impairment in the classroom related to ADHD symptoms. There are now several more detailed measures of specific types of impairment, including scales such as the ADHD Impact Module [50], Impairment Rating Scale (IRS), Life Participation Scale [51], and the Weiss Functional Impairment Rating Scale. Fabiano and colleagues developed the IRS [34].

Impairments in adaptive and social functioning can be assessed using semi-structured interviews such as the Social Adjustment Inventory for Children and Adolescents (SAICA) [52, 53] or Vineland Scales of Adaptive Behavior. These measures are utilized for both diagnostic purposes, treatment planning, and as outcome measures. The Vineland is an interview measure of adaptive functioning, and children with ADHD are markedly deficient relative to their IQ [54]. Moreover, weaknesses and strengths can suggest specific areas to focus on or enhance. Unlike the global measures, sensitivity to treatment is unknown as they are seldom utilized as treatment outcome measures. Unlike the rating scale measures of impairment, these measures take time to administer and require specialized training.

Rating scales for specific purposes: adverse events

In addition to tracking changes in symptoms and impairment, rating scales can be used to track adverse events. It is crucial to measure adverse events in treatment outcome studies, as they are strongly related to adherence and often limit effective dosing. Frequently used scales include the Pittsburgh Side Effects Scale [55] and Side Effect Rating Scale (SERS) developed by Barkley et al. [56]. Of note, some of the items on side effect scales are strongly correlated with treatment response (e.g., talks less).

These scales have the advantage of systematically surveying numerous behaviors that reflect an adverse event. It is important to examine change from baseline, as items may reflect psychiatric comorbidity as well as treatment response.

A limitation of these rating scales is that it is often unclear how best to score them as there are many items and the psychometric characteristics have not been thoroughly examined. Several studies have utilized a cutoff score on the 9-point scale to indicate a severe side effect [53]. Recently, investigators have used factor analysis to empirically derive factors. For example, Gruber et al. [57] extracted three side effects factors, Emotionality, Somatic Complaints, and Over-focused, and examined genetic moderators of response. In another study, Sonuga-Bark and colleagues [44] identified six factors: emotionality, sleep/appetite, disengaged, dizzy, uninterested, and aches. Treatment effects were seen only for emotionality (which improved) and sleep and appetite (which worsened) with stimulant treatment.

Another weakness is that most of the items are associated primarily with stimulant medications. Now there are several approved non-stimulant medications that are associated with different adverse events, such as lethargy, somnolence and fatigue. Moreover, there have been concerns about suicidal behavior as an adverse event, and assessment of suicide is now included in most clinical trials. Finally, many side effects occur at specific time points in the medication trail. Some adverse events are most likely to occur during the induction phase (e.g., insomnia, stomachache), while others occur as medication wears off (e.g., rebound irritability in late afternoons), or with long-term use (e.g., weight loss). Clearly, there is a need for developing rating scales and other instruments that can address these limitations and aid clinicians and researchers in assessing adverse events during specific times during the course of treatment.

Diagnostic interviews

Although rating scales are very helpful diagnostic tools, the gold standard for diagnosis is the diagnostic interview. However, the efficiency of the clinical interview is greatly enhanced when augmented with information from behavior rating scales which can indicate areas of concern which require additional probing.

Structured interviews are used in research studies to insure that relevant areas are probed. Both highly structured, respondent-based parent interviews, such as the Diagnostic Interview for Children-IV (DISC-IV) and semi-structured, interviewer-based instruments, such as the Schedule for Affective Disorders and Schizophrenia for School Age Children (K-SADS) have demonstrated good to excellent reliability for diagnosing ADHD and disruptive behavior disorders [58]. Of note, child or adolescent interviews have only modest reliability relative to parent interviews for disruptive behavior disorders, such as ADHD [59]. For mood symptoms and internalizing disorders, however, the parent may not necessarily be the best informant and both parent and child should be interviewed.

Description of diagnostic interviews

The K-SADS has several versions and is used to assess current and lifetime psychiatric disorders. The clinician rates current and lifetime symptoms for a number of DSM-IV disorders. There is an unstructured part, a medical and treatment history component, and a screening interview along with several supplements, including a disruptive behavior module which includes ADHD, ODD, and conduct disorder. The K-SADS is meant to be administered by a clinician who has received specific training, and has a skip-out structure so that the entire interview does not need to be administered. As a semi-structured interview, the clinician has considerable latitude in querying different symptoms. The clinician provides a summary judgment for each symptom after interviewing the parent and the child, and the interview can take 45–90 minutes. A strength of the K-SADS for ADHD is in identifying psychiatric comorbidity,

especially mood disorders. A weakness, however, is that there is not a module for autism spectrum disorders, which often can present as ADHD.

Specific diagnostic interviews used to assess ADHD are described in Table 19.2.

In contrast to the semi-structured K-SADS, the DISC-IV [60], is highly structured and can be administered by a research assistant. There is also a computerized administration. There are six major sections and 20 diagnostic modules, including an ADHD module that can be administered separately. The DISC-IV can be used to gather lifetime information, past year information, or information from the past 4 weeks. The reliability of the parents' reports on the DISC-Revised (DISC-R) was good to excellent for ADHD [60, 61].

In choosing a structured diagnostic interview, the decision of whether to use a structured versus a semi-structured interview depends to some extent on the purpose of the study. Semi-structured interviews are more appropriate for clinical purposes, whereas highly structured interviews are generally more appropriate for epidemiological studies.

Special issues in ADHD assessment: adolescents

Assessment of adolescents is more complex than that of school-age children. Some adolescents, especially those with ADHD Inattentive type, may first present for evaluation at this age as symptoms may have been more subtle or obscured by other factors (e.g., high IQ, compensatory strategies). However, ADHD may be more obvious as demands for independent work increase. Nonetheless, it may be more difficult to assess attention symptoms than behavioral symptoms using interviews and rating scales. In other cases of youth with comorbid externalizing disorders or long-standing academic and social failures, the ADHD may be overshadowed by more severe or prominent psychiatric comorbidity, such as substance use disorder, conduct disorder, and mood disorders. Assessment is also more complicated because of differences between parent, adolescent, and school informants. After middle school, it is not unusual for teachers, who spend less time with teenagers than with elementary school children, to be unaware of ADHD symptoms unless they are severe. Furthermore, differential diagnosis is complicated by the greater range and likelihood of other psychiatric diagnoses, such as schizophrenia, bipolar disorder, and substance use disorder, which often

Table 19.2. Diagnostic interviews

Diagnostic interview	Complete name	Description
K-SADS-P IVR [78, 79]	Schedule for Affective Disorders and Schizophrenia for School Age Children	The original version of K-SADS was the K-SADS-P IVR (present state), which also evaluates the worst episode during the past year and which was an extension of the adult Schedule for Affective Disorders and Schizophrenia and which focused on research diagnostic criteria. This was designed to be administrated by clinicians
K-SADS-E [80]	Schedule for Affective Disorders and Schizophrenia for School Age Children	E stands for Epidemiologic. Explores present episode of disorders and worst past episode. This version combines the present-episode and lifetime time frames
K-SADS-PL [81]	Schedule for Affective Disorders and Schizophrenia for School Age Children	PL stands for Present and Lifetime. This version is a cross between K-SADS-P and K-SADS-E. Explores lifetime histories of "worst" episodes. Symptom ratings reduced to 3-point scales
WASH-U K-SADS [82]	Washington University Schedule for Affective Disorders and Schizophrenia for School Age Children	Involves both present and lifetime time frames
Columbia K-SADS	Columbia University Schedule for Affective Disorders and Schizophrenia for School Age Children	Rates the current episode, the past 2 weeks, and the worst past episode
DISC [60]	Diagnostic Interview for Children-IV	Designed to asses over 30 of the most common psychiatric diagnoses in children and adolescents. The instrument was originally designed to be administered by clinically untrained interviewers. The current version is designed to be compatible with DSM-IV and International Classification of Disease-10 (ICD-10) and includes assessment for three time frames: the present (past 4 weeks), the last year, and "ever"

Source: Angold and Fischer [83].

appear in adolescents and whose symptoms overlap with ADHD.

Finally, there is the issue of adolescent self-report. It is well known that a social norm for young adolescents is to view themselves as not having any difficulties. As a result, self-report rating for ADHD may be less reliable in younger teenagers. However, in older teens, adolescent self-ratings appear to be more congruent with other ratings, and are sensitive to stimulant medication effects [45].

There are now several broad- and narrowband rating scales that have self-report versions. The Conners–Wells' Adolescent Self-Report was developed specifically for adolescents, and was normed on 12- to 17-year-olds [62]. The Conners–Wells' has demonstrated sensitivity to medication effects in clinical trials [45].

The Brown Attention Deficit Disorder Scales for Children and Adolescents [63] is a theoretically developed self-report scale to measure executive functioning deficits, and has norms for 12- to 18-year-olds. As noted by Collett *et al.* [35], the BADDS may detect qualitative nuances of ADHD that are not detected by DSM-IV scales. Also noteworthy is the Behavioral Rating Inventory of Executive Functioning (BRIEF) Adolescent version, which assesses executive functioning and ADHD symptoms through parent or adolescent self-report.

Adolescent self-report measures should be used cautiously, especially with younger adolescents who may be unwilling to admit to ADHD symptoms. In other situations, high school students may be anxious about college and wish to overstate symptoms to receive medication. Consequently, information from multiple sources should be obtained and reasons for differences between adolescent-, parent-, and teacher-provided information should be explored. In cases of diagnostic uncertainty, neuropsychological testing and review of previous school and medical records may provide confirmatory evidence.

Special issues in ADHD assessment: preschool children

Although the majority of children referred for ADHD are school age or above, with increasing recognition of ADHD more young children are referred. Several rating scales that have been reviewed have norms that extend to the preschool period, such as the CBCL, BASC, and Conners' Parent Rating Scale. However, behavior rating scales should be used cautiously, as developmental disorders that can be mistaken for ADHD are also often identified at this age (such as mental retardation or autism spectrum disorders). Because there is some overlap in symptoms, specificity of results may be diminished. The recently developed Conners' Early Childhood Scale is notable, in that it also contains scales to assess developmental milestones and validity of responses for 2- to 6-year-olds.

Summary and recommendations for clinical use

1. Rating scales and diagnostic interviews have a long history in ADHD and child psychopathology research and clinical practice.
2. Rating scales and diagnostic interviews help increase the reliability and validity of the diagnostic process.
3. It is advantageous to obtain information from home and school to address cross-situational DSM requirement as well as to understand differences in perceptions and behavior in home and school settings.
4. Broadband scales are best suited as diagnostic aides due to their broader content validity that includes symptoms of comorbid disorders.
5. Narrowband scales are less burdensome and are useful for monitoring treatment response.
6. There are few data on incremental validity of assessment measures and considerable overlap between rating scales and diagnostic interviews. Clinicians should work to develop an efficient process, such as having rating completed and reviewed prior to the interview for more detailed questioning, and to probe and resolve inconsistent or contradictory reports.
7. Both global and specific measures of impairment should be utilized to guide treatment intensity and duration.
8. Rating scales measures of adverse events are most useful when completed before and during treatment, so that changes from baseline can be assessed.
9. For assessing adolescents, self-ratings are necessary but not sufficient due to high risk of underreporting, especially in younger adolescents.
10. In preschool-age children, elevated behavior ratings are useful for screening purposes, but should be viewed cautiously due to poor specificity for ADHD and less stability over time.

In summary, assessment of ADHD in children and adolescents is multifaceted and involves a thorough evaluation of symptoms in the context of multiple settings. It is important to assess impairment of symptoms, possible comorbidities, social and family aspects, as well as risk factors and protective factors impacting the child. In order to obtain relevant information, rating scales and diagnostic interviews can be useful tools to aid a clinician as were discussed in this chapter. A clinician will need to consider the age of the patient as well as whether broader-band scales or more specific measures are desired to aid with a particular diagnostic situation. Due to the overlap between rating scales and diagnostic interviews, each clinician will need to develop an efficient process to elicit the necessary information before compiling the data and making an accurate diagnosis.

References

1. Castellanos FX, Tannock R. Neuroscience of attention-deficit/hyperactivity disorder: the search for endophenotypes. *Nat Rev Neurosci.* 2002;3(8):617–28.
2. American Psychiatric Association. *Diagnostic and Statistical Manual of Mental Disorders*, 5th edn. (DSM-5) Arlington, VA: American Psychiatric Publishing; 2013.
3. Cantwell DP, Baker L. Differential diagnosis of hyperactivity. *J Dev Behav Pediatr.* 1987;8(3):159–70.
4. Stein MA. Diagnosis of ADHD. In: Accardo PJ, Capute AJ, eds. *Neurodevelopmental Disorders of Childhood.* Baltimore, MD: Brookes. 2007; 639–56.
5. Stein MA. ADHD in primary care: overdiagnosed, underdiagnosed, and misunderstood. In: Rogers B, Montgomery T, Lock T, Accardo PJ, eds. *Attention Deficit Hyperactivity Disorder: The Clinican Spectrum.* Baltimore, MD: York Press. 2001; 51–72.
6. Stein MA, Efron L, Schiff W, Glanzman M. Attention deficits and hyperactivity. In: Batshaw M, ed. *Children with Disabilities*, 5th edn University of Michigan: Brookes Publishing. 2002; 389–416.
7. Conners CK, Rothschild G, Eisenberg L, Schwartz LS, Robinson E. Dextroamphetamine sulfate in children with learning disorders. Effects on perception, learning, and achievement. *Arch Gen Psychiatry.* 1969;21(2):182–90.

8. Conners CK, Sitarenios G, Parker JD, Epstein JN. The revised Conners' Parent Rating Scale (CPRS-R): factor structure, reliability, and criterion validity. *J Abnorm Child Psychol*. 1998;**26**(4): 257–68.

9. Conners CK. Rating scales in attention-deficit/hyperactivity disorder: use in assessment and treatment monitoring. *J Clin Psychiatry*. 1998; **59**(Suppl 7):24–30.

10. Conners CK. Psychological assessment of children with minimal brain dysfunction. *Ann N Y Acad Sci*. 1973;**205**:283–302.

11. Gomez R, Harvey J, Quick C, Scharer I, Harris G. DSM-IV AD/HD: confirmatory factor models, prevalence, and gender and age differences based on parent and teacher ratings of Australian primary school children. *J Child Psychol Psychiatry*. 1999; **40**(2):265–74.

12. Hartman CA, Hox J, Mellenbergh GJ, *et al*. DSM-IV internal construct validity: when a taxonomy meets data. *J Child Psychol Psychiatry*. 2001;**42**(6): 817–36.

13. Pliszka S, AACAP Working Group on Quality Issues. Practice parameter for the assessment and treatment of children and adolescents with attention-deficit/hyperactivity disorder. *J Am Acad Child Adolesc Psychiatry*. 2007;**46**(7):894–921.

14. Clinical practice guideline: diagnosis and evaluation of the child with attention-deficit/hyperactivity disorder. American Academy of Pediatrics. *Pediatrics*. 2000; **105**(5):1158–70.

15. American Academy of Pediatrics . Subcommittee on AttentionDeficit/Hyperactivity Disorder and Committee on Quality Improvement. Clinical practice guideline: treatment of the school-aged child with attention-deficit/hyperactivity disorder. *Pediatrics*. 2001;**108**(4):1033–44.

16. Brown RT, Amler RW, Freeman WS, *et al*. Treatment of attention-deficit/hyperactivity disorder: overview of the evidence. *Pediatrics*. 2005;**115**(6):e749–57.

17. Kollins SH, Sparrow EP. *Guide to Assessment Scales in Attention-deficit/Hyperactivity Disorder*, 2nd edn. London: Springer Healthcare Ltd.; 2010.

18. Hinshaw SP, Nigg JT. Behavior rating scales in the assessment of disruptive behavior problems in childhood. In: Shaffer D, Lucas CP, Richters JE, eds. *Diagnostic Assessment in Child and Adolescent Psychopathology*. New York, NY: Guilford Press. 1999; 91–126.

19. Dopfner M, Steinhausen HC, Coghill D, *et al*. Cross-cultural reliability and validity of ADHD assessed by the ADHD Rating Scale in a pan-European study. *Eur Child Adolesc Psychiatry*. 2006;**15**(Suppl 1): I46–55.

20. Goyette CH, Conners CK, Ulrich RF. Normative data on revised Conners Parent and Teacher Rating Scales. *J Abnorm Child Psychol*. 1978;**6**(2):221–36.

21. Shekim WO, Cantwell DP, Kashani J, *et al*. Dimensional and categorical approaches to the diagnosis of attention deficit disorder in children. *J Am Acad Child Psychiatry*. 1986;**25**(5):653–8.

22. Stein MA, O'Donnell JP. Classification of children's behavior problems: clinical and quantitative approaches. *J Abnorm Child Psychol*. 1985;**13**(2): 269–79.

23. Achenbach TM. Commentary: Definitely more than measurement error: but how should we understand and deal with informant discrepancies? *J Clin Child Adolesc Psychol*. 2011;**40**(1):80–6.

24. Zhang S, Faries DE, Vowles M, Michelson D. ADHD Rating Scale IV: psychometric properties from a multinational study as a clinician-administered instrument. *Int J Methods Psychiatr Res*. 2005;**14**(4): 186–201.

25. Servera M, Lorenzo-Seva U, Cardo E, Rodriguez-Fornells A, Burns GL. Understanding trait and sources effects in attention deficit hyperactivity disorder and oppositional defiant disorder rating scales: mothers', fathers', and teachers' ratings of children from the Balearic Islands. *J Clin Child Adolesc Psychol*. 2010; **39**(1):1–11.

26. Wender E. ADHD symptoms and parent-teacher agreement. *J Dev Behav Pediatr*. 2004;**25**(1):48–9; discussion 52.

27. Spencer TJ, Biederman J, Ciccone PE, *et al*. PET study examining pharmacokinetics, detection and likeability, and dopamine transporter receptor occupancy of short- and long-acting oral methylphenidate. *Am J Psychiatry*. 2006;**163**(3):387–95.

28. Cantwell DP. The diagnostic process and diagnostic classification in child psychiatry–DSM-III. *J Am Acad Child Psychiatry*. 1980;**19**(3):345–55.

29. Mash EJ, Hunsley J. Evidence-based assessment of child and adolescent disorders: issues and challenges. *J Clin Child Adolesc Psychol*. 2005;**34**(3):362–79.

30. De Los Reyes A, Kazdin AE. Informant discrepancies in the assessment of childhood psychopathology: a critical review, theoretical framework, and recommendations for further study. *Psychol Bull*. 2005;**131**(4):483–509.

31. Biederman J, Faraone SV, Doyle A, *et al*. Convergence of the Child Behavior Checklist with structured interview-based psychiatric diagnoses of ADHD children with and without comorbidity. *J Child Psychol Psychiatry*. 1993;**34**(7):1241–51.

32. Glow RA, Glow PH, Rump EE. The stability of child behavior disorders: a one year test-retest study of Adelaide versions of the Conners Teacher and Parent Rating Scales. *J Abnorm Child Psychol.* 1982;**10**(1): 33–60.

33. Saylor KE, Buermeyer CM, Spencer TJ, Barkley RA. Adaptive changes related to medication treatment of ADHD: listening to parents of children in clinical trials of a novel nonstimulant medication. *J Clin Psychiatry.* 2002;**63**(Suppl 12):23–8.

34. Fabiano GA, Pelham WE, Jr., *et al.* A practical measure of impairment: psychometric properties of the impairment rating scale in samples of children with attention deficit hyperactivity disorder and two school-based samples. *J Clin Child Adolesc Psychol.* 2006;**35**(3):369–85.

35. Collett BR, Ohan JL, Myers KM. Ten-year review of rating scales. V: scales assessing attention-deficit/ hyperactivity disorder. *J Am Acad Child Adolesc Psychiatry.* 2003;**42**(9):1015–37.

36. Pelham WE, Jr., Fabiano GA, Massetti GM. Evidence-based assessment of attention deficit hyperactivity disorder in children and adolescents. *J Clin Child Adolesc Psychol.* 2005;**34**(3):449–76.

37. Penny AM, Waschbusch DA, Klein RM, Corkum P, Eskes G. Developing a measure of sluggish cognitive tempo for children: content validity, factor structure, and reliability. *Psychol Assess.* 2009;**21**(3):380–9.

38. Ludwig HT, Matte B, Katz B, Rohde LA. Do sluggish cognitive tempo symptoms predict response to methylphenidate in patients with attention-deficit/ hyperactivity disorder-inattentive type? *J Child Adolesc Psychopharmacol.* 2009;**19**(4):461–5.

39. Martel MM. Research review: a new perspective on attention-deficit/hyperactivity disorder: emotion dysregulation and trait models. *J Child Psychol Psychiatry.* 2009;**50**(9):1042–51.

40. Anastopoulos AD, Smith TF, Garrett ME, *et al.* Self-regulation of emotion, functional impairment, and comorbidity among children with AD/HD. *J Atten Disord.* 2011;**15**(7):583–92.

41. Tripp G, Schaughency EA, Clarke B. Parent and teacher rating scales in the evaluation of attention-deficit hyperactivity disorder: contribution to diagnosis and differential diagnosis in clinically referred children. *J Dev Behav Pediatr.* 2006;**27**(3): 209–18.

42. Langberg JM, Vaughn AJ, Brinkman WB, Froehlich T, Epstein JN. Clinical utility of the Vanderbilt ADHD Rating Scale for ruling out comorbid learning disorders. *Pediatrics.* 2010;**126**(5):e1033–8.

43. Biederman J, Gao H, Rogers AK, Spencer TJ. Comparison of parent and teacher reports of

attention-deficit/hyperactivity disorder symptoms from two placebo-controlled studies of atomoxetine in children. *Biol Psychiatry.* 2006;**60**(10):1106–10.

44. Sonuga-Barke EJ, Coghill D, Wigal T, DeBacker M, Swanson J. Adverse reactions to methylphenidate treatment for attention-deficit/hyperactivity disorder: structure and associations with clinical characteristics and symptom control. *J Child Adolesc Psychopharmacol.* 2009;**19**(6):683–90.

45. Wilens TE, McBurnett K, Bukstein O, *et al.* Multisite controlled study of OROS methylphenidate in the treatment of adolescents with attention-deficit/ hyperactivity disorder. *Arch Pediatr Adolesc Med.* 2006;**160**(1):82–90.

46. Gordon M, Antshel K, Faraone S, *et al.* Symptoms versus impairment: the case for respecting DSM-IV's Criterion D. *J Atten Disord.* 2006;**9**(3): 465–75.

47. Buitelaar JK, Wilens TE, Zhang S, Ning Y, Feldman PD. Comparison of symptomatic versus functional changes in children and adolescents with ADHD during randomized, double-blind treatment with psychostimulants, atomoxetine, or placebo. *J Child Psychol Psychiatry.* 2009;**50**(3):335–42.

48. Guy W. *ECDEU Assessment Manual for Psychopharmacology.* Rockville, MD: U. S. Dept. of Health, Education and Welfare, Public Health Service, Alcohol, Drug Abuse, and Mental Health Administration, National Institute of Mental Health, Psychopharmacology Research Branch, Division of Extramural Research Programs; 1976.

49. Swanson JM. *School-based Assessments and Interventions for ADD Students.* Irvine, CA: KC Publishing; 1992.

50. Landgraf JM, Rich M, Rappaport L. Measuring quality of life in children with attention-deficit/hyperactivity disorder and their families: development and evaluation of a new tool. *Arch Pediatr Adolesc Med.* 2002;**156**(4):384–91.

51. Saylor K, Buermeyer C, Sutton V, *et al.* The Life Participation Scale for Attention-Deficit/Hyperactivity Disorder–Child Version: psychometric properties of an adaptive change instrument. *J Child Adolesc Psychopharmacol.* 2007;**17**(6):831–42.

52. John K, Gammon GD, Prusoff BA, Warner V. The Social Adjustment Inventory for Children and Adolescents (SAICA): testing of a new semistructured interview. *J Am Acad Child Adolesc Psychiatry.* 1987; **26**(6):898–911.

53. Stein MA, Sarampote CS, Waldman ID, *et al.* A dose-response study of OROS methylphenidate in children with attention-deficit/hyperactivity disorder. *Pediatrics.* 2003;**112**(5):e404.

54. Stein MA, Szumowski E, Blondis TA, Roizen NJ. Adaptive skills dysfunction in ADD and ADHD children. *J Child Psychol Psychiatry*. 1995;**36**(4): 663–70.

55. Spencer TJ, Greenbaum M, Ginsberg LD, Murphy WR. Safety and effectiveness of coadministration of guanfacine extended release and psychostimulants in children and adolescents with attention-deficit/hyperactivity disorder. *J Child Adolesc Psychopharmacol*. 2009;**19**(5):501–10.

56. Barkley RA, McMurray MB, Edelbrock CS, Robbins K. Side effects of methylphenidate in children with attention deficit hyperactivity disorder: a systemic, placebo-controlled evaluation. *Pediatrics*. 1990;**86**(2): 184–92.

57. Gruber R, Joober R, Grizenko N, *et al.* Dopamine transporter genotype and stimulant side effect factors in youth diagnosed with attention-deficit/hyperactivity disorder. *J Child Adolesc Psychopharmacol*. 2009;**19**(3): 233–9.

58. Shaffer D, Fisher P, Lucas CP, Dulcan MK, Schwab-Stone ME. NIMH Diagnostic Interview Schedule for Children Version IV (NIMH DISC-IV): description, differences from previous versions, and reliability of some common diagnoses. *J Am Acad Child Adolesc Psychiatry*. 2000;**39**(1): 28–38.

59. Jensen P, Roper M, Fisher P, *et al.* Test-retest reliability of the Diagnostic Interview Schedule for Children (DISC 2.1). Parent, child, and combined algorithms. *Arch Gen Psychiatry*. 1995;**52**(1):61–71.

60. Schwab-Stone M, Fisher P, Piacentini J, *et al.* The Diagnostic Interview Schedule for Children-Revised Version (DISC-R): II. Test-retest reliability. *J Am Acad Child Adolesc Psychiatry*. 1993;**32**(3):651–7.

61. Schwab-Stone M, Fallon T, Briggs M, Crowther B. Reliability of diagnostic reporting for children aged 6–11 years: a test-retest study of the Diagnostic Interview Schedule for Children-Revised. *Am J Psychiatry*. 1994;**151**(7):1048–54.

62. Conners CK, Wells KC, Parker JD, *et al.* A new self-report scale for assessment of adolescent psychopathology: factor structure, reliability, validity, and diagnostic sensitivity. *J Abnorm Child Psychol*. 1997;**25**(6):487–97.

63. Brown TE. *Brown Attention-Deficit Disorder Scales (Brown ADD Scales)*. San Antonio, TX: Psychological Corporation; 1996.

64. Hart EL, Lahey BB. General child behavior rating scales. In: Schaffer D, Lucas CP, Richters JE, eds. *Diagnostic Assessment in Child and Adolescent Psychopathology*. New York, NY: Guilford Press. 1999; 68–87.

65. DuPaul GJ, George J, Power TJ, Anastopoulos AD. *ADHD Rating Scale–IV: Checklists, Norms, and Clinical Interpretation*. New York, NY: Guilford Press; 1998.

66. Gadow KD, Sprafkin J. *ADHD Symptom Checklist-4 Manual*. Stonybrook, NY: Checkmate Plus; 1997.

67. Gadow KD, Sprafkin J. *Early Childhood Inventory-4 Norms Manual*. Stonybrook, NY: Checkmate Plus; 1997.

68. Sprafkin J, Gadow KD. *Early Childhood Symptom Inventories Manual*. Stonybrook, NY: Checkmate Plus; 1996.

69. Gadow KD, Sprafkin J. *Youth's Inventory-4 Manual*. Stonybrook, NY: Checkmate Plus; 1999.

70. Reynolds CR, Kamphaus RW. *The Clinician's Guide to Behavior Assessment System for Children*. New York, NY: Guilford Press; 2002.

71. Gioia GA, Isquith PK, Guy SC, Kenworthy L. Behavior rating inventory of executive function. *Child Neuropsychol*. 2000;**6**(3):235–8.

72. Gioia GA, Espy KA, Isquith PK. *Behavior Rating Inventory of Executive Function – Preschool Version*. Lutz, FL: Psychological Assessment Resources, Inc.; 2003.

73. Conners CK. *Conners Early Childhood*. North Tonawanda, NY: Multi-Health Systems, Inc.; 2009.

74. Conners CK. *Conners 3rd Edition (Conners 3)*. North Tonawanda, NY: Multi-Health Systems, Inc.; 2008.

75. Conners CK. *Conners Comprehensive Behavior Rating Scales*. North Tonawanda, NY: Multi-Health Systems, Inc.; 2008.

76. Pedigo TK, Pedigo KL, Scot VB, *et al. Pediatric Attention Disorders Diagnostic Screener*. Savannah, GA: Targeted Testing, Inc.; 2000.

77. Wolraich ML, Lambert W, Doffing MA, *et al.* Psychometric properties of the Vanderbilt ADHD diagnostic parent rating scale in a referred population. *J Pediatr Psychol*. 2003;**28**(8):559–67.

78. Puig-Antich J, Chambers W. *The Schedule for Affective Disorders and Schizophrenia for School-Age Children (K-SADS)*. New York, NY: New York State Psychiatric Institute; 1978.

79. Ambrosini PJ, Metz C, Prabucki K, Lee JC. Videotape reliability of the third revised edition of the K-SADS. *J Am Acad Child Adolesc Psychiatry*. 1989;**28**(5):723–8.

80. Orvaschel H, Puig-Antich J, Chambers W, Tabrizi MA, Johnson R. Retrospective assessment of prepubertal major depression with the Kiddie-SADS-e. *J Am Acad Child Psychiatry*. 1982;**21**(4):392–7.

81. Kaufman J, Birmaher B, Brent D, *et al.* Schedule for Affective Disorders and Schizophrenia for School-Age Children-Present and Lifetime Version (K-SADS-PL):

initial reliability and validity data. *J Am Acad Child Adolesc Psychiatry*. 1997;**36**(7):980–8.

82. Geller B, Zimmerman B, Williams M, Frazier J. *WASH-U KSADS*. St. Louis, MO: Department of Psychiatry, Washington University; 1996.

83. Angold A, Fischer PW. Interview-based interviews. In: Shaffer D, Lucas CP, Richters JE, eds. *Diagnostic Assessment in Child and Adolescent Psychopathology*. New York, NY: Guilford Press. 1999; 34–64.

Chapter 20

Stimulant medication in children and adolescents

Jonathan R. Stevens and Timothy E. Wilens

Introduction

Stimulants are among the most effective and most studied psychotropic medications in clinical use today. Over the past decade, with the increase in the diagnosis of attention-deficit hyperactivity disorder (ADHD), there has been a corresponding increase in the use of stimulants – the most commonly prescribed medications for this condition. This chapter explores contemporary issues of prescribing stimulants for children and adolescents with ADHD and examines specific areas in recent literature and clinical concerns that may persist.

Stimulant preparations overview

Two groups of stimulants are currently approved by the US Food and Drug Administration (FDA) for ADHD treatment of the pediatric population, methylphenidates (MPH) and amphetamines (AMPH). These medicines are available in both branded and generic formulations. Table 20.1 describes the names, preparations, strengths, and duration of behavioral effects of commonly available stimulants.

Since April 2000, several stimulant formulations have been approved – including extended-release preparations of oral MPH, transdermal MPH, extended-release dexmethylphenidate (d-MPH), lisdexamfetamine, and an oral solution of dextroamphetamine sulfate. By and large, these longer-acting forms of MPH and AMPH circumvent the short duration of action of the immediate-release stimulants (e.g., 3–5 hours of effectiveness for ADHD). The stimulants are classified by the FDA and Drug Enforcement Agency (DEA) as Schedule II agents.

Methylphenidate (MPH) preparations

Immediate-acting MPH comes in three preparations (i.e., tablet, chewable tablet, and oral solution). A sustained-release form of MPH (MPH sustained-release [SR]) and its branded generic (MPH extended-release [ER]) are essentially identical in that they are both MPH molecules mixed into a wax matrix. A chewable, extended-release MPH preparation is also available as a branded generic, offering MPH in a hydrophilic polymer.

d-MPH is the dextro-isomer of MPH. MPH, as a secondary amine, gives rise to four optical isomers: d-threo, l-threo, d-erythro, and l-erythro. The standard preparation of racemic MPH comprises d,l-threo-MPH. Further data suggest that the d-threo-MPH (d-MPH) isomer is the active form. A head-to-head study showed d-MPH to be similar in efficacy to immediate-release, racemic MPH when used in children with ADHD, though its duration of action was longer [1]. A longer-acting version of d-MPH (d-MPH XR) has been approved for pediatric and adult patients with ADHD.

Of the long-acting versions of MPH, osmotic-release oral system (OROS) MPII uses an osmotic pump mechanism that creates an ascending profile of MPH in the blood, providing effective treatment for up to 10–12 hours. OROS MPH tablets cannot be crushed without losing their prolonged action. While OROS MPH uses a pump technology, there are several extended-release MPH preparations – MPH controlled delivery (CD), MPH long acting (LA), and d-MPH XR – which use a beaded technology that contains spheres of active medication. These preparations contain anywhere from 30% (MPH CD) to 50% (MPH LA and d-MPH XR) of immediate-release MPH and

Attention-Deficit Hyperactivity Disorder in Adults and Children, ed. Lenard A. Adler, Thomas J. Spencer and Timothy E. Wilens.
Published by Cambridge University Press. © Cambridge University Press 2015.

Table 20.1. Stimulants: names, formulations, and strengths

Generic name	Brand name	Formulations and strengths	Duration of behavioral effect (hours)	Comments
Amphetamines				
D-amphetamine	Dexedrine Dexedrine Spansule ProCentra	Tablets: 5, 10 mg Spansules: 5, 10, 15 mg Oral Solution: 5 mg/5 mL	3–6	
Mixed amphetamine/ dextroamphetamine	Adderall Adderall XR	Tablets: 5, 7.5, 10, 12.5, 15, 20, 30 mg Capsules: 5, 10, 15, 20, 25, 30 mg	4–6 8–10	Capsule with 1:1 ratio of IR to DR beads
Lisdexamfetamine dimesylate	Vyvanse	Capsules: 20, 30, 40, 50, 60, 70 mg		Inactive prodrug in which l-lysine is chemically bonded to d-amphetamine
D-methamphetamine	Desoxyn	Tablet: 5 mg		
Methylphenidates				
Methylphenidate	Ritalin Methylin Ritalin SR Ritalin LA Metadate ER Metadate CD Concerta Daytrana	Tablets: 5, 10, 20 mg Tablets, chewable: 2.5, 5, 10 mg Oral solution: 5 mg/5 mL, 10 mg/5 mL (500 mL) Tablet: 20 mg Capsules: 10, 20, 30, 40 mg Tablets: 10, 20 mg Capsules: 10, 20, 30 mg Tablets: 18, 27, 36, 54 mg Transdermal patch: 10, 15, 20, 30 mg/9 hours	3–4 3–4 3–4 8–9 8–9 8–9 10–12 9	Capsule with 1:1 ratio of IR beads to DR beads Capsule with 3:7 ratio of IR beads to DR beads Ascending profile, OROS technology Delivery rate of 1.1, 1.6, 2.2, 3.3 mg/hour for the patches, respectively, based on 9-hour wear times in patients ages 6–12 years
	Quillivant XR	Oral suspension: 25 mg/5ml	10–12	
Dexmethylphenidate	Focalin Focalin XR	Tablets: 2.5, 5, 10 mg Capsules: 5, 10, 20 mg		d isomer of methylphenidate, twice as potent as racemic methylphenidate

Abbreviations: DR = delayed release, IR = immediate release, OROS = osmotic-release oral system.

provide a stimulant effect during the morning hours. These beaded preparations are useful for children who cannot or dislike taking pills as parents can open the capsules to sprinkle medicine on their child's food. There are also easier to ingest versions of immediate-release MPH, including a chewable tablet or liquid form. These latter two MPH forms have not yet been subject to large-scale clinical trials.

The MPH transdermal system (MTS) was approved in 2006, with a recommended wear time of 9 hours [2]. This patch can be applied to the skin (e.g., on the hip) prior to or upon awakening [3] and it is removed approximately 3 hours prior to the necessary duration of effect [4]. MTS is advantageous for patients (or their parents) who desire having an "off switch" for controlling the delivery of an active drug.

Amphetamine (AMPH) preparations

Amphetamines are manufactured in the dextro isomer, such as dextroamphetamine (d-AMPH), or in racemic forms with mixtures of d- and l-amphetamine (mixed amphetamine salts, MAS). An extended-release MAS formulation (MAS XR) is a dual-pulse capsule preparation that includes both immediate- and extended-release beads.

Lisdexamfetamine (LDX) is an inactive prodrug that converts to d-AMPH upon cleavage of the lysine portion of the molecule. Approved for use in both pediatric and adult groups with ADHD it was developed with the intention of creating a longer-lasting and more difficult to misuse version of d-AMPH. Intravenously and intranasally administered LDX produces effects comparable to orally administered LDX, therefore reducing the likelihood of abuse by these routes of administration [5].

Pharmacokinetics of stimulant preparations

After oral administration, both MPH and AMPH are almost completely absorbed [6], with food having little impact on this process [7]. Immediate-release MPH reaches a peak concentration at 1.5–2.5 hours and has an elimination half-life that is independent of the preparation of MPH (2.5–3.5 hours after oral administration). MPH undergoes extensive presystemic metabolism through hydrolysis or de-esterification with limited oxidation [6, 8]. Carboxylesterase-1A1 (CES-1), located in the stomach and liver, is the primary enzyme involved with first-pass MPH metabolism. Difference in an individual's hydrolyzing enzyme activity, linked to variants in human CES-1 gene [9], can lead to wide variations in MPH metabolism (and corresponding MPH blood concentrations) in certain persons. MTS avoids much of the first-pass metabolism through CES-1 [10], thereby producing potentially higher plasma MPH levels.

AMPH absorption is typically rapid, with peak plasma levels of AMPH generally observed 3 hours after oral ingestion [6]. Its half-life is considerably longer than that of MPH (approximately 7 hours). All of the AMPHs are metabolized hepatically by side-chain oxidative deamination and by ring hydroxylation. Because AMPHs are basic compounds, urinary excretion is highly dependent on urinary pH. Acidification of the urine increases urinary output of AMPHs [11]. Therefore, taking the medicine with ascorbic acid or fruit juice may decrease its absorption, while alkalinizing agents (e.g., sodium bicarbonate) may increase the absorption [12], although the clinical correlates of these alterations remain unclear.

Peak plasma concentrations for both MPH and AMPH may vary by four- to fivefold in children and adults, likely a result of inter-individual variability in metabolism and plasma clearance [6]. Inter-individual differences in pharmacokinetics may be less dramatic when stimulant dose is adjusted for body weight, using mg/kg as a general guide [13]. Inter-individual variability may also be an argument for examining the individual pharmacokinetics of stimulants for those patients who fail to respond to conventional dosing

strategies [14]. Laboratory testing for plasma stimulant levels (particularly for MPH) is increasingly available, but relatively uncommonly used in clinical practice.

Stimulant dosing and administration

Absolute dose limits (in mg) of stimulants do not adequately consider use in refractory cases, or adolescents. For example, the FDA recommends maximum daily MPH doses of up to 60 mg/day for short-acting forms and 72 mg/day for extended-release preparations. Others have proposed prescribing of 1 mg/kg/day [14] or even 2 mg/kg/day of racemic MPH [15].

Stevens et al. recently examined serum levels of MPH in patients receiving relatively higher doses of OROS MPH (mean of 169 mg; 3 mg/kg/day) and found acceptable blood pressure and pulse; serum levels were within the accepted levels of therapeutic (MPH levels < 50 ng/mL) [16]. In fact, no one in the study exceeded the general normative values for toxicity [16]. While measuring MPH levels can be helpful in patients receiving higher than FDA-approved doses of stimulants, results from several studies that have examined the association between plasma levels of stimulants and the reduction of ADHD symptoms have generally been equivocal. Monitoring of drug levels in blood may also be of some value for confirming compliance. These recommendations are tentative and further clinical research in this area is warranted.

When starting a psychostimulant, two early decision points involve choosing a stimulant class (e.g., MPH or AMPH), and then choosing the desired duration of action of a preparation (e.g., longer-acting versus short-acting). Contemporary guidelines suggest that once-daily preparations are preferred for most pediatric patients [17]. The dose for each child or adolescent should be individually optimized based on its therapeutic efficacy and side effects. Steady titration of treatment is advisable until an acceptable response is noted, with the addition of similar (or sculpted) afternoon doses dependent on breakthrough symptoms.

The starting dose for many preparations of MPH, AMPH compounds, and d-AMPH in most children is 2.5 to 5 mg, with a suggested target daily dose ranging from 0.3 to 1 mg/kg for AMPH and 0.6 to 2 mg/kg for MPH. Once pharmacotherapy is initiated, frequent contact with the patient and family is necessary during the initial phase of treatment to carefully monitor response and adverse effects. Apparent stimulant "ineffectiveness" may stem from excessively deliberate dose titration or medication underdosing. This underdosing may occur early in the course of a stimulant trial or months (or even years) later in treatment when a previously successful stimulant regimen loses its effectiveness because the child has grown and requires an increased dosage to compensate for improved stimulant metabolism and/or clearance. For instance, data would suggest that over the first 6 months of treatment, MPH is associated with a mild tolerance that may necessitate a 20–30% escalation of dose to maintain effectiveness [18].

Stimulant dosing often varies widely depending on the treatment setting. In the National Institute of Mental Health (NIMH) Multimodal Treatment of ADHD (MTA) study, mean daily MPH doses for children were significantly lower for patients receiving community care (18.7 mg/day) than for investigator-treated subjects (32.8 mg/day) [19]; the latter group had superior outcomes [20].

Medication interruptions, medication holidays

The appropriateness or merits of medication holidays remains unresolved. The symptoms of ADHD, although usually more noticeable in the school setting, are often disruptive to the child's family and social life. In cases in which important adverse effects are present, it may be necessary to allow for periodic drug holidays (either during weekends or the summer). In children whose major symptoms occur during school and who prefer to be treated during school days only, weekends and school vacations off medication may be appropriate. Conversely, in children who manifest symptoms predominantly in the home environment, medication-free holidays may be more problematic. Children should begin the academic year receiving an appropriate stimulant dose (initiated 1 or 2 weeks before the resumption of classes). Following a sufficient period of clinical stabilization (i.e., 6 to 12 months) it is prudent to re-evaluate the need for continued pharmacological intervention. Supervised discontinuation trials in the middle of the school year (as opposed to the summer months) may facilitate close assessment of a child's behavior and academic performance from multiple viewpoints.

Potential drug–drug interactions of stimulants

Interactions between stimulants and most prescription and non-prescription medications are generally mild. Stimulants appear to have few worrisome interactions with commonly prescribed medications (selective serotonin reuptake inhibitors [SSRIs], second-generation antipsychotics, atomoxetine, or alpha-2 (α_2)-adrenergic medications). Potential interactions with less common drug combinations may include increased plasma levels of tricyclic antidepressants (TCAs); increased plasma levels of phenobarbital, primidone, and phenytoin; increased prothrombin time on anticoagulants; attenuation or reversal of the guanethidine antihypertensive effect; and increased pressor responses to vasopressor drugs [21]. The relative lack of drug–drug interactions of MPH and other psychostimulants in the context of more-complex medical regimens may be due to the low bioavailability of MPH (20–30%) in orally administered forms [8].

Stimulant efficacy

The efficacy and safety of stimulants for the treatment of pediatric ADHD treatment are based on a large number of studies of (primarily) latency-age children where the average response is 70% [20, 22, 23]. When clinical response is assessed quantitatively via rating scales, the effect size of stimulant treatment relative to placebo is robust (averaging about 1.0), one of the largest effects for any psychotropic medication [17, 24].

Treatment data for preschoolers (ages 3 to 5 years) are less robust, though existing literature suggests that this group may have a lower response rate to stimulants and may be more treatment-refractory or diagnostically heterogeneous [25]. Results from the largest preschool stimulant treatment study (Preschool ADHD Treatment Study [PATS]) to date, a NIMH-sponsored multisite study of 165 children who tolerated study medication, 85% of patients were deemed to be MPH responders (versus 10% placebo responders) [26]. The effect sizes were smaller than in school-aged youth with improvement noted in both school and home settings. Findings from the PATS study support the results of earlier, smaller, controlled stimulant

Table 20.2. Possible strategies for stimulant side effects

Frequency of side effect	Stimulant side effect	Suggested interventions
• Common	• Decreased appetite	• Dose after meals. Encourage frequent snacks. Drug holidays. Decrease dose
	• Behavioral rebound	• Try a sustained-release stimulant. Add reduced dose in late afternoon
	• Irritability/dysphoria	• Try another stimulant medication. Consider coexisting conditions (e.g., depression) or medications (e.g., antidepressants)
	• Sleep problems	• Institute a bedtime routine. Reduce or eliminate afternoon dose. Reduce overall dose. Restrict or eliminate caffeine
• Rare	• Exacerbation of tics	• Observe. Try another stimulant or class of ADHD medications (e.g., α-adrenergic drugs)
	• Psychosis/euphoria/mania/ depression	• Stop treatment with stimulants. Refer to mental health specialist

studies in preschoolers, showing mostly modest-to-robust response and improvements in mother–child interactions, behavior, and structured tasks [27].

As with preschoolers, there is a smaller body of research of stimulants in adolescents [28, 29]. The majority of existing studies report at least moderate response to treatment without tolerance or evidence of misuse or abuse. For instance, two multisite studies demonstrated the efficacy of OROS MPH and MAS XR for ADHD. In a controlled study of 177 adolescents with ADHD treated with OROS MPH, over a third (37%) required the highest FDA-approved dose (72 mg) for outcome [28]. In another controlled study of 318 adolescents with ADHD, MAS XR resulted in significant improvements in mean ADHD measures of inattentive and hyperactive/impulsive subscales versus placebo [29]. In the majority of stimulant studies previously cited, the most common study drug was MPH, followed by AMPH. A review of the existing literature provides little evidence of a differential response to the various stimulants. Moreover, in many stimulant studies a crossover design was used and the study lengths were brief (ranging from a few days to a few weeks) [28]. Most studies were conducted on white males; there have been less data on the safety and efficacy of stimulants in females and various minority groups [30].

Common or expected stimulant-related adverse effects

Common adverse effects during stimulant treatment in the pediatric population include delay of sleep onset, headache, appetite suppression, transient headache, transient stomachache, and behavioral rebound (i.e., sudden or pronounced recurrence of ADHD symptoms). Less frequently observed outcomes include mood dysregulation or tics. Charach *et al.* collected side effect data during a 5-year period in children with ADHD who were initially randomized to stimulant or to no medication [31]. The most common sustained side effect reported was loss of appetite. At least one physiological adverse effect (e.g., headache, appetite loss, abdominal pain) was reported by half of the children by the end of the fifth year of monitoring. More importantly, children continued to use the medication, suggesting that the adverse events were mild and of minor health concern. Although AMPH and MPH are equally likely to produce an improvement in ADHD symptoms, the occurrence of stimulant-related side effects may be greater with the use of AMPH (or d-AMPH) compared with MPH (10% versus 6%, $p < 0.05$), although idiosyncratic patterns were noted for individual children [32].

Table 20.2 delineates suggested strategies for managing common stimulant-related adverse effects. Attempts should be made to manage adverse effects that occur in the context of a satisfactory clinical response to stimulants. In cases of stimulant-induced medical (headaches) or psychiatric symptoms (i.e., dysphoria, anxiety), it is necessary to assess whether these symptoms develop 1 to 2 hours post administration (acute phase) or during the wear-off phase. Acute effects generally indicate the need to reduce the maximum concentration in the blood by reducing the dose or release mechanism of the stimulant (e.g., changing from immediate-release to extended-release forms), whereas wear-off symptoms necessitate reducing the stimulant decay curve by adding a stimulant just before symptom onset or changing to a more extended-release agent.

Long-term or unexpected stimulant effects

Height and weight changes

Numerous studies have investigated abnormalities in the growth process related to ADHD, but controversies remain concerning both the direction of deviation from the norm and the cause of that deviation. Even with the plethora of studies conducted in this area, myriad methodological difficulties interfere with drawing a simple conclusion (e.g., the absence of a comparable control group [untreated children with ADHD] or an ADHD group receiving medication treatment with psychotropics other than stimulants).

In the past 10 years, several investigations have confirmed that reduction of growth is stimulant related [33–36], whereas others have failed to show any statistically significant growth delay during treatment. Growth slowdown for height and weight was reported with children with ADHD (ages 7–10) who were treated with MPH at a mean dosage of 30 mg/kg/day in the MTA study [35]. School-age children grew 1.0 cm less and gained 2.5 kg less than predicted by the Centers for Disease Control and Prevention growth charts. Similar effects were observed for preschool children [37], who grew 1.5 cm less in height and gained 2.5 kg less weight than predicted while being treated with MPH at a mean dosage of 14 mg/kg/day.

Spencer *et al.* formulated the disorder-related delay hypothesis suggesting that the observed growth deficit may be connected with ADHD, rather than with stimulant medication [38]. Children with ADHD could develop more slowly than the norm, and the consequence of this would be lower rates of growth in succeeding years than expected and the later achievement of biological maturity than in their healthy peers. Others have reported dissimilar findings [33] and have shown that unmedicated children with ADHD were taller than medicated children.

The aggregate literature seems to suggest small but largely clinically insignificant reductions in weight over time. Height may be negatively influenced over the first year to two of treatment; however, catch-up or rebound in height to expected values appears operant with chronic treatment [39]. Monitoring of growth in

height and weight should be part of the management of youth with ADHD receiving stimulants.

Tics

Stimulant use in children with mild to moderate tics remains of concern. Most studies have failed to confirm the hypothesis that stimulant drug therapy exacerbates tic severity in ADHD youth [40, 41]. For example, Palumbo and colleagues pooled data from three placebo-controlled trials (total n = 416), and two open-label studies involving patients receiving OROS MPH, MPH, or placebo [42]. Though approximately 13% of patients in each of the three groups had a history of tics, there was no significant difference between the three groups of the number of children that experienced tics. Double-blind clinical trials of both immediate-release and long-acting stimulants have not found that stimulants increase the rate of tics relative to placebo [43, 44]. Children with comorbid ADHD and tic disorders, on average, show a decline in tics when treated with a stimulant that persists even after a year of treatment [45].

If a patient has treatment-emergent tics during a trial of a given stimulant, an alternative stimulant or a non-stimulant should be tried. If the patient's ADHD symptoms respond adequately only to a stimulant medication that induces tics, then combined pharmacotherapy of the stimulant and an α agonist (clonidine or guanfacine) is recommended [46]. Withdrawal of stimulants in placebo-controlled double-blind fashion did not change frequency or severity of tics in series of 19 children with ADHD and vocal or motor tics who were on stimulants for a long time [47].

Sudden death and cardiac complications

The potential cardiovascular effects of medications used to treat ADHD, and whether such stimulants might be associated with sudden death, has been a source of great concern and publicity in recent years. The literature has been summarized by Wilens *et al.* [48] and a commentary has been provided by the FDA [49]. Wilens and colleagues cited the >300 controlled trials of stimulant medication involving more than 5000 subjects, none of which observed sudden death. Moreover, the anatomical characteristics in autopsies in subjects who have had sudden death during stimulant treatment were similar to those reported in sudden death in the general population. However, Gould *et al.* found a significant association between stimulant

Table 20.3. Massachusetts General Hospital Cardiovascular Screen

Cardiovascular history	Yes	No	Comment
A) Personal history			
1) Congenital or acquired cardiac disease	○	○	
2) Coronary artery disease	○	○	
3) Chest pain	○	○	
4) Palpitations	○	○	
5) Shortness of breath	○	○	
6) Dizziness	○	○	
7) Syncope	○	○	
B) Family history (<30 years of age)			
1) History of early myocardial infarction	○	○	
2) History of cardiac death	○	○	
3) History of significant arrthymias?	○	○	
4) History of long QT syndrome	○	○	
C) Objective			
1) Baseline (off medication) blood pressure and heart rate within normal limits	○	○	

If positive on an item, recommend referral to primary care physician or pediatric cardiology for further assessment prior to initiating medication.

use and sudden death in a matched case–control study of 564 cases of sudden unexplained death in youth and a comparison group (who died as passengers in motor vehicle traffic accidents) [50]. Ten of the subjects (1.8%) in the sudden unexplained death group were taking MPH, whereas only two (0.4%) of the comparison group of young people who died in road traffic accidents were taking stimulants (odds ratio [OR] = 7.4; 95% confidence interval [CI] 1.4, 74.9). As a case–control study, this analysis could not determine causation directly. Referring to this study, in 2009 the FDA commented that it was "unable to conclude that these data affect the overall risk and benefit profile of stimulant medication used to treat ADHD in children" [49].

At this stage, it appears that sudden death is a rare event in children with ADHD and there are insufficient data to establish a causal link with stimulant medication used to treat this condition [51]. Nevertheless, it would be prudent to follow the guidelines of the use of stimulants in children – monitoring risk factors and measuring blood pressure and pulse – although EKG is not mandatory [52, 53]. Pertinent questions that should be asked with regard to family history of premature sudden death and a personal history of cardiovascular symptoms are summarized in Table 20.3.

Patients answering any of these questions affirmatively should be examined and investigated more carefully.

Psychosis or mania

Psychosis or mania may be a rare adverse effect of stimulant (and non-stimulant) therapy for ADHD. A recent pooled analysis of 49 randomized trials in children and >800 reports in over 800 adults and children treated for ADHD (some with non-stimulants, including atomoxetine) found a rate of psychotic/manic events of 1.48 per 100 person-years in the pooled drug group compared to none in the placebo group [54]. In approximately 90% of the cases, there was no history of a similar psychiatric condition prior to ADHD treatment. Hallucinations involving visual and/or tactile sensations of insects, snakes, or worms were common in cases involving children. In reviewing several trials, the FDA found that stimulant-associated psychotic-like and manic-like symptoms occurred rarely – in approximately 0.25% of children treated with stimulants. In 55 of 60 reported cases of psychotic-like or manic-like symptoms in response to stimulants, the symptoms resolved when the stimulant was discontinued. In the five cases that persisted, the patients were rediagnosed with schizophrenia or bipolar disorder. The occurrence of psychosis and other pronounced mood dysregulation with stimulant treatment generally warrants consideration of an alternative agent. In some cases, children may tolerate a carefully monitored rechallenge of stimulant at a lower dose.

Carcinogenic effects

In 2005, El-Zein and colleagues reported "chromosomal breaks" in the peripheral lymphocytes of children taking therapeutic MPH [55]. This study added to a sparse body of animal literature that showed increased hepatic tumors in rodents treated with very high (4 to 47 mg/kg) oral doses of MPH [56]. However, the preponderance of data seems to suggest a lack of association between stimulants and cancer. For instance, an older study of pharmacy records that suggested the number of cancers in patients receiving stimulants was actually less than expected [57]. Moreover, a large systematic review found either negative or weakly positive results for chromosomal changes in rodent assay systems [58]. In what is likely to be one of many follow-up studies addressing this pressing issue, Ponsa *et al.* [59] followed a similar strategy as El-Zein *et al.* and found no evidence of an increased frequency of micronuclei (indicative of genomic damage). In the three end points studied (i.e., a cytokinesis-block micronucleus assay, a sister chromated exchange analysis, and a determination of chromosome aberrations), the results did not support a potential increased risk of cancer after exposure.

Risk of substance abuse

Wilens *et al.* performed a meta-analysis and reported that the use of stimulants did not increase the risk for later substance use disorders (SUD) in either adolescents or adults [60]. Subsequently Katusic *et al.* [61] and Wilens *et al.* [62] reported a protective effect of stimulants into young adulthood whereas Biederman *et al.* [63] and Mannuzza *et al.* [64] simultaneously reported that early stimulant treatment neither increased nor decreased the risk for subsequent SUD in young adulthood. The waning of the protective effect in adults may be a reflection of findings in adolescents not spanning the full age of risk of SUD or that most adolescents have stopped their ADHD treatment, thus losing the protective effect of stimulants.

Issues of misuse and diversion

There has been substantial interest in misuse and diversion of stimulants prescribed for ADHD (for review see Wilens *et al.* [65]). While the majority of individuals treated for their ADHD use their medications appropriately [65, 66], a group appear to misuse the stimulants. Survey studies have indicated that approximately 5% of college students have misused stimulants [67, 68] and that misuse is more common in competitive colleges, and that stimulants are more often misused for their pro-cognitive effects than for euphoria [68]. Data regarding those to whom the stimulants were diverted show that these individuals misused the stimulants in context with other substances of abuse [69] and other psychopathology such as depression [70] and conduct disorder [68].

Special populations

The use of stimulants in the treatment of children with ADHD and common comorbid conditions is important clinically. The lifetime prevalence of comorbid psychiatric or learning disorders is estimated to be as high as 80% [71, 72]. Common comorbid diagnoses in children with ADHD include mood disorders (e.g.,

major depression, bipolar disorder, dysthymia), anxiety disorders, and substance abuse disorders. Some medical conditions (e.g., epilepsy) are more likely to be comorbid with ADHD. The presence of comorbidities often worsens the prognosis of these patients and complicates their treatment, thereby warranting special mention.

Bipolar disorder

The majority of youth with bipolar disorder have co-occurring psychiatric illnesses. Among these, ADHD is by far the most common comorbidity with pediatric bipolar disorder [73]. Clinical studies generally demonstrate high rates of ADHD in patients who have bipolar disorder, ranging from 60% to 90% [74]. Likewise, cross-sectional studies have found rates of bipolar disorder ranging from 11% to 23% in youth who have ADHD [75].

Two controlled trials suggest that stimulants are effective in treating comorbid ADHD without precipitating hypomania or mania in mood-stabilized bipolar disorder youth. In 2005, Scheffer and colleagues performed a double-blind, placebo-controlled trial of pediatric patients diagnosed with bipolar disorder and ADHD [76]. In this study of 31 children, treatment with divalproex sodium (mean dose: 750 mg daily) reduced manic symptoms in 80% of participants, but reduced ADHD symptoms in only 7.5% of participants. With the addition of MAS, the subsequent improvement in ADHD was significantly greater than with placebo. Findling and colleagues reported that in youth stabilized with a stable dose of at least one mood stabilizer, concomitant treatment with MPH improved ADHD in a dose-dependent manner without mood destabilization [77]. Therefore, for bipolar youth with co-occurring ADHD, mood stabilization with a traditional mood stabilizer or an atypical antipsychotic medication is recommended before starting stimulant therapy [78]. Clinicians must take into account the risk of adverse effects or potential mood destabilization from stimulants and discuss this with families, but not overvalue potential risks when making a recommendation.

Developmental disorders

The recent rise in the diagnosis of autistic spectrum disorder and other pervasive developmental disorders (PDD) in children has refocused attention on

Table 20.4. Representative studies (controlled) of stimulants in children and adolescents with pervasive developmental disorders

Study	Findings
Quintana *et al.* (1995) [79] Double-blind, placebo-controlled, crossover study (n = 10) Treatment: immediate-release MPH, placebo Dosage: 18 to 54 mg/day Duration: 10 weeks	• MPH more efficacious than placebo • No significant side effects noted
Handen *et al.* (2000) [80] Double-blind, placebo-controlled, crossover study (n = 13) Treatment: immediate-release MPH, placebo Dosage: 0.3 or 0.6 mg/kg per dose Duration: 1 week	• 8 of 13 children (62%) were MPH responders (based on >50% decrease on the Teacher Conners' Hyperactivity Index) • Ratings of stereotypy and inappropriate speech also decreased • Adverse events included social withdrawal and irritability, especially at the 0.6 mg/kg dose
RUPP Autism Network (2005) [81] Double-blind, placebo-controlled, crossover study followed by open-label continuation (n = 72) Dosage: 7.5 to 50 mg/day Duration: 12 weeks	• MPH superior to placebo on hyperactivity scale rated by parents and teachers • 35 of 72 participants (49%) considered MPH responders • 13 of 72 subjects (18%) were withdrawn as a result of adverse effects (e.g., irritability)
Posey *et al.* (2007) [82] Double-blind, placebo-controlled, crossover study (n = 66) Treatment: immediate-release MPH, placebo Dosage: 0.125, 0.25, and 0.5 mg/kg per dose, twice daily, with an additional half-dose in the afternoon Duration: 4 weeks	• MPH associated with significant improvement • Improvement most evident at the 0.25- and 0.5-mg/kg doses • Hyperactive and impulsive symptoms improved more than inattention • No significant effects on ODD or stereotyped and repetitive behavior

stimulants as a possible therapeutic option for children with functionally impairing hyperactivity, distractibility, and impulsiveness.

Several randomized, controlled studies have supported the appropriateness of stimulant use in PDD children (see Table 20.4) [79–82]. These studies contradict the results of a retrospective review of stimulant use in 195 patients with PDD [83], which suggested a low rate of treatment success and frequent side effects (e.g., irritability and increased stereotypic movements). A preponderance of the evidence suggests that symptoms of ADHD are common in PDD and that MPH is an empirically supported treatment to target ADHD symptoms in PDD. However, tolerability remains a problem, and caregivers should be cautioned to be watchful for potential adverse effects. With the increasing recognition of autistic spectrum disorders in young children, further studies are needed to clarify the roles of AMPH and non-stimulant medications in the treatment of ADHD symptoms in children with PDD.

Seizure disorders

Studies in pediatric epilepsy have found a 2.5-fold to 5.5-fold increased risk of ADHD compared with healthy controls [84, 85]. Although not a contraindication, the physician's desk reference discourages the use

of stimulants in children with seizure disorder because stimulants lower the seizure threshold. Baptista-Neto and colleagues have reviewed this topic [86], citing retrospective chart reviews, open-label trials, and controlled trials of MPH in patients with epilepsy and ADHD showing significant improvements in ADHD symptoms without an exacerbation of seizures or an adverse effect on antiepileptic drug serum levels. Moreover, a large retrospective cohort study of >30 000 pediatric patients found no statistically significant association between the use of stimulants and seizure risk in children with ADHD and without prior seizure disorder [87]. Recently, a pilot randomized controlled trial of OROS MPH to treat ADHD plus epilepsy (n = 31) found that stimulant treatment reduced ADHD symptoms more than placebo treatment [88]. However, there were too few seizures during the active (5) and placebo arms (3) to assess seizure risk. These recent works suggest that stimulants may be a safe and effective treatment in certain children with seizure disorders.

Can stimulants protect against the development of psychiatric disorders?

One of the newest areas of interest in the stimulant literature concerns whether treatment with stimulants modifies long-term outcomes. Daviss and colleagues examined the association between stimulant treatment for ADHD and the risk for subsequent major depression by comparing the rates of pharmacotherapy of youth (11–18 years old) with ADHD and histories of major depression disorder (MDD; n = 36) to those with ADHD without a lifetime history of MDD (n = 39) [89]. These investigators found that stimulants protected youth against subsequent development of major depression. More recently, a case–control, 10-year prospective follow-up study of white males with (n = 140) and without ADHD was conducted [90]. At the 10-year follow-up, participants with ADHD who were treated with stimulants were significantly less likely to develop depressive and anxiety disorders and disruptive behavior and less likely to repeat a grade compared with participants with ADHD who were not treated. This study highlights additional protective effects (e.g., lower risk for the subsequent development of psychopathology and grade retention).

Conclusion

Pharmacotherapy with stimulants is a mainstay of evidence-based treatment for children and adolescents with ADHD and comorbid conditions. The use of stimulants should follow a careful evaluation of the child and his or her family, including psychiatric, social, cognitive, and educational evaluations. Early therapeutic intervention is important before complications, chronicity, and social incapacitation occur. Otherwise, the challenge of treatment and restabilization of functional life habits becomes more difficult. The family and the child need to be made familiar with the risks and benefits of such intervention, the availability of alternative treatments, and the likely short- and long-term adverse effects. Certain adverse effects can be anticipated based on known pharmacological properties of the drug (i.e., decreased appetite, insomnia), whereas others are idiosyncratic and are difficult to anticipate based on the drug properties. Short-term adverse effects can be minimized by introducing the medication at low initial doses and titrating upward steadily. Long-term side effects require monitoring of potential adverse effects such as growth impairment. Idiosyncratic adverse effects generally require drug discontinuation and selection of alternative treatment modalities. Special attention must be given to issues of comorbidity with other psychiatric and medical disorders.

Disclosures

Dr. Stevens has no conflicts of interest or financial ties to disclose. Dr. Wilens receives grant support from Abbott, McNeil, Eli Lilly, NIH (NIDA), Merck, and Shire; has been a speaker for Eli Lilly, McNeil, Novartis, and Shire, and is a consultant for Abbott, McNeil, Eli Lilly, NIH, Novartis, Merck, and Shire.

References

1. Wigal S, Swanson JM, Feifel D, *et al*. A double-blind, placebo-controlled trial of dexmethylphenidate hydrochloride and d,l-threo-methylphenidate hydrochloride in children with attention-deficit/hyperactivity disorder. *J Am Acad Child Adolesc Psychiatry*. 2004;**43**(11):1406–14.

2. Findling RL, Lopez FA, eds. Efficacy of transdermal methylphenidate with reference to Concerta in ADHD. 52nd Annual Meeting of American Academy of Child and Adolescent Psychiatry; 2005 October 18–23; Toronto, Canada; 2005.

3. Wilens TE, Hammerness P, Martelon M, *et al*. A controlled trial of the methylphenidate transdermal system on before-school functioning in children with attention-deficit/hyperactivity disorder. *J Clin Psychiatry*. 2010;**71**(5):548–56.

4. Wilens TE, Boellner SW, Lopez FA, *et al*. Varying the wear time of the methylphenidate transdermal system in children with attention-deficit/hyperactivity disorder. *J Am Acad Child Adolesc Psychiatry*. 2008; **47**(6):700–8.

5. Jasinski DR, Krishnan S. Human pharmacology of intravenous lisdexamfetamine dimesylate: abuse liability in adult stimulant abusers. *J Psychopharmacol*. 2009;**23**(4):410–18.

6. Patrick KS, Markowitz JS. Pharmacology of methylphenidate, amphetamine enantiomers and pemoline in attention-deficit hyperactivity disorder. *Hum Psychopharmacol*. 1997;**12**:527–46.

7. Gualtieri CT, Wargin W, Kanoy R, *et al*. Clinical studies of methylphenidate serum levels in children and adults. *J Am Acad Child Psychiatry*. 1982;**21**(1): 19–26.

8. Markowitz JS, Patrick KS. Differential pharmacokinetics and pharmacodynamics of methylphenidate enantiomers: does chirality matter? *J Clin Psychopharmacol*. 2008;**28**(3): S54–61.

9. Zhu HJ, Patrick KS, Yuan HJ, *et al*. Two CES1 gene mutations lead to dysfunctional carboxylesterase 1 activity in man: clinical significance and molecular basis. *Am J Hum Genet*. 2008;**82**(6):1241–8.

10. Zhu H, Wang JS, Donovan JL, *et al.* Interactions of attention-deficit/hyperactivity disorder therapy agents with the efflux transporter P-glycoprotein. *Eur J Pharmacol.* 2008;**578**:148–58.

11. Greenhill LL, Pliszka S, Dulcan MK, *et al.* Practice parameter for the use of stimulant medications in the treatment of children, adolescents, and adults. *J Am Acad Child Adolesc Psychiatry.* 2002;**41**(2 Suppl): 26S–49S.

12. Vitiello B. Research in child and adolescent psychopharmacology: recent accomplishments and new challenges. *Psychopharmacology.* 2007;**191**: 5–13.

13. Angrist B, Corwin J, Bartlik B. Early pharmacokinetics and clinical effects of oral d-amphetamine in normal subjects. *Biol Psychiatry.* 1987;**22**:1357–68.

14. Sachdev P, Troller J. How high a dose of stimulant medication in adult attention deficit hyperactivity disorder? *Aust N Z J Psychiatry.* 2000;**34**:645–50.

15. Biederman J, Mick E, Surman C, *et al.* A randomized, placebo-controlled trial of OROS methylphenidate in adults with attention-deficit/hyperactivity disorder. *Biol Psychiatry.* 2006;**59**(9):829–35.

16. Stevens JR, George RA, Fusillo S, Stern TA, Wilens TE. Plasma methylphenidate concentrations in youths treated with high-dose osmotic release oral system formulation. *J Child Adolesc Psychopharmacol.* 2010;**20**(1):49–54.

17. Pliszka S. Practice parameter for the assessment and treatment of children and adolescents with attention-deficit/hyperactivity disorder. *J Am Acad Child Adolesc Psychiatry.* 2007;**46**(7):894–921.

18. Wilens T, Pelham W, Stein M, Conners CK, Abikoff H. ADHD treatment with a once-daily formulation of methylphenidate hydrochloride: a two-year study. 156th Annual Meeting of the American Psychiatric Association, San Francisco, CA; 2003.

19. Jensen P, Hinshaw SP, Swanson JM, *et al.* Findings from the NIMH multimodal treatment study of ADHD: implications and applications for the primary care providers. *J Dev Behav Pediatr.* 2001;**22**:60–73.

20. MTA Cooperative Group. A 14-month randomized clinical trial of treatment strategies for attention-deficit/hyperactivity disorder. The MTA Cooperative Group. Multimodal Treatment Study of Children with ADHD [see comments]. *Arch Gen Psychiatry.* 1999; **56**(12):1073–86.

21. Stevens JR, Alpert JE, Fava M, Rosenbaum J. Psychopharmacology in the medical setting. In: Stern TA, Fricchione GH, eds. *Massachusetts General Hospital Handbook of General Hospital Psychiatry.* Amsterdam: Elsevier Science Publishers. 2010; 441–66.

22. Spencer T, Biederman J, Wilens T, *et al.* Pharmacotherapy of attention deficit disorder across the life cycle. *J Am Acad Child Adolesc Psychiatry.* 1996;**35**(4):409–32.

23. Spencer T, Biederman J, Wilens T. Pharmacotherapy of ADHD: A life span perspective. In: Oldham J, Riba M, eds. *American Psychiatric Press Review of Psychiatry.* Washington, DC: American Psychiatric Association. 1997; 87–128.

24. Faraone SV, Biederman J, Spencer T, Aleardi M. Comparing the efficacy of medications for ADHD using meta-analysis. *Med Gen Med.* 2006;**8**(4):4.

25. Byrne JM, Bawden HN, DeWolfe NA, Beattie TL. Clinical assessment of psychopharmacological treatment of preschoolers with ADHD. *J Clin Exp Neuropsychol.* 1998;**20**(5):617–27.

26. Greenhill LL, Abikoff H, Kollins S, Wigal S, Swanson J, Group PCS. Outcome results from the NIMH multi-site Preschool ADHD Treatment Study (PATS). 51st Annual Meeting of the American Academy of Child and Adolescent Psychiatry; 2004 October 19–24; Washington, DC; 2004.

27. Wilens TE. Treatment and assessment of ADHD in children and adolescents. In: Biederman JB, ed. *ADHD Across the Lifespan: An Evidence-Based Understanding from Research to Clinical Practice.* Hasbrouck Heights, NJ: Veritas Institute for Medical Education. 2006; 176–206.

28. Wilens T, McBurnett K, Bukstein O, *et al.* Multisite, controlled trial of OROS® methylphenidate (CONCERTA®) in the treatment of adolescents with attention-deficit/hyperactivity disorder. *Arch Pediatr Adolesc Med.* 2006;**160**(1):82–90.

29. Grcevich S. SLI381: a long-acting psychostimulant preparation for the treatment of attention-deficit hyperactivity disorder. *Expert Opin Investig Drugs.* 2001;**10**(11):2003–11.

30. Pelham WE, Walker JL, Sturges J, Hoza J. Comparative effects of methylphenidate on ADD girls and boys. *J Am Acad Child Adolesc Psychiatry.* 1989;**28**(5):773–6.

31. Charach A, Ickowicz A, Schachar R. Stimulant treatment over five years: adherence, effectiveness, and adverse effects. *J Am Acad Child Adolesc Psychiatry.* 2004;**43**(5):559–67.

32. Barbaresi WJ, Katusic SK, Colligan RC, *et al.* Long-term stimulant medication treatment of attention-deficit/hyperactivity disorder: results from a population-based study. *J Dev Behav Pediatr.* 2006; **27**(1):1–10.

33. Swanson JM, Elliott GR, Greenhill LL, *et al.* Effects of stimulant medication on growth rates across 3 years in the MTA follow-up. *J Am Acad Child Adolesc Psychiatry.* 2007;**46**(8):1015–27.

34. Poulton A, Cowell CT. Slowing of growth in height and weight on stimulants: a characteristic pattern. *J Paediatr Child Health.* 2003;**39**:180–5.

35. MTA Cooperative Group. National Institute of Mental Health multimodal treatment study of ADHD follow-up: changes in effectiveness and growth after the end of treatment. *Pediatrics.* 2004;**113**:762–9.

36. Lisska MC, Rivkees SA. Daily methylphenidate use slows the growth of children: a community based study. *J Pediatr Endocrinol Metab.* 2003;**16**(5):711–18.

37. Swanson J, Greenhill L, Wigal T, *et al.* Stimulant-related reductions of growth rates in the PATS. *J Am Acad Child Adolesc Psychiatry.* 2006;**45**(11):1304–13.

38. Spencer TJ, Biederman J, Harding M, *et al.* Growth deficits in ADHD children revisited: evidence for disorder-associated growth delays? *J Am Acad Child Adolesc Psychiatry.* 1996;**35**(11):1460–9.

39. Faraone SV, Biederman J, Morley CP, Spencer TJ. Effect of stimulants on height and weight: a review of the literature. *J Am Acad Child Adolesc Psychiatry.* 2008;**47**(9):994–1009.

40. Pidsosny IC, Virani A. Pediatric psychopharmacology update: psychostimulants and tics – past, present, and future. *J Can Acad Child Adolesc Psychiatry.* 2006;**15**(2):84–6.

41. Law SF, Schachar RJ. Do typical clinical doses of methylphenidate cause tics in children treated for attention-deficity hyperactivity disorder? *J Am Acad Child Adolesc Psychiatry.* 1999;**38**(8):944–51.

42. Palumbo D, Spencer T, Lynch J, Co-Chien H, Faraone SV. Emergence of tics in children with ADHD: impact of once-daily OROS methylphenidate therapy. *J Child Adolesc Psychopharmacol.* 2004;**14**(2):185–94.

43. Biederman J, Lopez FA, Boellner SW, Chandler MC. A randomized, double-blind, placebo-controlled, parallel-group study of SLI381 in children with attention deficit hyperactivity disorder. *Pediatrics.* 2002;**110**(2):258–66.

44. Wolraich ML, Greenhill LL, Pelham W, *et al.* Randomized, controlled trial of oros methylphenidate once a day in children with attention-deficit/hyperactivity disorder. *Pediatrics.* 2001;**108**(4):883–92.

45. Gadow KD, Sverd J, Sprafkin J, Nolan EE, Grossman S. Long-term methylphenidate therapy in children with comorbid attention-deficit hyperactivity disorder and chronic multiple tic disorder. *Arch Gen Psychiatry.* 1999;**56**:330–6.

46. Tourette's Syndrome Study Group. Treatment of ADHD in children with tics: a randomized controlled trial. *Neurology.* 2002;**58**:527–36.

47. Nolan EE, Gadow KD, Sprafkin J. Stimulant medication withdrawal during long-term therapy in children with comorbid attention-deficit hyperactivity disorder and chronic multiple tic disorder. *Pediatrics.* 1999;**103**(4):730–7.

48. Wilens T, Spencer T, Prince J, Biederman J. Stimulants and sudden death: what is a physician to do? *Pediatrics.* 2006;**118**(3):1215–19.

49. FDA. Communication about an ongoing safety review of stimulant medication used in children with attention-deficit/hyperactivity disorder (ADHD). In: FDA US, ed.; 2009.

50. Gould MS, Walsh TB, Munfakh JL, *et al.* Sudden death and use of stimulant medications in youths. 2009 [updated 2009; cited 2009 Aug 28]; 922–1001]. Available from: http://ajp.psychiatryonline.org/cgi/reprint/ajp;166/9/992.

51. Besag FM. Is suicidality serious? *Curr Drug Saf.* 2009;**4**(2):95–6.

52. Perrin JM, Friedman RA, Knilans TK. Cardiovascular monitoring and stimulant drugs for attention-deficit/hyperactivity disorder. *Pediatrics.* 2008;**122**(2):451–3.

53. Vetter VL, Elia J, Erickson C, *et al.* Cardiovascular monitoring of children and adolescents with heart disease receiving medications for attention deficit/hyperactivity disorder [corrected]. A scientific statement from the American Heart Association Council on Cardiovascular Disease in the Young Congenital Cardiac Defects Committee and the Council on Cardiovascular Nursing. *Circulation.* 2008;**120**(7):e55–9.

54. Mosholder AD, Gelperin K, Hammad TK, Phelan K, Johann-Liang R. Hallucinations and other psychotic symptoms associated with the use of attention-deficit/hyperactivity disorder drugs in children. *Pedatrics.* 2009;**123**:611–16.

55. El-Zein RA, Abdel-Rahman SZ, Hay MJ, *et al.* Cytogenetic effects in children treated with methylphenidate. *Cancer Lett.* 2005;**230**(2):284–91.

56. Dunnick JK, Hailey JR. Experimental studies on the long-term effects of methylphenidate hydrochloride. *Toxicology.* 1995;**103**:77–84.

57. Selby JV, Friedman GD, Fireman BH. Screening prescription drugs for possible carcinogenicity: eleven to fifteen years of follow-up. *Cancer Res.* 1989;**49**(20):5736–47.

58. Center for the Evaluation of Risks to Human Reproduction NTP. NTP-CERHR monograph on the potential human reproductive and developmental effects of methylphenidate. NIH Publication No. 05–4473; 2005.

59. Ponsa I, Ramos-Quiroga JA, Ribases M, *et al.* Absence of cytogenetic effects in children and adults with

attention-deficit/hyperactivity disorder treated with methylphenidate. *Mutat Res.* 2009;**666**(1–2):44–9.

60. Wilens T, Faraone S, Biederman J, Gunawardene S. Does stimulant therapy of ADHD beget later substance abuse: a meta-analytic review of the literature. *Pediatrics.* 2003;**11**(1):179–85.

61. Katusic SK, Barbaresi WJ, Colligan RC, *et al.* Psychostimulant treatment and risk for substance abuse among young adults with a history of attention-deficit/hyperactivity disorder: a population-based, birth cohort study. *J Child Adolesc Psychopharmacol.* 2005;**15**(5):764–76.

62. Wilens T, Adamson J, Monuteaux MC, *et al.* Effect of prior stimulant treatment for attention-deficit hyperactivity disorder on subsequent risk for cigarette smoking and alcohol and drug use disorders in adolescents. *Arch Pediatr Adolesc Med.* 2008;**162**(10):916–21.

63. Biederman J, Monuteaux MC, Spencer T, *et al.* Stimulant therapy and risk for subsequent substance use disorders in male adults with ADHD: a naturalistic controlled 10-year follow-up study. *Am J Psychiatry.* 2008;**165**(5):597–603.

64. Mannuzza S, Klein RG, Truong NL, *et al.* Age of methylphenidate treatment initiation in children with ADHD and later substance abuse: prospective follow-up into adulthood. *Am J Psychiatry.* 2008;**165**(5):604–9.

65. Wilens TE, Adler LA, Adamson J, *et al.* Misuse and diversion of stimulants prescribed for ADHD: a systematic review of the literature. *J Am Acad Child Adolesc Psychiatry.* 2008;**47**(1):21–31.

66. Wilens TE, Gignac M, Swezey A, Monuteaux MC, Biederman J. Characteristics of adolescents and young adults with ADHD who divert or misuse their prescribed medications. *J Am Acad Child Adolesc Psychiatry.* 2006;**45**(4):408–14.

67. McCabe SE, Knight JR, Teter CJ, Wechsler H. Non-medical use of prescription stimulants among US college students: prevalence and correlates from a national survey. *Addiction.* 2005;**99**(1):96–106.

68. Teter CJ, McCabe SE, LaGrange K, Cranford JA, Boyd CJ. Illicit use of specific prescription stimulants among college students: prevalence, motives, and routes of administration. *Pharmacotherapy.* 2006;**26**(10):1501–10.

69. McCabe SE, Teter CJ, Boyd CJ. The use, misuse and diversion of prescription stimulants among middle and high school students. *Subst Use Misuse.* 2004;**39**(7):1095–116.

70. Poulin C. From attention-deficit/hyperactivity disorder to medical stimulant use to the diversion of prescribed stimulants to non-medical stimulant use: connecting the dots. *Addiction.* 2007;**102**(5):740–51.

71. Biederman J, Faraone SV, Spencer T, *et al.* Patterns of psychiatric comorbidity, cognition, and psychosocial functioning in adults with attention deficit hyperactivity disorder. *Am J Psychiatry.* 1993;**150**:1792–8.

72. Willoughby MT, Curran PJ, Costello EJ, Angold A. Implications of early versus late onset of attention-deficit/hyperactivity disorder symptoms. *J Am Acad Child Adolesc Psychiatry.* 2000;**39**(12):1512–19.

73. Nandagopal JJ, DelBello MP, Kowatch R. Pharmacologic treatment of pediatric bipolar disorder. *Child Adolesc Psychiatr Clin N Am.* 2003;**18**:455–69.

74. Joshi G, Wilens T. Comorbidity in pediatric bipolar disorder. *Child Adolesc Psychiatr Clin N Am.* 2009;**18**(2):291–319, vii–viii.

75. Wozniak J, Biederman J, Kiely K, *et al.* Mania-like symptoms suggestive of childhood-onset bipolar disorder in clinically referred children. *J Am Acad Child Adolesc Psychiatry.* 1995;**34**:867–76.

76. Scheffer RE, Kowatch RA, Carmody T, Rush AJ. Randomized, placebo-controlled trial of mixed amphetamine salts for symptoms of comorbid ADHD in pediatric bipolar disorder after mood stabilization with divalproex sodium. *Am J Psychiatry.* 2005;**162**:58–64.

77. Findling RL, Short EJ, McNamara NK, *et al.* Methylphenidate in the treatment of children and adolescents with bipolar disorder and attention-deficit/hyperactivity disorder. *J Am Acad Child Adolesc Psychiatry.* 2007;**46**(11):1445–53.

78. DelBello MP, Soutullo CA, Hendricks W, *et al.* Prior stimulant treatment in adolescents with bipolar disorder: association with age at onset. *Bipolar Disord.* 2001;**3**(2):53–7.

79. Quintana H, Birmaher B, Stedge D, *et al.* Use of methylphenidate in the treatment of children with autistic disorder. *J Autism Dev Disord.* 1995;**25**(3):283–94.

80. Handen BL, Johnson CR, Lubetsky M. Efficacy of methylphenidate among children with autism and symptoms of attention-deficit hyperactivity disorder. *J Autism Dev Disord.* 2000;**30**(3):245–55.

81. Research Units on Pediatric Psychopharmacology Autism Network. Randomized, controlled, crossover trial of methylphenidate in pervasive developmental disorders with hyperactivity. *Arch Gen Psychiatry.* 2005;**62**(11):1266–74.

82. Posey DJ, Aman MG, McCracken JT, *et al.* Positive effects of methylphenidate on inattention and hyperactivity in pervasive developmental disorders: an

analysis of secondary measures. *Biol Psychiatry.* 2007;**61**(4):538–44.

83. Stigler KA, Desmond LA, Posey DJ, Wiegand RE, McDougle CJ. A naturalistic retrospective analysis of psychostimulants in pervasive developmental disorders. *J Child Adolesc Psychopharmacol.* 2004;**14**(1):49–56.

84. Davies S, Heyman I, Goodman R. A population survey of mental health problems in children with epilepsy. *Dev Med Child Neurol.* 2003;**45**:292–5.

85. Herman BH, Jones J, Dabbs K, *et al.* The frequency, complications, and aetiology of ADHD in new onset paediatric epilepsy. *Brain.* 2007;**130**:3135–48.

86. Baptista-Neto L, Dodds A, Rao S, *et al.* An expert opinion on methylphenidate treatment for attention deficit hyperactivity disorder in pediatric patients with epilepsy. *Expert Opin Investig Drugs.* 2008;**17**(1): 77–84.

87. McAfee AT, Holdridge KC, Johannes CB, Hornbuckle K, Walker AM. The effect of pharmacotherapy for attention deficit hyperactivity disorder on risk of seizures in pediatric patients as assessed in an insurance claims data. *Curr Drug Saf.* 2008;**3**(2): 123–31.

88. Gonzalez-Heydrich J, Waber J, Waber D, *et al.* Adaptive phase I study of OROS methylphenidate treatment of attention deficit hyperactivity disorder with epilepsy. *Epilepsy Behav.* 2010;**18**(3):229–37.

89. Daviss WB, Birmaher B, Diler RS, Mintz J. Does pharmacotherapy for attention-deficit/hyperactivity disorder predict risk of later major depression? *J Child Adolesc Psychopharmacol.* 2008;**18**(3):257–64.

90. Biederman J, Monuteaux MC, Spencer T, Wilens TE, Faraone SV. Do stimulants protect against psychiatric disorders in youth with ADHD? A 10-year follow-up study. *Pediatrics.* 2009;**124**(1):71–8.

Chapter 21

Non-stimulant treatment of ADHD

Juan D. Pedraza and Jeffrey H. Newcorn

Introduction and rationale

The psychostimulants, primarily methylphenidate (MPH) and amphetamine (AMPH), are the most effective and frequently prescribed medications for attention-deficit hyperactivity disorder (ADHD). Hundreds of controlled clinical trials have established the utility of these medications in reducing the over-activity, impulsivity, and inattention characteristic of children with ADHD, leading to improvement in a wide variety of associated behaviors, including academic performance, social functioning, and disruptive behavior. The effect size of stimulant medication for treatment of core ADHD symptoms is considered to be large, making these medications among the most effective treatments in psychiatric practice. Moreover, the tolerability profile of stimulants is considered to be quite agreeable. Yet, despite their overall robust efficacy and reasonable tolerability profile, stimulant treatments have their limitations, as outlined below.

Response. Some patients do not tolerate stimulant treatments well or do not achieve optimal symptom reduction with these medications. For example, in the Multimodal Treatment Study of Children with ADHD (i.e., MTA study), only 56% of patients had an optimal response (defined as a composite rating of "1" on a composite scale comprising symptoms of ADHD and oppositional defiant disorder [ODD]) to well-titrated medication treatment, primarily stimulants (and almost exclusively immediate-release formulations, since the MTA study was conducted in the mid to late 1990s), using all available compounds and formulations; approximately 20% of the patients did not respond to treatment with either stimulant class [1]. In addition, while the 14-month MTA findings [2] clearly established the relative superiority of assignment to the MTA medication algorithm over behavior

interventions over the course of 1 year (i.e., relatively long-term improvement), findings from the 36- and 72-month follow-up assessments suggest that the superiority of intensive, carefully monitored medication management gradually dissipates when children are returned to community treatment. While this result does not contradict the findings of robust efficacy of acute stimulant treatment, it does suggest the importance of considering multiple perspectives regarding intervention [3, 4].

Tolerability. The side effects of stimulant treatment are similar whether MPH or AMPH formulations are used [5]. The most frequently occurring adverse effects are decreased appetite and insomnia, but changes in affective function and mood regulation can be observed – particularly when the medication wears off. While more serious side effects of stimulants, such as psychosis, obsessive ruminations, and movement disorders, are infrequent and usually abate if the medication dose is lowered or stopped, tolerability concerns do appear to limit treatment in selected individuals [5]. It is presumed that issues regarding tolerability affect adherence to treatment, and it has been well established that long-term adherence to stimulant treatment is relatively poor [5].

Growth. Adverse consequences of stimulants on growth have been attributed to either decreased appetite or the direct effects of stimulant medication on dopaminergic neurons in the pituitary, with resultant effects on growth hormone. Initial studies of growth delay following stimulant treatment concluded that loss in expected weight and height was relatively small, drug discontinuation resulted in growth rebound [6–8], and patients treated continuously for up to 5 years until the age of 13 showed no difference in height when compared to untreated peers [9].

Attention-Deficit Hyperactivity Disorder in Adults and Children, ed. Lenard A. Adler, Thomas J. Spencer and Timothy E. Wilens.
Published by Cambridge University Press. © Cambridge University Press 2015.

However, recent findings from the MTA study suggesting decreased growth velocity and attainment in children consistently treated with stimulants have generated renewed interest in the potential adverse effects of stimulants on growth [10–12].

Cardiovascular effects. In addition to their desired therapeutic effects, the noradrenergic properties of stimulants are known to affect cardiovascular indices. Virtually all studies report small to moderate increases in pulse and blood pressure, with larger increases noted in selected individuals and at certain times of day (i.e., in relation to blood level of drug). While the degree of stimulant-induced risk for frank central nervous system toxicity is considered to be extremely low, and may not exceed the level observed in the general population [13–15], the potential for increased cardiac risk with treatment remains a concern. This is especially true in adults, in whom the high rate of hypertension [13] represents an important consideration. Thus, identification of non-stimulant treatments that minimize cardiovascular risk remains a priority.

Tics. Tic disorders are considered a relative contraindication for stimulant use despite the fact that the relationship between stimulant treatment and tic emergence or exacerbation is not straightforward. Recent data indicate that many patients with comorbid tic disorder and ADHD can be treated safely with stimulants, with either improvement in ADHD and no worsening of tics [16–18], or even improvement in tics [19]; however, it is also clear that stimulants can exacerbate tics in at least some individuals [16]. Consequently, it stands to reason that the availability of non-stimulants that may reduce the risk for tic emergence or exacerbation would represent an advantage for some patients.

Abuse potential. AMPH and MPH are Class II controlled substances, and both preclinical and clinical studies have documented the potential for abuse of these agents [20, 21]. Both stimulant classes have been associated with a higher degree of likeability and euphorogenic effects than non-scheduled agents [22, 23], and a 2005 survey found that 1.1 million Americans reported non-medical use of stimulants in the past month [24]. A recent meta-analysis [24] of 21 studies with over 100 000 subjects found that between 5% and 35% of college-age adults took non-prescribed stimulant medications; lifetime diversion rates for stimulants in this population ranged between 16% and 29%. Although results of a 2006 survey suggest that this behavior may have peaked [25, 26], the

magnitude of illicit use in certain segments of the population (e.g., high school and college students) is disturbing. Therefore, identification of effective, non-abusable treatments for ADHD remains a high priority.

Neurobiological rationale for non-stimulant treatment of ADHD. Brain regions most often implicated in the pathophysiology of ADHD include the prefrontal cortex (PFC), primarily the dorsolateral (DLPFC) and ventrolateral (VLPFC) regions, anterior cingulate gyrus (ACG), striatum (caudate in particular), and cerebellum [27–30]. The fact that many of these regions are characterized by high levels of dopaminergic and/or noradrenergic neurotransmission [28, 29], coupled with the fact that stimulant medications are highly efficacious in reducing ADHD symptoms [30], has supported the view of ADHD as a catecholaminergic condition [31–33]. Until recently, the preponderance of research has focused on the dopaminergic effects of stimulants. The striatum, in particular, has received considerable attention, because it contains large numbers of dopamine transporters (DAT) [34, 35], and DAT inhibition through competitive binding is thought to represent a primary mechanism of stimulant treatment [36–39]. However, many of the brain regions implicated in ADHD are also known to receive dense noradrenergic innervation (for example, VLPFC, ACG) [40, 41], and it is well established that norepinephrine (NE) plays an important role in the regulation of attention, particularly the ability to focus on salient stimuli [41, 42]. These findings, coupled with the long-recognized observation that virtually all medications known to improve ADHD symptoms (including the psychostimulants) have facilitating effects on NE neurotransmission [30, 35], form the basis of the noradrenergic hypothesis of ADHD [27, 31, 43, 44]. Nevertheless, single neurotransmitter models clearly cannot capture the complexity of the neural circuitry subserving broad regulatory functions such as attention and executive control, or the pathophysiology of ADHD, and more recent conceptualizations have focused on interactive properties of dopamine (DA) and NE neurotransmission [27, 31] as well as the modulating roles of other neurotransmitter systems. The fact that all US Food and Drug Administration (FDA)-approved agents – including stimulants and non-stimulants alike – are believed to potentiate the function of central catecholamines (i.e., NE and DA) in regions within the fronto-striatal attention circuit provides a unifying explanation for treatment efficacy.

This research provides a neurobiological rationale for the use of non-stimulant agents (most of which target NE neurotransmission) in the treatment of ADHD.

This chapter reviews current non-stimulant medication treatment options for ADHD. We present information regarding mechanism of action, pharmacokinetics, efficacy, tolerability and safety profile, and additionally discuss issues related to treatment selection and guidelines for titrating and monitoring treatment. In addition to the FDA-approved non-stimulants, we also discuss medications which are not FDA approved but may have a role in clinical practice. We also discuss the atypical stimulant modafinil, since modafinil is a Schedule IV medication which is somewhat less heavily regulated, and is often discussed in reviews of non-stimulant treatments for ADHD.

Non-stimulants used in ADHD

At present, there are only two classes of FDA-approved non-stimulant agents: the selective norepinephrine reuptake inhibitors (e.g., atomoxetine) and the alpha-2 (α_2) agonists (e.g., guanfacine extended-release [GXR] and clonidine extended-release [CXR]). Both of these drug classes target noradrenergic neurotransmission preferentially. Atomoxetine is approved in children 6 years of age and older, as well as adults. GXR and CXR are only approved for use in children and adolescents, but they are approved for combined treatment with stimulants as well as monotherapy for ADHD. The main clinical differences between these agents and the stimulants are their non-controlled status, potential for "24/7" duration of activity (though comparator pharmacokinetic/pharmacodynamic studies have not been undertaken), and generally slower onset of action (often at least several weeks).

Non-FDA-approved agents most often used in the clinical setting include the immediate-release/short-acting α_2 agonists, clonidine and guanfacine, the mixed noradrenergic/dopaminergic agonist bupropion, the mixed serotonin/norepinephrine reuptake inhibitors (SNRIs) venlafaxine and desvenlafaxine, and the partial DA agonist and serotonin (5-HT) antagonist buspirone. There are also considerable data on the noradrenergic reuptake inhibiting tricyclic antidepressants (TCAs) and the monoamine oxidase inhibitors (MAOIs), and emerging data on the N-methyl D-aspartate (NMDA) receptor antagonist amantadine. Although these latter medications are rarely used and should only be considered in unusual cases after other options have been exhausted, they are presented here for their historical and heuristic value.

Atomoxetine

Atomoxetine (ATMX) binds selectively to the NE transporter (NET), thereby increasing synaptic NE diffusely and DA in the PFC. The latter effect is due to the fact that NET, which are relatively abundant in the PFC while DAT are sparse [45, 46], regulate reuptake of prefrontal DA in the PFC. Thus, ATMX facilitates both noradrenergic and dopaminergic neurotransmission in the PFC [47]. The lack of dopaminergic activity in the nucleus accumbens and striatum suggests the decreased likelihood of drug abuse liability and motoric effects that can be seen with the psychostimulants. ATMX is well absorbed after oral administration and is metabolized primarily through the cytochrome P 450 2D6 (CYP2D6) pathway, so that co-administration with some selective serotonin reuptake inhibitors (SSRIs) (e.g., paroxetine and to a lesser extent fluoxetine) can elevate serum ATMX levels. However, ATMX does not induce CYP2D6 enzymatic function, so it does not alter the kinetics of SSRIs and hence, the two classes of medications can be used together when this is indicated.

The efficacy of ATMX has been well documented in short- and long-term studies [33, 48–50]; the effect size of treatment is approximately 0.7 across multiple studies, with multiple informants, though one study in youth with ADHD + comorbid anxiety disorders produced an effect size of 1.0 for ADHD symptoms. Full therapeutic effect can take up to 6–8 weeks, but responders typically show some degree of improvement by 4 weeks [48, 51]. The adverse effect profile of ATMX is generally benign (with some noteworthy exceptions; see below), with symptoms such as somnolence (most often occurring early in treatment), decreased appetite, and nausea and vomiting (the latter is less common) seen. Insomnia, irritability, and mood swings are less frequent though potentially more problematic. Small reductions in height and weight can also occur, though probably less than with stimulants. Small, statistically significant changes have been observed in heart rate and pulse with ATMX [52], similar or even slightly greater (in the case of heart rate) to what is seen with stimulants.

ATMX has been reported to improve ADHD symptoms in patients with comorbidities such as oppositional defiant disorder, conduct disorder, and anxiety disorders [48, 53–56], and may have beneficial effects on some of these comorbid conditions as well. ATMX does not worsen tics in patients with tic disorders + ADHD [57–59], and there was a suggestion of improvement in tic symptoms in a subgroup of patients with Tourette syndrome. Preliminary studies have shown that ATMX is effective in treating children with autism spectrum disorders (ASD) and ADHD symptoms, but the response seems to be lower than in normally developing children with ADHD [60]. Recent analyses have generated interest in the potential role of ATMX in adults with ADHD and comorbid alcohol use disorders [61], as ADHD symptom improvement was correlated with a reduction of alcohol cravings in patients treated with ATMX in comparison to placebo [61]. However, other studies have found negative results when comparing ATMX with placebo in adolescents with ADHD and comorbid non-tobacco substance use disorders [62, 63] or ASD [60, 64, 65]. Although initially formulated to be an antidepressant, ATMX does not seem to exert an effect on symptoms of comorbid depression [66]. ATMX has been shown to be effective in longer-term treatment of ADHD in children and adolescents [67], with efficacy demonstrated out to 2 years [68].

Multiple studies have demonstrated that ATMX is an effective and generally well-tolerated treatment for adults with ADHD. It was the first ADHD treatment to be approved specifically for adult use based on efficacy in well-controlled adult trials [69]. A wide variety of studies have evaluated the use of ATMX alone and in combination with a stimulant for the treatment of ADHD with and without comorbidities [70–72]. ATMX has been found to be helpful for adult patients with ADHD and emotional dysregulation [73] and also for patients with ADHD and executive function deficits [74]. Further, there is documented improvement of ADHD symptoms in patients with comorbid alcohol abuse [61, 75] and social anxiety disorder [76]. Studies have shown that once- and twice-daily dosing is efficacious for adults with ADHD, although the incidence of adverse effects is not higher and may be slightly lower with twice-daily dosing [77].

Despite considerable potential advantages over stimulants – e.g., lower risk for abuse, apparently long-lasting therapeutic effects, and non-controlled status – there are also limitations to be considered. Comparator studies in youth with ADHD have demonstrated the effect size for ATMX to be somewhat lower than

for MPH in the largest head-to-head comparison [32], and substantially lower than AMPH in a smaller comparator trial [78]. In addition, there has been concern about potential for liver toxicity and suicidal behavior, resulting in a box warning for suicidality. Patients and their families should be educated about these issues and patients should be monitored for suicidality during the first few months of treatment and following any dose changes. Despite these limitations, ATMX can be considered a first-line treatment in children and adolescents with a history of substance abuse or dependence, in those with significant anxiety symptoms, and in selected individuals based on prior treatment experience, family preference, and possibly duration of effects (i.e., throughout the day). Ongoing research is attempting to more comprehensively evaluate the role of ATMX within the ADHD medication armamentarium, and, in particular, whether there is evidence that some patients may respond preferentially to ATMX over stimulants.

Strattera is manufactured in capsules containing 10, 18, 25, 40, 60, 80, or 100 mg of atomoxetine hydrochloride. Titration follows a sequential, weight-based approach. Individuals weighing 70 kg or less generally begin at a dose of 0.5 mg/kg/day, which can be increased after a minimum of 3 days to a target dose of 1.2 mg/kg/day (although it is often prudent to increase the dose at a slower rate, and not go as high as 1.2 mg/kg immediately). The maximum recommended dosage is 1.4 mg/kg/day or 100 mg/day (whichever is less); however, most of the pre-marketing studies in children and adolescents studied doses up to 1.8 mg/kg/day and did not find undue tolerability concerns at higher doses. The medication can be administered either twice daily or once daily; initial studies followed a twice-daily dosing schedule but more recent studies used a once-daily administration schedule. Recent data indicate that tolerability during titration is generally better when the medication is administered in divided doses, and adverse effects, when present, do not last as long [79]. Consequently, it is often advisable to titrate on a BID schedule, or to extend the duration of medication exposure before raising doses, if administering the drug once daily. Administering the medication in the evening during titration is another method of limiting sedative adverse effects. However, while the medication is effective and generally better tolerated when administered in the evening, the observed magnitude of improvement is not as great [79], so it is prudent to move the dose to the AM once tolerability stabilizes.

ATMX undergoes extensive biotransformation; it is mainly metabolized via the CYP2D6 enzymatic pathway, in which ATMX is oxidized to form 4-hydroxyatomoxetine (the major metabolite). Poor metabolizers (approximately 7% of the population) have a much higher plasma level at the same dose, and the drug half-life is considerably longer (approximately 19 hours vs. 4.5 hours). However, poor metabolizers can be titrated using the same sequential dose-escalating approach described above, so genotyping is not required. Extensive metabolizers with moderate or severe hepatic insufficiency have increased ATMX exposure compared with healthy volunteers; therefore, dosage reduction is recommended in these patients. No dosage adjustment is required for patients with end-stage renal disease or lesser degrees of renal insufficiency. ATMX pharmacokinetics are not influenced by sex or ethnic origin, with the one exception that Whites have a higher likelihood of being poor metabolizers [51]. ATMX can be administered with or without food; however, it is often recommended that it be given with food to protect against nausea. When given without food, absorption proceeds at a faster rate.

Alpha-2 agonists: clonidine and guanfacine

The early success of clonidine and guanfacine used off-label for the treatment of ADHD generated interest in the development and systematic study of extended-release formulations of these medications. In 2009, Intuniv (i.e., guanfacine extended-release [GXR]) received FDA approval for the treatment of ADHD in children and adolescents; this was followed by the approval of Kapvay (i.e., clonidine extended-release [CXR]) in 2010. Both CXR and GXR are approved in the USA as monotherapy or as adjunctive therapy to stimulant medications [80–84]. Efficacy of clonidine and guanfacine is primarily attributable to postsynaptic α_2 agonist effects, which result in enhanced noradrenergic neurotransmission. Presynaptic α_2 agonist effects may also contribute to therapeutic benefit, due to suppression of spontaneous locus coeruleus activity thought to be implicated in the over-arousal, hyperactivity, and excitability seen in individuals with ADHD. Suppression of spontaneous locus coeruleus activity is thought to promote stimulus-driven locus coeruleus firing associated with optimal task performance, with

additional cognitive enhancing effects attributable to effects on target pyramidal neurons in the PFC [85].

The main difference between clonidine and guanfacine is that clonidine is less specific for α_{2A} receptors than guanfacine [86], and additionally binds to a variety of receptors other than α_2. While the clinical significance of these differences in binding profile remains uncertain, differences in underlying neurobiological effects suggest that some patients may respond preferentially to one or the other medication. Because guanfacine and clonidine are similar medications in the same class, in the following section we will describe pharmacokinetic and pharmacodynamic properties, efficacy, dosing, and adverse effects of these medications together.

Pharmacokinetic and pharmacodynamic properties

Clonidine

Clonidine, or 2-(2,6-dichlorophenylamino)-2-imidazoline, is highly lipid soluble and is completely absorbed after oral administration, with peak plasma levels occurring within 3 to 5 hours. Clonidine has a half-life of 12 to 16 hours in adults and 8 to 12 hours in children. Elimination of clonidine is 65% by renal excretion and 35% by liver metabolism. Because the behavioral effects of immediate-release clonidine (CIR) last only 3 to 6 hours, the oral formulation is usually given on a TID or QID schedule [87, 88]. CXR is a stable matrix tablet formulation which releases clonidine gradually over a 12-hour period; hence, twice-daily administration is recommended. After administration of CXR, maximum clonidine concentrations were approximately 50% that of CIR, and occurred approximately 5 hours later. Similar elimination half-lives for CIR and CXR were observed and total systemic bioavailability following CXR was approximately 89% of that following CIR. Food had no effect on plasma concentrations, bioavailability, or elimination half-life [89].

The efficacy of CXR in the treatment of patients with ADHD has been assessed in two randomized double-blind placebo-controlled phase three trials [84, 90], with demonstrated efficacy in reducing ADHD symptoms in children and adolescents when compared with placebo. Recent studies have also shown that the medication is effective as an adjunctive treatment to stimulants in children and adolescents with ADHD who have partial response to stimulant monotherapy [83]. Clinical trials have shown that symptom improvement can be seen as soon as 2 weeks after starting treatment with CXR [84, 90]. The effectiveness of CXR for longer-term use (more than 5 weeks) has not been systematically evaluated in controlled trials [89].

CIR is manufactured in 0.1, 0.2, and 0.3 mg tablets. There is also a transdermal therapeutic system (i.e., clonidine patch), available in equivalent doses (e.g., 0.1, 0.2, and 0.3 mg), which provides more sustained coverage and eliminates the need for frequent oral doses per day. Each patch lasts about 5–6 days although the product labeling indicates 1-week activity [91]. When using the clonidine transdermal system, it is generally recommended to adjust the dose of oral clonidine and switch to the transdermal system once the optimal dose is determined. Combination of transdermal and oral forms may be used in some cases. When used to treat ADHD, clonidine is generally dosed at 3–5 mcg/kg/day [92], with a range of 0.15 to 0.3 mg/day. Some studies have used doses as high as 0.4 mg to 0.5 mg [93] but the risk of adverse effects may increase at higher doses. It is usually recommended to begin with low doses and increase slowly to minimize the possibility of sedation and adverse cardiovascular effects. A general rule is to not increase the dose more than 0.05 mg every 3 days.

CXR is available as 0.1 or 0.2 mg tablets which should be swallowed whole and not crushed, chewed, or broken; the medication may be taken with or without food [89]. The extended-release and immediate-release formulations should not be used interchangeably because of the different kinetics. Dosing should be initiated with one 0.1 mg tablet at bedtime, then 0.1 mg BID. The dosage should be adjusted in increments of 0.1 mg/day at weekly intervals until the desired response is achieved. As a rule, the medication should be taken twice a day, with either an equal or higher split dosage being given at bedtime [89].

Guanfacine

Guanfacine, or N-amidino-2-(2,6-dichlorophenyl) acetamide, is more specific in its effects on α_{2A} receptors compared with clonidine. Guanfacine is 10 times less potent than clonidine in reducing presynaptic NE release in the locus coeruleus (LC) or inhibiting LC firing [94], although this relative difference in potency is accounted for in the dosing. The plasma half-life of immediate-release guanfacine (GIR) is approximately 17 hours (range = 10 to 30 hours) in healthy adults, but tends to be shorter in younger individuals (range = 13 to 14 hours). Guanfacine and its metabolites are excreted primarily in the urine, with approximately 50% excreted as unchanged drug. Differences in the pharmacodynamic effects of GIR and GXR are primarily accounted for by the prolonged rate of dissolution of GXR [95], since the half-life of the two formulations is fairly similar. The time required to reach maximal plasma concentration (T_{max}) is considerably longer for GXR than GIR (2.5–3 hours for GIR and 5–6 hours GXR) [96]; additionally, GXR has a 40% lower maximum plasma concentration (C_{max}). The more gradual and prolonged onset of effects of GXR provides the basis for the extended duration of behavioral effects using a daily dosing strategy. GXR has been shown to be efficacious in decreasing both inattentive and hyperactive/impulsive ADHD symptoms [82, 97], and co-administration of GXR and MPH has been demonstrated to be safe and effective [98]. Open-label continuation studies indicate sustained drug effectiveness and safety with GXR monotherapy [97, 99] and co-administration of GXR and MPH [100] through 24 months.

GIR is available in 1 mg and 2 mg tablets. Because guanfacine is 10 times less potent than clonidine, 1 mg of guanfacine is comparable in potency and physiological effect to 0.1 mg of clonidine. Dosing of guanfacine reflects its lower potency and longer duration of action, with doses ranging from 0.5 mg (for GIR) to 4 mg/day. The half-life of guanfacine is somewhat longer than for clonidine, and GIR is generally given on a BID or TID schedule, with 0.5 mg dose increases every 3 to 4 days. Multiple studies have used doses ranging from 1.5 to 3.2 mg/day [101, 103] given between twice and four times daily. GXR tablets are available in 1 mg, 2 mg, 3 mg, and 4 mg doses. Because GXR is a sustained-release formulation, intended and labeled for once daily administration, tablets should be swallowed whole and not crushed, chewed, or broken. Also, GXR should not be administered with high-fat meals, due to increased exposure to the medication [104].

Titration of GXR in pre-marketing ADHD clinical trials [97, 100] was achieved using a weekly dose-escalating strategy, with 1 mg increments weekly. Although these studies used an absolute dosing approach, post-hoc analyses indicated that response may be optimized using a weight-adjusted approach. Clinically relevant improvements were observed beginning at doses in the range of 0.05–0.08 mg/kg, with potential for further improvement in doses up to 0.12 mg/kg. Clinical trials have shown that clinical improvement can be seen between 2 and 4 weeks after starting treatment with GXR [84, 90, 105]. As with clonidine, switching from GIR to GXR should not assume that an equivalent daily dose will be required, because of the differing pharmacokinetic profiles of the two formulations.

Adverse effects

The adverse effect profiles of guanfacine and clonidine are similar, with the exception that dry mouth, sedation, bradycardia, and syncope are reported to be less common with guanfacine [99, 100, 106]. The sedative effects, when present, typically begin within the first weeks of treatment and resolve by the end of titration [97, 100]. Given that the α_2 agonists are approved antihypertensives, the potential for adverse cardiovascular events has been carefully examined. Although prolongation of PR and QTc intervals has been reported in some individuals with clonidine, systematic investigation has not supported consistent medication effects on EKG [99, 107, 108]. This is also true for guanfacine. Similarly, studies have not found differences in blood pressure in children with ADHD, though decreased blood pressure was seen early in treatment [103]. In some cases, light-headedness or syncope may occur, so it is important to hydrate well. Irritability has been reported with GIR in children with pervasive developmental disorder [109]. Dermatitis may develop when the adhesive formulation of clonidine is used, although this can often be managed by premedicating with hydrocortisone cream.

Treatment discontinuation

Potential discontinuation effects of guanfacine have been reasonably well studied using the extended-release formulation. Numerically greater mean increases in systolic and diastolic blood pressure and heart rate were reported following abrupt discontinuation compared to tapering, though these differences were not statistically significant. However, since these data do not rule out the possibility that rebound hypertension may occur, it is advised that GXR be tapered in decrements of no more than 1 mg every 3 to 7 days. As with guanfacine, abrupt discontinuation of CXR is not advised; rather, the dose should be tapered by a reduction of no more than 0.1 mg every 3 to 7 days to reduce the potential for withdrawal effects [97]. If the medication has been used for only

1 week, it can be discontinued immediately; if it has been prescribed for 1–4 weeks, it can be tapered by 0.05 mg each day; if it has been prescribed for over 4 weeks, it must be tapered by 0.05 mg every third day [91]. Tachycardia, tachypnea with or without fever, anxiety, panic attacks, and acute mental status changes may be seen with missed doses or abrupt discontinuation of clonidine.

Bupropion

Bupropion hydrochloride, an antidepressant of the aminoketone class, is chemically unrelated to tricyclic, tetracyclic, selective serotonin reuptake inhibiting, or other known antidepressant agents. Bupropion is a relatively weak inhibitor of the neuronal uptake of NE, serotonin, and DA, and does not inhibit monoamine oxidase. The mechanism of action of bupropion is unknown, but it is presumed that its therapeutic activity is mediated by noradrenergic and/or dopaminergic mechanisms. The mean elimination half-life of bupropion after chronic dosing is 21 ($\pm$9) hours, and steady-state plasma concentrations of bupropion are reached within 8 days. Bupropion is extensively metabolized by CYP2B6, and there is potential for drug–drug interactions with medications that are metabolized by this isoenzyme. The most common side effects are agitation, anxiety, and insomnia [110]. There is a slight increased risk for drug-induced seizures at doses >450 mg/day, and exacerbation of tic disorders has been reported. On the other hand, weight gain and sexual dysfunction are minimal [111, 112]. The medication is available as an IR formulation, a sustained-release (SR) preparation, and a long-acting (XL) formulation; the former can be administered twice daily and the latter two once daily. Alternative formulations of extended-release bupropion are available as branded generic medications (i.e., Aplenzin, Fortivo).

Bupropion has been used off-label for the treatment of ADHD for at least two decades, and there have been several controlled trials, including fairly large multisite trials in youth [113] and adults [114]. Results of all randomized controlled studies of bupropion were evaluated in a random effects meta-analysis measuring efficacy using the physician-based Clinical Global Impression Improvement (CGI-I) scale (the measure in common across studies), with a pooled odds ratio (OR) of 2.42 (95% confidence intervals [CI] 1.09–5.36) favoring bupropion [115]. The XL formulation of bupropion utilizes a diffusion-controlled vehicle, providing sustained benefit throughout the day, as demonstrated by significant findings on Conners' Adult ADHD Rating Scale-Self Report (CAARS-S:S) total scores at 10:00 am, 4:00 pm, and 10:00 pm in the adult ADHD multisite trial [116].

Several small n studies have examined the role of bupropion in the treatment of comorbid ADHD and substance use disorders, and suggest that bupropion may have a role in treating this population [114, 117]; however, there has been considerable variability in findings across studies. For example, one study examining the effects of bupropion, MPH, and placebo in adults with ADHD + substance use disorders enrolled in a methadone clinic found no beneficial effects of either medication [118]. However, other studies had positive findings in the treatment of adolescents with ADHD and comorbid depressive disorders and adults with ADHD and comorbid bipolar disorder [119, 120].

Buspirone

Buspirone is an anxiolytic agent which displays high affinity and selectivity for the serotonin 5-HT_{1A} and 5-HT_2 receptors [121, 122]. Buspirone has a modest impact on the DA system by acting as an agonist of D_2 autoreceptors [123, 124]. Because of its dopaminergic effects, and the role of 5-HT_{1A} receptors in the regulation of impulse control, there have been several studies of buspirone for the treatment of ADHD. Two open-label trials evaluated efficacy in a small number of patients, finding significant improvement in ADHD symptoms [125, 126]. More recently, three randomized double-blind placebo-controlled trials have been conducted. Two randomized trials compared the effects of buspirone with those of MPH, finding only relatively modest effects of buspirone. The incidence of side effects did not differ significantly except for decreased appetite in the MPH group [127, 128]. One study assessed the efficacy of atomoxetine combined with buspirone versus atomoxetine monotherapy and placebo in adult ADHD, finding no statistical significance between the two active treatment groups [129]. Even though the studies that have been conducted with buspirone are small and the effects on ADHD symptoms have been modest, this medication may have a role in the treatment of patients with ADHD and comorbid anxiety.

Venlafaxine

Venlafaxine is a mixed SNRI approved by the FDA for the treatment of major depressive disorder (MDD), generalized anxiety disorder, and comorbid depression–anxiety. At low doses (<150 mg/day), venlafaxine acts only on serotonergic transmission. At moderate doses (>150 mg/day), it acts on serotonergic and noradrenergic systems, whereas at high doses (>300 mg/day), it also affects dopaminergic neurotransmission. Because of its partial noradrenergic mechanism of action, venlafaxine has been studied in the treatment for ADHD in children and adults. Improvement in ADHD symptoms has been seen on both parent and teacher ratings, with a generally agreeable side effect profile. Most trials have been open label and conducted in small samples; results have been promising but not totally convincing [130–133]. One double-blind, parallel group trial showed that venlafaxine had a comparable response to MPH in children [131], but this is not likely the case. All antidepressants, including venlafaxine, carry a black box warning regarding possible risk for suicidal behavior in youth and young adults.

Modafinil

Modafinil (i.e., Provigil) is an atypical Schedule IV stimulant that is FDA-approved for excessive sleepiness associated with narcolepsy, obstructive sleep apnea syndrome, and shift work sleep disorder. Preclinical studies of modafinil have demonstrated an increase in activity of the PFC without widespread central nervous system activation, with considerable activity in the tuberomammillary nucleus of the hypothalamus. Studies using positron emission tomography (PET) have shown that modafinil occupies a significant proportion of DAT and NET sites in monkey striatum and thalamus in vivo after intravenous administration [134], and its pharmacological effects are abolished or attenuated by a range of manipulations that decrease catecholaminergic functions, particularly those that are α1-adrenoceptor-mediated [135]. Multiple clinical studies have evaluated the efficacy of modafinil in the treatment of ADHD in children and adults, with positive findings vs. placebo demonstrated in multiple well-conducted studies [136, 137], with no withdrawal or rebound symptoms after abrupt discontinuation [138, 139]. Modafinil has also been evaluated in the treatment of adult ADHD, with reasonable tolerability but surprising lack of efficacy reported [140].

Tricyclic antidepressants (TCAs)

Among the oldest of the non-FDA-approved non-stimulant agents for ADHD are the noradrenergic TCAs (e.g., desipramine, imipramine, and nortriptyline). TCAs are heterocyclic chemical compounds which act as SNRIs by blocking the serotonin transporter (SERT) and the NET, respectively, which results in elevated synaptic concentrations of these neurotransmitters [141] (note that the proportion of blockade of SERT and NET differs across the various TCA medications). TCAs have been largely replaced in clinical use by newer antidepressants such as the SSRIs and SNRIs, which typically have more favorable side effect profiles. However, the SSRIs do not affect NE and generally are not effective in ADHD; in contrast, a fairly large literature supports the efficacy of the more noradrenergic TCAs in ADHD. In several double-blind, placebo-controlled studies [142, 143], desipramine was found to be effective in the management of children with ADHD, including patients who failed to respond to stimulants. However, although treatment with this medication produced significant improvement, patients treated with desipramine were found to have increased risk for elevated diastolic blood pressure and heart rate (mainly sinus tachycardia), and electrocardiographic evidence of intraventricular conduction defects [142, 143]. For this reason, noradrenergic non-stimulant alternatives to the TCAs were sought, ultimately leading to the testing and approval of atomoxetine for ADHD. One important benefit of the TCAs in the treatment of ADHD is the positive effect on frequently occurring comorbid conditions, including anxiety, depression, and tic disorders. However, the side effect profile of the TCAs – especially the potentially adverse cardiovascular profile – and the availability of other effective non-stimulants have made the use of this group of medications very infrequent.

Monoamine oxidase inhibitors (MAOIs)

Although they are rarely used in clinical practice, a moderately sized database attests to the efficacy of MAOIs in the treatment of children and adults with ADHD. Research conducted at the National Institute of Mental Health (NIMH) in the 1980s examined the potential utility of MAOIs to test the multisystem model of ADHD, since MAOIs affect neurotransmission of multiple neurotransmitters, including the catecholamines and serotonin (5-HT). Comparable efficacy of MAOIs (clorgyline or tranylcypromine) and dextroamphetamine was demonstrated in a crossover trial of 14 prepubertal boys with ADHD [144]. Clinical improvement was not correlated with medication-induced changes in plasma and/or urinary catecholamine metabolites such as MHPG (breakdown product of NE), which the authors interpreted as indicating that improvement was not fully accounted for by catecholaminergic mechanisms [145]. Because MAO-A inhibiting drugs such as the ones studied initially require substantial dietary restrictions due to risk of hypertensive crisis, additional research was undertaken with the MAO-B inhibiting medication selegiline, which does not have the same dietary restrictions. However, change in ADHD ratings with selegiline was not found to differ from placebo in a small, parallel group study of adults with ADHD [146].

Amantadine

There are emerging data on the potential utility of glutamatergic agents such as amantadine in ADHD. Amantadine is an NMDA-receptor antagonist, which likely has indirect effects to enhance dopaminergic neurotransmission [147]. It also has direct dopaminergic effects through blockade of DA reuptake. Amantadine has been studied in two open-label trials [148, 149], and one comparison trial vs. MPH [150]. Both open studies found positive results of treatment and reasonable tolerability, although the medication was dosed very differently in the two studies; one [148] dosed amantadine at 150 mg/day while the other [149] studied much lower doses (10 and 20 mg, with the 20 mg dose performing much better). In the comparator trial [150], amantadine dosed at 100 or 150 mg/day (based on the subject's weight) produced improvement comparable to MPH; however, there was no placebo comparison group, and therefore no control over potential positive expectancy effects of treatment. Though potentially promising, the data on amantadine should be considered preliminary.

When should non-stimulants be used?

Because non-stimulants have a somewhat lower effect size than stimulants, the various professional guidelines [151, 152] and treatment algorithms indicate that stimulants should be used as the first-choice medication option for youth with ADHD [153]. However, non-stimulants can have an important role if there is poor response or tolerability to stimulants, or when certain comorbid disorders are present. For example, the presence of comorbid anxiety disorders might represent a good indication for atomoxetine, given the robust response to ADHD symptoms and the solid response to anxiety symptoms in this population. Alpha-2 agonists would potentially be a good choice for a patient with ADHD + comorbid for tic disorders and/or disruptive behavior disorders. Bupropion could be a parsimonious recommendation for someone with ADHD + comorbid depression, particularly if the first-choice treatment is an antidepressant. All of the non-stimulants could be options for individuals with ADHD + substance use disorders, as stimulant use is potentially problematic in this population. The α_2 agonists additionally have a labeled indication for adjunctive therapy, and can aid in mitigating the increases in heart rate and blood pressure that often accompany stimulant treatment. Importantly, non-stimulant medications can be used alone or in combination with stimulants to provide medication coverage throughout the day and into the evening, in some cases even when using once-daily dosing. This is particularly important because the time-action effects of stimulants (even the long-acting formulations) – i.e., rapid onset of effect but also a fairly rapid offset of effect – can be problematic for many patients. It should also be noted that as opposed to stimulants, patients treated with non-stimulants such as atomoxetine and α_2 agonists may not demonstrate clinical improvement until 2 to 4 weeks after starting treatment, and may take even longer to demonstrate the full effects. This should be taken into consideration when beginning treatment in patients who require acute stabilization of their symptoms, and patients should be counseled about the expected time course to improvement.

Summary

There are two classes of approved non-stimulant medications for ADHD – the selective noradrenergic reuptake inhibitors and the α_2-adrenergic agonists. In addition, several other medication classes have been used off-line with reported efficacy. While the non-stimulant medications are, on average, not as broadly or robustly effective as the psychostimulants, they can be extremely helpful in managing certain patients with ADHD – either as monotherapy or as adjunctive

agents. Currently, there is considerable interest among pharmaceutical companies to develop new classes of non-stimulant medications. It is anticipated that current and yet to be developed non-stimulants will have a prominent role in the treatment of selected subgroups of ADHD patients, as we learn more about the multiplicity of neural circuits and neurotransmitter systems that are implicated in the pathophysiology and/or maintenance of ADHD in the years ahead, and are better able to match treatment selection to individual patient characteristics.

References

1. Swanson JM, Kraemer HC, Hinshaw SP, et al. Clinical relevance of the primary findings of the MTA: success rates based on severity of ADHD and ODD symptoms at the end of treatment. *J Am Acad Child Adolesc Psychiatry*. 2001;**40**(2):168–79.

2. A 14-month randomized clinical trial of treatment strategies for attention-deficit/hyperactivity disorder. The MTA Cooperative Group. Multimodal Treatment Study of Children with ADHD. *Arch Gen Psychiatry*. 1999;**56**(12):1073–86.

3. Swanson J, Arnold LE, Kraemer H, et al. Evidence, interpretation, and qualification from multiple reports of long-term outcomes in the Multimodal Treatment Study of Children with ADHD (MTA): part I: executive summary. *J Atten Disord*. 2008;**12**(1):4–14.

4. Swanson J, Arnold LE, Kraemer H, et al. Evidence, interpretation, and qualification from multiple reports of long-term outcomes in the Multimodal Treatment Study of children with ADHD (MTA): Part II: supporting details. *J Atten Disord*. 2008;**12**(1):15–43.

5. Spencer T, Biederman J, Wilens T. Stimulant treatment of adult attention-deficit/hyperactivity disorder. *Psychiatr Clin North Am*. 2004;**27**(2):361–72.

6. Pizzi WJ, Rode E.C, Barnhart JE. Methylphenidate and growth: demonstration of a growth impairment and a growth-rebound phenomenon. *Dev Pharmacol Ther*. 1986;**9**(5):361–8.

7. Vincent J, Varley CK, Leger P. Effects of methylphenidate on early adolescent growth. *Am J Psychiatry*. 1990;**147**(4):501–2.

8. Spencer T, Biederman J, Wilens T. Growth deficits in children with attention deficit hyperactivity disorder. *Pediatrics*. 1998;**102**(2 Pt 3):501–6.

9. Spencer TJ, Biederman J, Harding M, et al. Growth deficits in ADHD children revisited: evidence for disorder-associated growth delays? *J Am Acad Child Adolesc Psychiatry*. 1996;**35**(11):1460–9.

10. Swanson JM, Elliott GR, Greenhill LL, et al. Effects of stimulant medication on growth rates across 3 years in

the MTA follow-up. *J Am Acad Child Adolesc Psychiatry*. 2007;**46**(8):1015–27.

11. Swanson JM, Hinshaw SP, Arnold LE, *et al*. Secondary evaluations of MTA 36-month outcomes: propensity score and growth mixture model analyses. *J Am Acad Child Adolesc Psychiatry*. 2007;**46**(8):1003–14.

12. MTA Cooperative Group. National Institute of Mental Health Multimodal Treatment Study of ADHD follow-up: changes in effectiveness and growth after the end of treatment. *Pediatrics*. 2004;**113**(4):762–9.

13. Westover AN, Halm EA. Do prescription stimulants increase the risk of adverse cardiovascular events?: a systematic review. *BMC Cardiovasc Disord*. 2012;**12**(1):41.

14. Habel LA, Cooper WO, Sox CM, *et al*. ADHD medications and risk of serious cardiovascular events in young and middle-aged adults. *JAMA*. 2011;**306**(24):2673–83.

15. Cooper WO, Habel LA, Sox CM, *et al*. ADHD drugs and serious cardiovascular events in children and young adults. *N Engl J Med*. 2011;**365**(20):1896–904.

16. Pringsheim T, Steeves T. Pharmacological treatment for Attention Deficit Hyperactivity Disorder (ADHD) in children with comorbid tic disorders. *Cochrane Database Syst Rev*. 2011;(4):CD007990.

17. Bloch MH, Panza KE, Landeros-Weisenberger A, Leckman JF. Meta-analysis: treatment of attention-deficit/hyperactivity disorder in children with comorbid tic disorders. *J Am Acad Child Adolesc Psychiatry*. 2009;**48**(9):884–93.

18. Poncin Y, Sukhodolsky DG, McGuire J, Scahill L. Drug and non-drug treatments of children with ADHD and tic disorders. *Eur Child Adolesc Psychiatry*. 2007;**16**(Suppl 1):78–88.

19. Tourette's Syndrome Study Group. Treatment of ADHD in children with tics: a randomized controlled trial. *Neurology*. 2002;**58**(4):527–36.

20. Vitiello B. Long-term effects of stimulant medications on the brain: possible relevance to the treatment of attention deficit hyperactivity disorder. *J Child Adolesc Psychopharmacol*. 2001;**11**(1):25–34.

21. Kollins SH, MacDonald EK, Rush CR. Assessing the abuse potential of methylphenidate in nonhuman and human subjects: a review. *Pharmacol Biochem Behav*. 2001;**68**(3):611–27.

22. Jasinski DR, Fraies DE, Moore RJ, Schuh LM, Allen AJ. Abuse liability assessment of atomoxetine in a drug-abusing population. *Drug Alcohol Depend*. 2008;**95**(1–2):140–6.

23. Wilens TE, Adler LA, Adams J, *et al*. Misuse and diversion of stimulants prescribed for ADHD: a systematic review of the literature. *J Am Acad Child Adolesc Psychiatry*. 2008;**47**(1):21–31.

24. National Institute on Drug Abuse. *Prescription Pain and Other Medications*. 2006.

25. Novak SP, Kroutil LA, Williams RL, Van Brunt DL. The nonmedical use of prescription ADHD medications: results from a national Internet panel. *Subst Abuse Treat Prev Policy*. 2007;**2**:32.

26. Kaye S, Darke S. The diversion and misuse of pharmaceutical stimulants: what do we know and why should we care? *Addiction*. 2012;**107**(3):467–77.

27. Durston S, Casey BJ. A shift from diffuse to focal cortical activity with development: the authors' reply. *Dev Sci*. 2006;**9**(1):18–20.

28. Epstein JN, Casey BJ, Tonev ST, *et al*. ADHD- and medication-related brain activation effects in concordantly affected parent-child dyads with ADHD. *J Child Psychol Psychiatry*. 2007;**48**(9):899–913.

29. Vaidya CJ, Austin G, Kirkorian G, *et al*. Selective effects of methylphenidate in attention deficit hyperactivity disorder: a functional magnetic resonance study. *Proc Natl Acad Sci U S A*. 1998;**95**(24):14494–9.

30. Dickstein SG, Bannon K, Castellanos FX, Milham MP. The neural correlates of attention deficit hyperactivity disorder: an ALE meta-analysis. *J Child Psychol Psychiatry*. 2006;**47**(10):1051–62.

31. Winterstein AG, Gerhard T, Shuster J, *et al*. Utilization of pharmacologic treatment in youths with attention deficit/hyperactivity disorder in Medicaid database. *Ann Pharmacother*. 2008;**42**(1):24–31.

32. Newcorn JH, Kratochvil CJ, Allen AJ, *et al*. Atomoxetine and osmotically released methylphenidate for the treatment of attention deficit hyperactivity disorder: acute comparison and differential response. *Am J Psychiatry*. 2008;**165**(6):721–30.

33. Wang Y, Zheng Y, Du Y, *et al*. Atomoxetine versus methylphenidate in paediatric outpatients with attention deficit hyperactivity disorder: a randomized, double-blind comparison trial. *Aust N Z J Psychiatry*. 2007;**41**(3):222–30.

34. Mason MF, Norton MI, Van Horn JD, *et al*. Wandering minds: the default network and stimulus-independent thought. *Science*. 2007;**315**(5810):393–5.

35. Fassbender C, Zhang H, Buzy WM, *et al*. A lack of default network suppression is linked to increased distractibility in ADHD. *Brain Res*. 2009;**1273**:114–28.

36. Fair DA, Posner J, Nagel BJ, *et al*. Atypical default network connectivity in youth with attention-deficit/hyperactivity disorder. *Biol Psychiatry*. 2010;**68**(12):1084–91.

37. Uddin LQ, Kelly AM, Biswal BB, *et al*. Network homogeneity reveals decreased integrity of

default-mode network in ADHD. *J Neurosci Methods.* 2008;**169**(1):249–54.

38. Kelly AM, Uddin LQ, Biswal BB, Castellanos FX, Milham MP. Competition between functional brain networks mediates behavioral variability. *Neuroimage.* 2008;**39**(1):527–37.

39. Halperin JM, Schulz KP. Revisiting the role of the prefrontal cortex in the pathophysiology of attention-deficit/hyperactivity disorder. *Psychol Bull.* 2006;**132**(4):560–81.

40. Willcutt EG, Doyle AE, Nigg JT, Faraone SV, Pennington BF. Validity of the executive function theory of attention-deficit/hyperactivity disorder: a meta-analytic review. *Biol Psychiatry.* 2005; **57**(11):1336–46.

41. Conners CK. Forty years of methylphenidate treatment in Attention-Deficit/Hyperactivity Disorder. *J Atten Disord.* 2002;**6**(Suppl 1):S17–30.

42. Kuczenski R, Segal DS. Effects of methylphenidate on extracellular dopamine, serotonin, and norepinephrine: comparison with amphetamine. *J Neurochem.* 1997;**68**(5):2032–7.

43. Greenhill LL, Pliska S, Dulcan MK, *et al.* Practice parameter for the use of stimulant medications in the treatment of children, adolescents, and adults. *J Am Acad Child Adolesc Psychiatry.* 2002;**41**(2 Suppl): 26S–49S.

44. Barkley RA. International Consensus Statement on ADHD. *J Am Acad Child Adolesc Psychiatry.* 2002;**41**(12):1389.

45. Lewis DA, Sesack SR, Levey AI, Rosenberg DR. Dopamine axons in primate prefrontal cortex: specificity of distribution, synaptic targets, and development. *Adv Pharmacol.* 1998;**42**:703–6.

46. Sesack SR, Howry VA, Guido MA, Levey AI. Cellular and subcellular localization of the dopamine transporter in rat cortex. *Adv Pharmacol.* 1998; **42**:171–4.

47. Bymaster FP, Katner JS, Nelson DR, *et al.* Atomoxetine increases extracellular levels of norepinephrine and dopamine in prefrontal cortex of rat: a potential mechanism for efficacy in attention deficit/ hyperactivity disorder. *Neuropsychopharmacology.* 2002;**27**(5):699–711.

48. Newcorn JH, Spencer TJ, Biederman J, Milton DR, Michelson D. Atomoxetine treatment in children and adolescents with attention-deficit/hyperactivity disorder and comorbid oppositional defiant disorder. *J Am Acad Child Adolesc Psychiatry.* 2005;**44**(3): 240–8.

49. Newcorn JH, Kratochvil CJ, Allen AJ, *et al.* Atomoxetine and osmotically released methylphenidate for the treatment of attention deficit hyperactivity disorder: acute comparison and differential response. *Am J Psychiatry.* 2008;**165**(6):721–30.

50. Dittmann RW, Schacht A, Helsberg K, *et al.* Atomoxetine versus placebo in children and adolescents with attention-deficit/hyperactivity disorder and comorbid oppositional defiant disorder: a double-blind, randomized, multicenter trial in Germany. *J Child Adolesc Psychopharmacol.* 2011; **21**(2):97–110.

51. Garnock-Jones KP, Keating GM. Atomoxetine: a review of its use in attention-deficit hyperactivity disorder in children and adolescents. *Paediatr Drugs.* 2009;**11**(3):203–26.

52. Christman AK, Fermo JD. Markowitz JS. Atomoxetine, a novel treatment for attention-deficit-hyperactivity disorder. *Pharmacotherapy.* 2004;**24**(8):1020–36.

53. Biederman J, Spencer TJ, Newcorn JH, *et al.* Effect of comorbid symptoms of oppositional defiant disorder on responses to atomoxetine in children with ADHD: a meta-analysis of controlled clinical trial data. *Psychopharmacology (Berl).* 2007;**190**(1): 31–41.

54. Michelson D, Faries D, Wernicke J, *et al.* Atomoxetine in the treatment of children and adolescents with attention-deficit/hyperactivity disorder: a randomized, placebo-controlled, dose-response study. *Pediatrics.* 2001;**108**(5):E83.

55. Kratochvil CJ, Newcorn JH, Arnold LE, *et al.* Atomoxetine alone or combined with fluoxetine for treating ADHD with comorbid depressive or anxiety symptoms. *J Am Acad Child Adolesc Psychiatry.* 2005;**44**(9):915–24.

56. Geller D, Donnelly C, Lopez F, *et al.* Atomoxetine treatment for pediatric patients with attention-deficit/ hyperactivity disorder with comorbid anxiety disorder. *J Am Acad Child Adolesc Psychiatry.* 2007;**46**(9): 1119–27.

57. Allen AJ, Kurlan RM, Gilbert DL, *et al.* Atomoxetine treatment in children and adolescents with ADHD and comorbid tic disorders. *Neurology.* 2005;**65**(12): 1941–9.

58. Feldman PD, Ruff DD, Allen AJ. Atomoxetine and tics in ADHD. *J Am Acad Child Adolesc Psychiatry.* 2005;**44**(5):405–6.

59. Spencer TJ, Sallee FR, Gilbert DL, *et al.* Atomoxetine treatment of ADHD in children with comorbid Tourette syndrome. *J Atten Disord.* 2008;**11**(4): 470–81.

60. Arnold LE, Aman MG, Cook AM, *et al.* Atomoxetine for hyperactivity in autism spectrum disorders: placebo-controlled crossover pilot trial. *J Am Acad Child Adolesc Psychiatry.* 2006;**45**(10):1196–205.

61. Wilens TE, Adler LA, Tanaka Y, *et al.* Correlates of alcohol use in adults with ADHD and comorbid alcohol use disorders: exploratory analysis of a placebo-controlled trial of atomoxetine. *Curr Med Res Opin.* 2011;**27**(12):2309–20.

62. Thurstone C, Riggs PD, Salomonsen-Sautel S, Mikulich-Gilbertson SK. Randomized, controlled trial of atomoxetine for attention-deficit/hyperactivity disorder in adolescents with substance use disorder. *J Am Acad Child Adolesc Psychiatry.* 2010;**49**(6): 573–82.

63. McRae-Clark AL, Carter RE, Killeen TK, *et al.* A placebo-controlled trial of atomoxetine in marijuana-dependent individuals with attention deficit hyperactivity disorder. *Am J Addict.* 2010;**19**(6): 481–9.

64. Harfterkamp M, van de Loo-Neus G, Minderaa RB, *et al.* A randomized double-blind study of atomoxetine versus placebo for attention-deficit/hyperactivity disorder symptoms in children with autism spectrum disorder. *J Am Acad Child Adolesc Psychiatry.* 2012; **51**(7):733–41.

65. Ghanizadeh A. Atomoxetine for treating ADHD symptoms in autism: a systematic review. *J Atten Disord.* 2013;**17**(8):635–40.

66. Atomoxetine ADHD and Comorbid MDD Study Group; Bangs ME, Emslie GJ. Efficacy and safety of atomoxetine in adolescents with attention-deficit/hyperactivity disorder and major depression. *J Child Adolesc Psychopharmacol.* 2007;**17**(4): 407–20.

67. Buitelaar JK, Danckaerts M, Gillberg C, *et al.* A prospective, multicenter, open-label assessment of atomoxetine in non-North American children and adolescents with ADHD. *Eur Child Adolesc Psychiatry.* 2004;**13**(4):249–57.

68. Wilens TE, Newcorn JH, Kratochvil CJ, *et al.* Long-term atomoxetine treatment in adolescents with attention-deficit/hyperactivity disorder. *J Pediatr.* 2006;**149**(1):112–19.

69. Simpson D, Plosker, GL. Atomoxetine: a review of its use in adults with attention deficit hyperactivity disorder. *Drugs.* 2004;**64**(2):205–22.

70. Michelson D, Adler L, Spencer T, *et al.* Atomoxetine in adults with ADHD: two randomized, placebo-controlled studies. *Biol Psychiatry.* 2003;**53**(2): 112–20.

71. Faraone SV, Biederman J, Spencer T, *et al.* Efficacy of atomoxetine in adult attention-deficit/hyperactivity disorder: a drug-placebo response curve analysis. *Behav Brain Funct.* 2005;**1**:16.

72. Adler LA, Spencer T, Brown TE, *et al.* Once-daily atomoxetine for adult attention-deficit/hyperactivity disorder: a 6-month, double-blind trial. *J Clin Psychopharmacol.* 2009;**29**(1):44–50.

73. Reimherr FW, Marchant BK, Strong RE, *et al.* Emotional dysregulation in adult ADHD and response to atomoxetine. *Biol Psychiatry.* 2005;**58**(2):125–31.

74. Brown TE, Holdnack J, Saylor K, *et al.* Effect of atomoxetine on executive function impairments in adults with ADHD. *J Atten Disord.* 2011;**15**(2): 130–8.

75. Wilens TE, Adler LA, Weiss MD, *et al.* Atomoxetine treatment of adults with ADHD and comorbid alcohol use disorders. *Drug Alcohol Depend.* 2008; **96**(1–2):145–54.

76. Adler LA, Liebowitz M, Kronenberger W, *et al.* Atomoxetine treatment in adults with attention-deficit/hyperactivity disorder and comorbid social anxiety disorder. *Depress Anxiety.* 2009;**26**(3): 212–21.

77. Adler L, Dietrich A, Reimherr FW, *et al.* Safety and tolerability of once versus twice daily atomoxetine in adults with ADHD. *Ann Clin Psychiatry.* 2006; **18**(2):107–13.

78. Wigal SB, McGough JJ, McCracken JT, *et al.* A laboratory school comparison of mixed amphetamine salts extended release (Adderall XR) and atomoxetine (Strattera) in school-aged children with attention deficit/hyperactivity disorder. *J Atten Disord.* 2005;**9**(1):275–89.

79. Waxmonsky JG, Waschbusch DA, Akinnusi O, Pelham WE. A comparison of atomoxetine administered as once versus twice daily dosing on the school and home functioning of children with attention-deficit/hyperactivity disorder. *J Child Adolesc Psychopharmacol.* 2011;**21**(1):21–32.

80. Wilens TE, Bukstein O, Brams M, *et al.* A controlled trial of extended-release guanfacine and psychostimulants for attention-deficit/hyperactivity disorder. *J Am Acad Child Adolesc Psychiatry.* 2012;**51**(1):74–85.e2.

81. Connor DF, Findling RL, Kollins SH, *et al.* Effects of guanfacine extended release on oppositional symptoms in children aged 6–12 years with attention-deficit hyperactivity disorder and oppositional symptoms: a randomized, double-blind, placebo-controlled trial. *CNS Drugs.* 2010;**24**(9): 755–68.

82. Biederman J, Melmed RD, Patel A, *et al.* A randomized, double-blind, placebo-controlled study of guanfacine extended release in children and adolescents with attention-deficit/hyperactivity disorder. *Pediatrics.* 2008;**121**(1):e73–84.

83. Kollins SH, Jain R, Brams M, *et al.* Clonidine extended-release tablets as add-on therapy to

psychostimulants in children and adolescents with ADHD. *Pediatrics*. 2011;**127**(6):e1406–13.

84. Jain R, Segal S, Kollins SH, Khayrallah M. Clonidine extended-release tablets for pediatric patients with attention-deficit/hyperactivity disorder. *J Am Acad Child Adolesc Psychiatry*. 2011;**50**(2):171–9.

85. Arnsten AF, Pliszka SR. Catecholamine influences on prefrontal cortical function: relevance to treatment of attention deficit/hyperactivity disorder and related disorders. *Pharmacol Biochem Behav*. 2011; **99**(2):211–16.

86. Newcorn JH, Schulz K, Harrison M, *et al*. Alpha 2 adrenergic agonists. Neurochemistry, efficacy, and clinical guidelines for use in children. *Pediatr Clin North Am*. 1998;**45**(5):1099–22, viii.

87. Hunt RD, Minderaa RB, Cohen DJ. Clonidine benefits children with attention deficit disorder and hyperactivity: report of a double-blind placebo-crossover therapeutic trial. *J Am Acad Child Psychiatry*. 1985;**24**(5):617–29.

88. Steingard R, Biederman J, Spencer T, Wilens T, Gonzalez A. Comparison of clonidine response in the treatment of attention-deficit hyperactivity disorder with and without comorbid tic disorders. *J Am Acad Child Adolesc Psychiatry*. 1993;**32**(2): 350–3.

89. Shionogi Inc., S.P. *Kapvay (clonidine hydrochloride) extended-release tablets: prescribing information [online]*.

90. Croxtall D. Clonidine extended-release: in attention-deficit hyperactivity disorder. *Paediatr Drugs*. 2011;**13**(5):329–36.

91. Hunt RD, Capper L, O'Connell P. Clonidine in child and adolescent psychiatry. *J Child Adolesc Psychopharmacol*. 1990;**1**(1):87–102.

92. Singer HS, Brown J, Quaskey S, *et al*. The treatment of attention-deficit hyperactivity disorder in Tourette's syndrome: a double-blind placebo-controlled study with clonidine and desipramine. *Pediatrics*. 1995;**95**(1):74–81.

93. Wilens TE, Biederman J, Spencer T. Clonidine for sleep disturbances associated with attention-deficit hyperactivity disorder. *J Am Acad Child Adolesc Psychiatry*. 1994;**33**(3):424–6.

94. Engberg G, Eriksson E. Effects of alpha 2-adrenoceptor agonists on locus coeruleus firing rate and brain noradrenaline turnover in N-ethoxycarbonyl-2-ethoxy-1,2-dihydroquinoline (EEDQ)-treated rats. *Naunyn Schmiedebergs Arch Pharmacol*. 1991;**343**(5):472–7.

95. Swearingen D, Pennick M, Shojaei A, Lyne A, Fiske K. A phase I, randomized, open-label, crossover study of the single-dose pharmacokinetic properties of

guanfacine extended-release 1-, 2-, and 4-mg tablets in healthy adults. *Clin Ther*. 2007;**29**(4): 617–25.

96. Boellner SW, Pennick M, Fiske K, Lyne A, Shojaei A. Pharmacokinetics of a guanfacine extended-release formulation in children and adolescents with attention-deficit-hyperactivity disorder. *Pharmacotherapy*. 2007;**27**(9):1253–62.

97. Sallee FR, McGough J, Wigal T, *et al*. Guanfacine extended release in children and adolescents with attention-deficit/hyperactivity disorder: a placebo-controlled trial. *J Am Acad Child Adolesc Psychiatry*. 2009;**48**(2):155–65.

98. Spencer TJ, Greenbaum M, Ginsberg LD, Murphy WR. Safety and effectiveness of coadministration of guanfacine extended release and psychostimulants in children and adolescents with attention-deficit/ hyperactivity disorder. *J Child Adolesc Psychopharmacol*. 2009;**19**(5):501–10.

99. Biederman J, Melmed RD, Patel A, *et al*. Long-term, open-label extension study of guanfacine extended release in children and adolescents with ADHD. *CNS Spectr*. 2008;**13**(12):1047–55.

100. Sallee FR, Lyne A, Wigal T, McGough JJ. Long-term safety and efficacy of guanfacine extended release in children and adolescents with attention-deficit/ hyperactivity disorder. *J Child Adolesc Psychopharmacol*. 2009;**19**(3):215–26.

101. Hunt RD, Arnsten AF, Asbell MD. An open trial of guanfacine in the treatment of attention-deficit hyperactivity disorder. *J Am Acad Child Adolesc Psychiatry*. 1995;**34**(1):50–4.

102. Chappell PB, Riddle MA, Scahill L, *et al*. Guanfacine treatment of comorbid attention-deficit hyperactivity disorder and Tourette's syndrome: preliminary clinical experience. *J Am Acad Child Adolesc Psychiatry*. 1995;**34**(9):1140–6.

103. Scahill L, Chappell PB, Kim YS, *et al*. A placebo-controlled study of guanfacine in the treatment of children with tic disorders and attention deficit hyperactivity disorder. *Am J Psychiatry*. 2001; **158**(7):1067–74.

104. Shire. *INTUNIV® (guanfacine) Extended-Release Tablets*. 2011; http://pi.shirecontent.com/PI/PDFs/ Intuniv_USA_ENG.pdf.

105. Sallee FR, Kollins SH, Wigal TL. Efficacy of guanfacine extended release in the treatment of combined and inattentive only subtypes of attention-deficit/ hyperactivity disorder. *J Child Adolesc Psychopharmacol*. 2012;**22**(3):206–14.

106. Wilson MF, Haring O, Lewin A, *et al*. Comparison of guanfacine versus clonidine for efficacy, safety and occurrence of withdrawal syndrome in step-2

treatment of mild to moderate essential hypertension. *Am J Cardiol.* 1986;**57**(9):43E–49E.

107. Kofoed L, Tadepalli G, Oesterheld JR, Awadallah S, Shapiro R. Case series: clonidine has no systematic effects on PR or QTc intervals in children. *J Am Acad Child Adolesc Psychiatry.* 1999;**38**(9): 1193–6.

108. Connor DF, Barkley RA, Davis HT. A pilot study of methylphenidate, clonidine, or the combination in ADHD comorbid with aggressive oppositional defiant or conduct disorder. *Clin Pediatr (Phila).* 2000; **39**(1):15–25.

109. Scahill L, Aman MG, McDougle CJ, et al. A prospective open trial of guanfacine in children with pervasive developmental disorders. *J Child Adolesc Psychopharmacol,* 2006;**16**(5):589–98.

110. *PRESCRIBING INFORMATION WELLBUTRIN (bupropion hydrochloride extended-release tablets).* 2004; http://www.biopsychiatry.com/bupropion/ bupropion-wellbutrin.pdf.

111. Wilens TE, Dodson W. A clinical perspective of attention-deficit/hyperactivity disorder into adulthood. *J Clin Psychiatry.* 2004;**65**(10): 1301–13.

112. Demyttenaere K, Jaspers L. Review: bupropion and SSRI-induced side effects. *J Psychopharmacol.* 2008;**22**(7):792–804.

113. Conners CK, Casat CD, Gualtieri CT, et al. Bupropion hydrochloride in attention deficit disorder with hyperactivity. *J Am Acad Child Adolesc Psychiatry.* 1996;**35**(10):1314–21.

114. Riggs PD, Leon SL, Mikulich SK, Pottle LC. An open trial of bupropion for ADHD in adolescents with substance use disorders and conduct disorder. *J Am Acad Child Adolesc Psychiatry.* 1998;**37**(12):1271–8.

115. Verbeeck W, Tuinier S, Bekkering GE. Antidepressants in the treatment of adult attention-deficit hyperactivity disorder: a systematic review. *Adv Ther.* 2009;**26**(2): 170–84.

116. Wilens TE, Haight BR, Horigan JP, et al. Bupropion XL in adults with attention-deficit/hyperactivity disorder: a randomized, placebo-controlled study. *Biol Psychiatry.* 2005;**57**(7):793–801.

117. Solhkhah R, Wilens TE, Daly J, et al. Bupropion SR for the treatment of substance-abusing outpatient adolescents with attention-deficit/hyperactivity disorder and mood disorders. *J Child Adolesc Psychopharmacol.* 2005;**15**(5):777–86.

118. Levin FR, Evans SM, Brooks DJ, et al. Treatment of methadone-maintained patients with adult ADHD: double-blind comparison of methylphenidate, bupropion and placebo. *Drug Alcohol Depend.* 2006;**81**(2):137–48.

119. Daviss WB, Bentivoglio P, Racusin R, et al. Bupropion sustained release in adolescents with comorbid attention-deficit/hyperactivity disorder and depression. *J Am Acad Child Adolesc Psychiatry.* 2001;**40**(3):307–14.

120. Wilens TE, Prince JB, Spencer T, et al. An open trial of bupropion for the treatment of adults with attention-deficit/hyperactivity disorder and bipolar disorder. *Biol Psychiatry.* 2003;**54**(1): 9–16.

121. Temple DL, Jr., Yevich JP, New JS. Buspirone: chemical profile of a new class of anxioselective agents. *J Clin Psychiatry.* 1982;**43**(12 Pt 2):4–10.

122. Taylor DP, Hyslop DK. Chronic administration of buspirone down-regulates 5-HT2 receptor binding sites. *Drug Dev Res.* 1991;**24**:93–105.

123. Tunnicliff G, Brokaw JJ, Hausz JA, Matheson GK, White GW. Influence of repeated treatment with buspirone on central 5-hydroxytryptamine and dopamine synthesis. *Neuropharmacology.* 1992;**31**(10):991–5.

124. Fuller RW, Perry KW. Effects of buspirone and its metabolite, 1-(2-pyrimidinyl)piperazine, on brain monoamines and their metabolites in rats. *J Pharmacol Exp Ther.* 1989;**248**(1):50–6.

125. Niederhofer H. An open trial of buspirone in the treatment of attention-deficit disorder. *Hum Psychopharmacol.* 2003;**18**(6):489–92.

126. Malhotra S, Santosh PJ. An open clinical trial of buspirone in children with attention-deficit/ hyperactivity disorder. *J Am Acad Child Adolesc Psychiatry.* 1998;**37**(4):364–71.

127. Mohammadi MR, Hafezi P, Galeiha A, Hajiaghaee R, Akhondzadeh S. Buspirone versus methylphenidate in the treatment of children with attention-deficit/ hyperactivity disorder: randomized double-blind study. *Acta Med Iran.* 2012;**50**(11):723–8.

128. Davari-Ashtiani R, Shahrbabaki ME, Razjouyan K, Amini H, Mazhabdar H. Buspirone versus methylphenidate in the treatment of attention deficit hyperactivity disorder: a double-blind and randomized trial. *Child Psychiatry Hum Dev.* 2010;**41**(6):641–8.

129. Sutherland SM, Adler LA, Chen C, Smith MD, Feltner DE. An 8-week, randomized controlled trial of atomoxetine, atomoxetine plus buspirone, or placebo in adults with ADHD. *J Clin Psychiatry.* 2012; **73**(4):445–50.

130. Findling RL, Greenhill LL, McNamara NK, et al. Venlafaxine in the treatment of children and adolescents with attention-deficit/hyperactivity disorder. *J Child Adolesc Psychopharmacol.* 2007;**17**(4):433–45.

131. Zarinara AR, Mohammadi MR, Hazrati N, *et al.* Venlafaxine versus methylphenidate in pediatric outpatients with attention deficit hyperactivity disorder: a randomized, double-blind comparison trial. *Hum Psychopharmacol.* 2010;**25**(7–8): 530–5.

132. Amiri S, Farhang S, Ghoreishizadeh MA, Malek A, Mohammadzadeh S. Double-blind controlled trial of venlafaxine for treatment of adults with attention deficit/hyperactivity disorder. *Hum Psychopharmacol.* 2012;**27**(1):76–81.

133. Mukaddes NM, Abali O. Venlafaxine in children and adolescents with attention deficit hyperactivity disorder. *Psychiatry Clin Neurosci.* 2004;**58**(1):92–5.

134. Madras BK, Xie Z, Lin Z, *et al.* Modafinil occupies dopamine and norepinephrine transporters in vivo and modulates the transporters and trace amine activity in vitro. *J Pharmacol Exp Ther.* 2006; **319**(2):561–9.

135. Heal DJ, Cheetham SC, Smith SL. The neuropharmacology of ADHD drugs in vivo: insights on efficacy and safety. *Neuropharmacology.* 2009;**57**(7–8):608–18.

136. Biederman J, Swanson JM, Wigal SB, *et al.* A comparison of once-daily and divided doses of modafinil in children with attention-deficit/ hyperactivity disorder: a randomized, double-blind, and placebo-controlled study. *J Clin Psychiatry.* 2006;**67**(5):727–35.

137. Greenhill LL, Biederman J, Boellner SW, *et al.* A randomized, double-blind, placebo-controlled study of modafinil film-coated tablets in children and adolescents with attention-deficit/hyperactivity disorder. *J Am Acad Child Adolesc Psychiatry.* 2006;**45**(5):503–11.

138. Swanson JM, Greenhill LL, Lopez FA, *et al.* Modafinil film-coated tablets in children and adolescents with attention-deficit/hyperactivity disorder: results of a randomized, double-blind, placebo-controlled, fixed-dose study followed by abrupt discontinuation. *J Clin Psychiatry.* 2006;**67**(1):137–47.

139. Wigal SB, Biederman J, Swanson JM, Yang R, Greenhill LL. Efficacy and safety of modafinil film-coated tablets in children and adolescents with or without prior stimulant treatment for attention-deficit/hyperactivity disorder: pooled analysis of 3 randomized, double-blind, placebo-controlled studies. *Prim Care Companion J Clin Psychiatry.* 2006;**8**(6):352–60.

140. Arnold VK, Feifel D, Earl CQ, Yang R, Adler LA. A 9-week, randomized, double-blind, placebo-controlled, parallel-group, dose-finding study to evaluate the efficacy and safety of modafinil as treatment for adults with ADHD. *J Atten Disord.* 2012;**18**(2):133–44.

141. Tatsumi, M, Groshan K, Blakely RD, Richelson E. Pharmacological profile of antidepressants and related compounds at human monoamine transporters. *Eur J Pharmacol.* 1997;**340**(2–3): 249–58.

142. Biederman J, Baldessarini RJ, Wright V, Knee D, Harmatz JS. A double-blind placebo controlled study of desipramine in the treatment of ADD: I. Efficacy. *J Am Acad Child Adolesc Psychiatry.* 1989;**28**(5): 77–84.

143. Biederman J, Baldessarini RJ, Wright V, *et al.* A double-blind placebo controlled study of desipramine in the treatment of ADD: II. Serum drug levels and cardiovascular findings. *J Am Acad Child Adolesc Psychiatry.* 1989;**28**(6):903–11.

144. Zametkin A, Rapoport JL, Murphy DL, Linnoila M, Ismond D. Treatment of hyperactive children with monoamine oxidase inhibitors. I. Clinical efficacy. *Arch Gen Psychiatry.* 1985;**42**(10):62–6.

145. Zametkin A, Rapoport JL, Murphy DL, *et al.* Treatment of hyperactive children with monoamine oxidase inhibitors. II. Plasma and urinary monoamine findings after treatment. *Arch Gen Psychiatry.* 1985;**42**(10):969–73.

146. Ernst M, Liebenauer LL, Jons PH, *et al.* Selegiline in adults with attention deficit hyperactivity disorder: clinical efficacy and safety. *Psychopharmacol Bull.* 1996;**32**(3):327–34.

147. Russell VA. Increased AMPA receptor function in slices containing the prefrontal cortex of spontaneously hypertensive rats. *Metab Brain Dis.* 2001;**16**(3–4):143–9.

148. Donfrancesco R, Calderoni D, Vitiello B. Open-label amantadine in children with attention-deficit/ hyperactivity disorder. *J Child Adolesc Psychopharmacol.* 2007;**17**(5):657–64.

149. Findling RL, McNamara NK, Stansbrey RJ, *et al.* A pilot evaluation of the safety, tolerability, pharmacokinetics, and effectiveness of memantine in pediatric patients with attention-deficit/hyperactivity disorder combined type. *J Child Adolesc Psychopharmacol.* 2007;**17**(1):19–33.

150. Mohammadi MR, Kazemi MR, Zia E, *et al.* Amantadine versus methylphenidate in children and adolescents with attention deficit/hyperactivity disorder: a randomized, double-blind trial. *Hum Psychopharmacol.* 2010;**25**(7–8):560–5.

151. Hughes CW, Emslie GJ, Crismon ML, *et al.* Texas Children's Medication Algorithm Project: update from Texas Consensus Conference Panel on Medication Treatment of Childhood Major Depressive Disorder. *J Am Acad Child Adolesc Psychiatry.* 2007;**46**(6): 667–86.

152. Mahajan R, Bernal MP, Panzer R, *et al.* Clinical practice pathways for evaluation and medication choice for attention-deficit/hyperactivity disorder symptoms in autism spectrum disorders. *Pediatrics.* 2012;**130**(Suppl 2):S125–38.

153. Pliszka S; AACAP Work Group on Quality Issues. Practice parameter for the assessment and treatment of children and adolescents with attention-deficit/hyperactivity disorder. *J Am Acad Child Adolesc Psychiatry.* 2007;**46**(7):894–921.

Chapter 22

Pharmacotherapy of ADHD in adults

Jefferson B. Prince, Nicholas R. Morrison, and Timothy E. Wilens

Introduction

Despite increased recognition that children with attention-deficit hyperactivity disorder (ADHD) commonly grow up to be adults with the same disorder, evidence-based guidelines on the treatment of adults with ADHD are lacking. Support groups (e.g., www.chadd.org and www.add.org) assist the newly diagnosed adult by providing education, an overview of treatment options, available resources, and peer support. Recently the World Health Organization supported the development of an easy to use screen tool for ADHD in adults. This tool has been validated [1] and is easy to access and use. Fortunately over the past several years, several organizations including the American Academy of Child and Adolescent Psychiatry, the Center for ADHD Advocacy, Canada, and the European Network Adult ADHD have published guidelines which provide clinicians with a thorough description of the clinical features of ADHD across the lifespan and outline principles for the assessment, diagnosis, and recognition of common comorbid disorders and treatment of ADHD. Once a reliable and valid diagnosis has been established the treatment of ADHD in adults relies on three foundations: psychoeducation, pharmacotherapy, and psychosocial treatments.

It is important to set clear realistic treatment goals with the adult and identify specific symptoms and problematic areas of functioning as targets of treatment. Response-based rating scales such as the ADHD Rating Scale (ADHD-RS), the Conners' Adult ADHD Rating Scale (CAARS), the Wender–Reimherr Adult ADHD Rating Scale, and the Brown Adult ADHD Rating Scale can be used to help assess symptoms and monitor outcome (for review see Adler and Cohen [2] and Murphey and Adler [3]). Additional

therapies often complement the effects of medication. As with children, college students and adults returning to school may benefit from additional educational supports. Coaching and organization training appear useful but remain understudied [4, 5].

Over the course of the past decade the database on the safety, tolerability, and efficacy of medications to treat adults with ADHD has significantly expanded. A recent review supports the practice that medications appear to be a cornerstone of treatment for adults with ADHD [6]. Presently there are three medication classes specifically approved for the treatment of ADHD in adults; atomoxetine (ATMX), amphetamine (AMPH), and methylphenidate (MPH). The administration of medication in adults with ADHD should be undertaken as a collaborative effort between the patient and the practitioner guiding the use and management of effective anti-ADHD agents. The use of medication should follow a careful evaluation of the adult including neurodevelopmental, psychiatric, medical, social, environmental, and cognitive assessments. Since many adults with ADHD suffer comorbid psychiatric disorders, it is necessary to prioritize treatment if clinically significant psychiatric comorbidities are present; typically sequencing initial treatment for the more severe disorder. In the following sections, guidelines for pharmacotherapy will be delineated, the available information on the use of medications for adult ADHD will be reviewed, and pharmacological strategies will be suggested for the management of ADHD symptoms with accompanying comorbid conditions.

Stimulants

Stimulants remain the best-studied and most frequently used treatment for ADHD in children,

Attention-Deficit Hyperactivity Disorder in Adults and Children, ed. Lenard A. Adler, Thomas J. Spencer and Timothy E. Wilens. Published by Cambridge University Press. © Cambridge University Press 2015.

adolescents, and adults. Over 300 controlled studies of pediatric ADHD have shown stimulants to be safe, well tolerated and efficacious in reducing ADHD symptoms in the short term as well as improving self-esteem, cognition, and social/family functioning [7]. Although the data in adults with ADHD are less extensive, adults appear to tolerate stimulant medication similarly to children.

To date we are aware of at least 25 short-term controlled studies (n = 2804 subjects) and at least 15 longer-term studies (n = 1989 subjects) of adults receiving either MPH or AMPH-based medications (mixed AMPH salts – MAS) (for review see Wilens *et al.* [6]). Of these, 29 controlled studies were with MPH and 12 controlled studies were with AMPH-based compounds.

In contrast to consistent robust responses to stimulants in children and adolescents of approximately 70% [7–9] controlled studies in adults have shown more equivocal responses to stimulants, ranging from 25% [10] to 88% [11] (see Table 22.1). Variability in the response rate appears to be related to several factors, including the diagnostic criteria utilized to determine ADHD, varying stimulant doses, comorbidity, and differing methods of assessing overall response. Dosing of the stimulants appears important in outcome: (1) controlled investigations using higher stimulant dosing (>1.0 mg/kg/day of MPH or >0.5 mg/kg/day of AMPH) generally resulted in more robust outcomes than those using lower stimulant dosing (<0.7 mg/kg/day) and (2) several studies utilizing a dose-ranging paradigm found a dose-dependent response to stimulants in adults with ADHD. For instance, Spencer *et al.* showed 40 mg of d-MPH XR resulted in a larger response rate than the 20 mg dose [12]. Medori *et al.* showed a similar pattern with osmotic-release oral system MPH (OROS MPH) [13]. Along the same lines, an older meta-analysis of six double-blind placebo-controlled studies comparing treatment of adults with ADHD with MPH (n = 140) to placebo (n = 113) found a mean effect size of 0.9 which was nearly double (1.3) in those studies using higher dosing of MPH (mean dose 70 mg/day or 1.05 mg/kg/day) compared to those studies using lower doses (effect size 0.7; mean dose 44 mg/day or 0.63 mg/kg/day) [14].

There are limited data available to guide the dosing parameters of the stimulants. US Food and Drug Administration (FDA) guidelines for dosing reflect general cautiousness and should not be the only guide

for clinical practice. The dose should be individually titrated based on therapeutic efficacy and side effects. Similar to pediatric groups with ADHD, in adults treatment may be started with either immediate-release (IR) or extended-release (ER) preparations at the lowest possible dose [7]. The stimulants have an immediate onset of action and may last from 3 to 12 hours based on the formulation of the agent (IR, ER). Initiation of treatment with once-daily dosing in the morning is advisable until an acceptable response is noted. Treatment with IR preparations generally starts at 5 mg of MPH or AMPH once daily and is titrated upward every 3 to 5 days until an effect is noted or adverse effects emerge. Repeat dosing of IR stimulants through the day is dependent on duration of effectiveness, wear off, and side effects. Typically, the behavioral half-life of the IR stimulants necessitates at least twice-daily dosing with the addition of similar or reduced afternoon doses dependent on breakthrough symptoms. In a typical adult, dosing of IR MPH is generally up to 30 mg three to four times daily or AMPH 15 to 20 mg three to four times a day. Stimulants are generally dosed in an absolute manner (e.g., mg/day). However, absolute dose limits (in mg) may not adequately consider a patient's height, weight, and use in refractory cases. Furthermore, it appears that for stimulants to be most effective, doses of 0.5–1 mg/kg/day of MPH (lower for d-MPH) or up to 0.5 mg/kg/day of AMPH seem necessary for efficacy [15]. Currently, most adults with ADHD treated with a stimulant are prescribed extended delivery preparations such as MAS-XR, OROS MPH, mixed AMPH salts extended release (MAS-ER), lisdexamfetamine (LDX), or one of the beaded MPH preparations (e.g., d-MPH). It is notable that comparable findings between response rates and adverse effects have been reported between ER and IR stimulants. For instance, Spencer *et al.* reported similar response rates and adverse effects using similar dosing of three times daily IR MPH and once-daily ER OROS MPH [16].

There is a paucity of longer-term data related to stimulants for ADHD. We located eight open (n = 1023 subjects) and seven controlled (n = 1136 subjects) studies of at least 12 weeks duration (see Table 22.2). The majority of longer-term studies are the continuation of controlled trials where subjects are followed openly. In one of the largest controlled long-term studies, Weiss and Hechtman demonstrated continued improvement with dextroamphetamine (d-AMPH) alone or in combination with paroxetine (64%

Table 22.1. Representative short-term controlled clinical studies of stimulants in adults with ADHD*

Study (year)	N	Design	Medication	Duration	Total dose mean and/or range	Outcome	Comments
Wood et al. (1976) [98]	15	Double-blind, placebo crossover	MPH	4 weeks	27 mg/day	73% response rate	Dx criteria not well defined; mild side effects
Mattes et al. (1984) [10]	61	Double-blind, placebo crossover	MPH	6 weeks	48 mg/day	25% response rate	Moderate rate of comorbidity; mild side effects
Wender et al. (1985) [99]	37	Double-blind, placebo crossover	MPH	5 weeks	43 mg/day	57% response rate (11% placebo)	68% dysthymia; 22% cyclothymia; mild side effects
Gualtieri and Hicks (1985) [100]	22	Double-blind, placebo crossover	MPH	2 weeks	42 mg/day	Mild to moderate response	No plasma level–response associations
Spencer et al. (1995) [101]	23	Double-blind, placebo crossover	MPH	7 weeks	1.0 mg/kg/day	78% response rate, dose relationship (4% placebo)	No plasma level associations; no effect of gender or comorbidity
Iaboni et al. (1996) [102]	30	Double-blind, placebo crossover	MPH	4 weeks	30–45 mg/day	Moderate response	Improvement in neuropsych and anxiety
Paterson et al. (1999) [103]	45	Double-blind, parallel	d-AMPH	6 weeks	23 mg/day	58% response rate	Weight loss only major adverse effect
Spencer et al. (2001) [104]	27	Double-blind, placebo crossover	AMPH salts	7 weeks	54 mg/day 20–60 mg/day	70% response rate, dose relationship (7% placebo)	No effect of comorbidity or gender on response; well tolerated
Taylor (2000) [105, 106]	39	Double-blind, placebo crossover	d-AMPH	7 weeks	22 mg/day	48% response rate	Used as comparator in two studies of non-stimulants; response >30% reduction in scales
Kooij et al. (2004) [107]	45	Double-blind, randomized crossover	MPH	3 weeks	0.5–1.0 mg/kg/day	38–51% response rate (7–18% placebo)	Higher rate of side effects for MPH and placebo
Carpentier et al. (2005) [108]	25	Double-blind, placebo crossover	MPH	8 weeks	15–45 mg/day	58% response rate on CGI (32% placebo)	SUD study; positive response to tx not significantly higher than placebo
Spencer et al. (2005) [109]	146	Double-blind, placebo parallel	MPH	6 weeks	1.1 mg/kg/day	76% response rate (19% placebo)	Tx well tolerated despite higher dose
Biederman et al. (2006) [110]	141	Double-blind, placebo parallel	OROS MPH	6 weeks	81 mg/day	66% response rate (39% placebo)	Slight vital sign increases
Weisler et al. (2006) [111]	255	Double-blind, placebo parallel	MAS XR	4 weeks	20, 40, or 60 mg/day	55% response rate on CGI (27% placebo)	MAS XR 60 mg group had greatest improvement on ADHD-RS
Spencer et al. (2007) [12]	221	Double-blind, fixed dose, placebo parallel	d-MPH ER	5 weeks	20, 30, or 40 mg/day	54–61% response rate on ADHD-RS (34% placebo)	Inconsistent dose response
Reimherr et al. (2007) [112]	45	Double-blind, placebo crossover	OROS MPH	8 weeks	57 mg/day (tx responder mean) 75 mg/day (tx non-responder mean)	54% response rate on CGI (22% placebo)	Total ADHD-RS score decrease of 41% (vs. 14%)

Table 22.1. (cont.)

Study (year)	N	Design	Medication	Duration	Total dose mean and/or range	Outcome	Comments
Jain et al. (2007) [113]	39	Double-blind, placebo crossover	MLR MPH	5–11 weeks	58 mg/day (mean) MLR MPH 65 mg/day (mean) placebo	49% response rate on CGI (23% placebo)	MLR MPH minimal side effects; short trial
Adler et al. (2008) [114]; Weber and Siddiqui (2009) [115]	420	Double-blind, placebo (2:2:2:1) parallel	LDX	4 weeks	30, 50, or 70 mg/day	Response rate on CGI: 57%, 62%, and 61% respectively (29% placebo)	Incidence of AEs highest in first week of LDX tx
Medori et al. (2008) [13]	401	Double-blind, placebo parallel	Prolonged release OROS MPH	5 weeks	18, 36, or 72 mg/day	Responders were 51%, 49%, and 60% respectively (27% placebo)	AE rates 75%, 76%, and 82% vs. 66% in placebo; most common decreased appetite and headache
Chronis-Tuscano et al. (2008) [116]	23	Double-blind, placebo-controlled	OROS MPH	7 weeks	36, 54, 72, or 90 mg/day (mean 84 mg/day)	Significant reduction in CGI scores at all doses	Few AEs
Adler et al. (2009) [117]	226	Double-blind, placebo parallel	OROS MPH	7 weeks	68 mg/day OROS MPH (mean) 87 mg/day placebo (mean)	37% response rate on CGI and AISRS (21% placebo)	Mild to moderate AE rate, 85% MPH vs. 64% placebo; OROS MPH overall effective and well tolerated in dose escalation
Winhusen et al. (2010) [118]	255	Double-blind, placebo parallel	OROS MPH	11 weeks	18–72 mg/day	71% response rate on CGI (44% placebo)	Cigarette cessation study; cigarette smoking abstinence not significantly different between groups
Wigal et al. (2010) [119]	105	Double-blind, crossover	LDX	2 weeks	30, 50, or 70 mg/day	77% response on CGI (23% placebo)	After open-label dose optimization (4 weeks), subjects entered 2-week crossover phase
Spencer et al. (2011) [16]	53	Single-blind, parallel	OROS MPH or IR MPH	6 weeks	77 mg/day IR MPH (mean) 80 mg/day OROS MPH (mean)	OROS once a day equal to IR MPH TID	OROS well tolerated and similar safety indices as IR; increased adherence with OROS
Wender et al. (2010) [19]	105	Double-blind, placebo crossover	MPH	2 weeks	45 mg/day 10–60 mg/day	74% experienced at least a 50% reduction on WRAADDS sx score (22% placebo)	Participants who improved on MPH IR entered a 12-month, open-label trial
TOTAL (n = 25)	n = 2804 15–420 (range)	Single: 1 Double: 24	MPH: 19 AMPH: 4 LDX: 2	2–11 weeks	MPH: 10–90 mg/day AMPH: 20–60 mg/day LDX: 30–70 mg/day	MPH, AMPH, and LDX improved ADHD sxs	AEs mild to moderate in severity

* Up to 11 weeks.
Response rate refers to subject reported much to very much improved (i.e., by clinical global improvement; CGI) or with clinically significant reduction in symptoms on ADHD rating scales.
Abbreviations: ADHD = attention-deficit hyperactivity disorder, AE = adverse event, AISRS = ADHD Investigator Symptom Report Scale, AMPH = amphetamine, CGI = Clinical Global Impression, d-AMPH = dexamphetamine, d-MPH = dexmethylphenidate, Dx = diagnosis, ER = extended release, IR = immediate release, LDX = lisdexamfetamine, MAS = mixed amphetamine salt, MAS XR = mixed amphetamine salt extended release, MLR = Multilayer Release, MPH = methylphenidate, OROS MPH = osmotic-release oral system methylphenidate, RS = Rating Scale, SR = sustained release, SUD = substance use disorder, sx = symptom, tx = treatment, WRAADDS = Wender–Reimherr Adult Attention Deficit Disorder Scale.

Table 22.2. Representative longer-term studies of stimulants in adults with ADHD*

Study (year)	N	Design	Medication	Duration	Total dose mean and/or range	Outcome	Comments
Levin et al. (1998) [120]	12	Open	MPH SR	12 weeks	68 mg/day 40–80 mg/day	Improved ADHD and cocaine use	Cocaine abusers, 8/12 completed; no abuse of MPH
Horrigan and Barnhill (2000) [121]	24	Open	AMPH salts	16 weeks	11 mg/day	54% response rate on CGI	Low doses used; retrospectively analyzed
Schubiner et al. (2002) [122]	48	Double-blind, placebo parallel	MPH	12 weeks	79 mg/day 30–90 mg/day	77% response rate on global improvement scale (21% placebo)	Comorbid cocaine dependence; CBT for both arms
Biederman et al. (2005) [123]; Weisler et al. (2005) [124]	223	Open	MAS XR	≤24 months	20, 40, and 60 mg/day	ADHD RS improved for all (p < 0.001)	AEs were mild to moderate, minimal cardiac effects; extension of controlled study
Weiss and Hechtman (2006) [17]	98	Double-blind, placebo factorial	Paroxetine and/or d-AMPH	20 weeks	Paroxetine (10, 20, 30, and 40 mg/day) d-AMPH (5, 10, 15, and 20 mg/day)	64% response rate to d-AMPH, 44% to paroxetine/d-AMPH, 17% to paroxetine, and 16% to placebo	Patients who received both d-AMPH and paroxetine had more severe AEs, but did not show greater improvement than patients treated with monotherapy
Levin et al. (2007) [125]	106	Double-blind, placebo parallel	MPH	14 weeks	40 mg/day 10–60 mg/day	47% response rate on AARS (55% placebo)	SUD study. Lower probability of cocaine in urine for MPH vs. placebo (p = 0.001)
Spencer et al. (2008) [126]	274	Double-blind, placebo parallel	Triple bead AMPH salts (MAS)	5 weeks (phase 1); 2 weeks (phase 2); 7 weeks (phase 3)	13, 25, 38, 50, 63, or 75 mg/day after dose optimization	52% response rate on CGI (21% placebo)	Mild to moderate AEs of insomnia, dry mouth, decreased appetite, headache, weight loss; improved quality of life >12-hour duration
Rösler et al. (2009) [18]	359	Double-blind, placebo parallel	MPH ER	6 months	41 mg/day	61% response rate (42% placebo)	Relatively low doses used; increased heart rate among MPH ER group
Weisler et al. (2009) [20]; Ginsberg et al. (2011) [11]	349	Open	LDX	12 months	30, 50, or 70 mg/day	84% improvement on CGI	Most AEs were mild to moderate in severity
Adler (2009) [127]**	170	Open	d-MPH ER	6 months	20–40 mg/day	95% response rate on CGI	Open-label extension of Spencer et al. [12]
Bejerot et al. (2010) [128]	133	Open	MPH d-AMPH	6- to 9-month follow-up	49 mg/day 18–90 mg/day 28 mg/day 15–70 mg/day	80% response rate	66 of 133 discontinued (38% before the 6- to 9-month time point)
Marchant et al. (2010) [21]	34	Open	OROS MPH	6 months	60 mg/day	85% response rate on CGI	Followed double-blind crossover phase; all 34 included for safety phase

Table 22.2. (*cont.*)

Study (year)	N	Design	Medication	Duration	Total dose mean and/or range	Outcome	Comments
Wender *et al.* (2010) [19]	78	Open	MPH	12 months	60 mg/day 30–100 mg/day	94% response rate on CGI	Participants who improved on MPH IR double-blind phase entered the 12-month, open-label trial
Konstenius *et al.* (2010) [129]	24	Double-blind, placebo parallel	OROS MPH	13 weeks	18–72 mg/day	84% retention in treatment completers (59% placebo)	Study in AMPH abusers; both groups reduced ADHD sxs; no difference between groups in craving for amphetamine
Biederman *et al.* (2010) [15]	227	Double-blind, placebo parallel	OROS MPH	6 weeks (phase 1); 24 weeks (phase 2); 4 weeks (phase 3)	78 mg/day OROS MPH at phase 1 end point (mean)	62% response rate on CGI and AISRS (37% placebo)	Results include phase 1 end point response rates only
TOTAL (n = 15)	n = 1989 12–359 (range)	Double blind: 7 Open: 8	MPH: 10 AMPH: 5 LDX: 1	12 weeks– 12 months	MPH: 10–100 mg/ day AMPH: 5–75 mg/ day LDX: 30–70 mg/ day	Long-term effectiveness of MPH and AMPH documented	AEs mild to moderate in severity

* At least 12 weeks.
** Subjects not included in overall n.
Response rate refers to subject reported much to very much improved (i.e., by clinical global improvement; CGI) or with clinically significant reduction in symptoms on ADHD rating scales.
Abbreviations: AARS = Adult ADHD Rating Scale, ADHD = attention-deficit hyperactivity disorder, AE = adverse event, AISRS = ADHD Investigator Symptom Report Scale, AMPH = amphetamine, CBT = cognitive-behavioral therapy, CGI = Clinical Global Impression, d-AMPH = dexamphetamine, d-MPH = dexmethylphenidate, ER = extended release, IR = immediate release, LDX = lisdexamfetamine, MAS = mixed amphetamine salt, MAS XR = mixed amphetamine salt extended release, MPH = methylphenidate, OROS MPH = osmotic-release oral system methylphenidate, RS = Rating Scale, SR = sustained release, SUD = substance use disorder, sx = symptoms.

and 44% response rates vs. 16% placebo, respectively) over a 20-week study [17]. Rösler *et al.* showed that MPH ER significantly improved ADHD (61% vs. 42% placebo) and related symptoms over the 24 weeks of the study [18]. Wender *et al.* studied 78 subjects who were part of a controlled trial for 12 months and found that those who responded to MPH in the short term responded to longer-term treatment with improvement in ADHD [19]. These data seem to suggest response to stimulants is sustained at the 24 to 72 weeks follow-up end points.

Open-label studies have also shown the effectiveness of long-term stimulants in adults with ADHD. Weisler *et al.* in a 12-month study following a double-blind, placebo-controlled trial of initially 349 subjects receiving 30–70 mg/day of LDX reported 84% improvement at end point, and most adverse events

were mild to moderate in severity [20]. In a similar 6-month, open-label study following a randomized, placebo-controlled trial of OROS MPH, Marchant *et al.* found a similar response rate of 85% of the 34 enrolled subjects demonstrated improvement [21]. These aggregate data seem to support the longer-term effectiveness and tolerability of stimulants in adults.

Side effects of stimulants

Stimulants can cause clinically significant anorexia, nausea, difficulty falling asleep, obsessiveness, headaches, dry mouth, rebound phenomena, anxiety, nightmares, dizziness, irritability, dysphoria, and weight loss [7]. Occasionally, stimulants may elicit a depressive reaction or psychosis. However, no cases of stimulant-related psychosis at therapeutic doses have been reported in adults [8]. Stimulant use may exacerbate tics or Tourette syndrome. While a physical withdrawal is not associated with stimulants, patients who have used high doses for a prolonged time may experience fatigue, hypersomnia, hyperphagia, dysphoria, and depression upon discontinuation. Given the abuse potential of these medications, it is important to inquire about concomitant use of drugs and alcohol. Although reduced appetite and difficulty initiating sleep are reported during the initial phases of treatment, they tend to dissipate with chronic care. Dry mouth is the most commonly reported symptom over time [20]. In patients who feel edgy during treatment with stimulants, administration of a low-dose beta-blocker (i.e., propanolol at 10 mg up to three times daily) or buspirone (5 to 10 mg up to three times daily) may be helpful in reducing the edginess/agitation associated with stimulant administration [22].

The stimulants also are associated with small increases in heart rate and blood pressure that are weakly correlated with dose. In part related to vital sign changes and their biological plausibility, there has been controversy as to cardiovascular risk in subjects receiving stimulants [23]. However, recent work has shed light on the cardiovascular risk of stimulants in adults. For instance, a recent retrospective study by Habel et al. [24], from four study sites in 25- to 64-year-old adults in 443 198 total medication users and non-users, examined serious cardiovascular events with comparison between current or new users and remote users to account for potential healthy-user bias. The authors reported on 806 182 person-years of follow-up (median, 1.3 years per person), and found no relationship between past or current ADHD medication use and serious cardiovascular or stroke outcomes. As highlighted by these authors, among young and middle-aged adults, current or new use of ADHD medications, compared with non-use or remote use, was not associated with an increased risk of serious cardiovascular events [24]. These data mirror the findings of a similarly designed study in youth with ADHD [25] and a recent review of the cardiovascular literature related to stimulant exposure in ADHD [26] and seem to suggest that the vital sign changes seen acutely and chronically in adults are not clinically significant.

These studies, along with more general guidelines on the use of stimulants [27, 28], suggest checking vital signs at premedication baseline and periodically thereafter especially in patients at elevated risk of hypertension [29]. These guidelines also recommend monitoring patients for clinical symptoms referrable to underlying cardiovascular disturbance and/or deleterious cardiovascular interactions with the medication and include palpitations, chest discomfort/pain, syncopal episodes, and shortness of breath [26]. For subjects with preexisting hypertension, one small study indicated stability in blood pressure when stimulants were used concomitantly with antihypertensives [30] and the use of stimulants in patients with preexisting conditions such as hypertension does not appear to increase the risk for serious cardiovascular outcomes [24, 25].

Adults with ADHD, with or without medication treatment, often experience sleep difficulties, including longer sleep-onset latency and lower sleep efficiency [31]. Various strategies have been suggested to help make it easier for ADHD patients to fall asleep, including sleep hygiene, behavioral modifications, adjusting timing or type of stimulant, and switching to an alternative ADHD treatment [32]. Complementary pharmacological treatments to consider include: melatonin (1–3 mg), clonidine (0.1–0.3 mg), diphenhydramine (25–50 mg), trazadone (25–50 mg), and mirtazapine (3.75–15 mg) [7, 33]. Interest persists in the use of melatonin, a hormone secreted by the pineal gland that helps regulate circadian rhythms [34]. Melatonin used alone [35] and in conjunction with sleep hygiene techniques [36] appears to improve sleep in ADHD youth – the results in adults have yet to be unveiled. In these two well-designed but small studies, the most concerning adverse events included migraine, nightmares, and aggression.

Medication interactions with stimulants

The interactions of stimulants with other prescription and non-prescription medications are generally mild and not a major source of concern [37, 38]. Concomitant use of sympathomimetic agents (e.g., pseudoephedrine) may potentiate the effects of both medications. Concurrent use of antihistamines may diminish the effects of stimulants. Likewise, excessive intake of caffeine may potentially compromise the effectiveness of the stimulants and exacerbate sleep difficulties. Although administering stimulants with ATMX is common clinical practice, and appears well tolerated and effective based upon open samples in pediatric samples [39, 40], this combination has not been tested systematically in adults. Although data on the co-administration of stimulants with tricyclic antidepressants (TCAs) suggest little interaction between these compounds [41], careful monitoring is warranted when prescribing stimulants with either TCAs or anticonvulsants. The stimulants and serotonin reuptake inhibitors can be co-adminstered. For instance, Weiss and Hechtman studied AMPH alone and in combination with paroxetine and the combination was well tolerated [17]. Co-administration of monoamine oxidase inhibitors (MAOIs) with stimulants may result in a hypertensive crisis and be potentially life-threatening. In fact, co-administration of stimulants with MAOIs is the only true contraindication.

Non-stimulants

Despite the increasing use of stimulants for adults with ADHD, up to 50% may not respond, have untoward side effects, or manifest comorbidity which stimulants may exacerbate or be ineffective in treating [42, 43]. To date, 47 studies of non-stimulant medications (n = 4571 subjects) have been reported including antidepressants, alpha (α) agonists, amino acids, wake promoting agents, and experimental agents for the treatment of ADHD in adults.

Atomoxetine

ATMX was the first medication approved by the FDA specifically for treating ADHD in adults (see Table 22.3). Unlike the stimulants, ATMX is not a controlled medication and therefore clinicians can call in prescriptions as well as provide samples and refills. ATMX specifically inhibits presynaptic norepinephrine reuptake, resulting similarly in increased synaptic norepinephrine [44]. ATMX exhibits little effect on serotonin reuptake and has minimal affinity for other receptors, neurotransmitters, or transporters. Because of its effects on norepinephrine, it is speculated that ATMX influences the posterior attentional systems that may result in disengagement from stimuli and the anterior attentional systems which include the analysis of data and response preparation [44, 45]. Unfortunately, unlike data with the relationship of dopamine (DA) with the DA transporter, little information is available on ligands with specific binding to the noradrenergic presynaptic reuptake protein. Despite the prominent inhibitory effects of ATMX on norepinephrine reuptake, preclinical data also show that the noradrenergic presynaptic reuptake protein

regulates DA in the frontal lobes and that by blocking this protein ATMX increases DA in the frontal lobes [44].

ATMX has been studied in at least eight controlled and six open studies constituting 3141 subjects. Initial 10-week studies of ATMX in 536 subjects resulted in reductions from baseline in CAARS scores of approximately 30% (versus 20% for placebo) with similar reductions in symptoms of inattention and hyperactivity/impulsivity. More recently, ATMX has been studied in another large short-term trial demonstrating continued efficacy for ADHD in adults [46].

Longer-term data also suggests ongoing effectiveness of ATMX in adults. In a large controlled 6-month study of ATMX, significant findings compared with placebo were noted acutely (6 weeks) and at the 6-month end point [47]. Adler et al. showed improved outcome in ADHD with >30% of symptoms compared with baseline at up to 221 weeks [47]. In this study of originally 384 adults, there were no new long-term adverse effects that emerged [47]. Similarly, Marchant et al. reported on a study of 384 adults treated openly for up to 156 weeks in which responders had significant improvement in ADHD and emotionality [48]. Interestingly, 39% of ATMX subjects enrolled in a double-blind non-responder study became responders during the open-label treatment [48].

ATMX is rapidly absorbed following oral administration and food does not appear to affect absorption. ATMX's maximum serum concentration (C_{max}) is 1–2 hours after dosing. ATMX is primarily metabolized via the hepatic cytochrome P450 system through the 2D6 enzyme (CYP2D6) to 4-hydroxyatomoxetine [49]. There are a number of alternative metabolic pathways, including the 2C19 enzyme. Although ATMX is metabolized by CYP2D6, it does not appear to either induce or inhibit CYP2D6 activity.

It is recommended that ATMX be initiated slowly at 0.5 mg/kg/day for 2 weeks and increased over a month to target dose of 1.2 mg/kg/day. Current dosing guidelines for ATMX recommend maximum dosage of 1.4 mg/kg/day or 100 mg/day, though increases up to 1.8 mg/kg/day may be necessary in refractory cases. Extensive testing was undertaken to look at the ability of patients with relatively slow metabolic activity at CYP2D6 (approximately 7% of the sample) to metabolize ATMX. These pediatric studies indicate that while patients with slow metabolizer status experienced increased rates of common side effects, these patients were generally able to tolerate ATMX.

Table 22.3. Representative clinical studies of non-stimulants in adults with ADHD

Study (year)	N	Medication	Design	Duration	Total dose mean and/or range	Outcome	Comments
Wood et al. (1982) [84]	8	L-DOPA (+ carbidopa)	Open	3 weeks	625 mg/day (62.5 mg/day)	No benefit	Side effects: nausea, sedation; low doses
Wender et al. (1983) [67]	22	Pargyline	Open	6 weeks	30 mg/day 10–50 mg/day	68% response rate	Delayed onset; brief behavioral action
Wender et al. (1985) [68]	11	Deprenyl	Open	6 weeks	30 mg/day	66% response rate	Amphetamine metabolite; 2 dropouts
Wood et al. (1985) [85]	19	Phenylalanine	Double-blind, placebo crossover	2 weeks	587 mg/day	46% response rate (15% placebo)	Transient mood improvement only
Mattes (1986) [130]	13	Propanolol	Open	Mean = 9 weeks (3–50 weeks)	528 mg/day 40–640 mg/day	85% response rate	Part of "temper" study
Reimherr et al. (1987) [86]	12	Tyrosine	Open	8 weeks	50–150 mg/kg/day	66% response rate	14-day onset of action; tolerance developed; 4 dropouts
Shekim et al. (1989) [131]	18	Nomifensine maleate	Open	4 weeks	50–300 mg/day	94% response rate	Immediate response; one patient with allergic reaction
Shekim et al. (1990) [132]	8	S-adenosyl-L-methionine	Open	4 weeks	≤2400 mg/day	75% response rate	Mild adverse effects
Wender and Reimherr (1990) [133]	19	BPR	Open	6–8 weeks	359 mg/day 150–450 mg/day	74% response rate	5 subjects could not tolerate lowest dose and dropped out; 10 subjects improved at 1 year
Wilens et al. (1995) [65]	37	Desipramine Nortriptyline	Open, retrospective	Mean = 50 weeks	183 mg/day 92 mg/day	68% response rate	Comorbidity unrelated to response; 60% on stimulants, 84% on concurrent meds; response sustained in 54% of patients
Adler et al. (1995) [134]	16	Venlafaxine	Open	8 weeks	110 mg/day 25–225 mg/day	83% response rate	4 subjects on other meds; 4 dropped out; 50% reduction in sxs
Hedges et al. (1995) [135]	18	Venlafaxine	Open	8 weeks	96 mg/day 50–150 mg/day	50% response rate	Side effects led to 39% dropout rate; study divided by med tolerance
Findling et al. (1996) [136]	10	Venlafaxine	Open	8 weeks	150 mg/day (7 of 9) 75–150 mg/day	70% response rate	Improved anxiety scores; 1 dropout
Wilens et al. (1996) [66]	43	Desipramine	Double-blind, placebo parallel	6 weeks	147 mg/day	68% response rate (0% placebo)	Comorbidity or levels not related to response
Ernst et al. (1996) [69]	24	Selegiline	Double-blind, placebo parallel	6 weeks	20 mg/day, followed by 60 mg/day	Mild improvement	High placebo response, mild side effects; three arms; 60 mg dose best
Spencer et al. (1998) [137]	22	(A)tomoxetine	Double-blind, placebo crossover	7 weeks	76 mg/day	50% response rate (9% placebo)	Noradrenergic agent; well tolerated

Table 22.3. *(cont.)*

Study (year)	N	Medication	Design	Duration	Total dose mean and/or range	Outcome	Comments
Wilens et al. (1999) [80]	32	ABT 418	Double-blind, placebo crossover	7 weeks	75 mg/day	40% response rate (13% placebo)	Nicotinic analog; attentional symptoms improved preferentially
Taylor and Russo (2000) [79]	22	Modafinil d-AMPH	Double-blind, placebo crossover	7 weeks	207 mg/day 22 mg/day	48% response rate 48% response rate	Improved neuropsychological functioning with both tx
Cephalon Inc. (2000) [138]	113	Modafinil	Double-blind, placebo crossover	7 weeks	100 and 400 mg/day	No difference vs. placebo	Cephalon report
Taylor and Russo (2001) [74]	17	Guanfacine d-AMPH	Double-blind, placebo crossover	7 weeks	1 mg/day 0.25–2 mg/day 10 mg/day 2.5–20 mg/day	Both tx improved vs. placebo	Well tolerated; neuropsychological profile improved
Wilens et al. (2001) [57]	40	BPR SR	Double-blind, placebo parallel	6 weeks	362 mg/day 100–400 mg/day	52% response rate (11% placebo)	Delayed onset of action; well tolerated
Upadhyaya et al. (2001) [139]	10	Venlafaxine	Open	12 weeks	75–300 mg/day	Improved ADHD and alcohol use	SUD study; 4/10 subjects completed 12 weeks
Kuperman et al. (2001) [140]	30	BPR SR MPH	Double-blind, placebo parallel	7 weeks	Maximum 300 mg/day Maximum 0.9 mg/kg/day	64% response rate BPR 50% response rate MPH (27% placebo)	Not statistically significant vs. placebo; n = 8–11/group
Levin et al. (2002) [61]	11	BPR	Single-blind	12 weeks	400 mg/day 250–400 mg/day	47% response rate	Cocaine abusers; reduced cocaine use
Wilens et al. (2003) [63]	36	BPR SR	Open	6 weeks	370 mg/day 200–400 mg/day	70% response rate by CGI	Bipolar + ADHD adults; no manic activation
Michelson et al. [54]; Simpson and Plosker (2004) [141]	536	ATMX	Double-blind, placebo parallel	10 weeks	60, 90, or 120 mg/day	58% response rate	Combination of two, separate multisite studies; improved functioning and less disability
Adler et al. (2005) [142]; Adler et al. (2008) [143]; Marchant et al. (2011) [48]	384	ATMX	Open	Mean = 40 weeks	99 mg/day	Decrease on CAARS 33.2%	Continuation of Michelson et al. [54]; safety and efficacy established in adults with ADHD
Wilens et al. (2005) [59]	162	BPR XL	Double-blind, placebo parallel	8 weeks	393 mg/day	53% response rate ADHD-RS (31% placebo)	Meds provided benefit throughout day vs. placebo; no serious or unexpected AEs
Wilens et al. (2005) [144]	6	Donepezil	Open	12 weeks	9 mg/day 2.5–10mg/day	55% improved on CGI	Not well tolerated
Reimherr et al. (2005) [58]	47	BPR SR	Double-blind, placebo parallel	6 weeks	298 mg/day 100–400 mg/day	41% response rate on CGI (22% placebo)	Not statistically significant vs. placebo

(cont.)

Table 22.3. (cont.)

Study (year)	N	Medication	Design	Duration	Total dose mean and/or range	Outcome	Comments
Adler et al. (2006) [145]	218	ATMX	Double-blind, multicenter	–	80 mg Q-D vs. 40 mg BID	Both treatments efficacious	Changes in dosing are not associated with greater AEs or safety risks. BID treatment had greater effect
Wilens et al. (2006) [81]	11	ABT-089	Double-blind, placebo crossover	8 weeks	4, 8, and 40 mg/day	ABT-089 improved CGI and CAARS	Nicotinic partial agonist; no safety or side effect profiles were observed; study interrupted
Biederman et al. (2006) [146]	28	Galantamine	Double-blind, placebo parallel	12 weeks	20 mg/day 8–24 mg/day	22% response rate on CGI (11% placebo)	Study did not support the use of galantamine; no statistically or clinically significant greater reduction in ADHD symptoms
Levin et al. (2006) [147]	98	MPH SR BPR SR	Double-blind, placebo parallel (MPH, BPR)	12 weeks	10–80 mg/day 100–400 mg/day	Response rates: 34% MPH and 49% BPR (46% placebo)	SUD study; MPH and BPR did not provide a clear advantage over placebo (AARS)
Wilens et al. (2008) [148]	126	NS2359	Double-blind, placebo parallel	8 weeks	0.5 mg/day	33% response rate on ADHD-RS (27% placebo)	Triple amine reuptake inhibitor; no serious AEs; some attentional improvement on neuropsychological testing; ADHD-RS not significant
Wilens et al. (2008) [52]	147	ATMX	Double-blind, placebo parallel	12 weeks	90 mg/day 25–100 mg/day	Improved ADHD & heavy drinking	SUD study; no serious AEs or specific drug–drug reactions related to current alcohol use; No effect on relapse rate vs. placebo
Levin et al. (2009) [149]	20	ATMX	Open	12 weeks	80 mg/day 20–100 mg/day	50% response rate on AARS	Cocaine abusers; little to no effect on cocaine abuse
Johnson et al. (2009) [150]	20	ATMX	Open	10 weeks-1 year	85 mg/day 40–100 mg/day	50% response rate on CGI	Side effects led to 95% dropout rate by 10 weeks; only one patient continued treatment for 1 year
Adler et al. (2009) [50]	442	ATMX	Double-blind, placebo parallel	14 weeks	83 mg/day 40–100 mg/day	ATMX improved sxs of ADHD and anxiety	Comorbid social anxiety disorder; Rates of insomnia, nausea, dry mouth, and dizziness were higher with ATMX than with placebo
Adler et al. (2009) [47]	501	ATMX	Double-blind, placebo parallel	6 months	85 mg/day 25–100 mg/day	ATMX was effective at 10 weeks and 6 months	Long-term study; AEs similar to previous trials

Table 22.3. *(cont.)*

Study (year)	N	Medication	Design	Duration	Total dose mean and/or range	Outcome	Comments
Wilens et al. (2010) [62]	32	BPR SR	Open	6 weeks	100–400 mg/day	66% response rate on ADHD RS	SUD study; 19/32 completed 6-week protocol; no clinically significant reductions observed in self-report of SUD or CGI SUD scores
Surman et al. (2010) [151]	45	ATMX	Open	6 weeks	79 mg/day 50–120 mg/day	64% response rate on CGI and AISRS	ADHD-NOS population, similar outcome vs. full ADHD; no serious AEs
Adler et al. (2010) [152]	18	ATMX	Open	10 weeks	25–120 mg/day	Improved ADHD, reduced cravings	SUD study; 12/18 completed
Takahashi et al. (2011) [153]	45	ATMX	Open	8 weeks	114 mg/day 40–120 mg/day	Improved CAARS and CGI scores	No serious AEs were reported
Young et al. (2011) [46]	502	ATMX	Double-blind, placebo-controlled	24 weeks	90 mg/day 40–100 mg/day	68% response rate (42% placebo)	AEs overall and for on-label or slow titration to ATMX were similar and consistent with previous adult ATMX studies
Arnold et al. (2012) [154]	330	Modafinil	Double-blind, placebo-controlled	9 weeks	225–510 mg/day	No benefit on ADHD sxs	Drug was reasonably tolerated
Sutherland et al. (2012) [155]	241	ATMX Buspirone	Double-blind, placebo-controlled	8 weeks	91 and 90 mg/day ATMX/buspirone and ATMX, respectively	Response rates of ATMX (69%) and ATMX/buspirone (78%)	Similar outcomes of ATMX and buspirone vs. ATMX monotherapy
TOTAL (n = 47)	n = 4571 6–536 (range)	BPR: 9 ATMX: 14 Others: 24	Double: 24 Single: 1 Open: 22	2 weeks– 1 year	BPR: 100–450 mg/day ATMX: 25–120 mg/day	Variable response	Some delay in therapeutic response – may be related to titration schedule. Response rates typically less than stimulants

Response rate refers to subject reported much to very much improved (i.e., by clinical global improvement; CGI) or with clinically significant reduction in symptoms on ADHD rating scales.

Abbreviations: AARS = Adult ADHD Rating Scale, ADHD = attention-deficit hyperactivity disorder, AE = adverse event, AISRS = Adult ADHD Investigator Symptom Rating Scale, ATMX = atomoxetine, BPR = bupropion, CAARS = Conners' Adult ADHD Rating Scale, CGI = Clinical Global Impression, d-AMPH = dextroamphetamine, MPH = methylphenidate, NOS = not otherwise specified, RS = Rating Scale, SR/XL = sustained release, SUD = substance use disorder, sx = symptom, tx = treatment.

In such situations or when ATMX is co-administered with medication known to inhibit CYP2D6 (e.g., fluoxetine, paroxetine), clinicians should consider reducing the dose. In addition to the treatment of both inattention and hyperactivity/impulsivity in adults with ADHD, ATMX may be particularly useful when anxiety, mood, or tics co-occur with ADHD. For example, Adler *et al.* in a large, 14-week multisite study of ATMX in adults with ADHD and social anxiety disorder reported clinically significant effects on both ADHD and on anxiety [50].

Although untested, because of its lack of abuse liability [51], ATMX may be particularly of use in adults with current substance use issues. For instance Wilens and associates demonstrated in a 12-week controlled trial that treatment with ATMX in recently abstinent alcoholics was associated with improved ADHD and reduced drinking although absolute abstinent rates were unaffected [52]. Moreover, ATMX has not been reported to have significant or serious drug interactions with alcohol or marijuana [53]. Since pharmacotherapy of ADHD is often chronic, missed doses of medication can be expected and may be problematic.

Although generally well tolerated, the most common side effects observed with ATMX appear reflective of increased noradrenergic tone. The most common side effects of ATMX include dry mouth, insomnia, nausea, decreased appetite, constipation, decreased libido, dizziness, and sweating [54]. Furthermore, 9.8% of ATMX-treated males experienced difficulty attaining or maintaining erections. During these trials, extensive laboratory testing suggested that ATMX causes no organ toxicity and there were no discontinuations in the clinical trials due to abnormal lab tests. However, there have been reports of hepatotoxicity in two patients taking ATMX (out of two million patients exposed to ATMX). Both patients recovered upon discontinuation of ATMX. ATMX should be discontinued in patients with jaudice, and patients should contact their doctors if they develop pruritis, jaundice, dark urine, right upper quadrant tenderness, and/or unexplained "flu-like" symptoms. Lab monitoring outside of routine medical care does not appear necessary. While the impact of ATMX on the cardiovascular system appears minimal [24, 55], ATMX was associated with mean increases in heart rate of 6 beats per minute, and increases in systolic and diastolic blood pressure of 1.5 mmHg. Adults should have their vital signs checked prior to initiating treatment with ATMX and periodically thereafter.

Antidepressants

Bupropion, a novel-structured antidepressant, has been reported to be moderately helpful in reducing ADHD symptoms in children [56]. There have been at least three open and six controlled trials using bupropion in adults with ADHD. In a 6-week double-blind placebo-controlled trial, bupropion at 200 mg sustained release (SR) BID (final mean dose 386 mg/day) resulted in a 42% reduction in the ADHD-RS with 52% of subjects treated with bupropion considered responders [57]. Similar results were found by Reimherr et al. [58] and using an alternative once-daily preparation [59]. Doses of 400 to 450 mg (SR or extended-release [XL] preparations) are usually necessary for best efficacy. Side effects include insomnia, edginess, and a theoretical risk for seizures with IR preparations. Despite

the small number of adults studied, bupropion may be helpful in ADHD, particularly when associated with comorbid depression [60], substance abuse [61, 62], bipolar disorder [63], or in adults with cardiac abnormalities [64]. Bupropion appears to be more stimulating than other antidepressants, and is associated with a higher rate of drug-induced seizures than other antidepressants [64]. These seizures appear to be dose related (>450 mg/day) and elevated in patients with bulimia or a previous seizure history. Bupropion has also been associated with excitement, agitation, increased motor activity, insomnia, tremors, and tics.

Despite an extensive experience in children and adolescents there are only two studies of TCAs in adult ADHD [65, 66]. Compared to the stimulants, TCAs have negligible abuse liability, single daily dosing, and efficacy for comorbid anxiety and depression. However, given concerns about potential overdose and the availability of ATMX, use of the TCAs has been significantly curtailed. Generally, TCA daily doses of 50 to 250 mg are required with a relatively rapid response to treatment (i.e., 2 weeks) when the appropriate dose is reached. TCAs should be initiated at 25 mg and slowly titrated upward within dosing and serum level parameters until an acceptable response or intolerable adverse effects are reported. Common side effects of the TCAs include dry mouth, constipation, blurred vision, weight gain, and sexual dysfunction. While cardiovascular effects of reduced cardiac conduction, and elevated blood pressure and heart rates are not infrequent, if monitored, they rarely prevent treatment. As serum TCA levels are variable, they are best used as guidelines for efficacy and to reduce central nervous system and cardiovascular toxicity.

The MAOI antidepressants have also been studied for the treatment of ADHD. Whereas open studies with pargyline and deprenyl in adult ADHD showed moderate improvements [67, 68], a controlled trial of selegiline (deprenyl) yielded less enthusiastic findings [69]. Ernst et al. reported dose-dependent improvements in ADHD symptoms on selegiline, which were not significant when compared to a high placebo response [69]. Although a pilot child-based study demonstrated efficacy of the reversible MAOI, moclobemide [70], data of its effectiveness for ADHD in adults are limited to case reports [71, 72]. The concerns of diet- or medication-induced hypertensive crisis limit the usefulness and safety of these medications, especially in a group of ADHD patients vulnerable to impulsivity. Additionally, other adverse effects associated with the MAOIs include agitation or lethargy, orthostatic hypotension, weight gain, sexual dysfunction, sleep disturbances, and edema, often leading to the discontinuation of these agents [64].

Miscellaneous medications

The α-adrenergic agonists clonidine and guanfacine have been used in childhood ADHD, especially in cases with a marked hyperactive or aggressive component [73]. There is a dearth of data on using the α agonists in adults with ADHD. Taylor and Russo reported results from 17 adults treated with either d-AMPH or guanfacine IR and found the active treatments produced similar reductions in ADHD symptoms compared with placebo [74]. To date, no studies of clonidine for ADHD have been completed in adults. Given the paucity of efficacy data for α agonists and concerns of their sedative and hypotensive effects, their use in adults remains unclear.

Modafinil, approved for the treatment of narcolepsy [75], has generated interest as a potential treatment for ADHD. Although controlled trials on the use of modafinil in children and adolescents with ADHD demonstrated efficacy [76, 77] modafinil did not receive approval from the FDA due to concerns about its safety, specifically related to its possible serious skin reactions, including erythema multiforme (EM), Stevens–Johnson syndrome (SJS), and toxic epidermal necrolysis (TEN) [78]. Although one double-blind placebo-controlled crossover design in 22 adults suggested improvements in ADHD symptoms [79], results of large company sponsored multisite trials in adults with ADHD have been negative (Table 22.3).

There was a burst of activity on the use of nicotinic agents for ADHD. Whereas smaller crossover studies of nicotinic analogs with either full or partial agonistic properties demonstrated efficacy in adults with ADHD [80–82], follow-up larger multisite parallel design studies failed to show a significant effect of the nicotinic analog ABT-089 on reducing ADHD symptomatology [83].

Trials with amino acids were in part undertaken with the assumptions that ADHD may be related to a deficiency in the catecholaminergic system, and that administration of precursors of these systems would reverse these deficits [84–86]. In these studies, transient improvement in ADHD was lost after 2 weeks of treatment. Therefore, amino acids have a limited role in the treatment of adults with

ADHD. Prohistaminergic agents, while appealing given the endogenous histamine effects on the attention arousal systems, have been disappointing [87]. Catecholamine-triamine reuptake inhibitors, and some pro-cognitive ampakines have also failed to demonstrate efficacy in controlled trials with adults with ADHD (see Table 22.3).

Suggested management strategies

Having received the diagnosis of ADHD, the adult needs to be familiarized with the risks and benefits of pharmacotherapy, the availability of alternative treatments, and the likely adverse effects. Patient expectations need to be explored and realistic goals of treatment need to be clearly delineated [88]. Likewise, the clinician should review with the patient the various pharmacological options available and that each will require systematic trials of the anti-ADHD medications for reasonable durations of time and at clinically meaningful doses. Treatment-seeking ADHD adults who manifest substantial psychiatric comorbidity, have residual symptomatology with treatment, or report psychological distress related to their ADHD (i.e., self-esteem issues, self-sabotaging patterns, interpersonal disturbances) should be directed to appropriate psychotherapeutic intervention with clinicians knowledgeable in ADHD treatment.

ADHD adults often require more comprehensive treatment for their ADHD given the sequelae associated with a chronic disorder, its effect on psychological development, and residual psychiatric and ADHD symptoms even with aggressive pharmacotherapy. To this end, the use of structured cognitive-based psychotherapies appears helpful especially when used conjointly with pharmacotherapy [89, 90]. For adults considering advanced schooling, educational planning and alterations in the school environment may be necessary.

The stimulant medications and ATMX are FDA approved and the most rigorously investigated pharmacotherapies (see Tables 22.1, 22.2, and 22.3) and are considered the first-line therapy for ADHD in adults. Although there are no evidence-based guidelines in selecting a first choice of medication for adults with ADHD, clinicians ought to base their recommendation after considering issues of comorbidity, tolerability, efficacy, and duration of action [7]. Older treatment guidelines recommend starting with longer-acting stimulant preparations in most cases [7].

Every few days the dose may be increased to optimize response. Frequently, patients benefit from adding IR AMPH or MPH in combination with longer-acting preparations in order to sculpt the dose to the patient's individual needs [91], although the efficacy of this practice is not well studied.

Consideration of another stimulant or ATMX is recommended if an ADHD adult is unresponsive or has intolerable side effects to the initial medication. Given their pharmacodynamic differences [92], if a MPH product was initially selected, then moving to an AMPH-based medication is appropriate. Although some adults are able to take ATMX once daily, many adults benefit from BID dosing [54]. Patients must also be made aware that the full benefits of ATMX may not occur for several weeks and they may not "feel" anything like they may have with the stimulants. Monitoring routine side effects, vital signs, and the misuse of the medication is warranted.

Adult ADHD is a heterogeneous disorder associated with considerable comorbidity with antisocial disorders, anxiety and mood disorders as well as substance use disorders [43, 93]. Adults with ADHD and comorbid mood or anxiety disorders may respond differently to ADHD pharmacotherapy, depending on the clinical state of their co-occurring disorders. The effects of stimulants on comorbid anxiety and depression have not been systematically assessed in adults with ADHD. While it is possible for stimulants to exacerbate anxiety and depression, patients may present with chronic anxiety/demoralization related to their untreated ADHD. Often in these cases, with treatment for their ADHD, symptoms of anxiety and demoralization diminish. Also, one can treat anxiety and ADHD simultaneously. Weiss and Hechtman found that adults receiving paroxetine or d-AMPH and paroxetine demonstrated greater improvement for mood and anxiety symptoms compared to adults receiving d-AMPH or placebo alone [17]. Likewise, patients presenting for treatment of depression may have their ADHD overlooked [94].

Other concurrent psychiatric disorders also need to be assessed, and if possible the relationship of the ADHD symptoms with these other disorders delineated. In subjects with ADHD plus bipolar mood disorders, for example, the risk of mania and/or hypomania needs to be addressed and closely monitored during the treatment of the ADHD [95]. In cases such as these, mood stabilization is the priority and usually involves both the introduction of anti-manic medications as well as discontinuing ADHD treatments as shown in children [96, 97]. Once the mood is euthymic, conservative introduction of anti-ADHD medications along with mood-stabilizing agents should be considered.

Treatment of refractory patients

Despite the availability of various agents for adults with ADHD, there appear to be a number of individuals who either do not respond, or are intolerant of adverse effects of medications used to treat their ADHD. In managing difficult cases, several therapeutic strategies are available. If psychiatric adverse effects develop concurrent with a poor medication response, alternate treatments should be pursued. Severe psychiatric symptoms that emerge during the acute phase can be problematic, irrespective of the efficacy of the medications for ADHD. These symptoms may require reconsideration of the diagnosis of ADHD and careful reassessment of the presence of comorbid disorders. For example, it is common to observe depressive symptoms in an ADHD adult, which are independent of the ADHD or treatment. If reduction of dose or change in preparation (i.e., IR vs. extended delivery) does not resolve the problem, consideration should be given to combined pharmacotherapies such as stimulants and non-stimulants or alternative treatments. Concurrent non-pharmacological interventions such as behavioral or cognitive therapy may assist with symptom reduction.

Summary

In summary, the aggregate literature supports that pharmacotherapy provides an effective treatment for adults with ADHD. Effective FDA-approved pharmacological treatments for ADHD adults to date have included the use of the stimulants and ATMX. Bupropion, TCAs, and modafinil have also been studied in the treatment of adult ADHD, and have a role in its treatment. Although interest remains high, data on the efficacy of cognitive enhancers remain minimal and their role is limited and research based at this point. Structured psychotherapy may be effective when used adjunctly with medications. Further controlled investigations assessing the efficacy of single and combination agents for adults with ADHD are necessary, with careful attention to diagnostics, comorbidity, symptom and neuropsychological outcome, long-term tolerability and efficacy, and use in specific ADHD subgroups.

References

1. Kessler RC, Adler LA, Gruber MJ, et al. Validity of the World Health Organization Adult ADHD Self-Report Scale (ASRS) Screener in a representative sample of health plan members. *Int J Methods Psychiatr Res.* 2007;**16**(2):52–65.

2. Adler L, Cohen J. Diagnosis and evaluation of adults with ADHD. *Psychiatr Clin North Am.* 2004;**27**: 187–201.

3. Murphy KR, Adler LA. Assessing attention-deficit/ hyperactivity disorder in adults: focus on rating scales. *J Clin Psychiatry.* 2004;**65**(Suppl 3):12–17.

4. Wilens TE, Dodson W. A clinical perspective of attention-deficit/hyperactivity disorder into adulthood. *J Clin Psychiatry.* 2004;**65**(10):1301–13.

5. Wilens TE, Faraone SV, Biederman J. Attention-deficit/hyperactivity disorder in adults. *JAMA.* 2004;**292**(5):619–23.

6. Wilens T, Morrison NR, Prince J. An update on the pharmacotherapy of attention-deficit/hyperactivity disorder in adults. *Expert Rev Neurother.* 2011;**11**(10): 1443–65.

7. Greenhill LL, Pliszka S, Dulcan MK, et al. Practice parameter for the use of stimulant medications in the treatment of children, adolescents, and adults. *J Am Acad Child Adolesc Psychiatry.* 2002;**41**(2 Suppl): 26S–49S.

8. Wilens TE, Spencer TJ. The stimulants revisited. *Child Adolesc Psychiatr Clin N Am.* 2000;**9**:573–603.

9. Spencer T. ADHD treatment across the life cycle. *J Clin Psychiatry.* 2004;**65**(Suppl 3):22–6.

10. Mattes JA, Boswell L, Oliver H. Methylphenidate effects on symptoms of attention deficit disorder in adults. *Arch Gen Psychiatry.* 1984;**41**(11):1059–63.

11. Ginsberg L, Katic A, Adeyi B, et al. Long-term treatment outcomes with lisdexamfetamine dimesylate for adults with attention-deficit/hyperactivity disorder stratified by baseline severity. *Curr Med Res Opin.* 2011;**27**(6):1097–107.

12. Spencer TJ, Adler LA, McGough JJ, et al. Efficacy and safety of dexmethylphenidate extended-release capsules in adults with attention-deficit/hyperactivity disorder. *Biol Psychiatry.* 2007;**61**(12):1380–7.

13. Medori R, Ramos-Quiroga JA, Casas M, et al. A randomized, placebo-controlled trial of three fixed dosages of prolonged release OROS methylphenidate in adults with attention-deficit/hyperactivity disorder. *Biol Psychiatry.* 2008;**63**(10):981–9.

14. Faraone SV, Spencer T, Aleardi M, Pagano C, Biederman J. Meta-analysis of the efficacy of methylphenidate for treating adult attention-deficit/ hyperactivity disorder. *J Clin Psychopharmacol.* 2004; **24**(1):24–9.

15. Biederman J, Mick E, Surman C, et al. A randomized, 3-phase, 34-week, double-blind, long-term efficacy study of osmotic-release oral system-methylphenidate in adults with attention-deficit/hyperactivity disorder. *J Clin Psychopharmacol.* 2010;**30**(5):549–53.

16. Spencer TJ, Mick E, Surman CB, et al. A randomized, single-blind, substitution study of OROS methylphenidate (Concerta) in ADHD adults receiving immediate release methylphenidate. *J Atten Disord.* 2011;**15**(4):286–94.

17. Weiss M, Hechtman L. A randomized double-blind trial of paroxetine and/or dextroamphetamine and problem-focused therapy for attention-deficit/ hyperactivity disorder in adults. *J Clin Psychiatry.* 2006;**67**(4):611–19.

18. Rösler M, Fischer R, Ammer R, Ose C, Retz W. A randomised, placebo-controlled, 24-week, study of low-dose extended-release methylphenidate in adults with attention-deficit/hyperactivity disorder. *Eur Arch Psychiatry Clin Neurosci.* 2009;**259**(2):120–9.

19. Wender PH, Reimherr FW, Marchant BK, et al. A one year trial of methylphenidate in the treatment of ADHD. *J Atten Disord.* 2010;**15**(1):36–45.

20. Weisler R, Young J, Mattingly G, et al. Long-term safety and effectiveness of lisdexamfetamine dimesylate in adults with attention-deficit/hyperactivity disorder. *CNS Spectr.* 2009;**14**(10):573–85.

21. Marchant BK, Reimherr FW, Halls C, Williams ED, Strong RE. OROS methylphenidate in the treatment of adults with ADHD: a 6-month, open-label, follow-up study. *Ann Clin Psychiatry.* 2010;**22**(3):196–204.

22. Ratey J, Greenberg M, Lindem KJ. Combination of treatments for attention deficit disorders in adults. *J Nerv Ment Dis.* 1991;**176**:699–701.

23. Nissen SE. ADHD drugs and cardiovascular risk. *N Engl J Med.* 2006;**354**(14):1445–8.

24. Habel LA, Cooper WO, Sox CM, et al. ADHD medications and risk of serious cardiovascular events in young and middle-aged adults. *JAMA.* 2011; **306**(24):2673–83.

25. Cooper WO, Habel LA, Sox CM, et al. ADHD drugs and serious cardiovascular events in children and young adults. *N Engl J Med.* 2011;**365**(20): 1896–904.

26. Hammerness P, Zusman R, Systrom D, et al. A cardiopulmonary study of lisdexamfetamine in adults with attention-deficit/hyperactivity disorder. *World J Biol Psychiatry.* 2013;**14**(4):299–306.

27. Gutgesell H, Atkins, D, Barst R, *et al*. Cardiovascular monitoring of children and adolescents receiving psychotropic drugs. A statement for healthcare professionals from the Committee on Congenital Heart Defects, Council on Cardiovascular Diseases in the young, American Heart Association. *Circulation* 1999;**99**(7):979–82.

28. Perrin JM, Friedman RA, Knilans TK, *et al*. Cardiovascular monitoring and stimulant drugs for attention-deficit/hyperactivity disorder. *Pediatrics*. 2008;**122**(2):451–3.

29. Wilens T, Hammerness P, Biederman J, *et al*. Blood pressure changes associated with medication treatment of adults with attention-deficit/hyperactivity disorder. *J Clin Psychiatry*. 2005;**66**(2):253–9.

30. Wilens TE, Zusman RM, Hammerness PG, *et al*. An open-label study of the tolerability of mixed amphetamine salts in adults with ADHD and treated primary essential hypertension. *J Clin Psychiatry*. 2006;**67**(5):696–702.

31. Van Veen MM, Kooij JJ, Boonstra AM, Gordijn MC, Van Someren EJ. Delayed circadian rhythm in adults with attention-deficit/hyperactivity disorder and chronic sleep-onset insomnia. *Biol Psychiatry*. 2010; **67**(11):1091–6.

32. Kratochvil CJ, Lake M, Pliszka SR, Walkup JT. Pharmacological management of treatment-induced insomnia in ADHD. *J Am Acad Child Adolesc Psychiatry*. 2005;**44**(5):499–501.

33. Prince J, Wilens T, Biederman J, Spencer TJ, Wozniak JR. Clonidine for sleep disturbances associated with attention-deficit hyperactivity disorder: a systematic chart review of 62 cases. *J Am Acad Child Adolesc Psychiatry*. 1996;**35**(5):599–605.

34. Macchi MM, Bruce JN. Human pineal physiology and functional significance of melatonin. *Front Neuroendocrinol*. 2004;**25**(3–4):177–95.

35. Tjon Pian Gi CV, Broeren JP, Starreveld JS, Versteegh FG. Melatonin for treatment of sleeping disorders in children with attention deficit/hyperactivity disorder: a preliminary open label study. *Eur J Pediatr*. 2003; **162**(7–8):554–5.

36. Weiss MD, Wasdell MB, Bomben MM, Rea KJ, Freeman RD. Sleep hygiene and melatonin treatment for children and adolescents with ADHD and initial insomnia. *J Am Acad Child Adolesc Psychiatry*. 2006; **45**(5):512–19.

37. Markowitz JS, Morrison SD, DeVane CL. Drug interactions with psychostimulants. *Int Clin Psychopharmacol*. 1999;**14**(1):1–18.

38. Markowitz JS, Patrick KS. Pharmacokinetic and pharmacodynamic drug interactions in the treatment of ADHD. *Clin Pharmacokinet*. 2001;**40**:753–72.

39. Hammerness P, Georgiopoulos A, Doyle RL, *et al*. An open study of adjunct OROS-methylphenidate in children who are atomoxetine partial responders: II. Tolerability and pharmacokinetics. *J Child Adolesc Psychopharmacol*. 2009;**19**(5):493–9.

40. Wilens TE, Hammerness P, Utzinger L, *et al*. An open study of adjunct OROS-methylphenidate in children and adolescents who are atomoxetine partial responders: I. Effectiveness. *J Child Adolesc Psychopharmacol*. 2009;**19**(5):485–92.

41. Cohen LG, Prince J, Biederman J, *et al*. Absence of effect of stimulants on the phamacokinetics of desipramine in children. *Pharmacotherapy*. 1999; **19**(6):746–52.

42. Shekim WO, Asarnow RF, Hess EB, Zaucha K, Wheeler N. A clinical and demographic profile of a sample of adults with attention deficit hyperactivity disorder, residual state. *Compr Psychiatry*. 1990; **31**:416–25.

43. Biederman J, Faraone SV, Spencer T. Patterns of psychiatric comorbidity, cognition, and psychosocial functioning in adults with attention deficit hyperactivity disorder. *Am J Psychiatry*. 1993;**150**: 1792–8.

44. Bymaster FP, Katner JS, Nelson DL, *et al*. Atomoxetine increases extracellular levels of norepinephrine and dopamine in prefrontal cortex of rat: a potential mechanism for efficacy in attention deficit/ hyperactivity disorder. *Neuropsychopharmacology*. 2002;**27**(5):699–711.

45. Pliszka S, McCracken J, Maas JW, *et al*. Catecholamines in attention-deficit hyperactivity disorder: current perspectives. *J Am Acad Child Adolesc Psychiatry*. 1996;**35**(3):264–72.

46. Young JL, Sarkis E, Qiao M, Wietecha L. Once-daily treatment with atomoxetine in adults with attention-deficit/hyperactivity disorder: a 24-week, randomized, double-blind, placebo-controlled trial. *Clin Neuropharmacol*. 2011;**34**(2):51–60.

47. Adler LA, Spencer T, Brown TE, *et al*. Once-daily atomoxetine for adult attention-deficit/hyperactivity disorder: a 6-month, double-blind trial. *J Clin Psychopharmacol*. 2009;**29**(1):44–50.

48. Marchant BK, Reimherr FW, Halls C, *et al*. Long-term open-label response to atomoxetine in adult ADHD: influence of sex, emotional dysregulation, and double-blind response to atomoxetine. *Atten Defic Hyperact Disord*. 2011;**3**(3): 237–44.

49. Ring BJ, Gillespie JS, Eckstein JA, Wrighton SA. Identification of the human cytochromes P450 responsible for atomoxetine metabolism. *Drug Metab Dispos*. 2002;**30**(3):319–23.

50. Adler LA, Liebowitz M, Kronenberger W, *et al.* Atomoxetine treatment in adults with attention-deficit/hyperactivity disorder and comorbid social anxiety disorder. *Depress Anxiety.* 2009;**26**(3): 212–21.

51. Heil SH, Holmes HW, Bickel WK, *et al.* Comparison of the subjective, physiological, and psychomotor effects of atomoxetine and methylphenidate in light drug users. *Drug Alcohol Depend.* 2002;**67**(2): 149–56.

52. Wilens TE, Adler LA, Weiss MD, *et al.* Atomoxetine treatment of adults with ADHD and comorbid alcohol use disorders. *Drug Alcohol Depend.* 2008;**96**(1–2): 145–54.

53. Adler L, Wilens T, Zhang S, *et al.* Retrospective safety analysis of atomoxetine in adult ADHD patients with or without comorbid alcohol abuse and dependence. *Am J Addict.* 2009;**18**(5):393–401.

54. Michelson D, Adler L, Spencer T, *et al.* Atomoxetine in adults with ADHD: two randomized, placebo-controlled studies. *Biol Psychiatry.* 2003;**53**:112–20.

55. Wernicke JF, Faries D, Girod D, *et al.* Cardiovascular effects of atomoxetine in children, adolescents, and adults. *Drug Saf.* 2003;**26**(10):729–40.

56. Casat CD, Pleasants DZ, Van Wyck Fleet J. A double blind trial of bupropion in children with attention deficit disorder. *Psychopharmacol Bull.* 1987;**23**:120–2.

57. Wilens TE, Spencer TJ, Biederman J, *et al.* A controlled clinical trial of bupropion for attention deficit hyperactivity disorder in adults. *Am J Psychiatry.* 2001;**158**(2):282–8.

58. Reimherr FW, Hedges DW, Strong RE, Marchant BK, Williams ED. Bupropion SR in adults with ADHD: a short-term, placebo-controlled trial. *Neuropsychiatr Dis Treat.* 2005;**1**(3):245–51.

59. Wilens TE, Haight BR, Horrigan JP, *et al.* Bupropion XL in adults with attention-deficit/hyperactivity disorder: a randomized, placebo-controlled study. *Biol Psychiatry.* 2005;**57**(7):793–801.

60. Daviss WB, Bentivoglio P, Racusin R, *et al.* Bupropion sustained release in adolescents with comorbid attention-deficit/hyperactivity disorder and depression. *J Am Acad Child Adolesc Psychiatry.* 2001;**40**(3):307–14.

61. Levin FR, Evans SM, McDowell DM, Brooks DJ, Nunes E. Bupropion treatment for cocaine abuse and adult attention-deficit/hyperactivity disorder. *J Addict Dis.* 2002;**21**(2):1–16.

62. Wilens TE, Prince JB, Waxmonsky J, *et al.* An open trial of sustained release bupropion for attention-deficit/hyperactivity disorder in adults with ADHD plus substance use disorders. *J ADHD Relat Disord.* 2010;**1**(3):25–35.

63. Wilens TE, Prince JB, Spencer T, *et al.* An open trial of bupropion for the treatment of adults with attention deficit hyperactivity disorder and bipolar disorder. *Biol Psychiatry.* 2003;**54**(1):9–16.

64. Gelenberg AJ, Bassuk EL. *The Practioner's Guide to Psychoactive Drugs.* New York, NY: Plenum Medical Book Company; 1991.

65. Wilens TE, Biederman J, Mick E, Spencer TJ. A systematic assessment of tricyclic antidepressants in the treatment of adult attention-deficit hyperactivity disorder. *J Nerv Ment Dis.* 1995;**183**:48–50.

66. Wilens T, Biederman J, Prince J, *et al.* Six-week, double blind, placebo-controlled study of desipramine for adult attention deficit hyperactivity disorder. *Am J Psychiatry.* 1996;**153**:1147–53.

67. Wender PH, Wood DR, Reimherr FW, Ward M. An open trial of pargyline in the treatment of attention deficit disorder, residual type. *Psychiatry Res.* 1983; **9**:329–36.

68. Wender PH, Wood DR, Reimherr FW, *et al.* Pharmacological treatment of attention deficit disorder residual type (ADD, RT, "minimal brain dysfunction", "hyperactivity") in adults. *Psychopharmacol Bull.* 1985;**21**:222–31.

69. Ernst M, Liebenauer L, Jons PH, *et al.* Selegiline in adults with attention deficit hyperactivity disorder: clinical efficacy and safety. *Psychopharmacol Bull.* 1996;**32**:327–34.

70. Trott GE, Friese HJ, Menzel M, Nissen G. Use of moclobemide in children with attention deficit hyperactivity disorder. *Psychopharmacology (Berl).* 1992;**106**(Suppl):S134–6.

71. Myronuk LD, Weiss M, Cotter L. Combined treatment with moclobemide and methylphenidate for comorbid major depression and adult attention-deficit/hyperactivity disorder. *J Clin Psychopharmacol.* 1996;**16**(6):468–9.

72. Vaiva G, De Lenclave MB, Bailly D. Treatment of comorbid opiate addiction and attention-deficit hyperactivity disorder (residual type) with moclobemide: a case report. *Prog Neuropsychopharmacol Biol Psychiatry.* 2002;**26**(3): 609–11.

73. Connor DF, Fletcher KE, Swanson JM, *et al.* A meta-analysis of clonidine for symptoms of attention-deficit hyperactivity disorder. *J Am Acad Child Adolesc Psychiatry.* 1999;**38**(12):1551–9.

74. Taylor FB, Russo J. Comparing guanfacine and dextroamphetamine for the treatment of adult attention-deficit/hyperactivity disorder. *J Clin Psychopharmacol.* 2001;**21**(2):223–8.

75. Randomized trial of modafinil for the treatment of pathological somnolence in narcolepsy. US Modafinil

in Narcolepsy Multicenter Study Group. *Ann Neurol.* 1998;**43**(1):88–97.

76. Biederman J, Swanson J, Wigal SB, *et al.* Efficacy and safety of modafinil film-coated tablets in children and adolescents with attention-deficit/hyperactivity disorder: results of a randomized, double-blind, placebo-controlled, flexible-dose study. *Pediatrics.* 2005;**116**:e777–84.

77. Wigal SB, Biederman J, Swanson JM, Young R, Greenhill LL. Efficacy and safety of modafinil film-coated tablets in children and adolescents with or without prior stimulant treatment for attention-deficit/hyperactivity disorder: pooled analysis of 3 randomized, double-blind, placebo-controlled studies. *Prim Care Companion J Clin Psychiatry.* 2006;**8**(6):352–60.

78. FDA. MODAFINIL. *Drug Saf Newslett.* 2007;**1**(1): 5–7.

79. Taylor FB, Russo J. Efficacy of modafinil compared to dextroamphetamine for the treatment of attention deficit hyperactivity disorder in adults. *J Child Adolesc Psychopharmacol.* 2000;**10**(4):311–20.

80. Wilens TE, Biederman J, Spencer TJ, *et al.* A pilot controlled clinical trial of ABT-418, a cholinergic agonist, in the treatment of adults with attention deficit hyperactivity disorder. *Am J Psychiatry.* 1999;**156**(12):1931–7.

81. Wilens T, Verlinden MH, Adler LA, Wozniak PJ, West SA. ABT-089, a neuronal nicotinic receptor partial agonist, for the treatment of attention-deficit/hyperactivity disorder in adults: results of a pilot study. *Biol Psychiatry.* 2006;**59**(11):1065–70.

82. Apostol G, Abi-Saab W, Kratochvil CJ, *et al.* Efficacy and safety of the novel alphabeta neuronal nicotinic receptor partial agonist ABT-089 in adults with attention-deficit/hyperactivity disorder: a randomized, double-blind, placebo-controlled crossover study. *Psychopharmacology (Berl).* 2012;**219**(3):715–25.

83. Wilens TE, Gault LM, Childress A, *et al.* Safety and efficacy of ABT-089 in pediatric attention-deficit/hyperactivity disorder: results from two randomized placebo-controlled clinical trials. *J Am Acad Child Adolesc Psychiatry.* 2011;**50**(1):73–84.e1.

84. Wood D, Reimherr F, Wender PH, *et al.* Effects of levodopa on attention deficit disorder, residual type. *Psychiatry Res.* 1982;**6**:13–20.

85. Wood DR, Reimherr FW, Wender PH. Treatment of attention deficit disorder with D,L-phenylalanine. *Psychiatry Res.* 1985;**16**:21–6.

86. Reimherr FW, Wender PH, Wood DR, Ward M. An open trial of L-tyrosine in the treatment of attention deficit hyperactivity disorder, residual type. *Am J Psychiatry.* 1987;**144**:1071–3.

87. Herring WJ, Adler LA, Baranak CC, *et al.* Effects of the histamine inverse agonist MK-0249 in adult attention deficit disorder: a randomized, controlled, crossover study. *Biol Psychiatry.* 2010;**67**(9):217S.

88. Haavik J, Halmoy A, Lundervold AJ, Fasmer OB. Clinical assessment and diagnosis of adults with attention-deficit/hyperactivity disorder. *Expert Rev Neurother.* 2010;**10**(10):1569–80.

89. Safren SA, Sprich S, Mimiaga MJ, *et al.* Cognitive behavioral therapy vs relaxation with educational support for medication-treated adults with ADHD and persistent symptoms: a randomized controlled trial. *JAMA.* 2010;**304**(8):875–80.

90. Solanto MV, Marks DJ, Wasserstein J, *et al.* Efficacy of meta-cognitive therapy for adult ADHD. *Am J Psychiatry.* 2010;**167**(8):958–68.

91. Adler LA, Reingold LS, Morrill MS, Wilens T. Combination pharmacotherapy for adult ADHD. *Curr Psychiatry Rep.* 2006;**8**(5):409–15.

92. Wilens T, Spencer T. Pharmacology of amphetamines. In: Tarter R, Ammerman R, Ott P, eds. *Handbook of Substance Abuse: Neurobehavioral Pharmacology.* New York, NY: Plenum Press. 1998; 501–13.

93. Biederman J. Impact of comorbidity in adults with attention-deficit/hyperactivity disorder. *J Clin Psychiatry.* 2004;**65**(Suppl 3):3–7.

94. Alpert J, Maddocks A, Nierenberg AA, *et al.* Attention deficit hyperactivity disorder in childhood among adults with major depression. *Psychiatry Res.* 1996; **62**:213–19.

95. Wilens T, Biederman J, Wozniak J, *et al.* Can adults with attention-deficit hyperactivity disorder be distinguished from those with comorbid bipolar disorder?: findings from a sample of clinically referred adults. *Biol Psychiatry.* 2003;**54**(1):1–8.

96. Scheffer RE, Kowatch RA, Carmody T, Rush RJ. Randomized, placebo-controlled trial of mixed amphetamine salts for symptoms of comorbid ADHD in pediatric bipolar disorder after mood stabilization with divalproex sodium. *Am J Psychiatry.* 2005;**162**(1): 58–64.

97. Findling RL, Short EJ, McNamara NK, *et al.* Methylphenidate in the treatment of children and adolescents with bipolar disorder and attention-deficit/hyperactivity disorder. *J Am Acad Child Adolesc Psychiatry.* 2007;**46**(11):1445–53.

98. Wood DR, Reimherr FW, Wender PH, Johnson GE. Diagnosis and treatment of minimal brain dysfunction in adults. *Arch Gen Psychiatry.* 1976;**33**:1453–60.

99. Wender PH, Reimherr FW, Wood D, Ward M. A controlled study of methylphenidate in the treatment of attention deficit disorder, residual type, in adults. *Am J Psychiatry.* 1985;**142**:547–52.

100. Gualtieri CT, Hicks RE. Neuropharmacology of methylphenidate and a neural substrate for childhood hyperactivity. *Psychiatr Clin North Am*. 1985;**8**: 875–92.

101. Spencer T, Wilens TE, Biederman J, *et al*. A double blind, crossover comparison of methylphenidate and placebo in adults with childhood onset attention deficit hyperactivity disorder. *Arch Gen Psychiatry*. 1995;**52**:434–43.

102. Iaboni F, Bouffard R, Minde K, Hechtman L. The efficacy of methylphenidate in treating adults with attention-deficit/hyperactivity disorder. Scientific Proceedings of the American Academy of Child and Adolescent Psychiatry, Philadelphia, PA, American Academy of Child and Adolescent Psychiatry. 1996.

103. Paterson R, Douglas C, Hallmayer J, Hagan M, Krupenia Z. A randomised, double-blind, placebo-controlled trial of dexamphetamine in adults with attention deficit hyperactivity disorder. *Aust N Z J Psychiatry*. 1999;**33**(4):494–502.

104. Spencer T, Biederman J, Wilens T, *et al*. Efficacy of a mixed amphetamine salts compound in adults with attention-deficit/hyperactivity disorder. *Arch Gen Psychiatry*. 2001;**58**(8):775–82.

105. Taylor FB. Comparing guanfacine and dextroamphetamine for adult ADHD: efficacy and implications. 153rd Annual Meeting of the American Psychiatric Association, Chicago, IL; 2000.

106. Taylor FB. Comparing modafinil to dextroamphetamine in the treatment of adult ADHD. 153rd Annual Meeting of the American Psychiatric Association, Chicago, IL; 2000.

107. Kooij JJ, Burger H, Boonstra AM, *et al*. Efficacy and safety of methylphenidate in 45 adults with attention-deficit/hyperactivity disorder. A randomized placebo-controlled double-blind cross-over trial. *Psychol Med*. 2004;**34**(6):973–82.

108. Carpentier PJ, de Jong CA, Dijkstra BA, Verbrugge CA, Krabbe PF. A controlled trial of methylphenidate in adults with attention deficit/hyperactivity disorder and substance use disorders. *Addiction*. 2005;**100**(12): 1868–74.

109. Spencer T, Biederman J, Wilens T, *et al*. A large, double-blind, randomized clinical trial of methylphenidate in the treatment of adults with attention-deficit/hyperactivity disorder. *Biol Psychiatry*. 2005;**57**(5):456–63.

110. Biederman J, Mick E, Surman C, *et al*. A randomized, placebo-controlled trial of OROS-methylphenidate in adults with attention-deficit/hyperactivity disorder. *Biol Psychiatry*. 2006;**59**(9):829–35.

111. Weisler RH, Biederman J, Spencer TJ, *et al*. Mixed amphetamine salts extended-release in the treatment

of adult ADHD: a randomized, controlled trial. *CNS Spectr*. 2006;**11**(8):625–39.

112. Reimherr FW, Williams ED, Strong RE, *et al*. A double-blind, placebo-controlled, crossover study of osmotic release oral system methylphenidate in adults with ADHD with assessment of oppositional and emotional dimensions of the disorder. *J Clin Psychiatry*. 2007;**68**(1):93–101.

113. Jain U, Hechtman L, Weiss M, *et al*. Efficacy of a novel biphasic controlled-release methylphenidate formula in adults with attention-deficit/hyperactivity disorder: results of a double-blind, placebo-controlled crossover study. *J Clin Psychiatry*. 2007;**68**(2):268–77.

114. Adler LA, Goodman DW, Kollins SH, *et al*.; 303 Study Group. Double-blind, placebo-controlled study of the efficacy and safety of lisdexamfetamine dimesylate in adults with attention-deficit/hyperactivity disorder. *J Clin Psychiatry*. 2008;**69**(9):1364–73.

115. Weber J, Siddiqui MA. Lisdexamfetamine dimesylate: in attention-deficit hyperactivity disorder in adults. *CNS Drugs*. 2009;**23**(5):419–25.

116. Chronis-Tuscano A, Seymour KE, Stein MA, *et al*. Efficacy of osmotic-release oral system (OROS) methylphenidate for mothers with attention-deficit/ hyperactivity disorder (ADHD): preliminary report of effects on ADHD symptoms and parenting. *J Clin Psychiatry*. 2008;**69**(12):1938–47.

117. Adler LA, Zimmerman B, Starr HL, *et al*. Efficacy and safety of OROS methylphenidate in adults with attention-deficit/hyperactivity disorder: a randomized, placebo-controlled, double-blind, parallel group, dose-escalation study. *J Clin Psychopharmacol*. 2009; **29**(3):239–47.

118. Winhusen TM, Somoza EC, Brigham GS, *et al*. Impact of attention-deficit/hyperactivity disorder (ADHD) treatment on smoking cessation intervention in ADHD smokers: a randomized, double-blind, placebo-controlled trial. *J Clin Psychiatry*. 2010;**71**(12): 1680–8.

119. Wigal T, Brams M, Gasior M, *et al*. Randomized, double-blind, placebo-controlled, crossover study of the efficacy and safety of lisdexamfetamine dimesylate in adults with attention-deficit/hyperactivity disorder: novel findings using a simulated adult workplace environment design. *Behav Brain Funct*. 2010;**6**: 34.

120. Levin FR, Evans SM, McDowell DM, Kleber HD. Methylphenidate treatment for cocaine abusers with adult attention-deficit/hyperactivity disorder: a pilot study. *J Clin Psychiatry*. 1998;**59**:300–5.

121. Horrigan J, Barnhill L. Low-dose amphetamine salts and adult attention-deficit/hyperactivity disorder. *J Clin Psychiatry*. 2000;**61**:414–17.

122. Schubiner H, Saules KK, Arfken CL, *et al.* Double-blind placebo-controlled trial of methylphenidate in the treatment of adult ADHD patients with comorbid cocaine dependence. *Exp Clin Psychopharmacol.* 2002;**10**(3):286–94.

123. Biederman J, Spencer TJ, Wilens TE, *et al.* Long-term safety and effectiveness of mixed amphetamine salts extended release in adults with ADHD. *CNS Spectr.* 2005;**10**(12 Suppl 20):16–25.

124. Weisler RH, Biederman J, Spencer TJ, Wilens TE. Long-term cardiovascular effects of mixed amphetamine salts extended release in adults with ADHD. *CNS Spectr.* 2005;**10**(12 Suppl 20):35–43.

125. Levin FR, Evans SM, Brooks DJ, Garawi F. Treatment of cocaine dependent treatment seekers with adult ADHD: double-blind comparison of methylphenidate and placebo. *Drug Alcohol Depend.* 2007;**87**(1): 20–9.

126. Spencer TJ, Landgraf JM, Adler LA, *et al.* Attention-deficit/hyperactivity disorder-specific quality of life with triple-bead mixed amphetamine salts (SPD465) in adults: results of a randomized, double-blind, placebo-controlled study. *J Clin Psychiatry.* 2008; **69**(11):1766–75.

127. Adler LA, Spencer T, McGough JJ, Hai J, Muniz R. Long-term effectiveness and safety of dexmethylphenidate extended-release capsules in adult ADHD. *J Atten Disord.* 2009;**12**(5):449–59.

128. Bejerot S, Ryden EM, Arlinde CM. Two-year outcome of treatment with central stimulant medication in adult attention-deficit/hyperactivity disorder: a prospective study. *J Clin Psychiatry.* 2010;**71**(12):1590–7.

129. Konstenius M, Jayaram-Lindstrom N, Beck O, Franck J. Sustained release methylphenidate for the treatment of ADHD in amphetamine abusers: a pilot study. *Drug Alcohol Depend.* 2010;**108**(1–2):130–3.

130. Mattes JA. Propanolol for adults with temper outbursts and residual attention deficit disorder. *J Clin Psychopharmacol.* 1986;**6**:299–302.

131. Shekim WO, Masterson A, Cantwell DP, Hanna GL, McCracken JT. Nomifensine maleate in adult attention deficit disorder. *J Nerv Ment Dis.* 1989;**177**:296–9.

132. Shekim WO, Antun F, Hanna GL, McCracken JT, Hess EB. S-adenosyl-l-methionine (SAM) in adults with ADHD, RS: preliminary results from an open trial. *Psychopharmacol Bull.* 1990;**26**:249–53.

133. Wender PH, Reimherr FW. Bupropion treatment of attention deficit hyperactivity disorder in adults. *Am J Psychiatry.* 1990;**147**:1018–20.

134. Adler LA, Resnick S, Kunz M, Devinsky O. Open label trial of venlafaxine in adults with attention deficit disorder. *Psychopharmacol Bull.* 1995;**31**:785–8.

135. Hedges D, Reimherr FW, Rogers A, Strong R, Wender PH. An open trial of venlafaxine in adult patients with attention deficit hyperactivity disorder. *Psychopharmacol Bull.* 1995;**31**(4):779–83.

136. Findling RL, Schwartz MA, Flannery DJ, Manos MJ. Venlafaxine in adults with attention-deficit/hyperactivity disorder: an open clinical trial. *J Clin Psychiatry.* 1996;**57**(5):184–9.

137. Spencer T, Biederman J, Wilens T, *et al.* Effectiveness and tolerability of tomoxetine in adults with attention deficit hyperactivity disorder. *Am J Psychiatry.* 1998; **155**(5):693–5.

138. Cephalon Inc. *Cephalon reports no benefit from Provigil in study of adults with ADHD.* West Chester, PA. 2000.

139. Upadhyaya HP, Brady KT, Sethuraman G, Sonne SC, Malcolm R. Venlafaxine treatment of patients with comorbid alcohol/cocaine abuse and attention-deficit/hyperactivity disorder: a pilot study. *J Clin Psychopharmacol.* 2001;**21**(1):116–18.

140. Kuperman S, Perry PJ, Gaffney GR, *et al.* Bupropion SR vs. methylphenidate vs. placebo for attention deficit hyperactivity disorder in adults. *Ann Clin Psychiatry.* 2001;**13**(3):129–34.

141. Simpson D, Plosker GL. Spotlight on atomoxetine in adults with attention-deficit hyperactivity disorder. *CNS Drugs.* 2004;**18**(6):397–401.

142. Adler LA, Spencer TJ, Milton DR, Moore RJ, Michelson D. Long-term, open-label study of the safety and efficacy of atomoxetine in adults with attention-deficit/hyperactivity disorder: an interim analysis. *J Clin Psychiatry.* 2005;**66**(3):294–9.

143. Adler LA, Spencer TJ, Williams DW, Moore RJ, Michelson D. Long-term, open-label safety and efficacy of atomoxetine in adults with ADHD: final report of a 4-year study. *J Atten Disord.* 2008;**12**(3): 248–53.

144. Wilens TE, Waxmonsky J, Scott M, *et al.* An open trial of adjunctive donepezil in attention-deficit/hyperactivity disorder. *J Child Adolesc Psychopharmacol.* 2005;**15**(6):947–55.

145. Adler L, Dietrich A, Reimherr FW, *et al.* Safety and tolerability of once versus twice daily atomoxetine in adults with ADHD. *Ann Clin Psychiatry.* 2006;**18**(2): 107–113.

146. Biederman J, Mick E, Faraone S, *et al.* A double-blind comparison of galantamine hydrogen bromide and placebo in adults with attention-deficit/hyperactivity disorder: a pilot study. *J Clin Psychopharmacol.* 2006; **26**(2):163–6.

147. Levin FR, Evans SM, Brooks DJ, *et al.* Treatment of methadone-maintained patients with adult ADHD: double-blind comparison of methylphenidate,

bupropion and placebo. *Drug Alcohol Depend.* 2006; **81**:137–48.

148. Wilens TE, Klint T, Adler L, *et al.* A randomized controlled trial of a novel mixed monoamine reuptake inhibitor in adults with ADHD. *Behav Brain Funct.* 2008;**4**(1):24.

149. Levin FR, Mariani JJ, Secora A, *et al.* Atomoxetine treatment for cocaine abuse and adult attention-deficit hyperactivity disorder (ADHD): a preliminary open trial. *J Dual Diagn.* 2009;**5**(1):41–56.

150. Johnson M, Cederlund M, Rastam M, Areskoug B, Gillberg C. Open-label trial of atomoxetine hydrochloride in adults with ADHD. *J Atten Disord.* 2010;**13**(5):539–45.

151. Surman C, Hammerness P, Petty C, *et al.* Atomoxetine in the treatment of adults with subthreshold and/or late onset attention-deficit hyperactivity disorder-not otherwise specified (ADHD-NOS): a prospective open-label 6-week study. *CNS Neurosci Ther.* 2010; **16**(1):6–12.

152. Adler L, Guida F, Irons S, Shaw D. Open label pilot study of atomoxetine in adults with ADHD and substance use disorder. *J Dual Diagn.* 2010;**6**(3–4): 196–207.

153. Takahashi M, Takita Y, Goto T, *et al.* An open-label, dose-titration tolerability study of atomoxetine hydrochloride in Japanese adults with attention-deficit/hyperactivity disorder. *Psychiatry Clin Neurosci.* 2011;**65**(1):55–63.

154. Arnold VK, Feifel D, Earl CQ, Yang R, Adler LA. A 9-week, randomized, double-blind, placebo-controlled, parallel-group, dose-finding study to evaluate the efficacy and safety of modafinil as treatment for adults with ADHD. *J Atten Disord.* 2014;**18**(2):133–44.

155. Sutherland SM, Adler LA, Chen C, Smith MD, Feltner DE. An 8-week, randomized controlled trial of atomoxetine, atomoxetine plus buspirone, or placebo in adults with ADHD. *J Clin Psychiatry.* 2012;**73**(4): 445–50.

Chapter 23

Psychosocial treatment of ADHD in adults

Mary V. Solanto

Introduction

Once thought to be a disorder limited to children, attention-deficit hyperactivity disorder (ADHD) is now known to persist to adulthood in approximately 50% of cases, resulting in an adult prevalence of 4% [1]. Longitudinal and cross-sectional studies have extensively documented significant impairment in virtually every major domain of functioning – academic, occupational, social, and emotional – for adults with ADHD [2], as well as high rates of comorbid conditions, including mood, anxiety, and substance abuse disorders [1].

Stimulant (methylphenidate, amphetamine) and non-stimulant (atomoxetine, guanfacine) medications are effective for adults as well as children in alleviating the core symptoms of inattention, hyperactivity, and impulsivity. However, response rates in adulthood are lower than those in childhood such that 20–50% of adults may have an unfavorable response with respect to efficacy or side effects [3]. Furthermore, there is little direct evidence that medications for ADHD enhance everyday self-management skills necessary for effective time management, organization, and planning. Indeed clinical observation strongly indicates that deficits in these functions persist in many adults even after medications are optimally titrated. These observations, taken together, point to the need for additional interventions to target these problems, as well as to address the difficulties in impulse control, emotional self-regulation, social functioning, and comorbidity, with which these patients frequently present. In this chapter, we will review the relevant literature, describe the development and components of our manualized psychosocial treatment for adult ADHD, describe the most recent controlled studies, and conclude with consideration of directions for future development and research.

Treatment literature before 2010

At the time we began this work in 1999, there were only a handful of published studies of psychosocial treatment of ADHD in adults. In the last 10 years, various approaches, including group-based and individual treatments, and various orientations (cognitive-behavioral, dialectical behavior therapy, behavioral analysis, mindfulness, and multimodal treatments) have been brought to bear on the functional difficulties experienced by adults with ADHD. Reviews of the research literature by Weiss and colleagues [4] and, Knouse and Safren [5] reveal variability in methodological rigor as well. The majority of studies were open trials, examining pre- to post-treatment change. Two studies included an untreated wait-list group [6, 7], which controls for spontaneous improvement over time but does not control for the non-specific effects of therapist attention and support. As will be described in the last section, the first two randomized trials that compared the active treatment with an active control for non-specific effects of treatment were published in 2010 [8, 9].

Studies prior to 2000

A search of the early published literature yielded two individual case studies [10], two small open trials of structured group treatment programs [11, 12], one small study of a group treatment with a wait-list control [13], and a systematic chart review of 26 individually treated cases [14] based on a cognitive treatment protocol by McDermott and Wilens [15] that mainly

---

Attention-Deficit Hyperactivity Disorder in Adults and Children, ed. Lenard A. Adler, Thomas J. Spencer and Timothy E. Wilens. Published by Cambridge University Press. © Cambridge University Press 2015.

targeted internalizing symptoms. All yielded promising results.

Open trials

In 2006, Rostain and colleagues published the results of an open trial of a 16-session multimodal treatment with 43 adults with ADHD [16]. The treatment consisted of medication for ADHD combined with individually rendered cognitive-behavioral therapy (CBT). The cognitive-behavioral treatment, described in detail in a book by these authors [17], focused on identification and modification of dysfunctional thoughts that underlie maladaptive coping and emotional disturbance and also imparted adaptive methods for coping with ADHD symptoms. Results yielded significant pre- to post-treatment change on self- and clinician-rated measures of ADHD and comorbid symptoms. However, since both medication and CBT were started simultaneously, it is not possible to differentiate the effects of the two interventions.

Following their initial pilot study of 11 patients [12], Philipsen and colleagues undertook a larger study of 72 individuals enrolled at four sites [18]. Given that patients with ADHD and those with borderline personality disorder share features of emotional dysregulation, poor impulse control, and low self-esteem, the treatment developed and provided by these authors was based on principles of both dialectical behavior therapy (DBT) and CBT. Treatment components included psychoeducation, behavioral analysis, emotional regulation, and mindfulness. In each of the 13 weekly 2-hour sessions, one broad topic was addressed, including: the neurobiology of ADHD, disorganization, emotion regulation, depression, impulse control, stress, addictive behaviors, and relationships. In both the earlier pilot study and the larger multisite study, results showed significant improvement from pre- to post-treatment on self-report on a *Diagnostic and Statistical Manual of Mental Disorders* (DSM)-IV checklist of ADHD symptoms and the Beck Depression Inventory. Given these promising results, this research group has now embarked on a randomized, placebo-controlled comparison of their structured skills training program and pharmacotherapy, separately and together, with support from the German Federal Ministry of Research and Education.

In 2008, we at Mount Sinai published the first study of our group CBT (originally termed "meta-cognitive therapy"), which is described in detail below. In that study, 38 adults diagnosed with AD/HD completed an 8- or 12-week manualized open trial. Twenty-six participants (68.4%) were concurrently receiving medication to treat ADHD. Treatment efficacy was measured using pre- and post-treatment self-report standardized measures (Conners' Adult ADHD Rating Scales – Self-Report: Long Version [CAARS-S:L] and Brown ADD Scales) and the ON-TOP, a novel measure, developed in our program, of time-management, organization, and planning competencies. General linear modeling revealed a robust post-treatment decline on the CAARS DSM-IV Inattentive symptom scale ($p < 0.001$), as well as improvement on the total Brown ADD score and on specific Brown scales of Activation, Memory, Effort, and Affect ($p < 0.001$), and also on the ON-TOP ($p < 0.001$). Effect sizes (partial eta squared) approached or exceeded 0.5 (large) for all measures. Categorical analysis of pre- to post-treatment change in ratings on CAARS DSM-IV Inattentive Symptoms revealed that 46.7% of participants decreased from the clinical range (T-score $\geq$ 65) to below the clinical threshold (T-score $<$ 65), a pattern that was not impacted by medication status.

Other open trials of group interventions are those by Virta *et al.* [19] of a 10- to 11-session "cognitive-behavioral rehabilitation program" and by Zylowska *et al.* [20] of an 8-week mindfulness meditation training. Like the studies by Hesslinger *et al.* [12] and Philipsen *et al.* [18] described above, the study by Virta *et al.* of 29 adults with ADHD addressed multiple themes, including motivation and initiation of activities, organization, attention, emotional regulation, memory, impulsivity, psychiatric comorbidity, and self-esteem [19]. Self-report ratings on the Brown ADD Scale reflected significant pre- to post-treatment changes on scales of Activation, Affect and Total symptoms. Although not specifically a study of a cognitive-behavioral intervention, it is interesting to note that Zylowska *et al.* showed pre- to post-treatment improvement in a sample of 24 adults and 8 adolescents on self-report ratings of ADHD symptoms, depression, and anxiety, as well as on performance on cognitive tests of attention and impulse control [20].

Studies with wait-list controls

The studies described thus far did not include a control for spontaneous improvement over time. Studies by

Stevenson *et al.* [6] and Safren *et al.* [7] addressed this issue by employing a wait-list control group, as follows: Stevenson and colleagues administered an eight-session group Cognitive Remediation Program to 22 adults with ADHD in weekly 2-hour sessions targeting the following seven functions: motivation, concentration, listening, impulsivity, organization, anger management, and self-esteem [6]. In addition, each participant was assigned a coach who accompanied the participant to the sessions, took notes, discussed problems with homework exercises, and contacted the patient at home at least once between sessions. Response of this group was compared to that of 21 adults randomly assigned to a wait-list control. Outcome on self-report measures revealed significant effects of treatment for ADHD symptoms, organization, and self-esteem. Thirty-six percent were considered responders immediately post-treatment with respect to ADHD symptoms, increasing to 55% at 2 months. Neither medication status nor internalizing disorders (anxiety or depression) impacted treatment outcomes.

Safren and colleagues conducted a study to address the question of whether CBT could add significantly to the benefits of pharmacotherapy for those who were suboptimally improved on medication [7]. CBT in this study focused on cognitive symptoms related to organization, planning, distractibility, and also included cognitive restructuring and optional modules addressing procrastination, anger management, assertiveness training, and communication skills, totaling 15 weekly sessions. Thirty-one patients with clinically significant ADHD symptoms despite stable medication treatment were randomly assigned either to receive CBT or to continue on medication only. A methodological advance that characterized this study is that pre- and post-treatment assessments were conducted by an independent (blind) evaluator (IE) and were also obtained via self-report measures. Results showed improvement in IE- and self-rated symptoms of ADHD and anxiety, as well as IE-rated depression. Responder rates were 56% to the combined intervention compared to 13% for continued pharmacotherapy alone.

The effect sizes for changes in total ADHD symptoms for the studies described above, as summarized by Knouse and Safren [5], were generally robust, ranging from 0.38 to 1.97 with an average of 1.12, signaling the potential utility of these interventions.

Development of the Mount Sinai CBT program for adult ADHD

Targets of treatment

In designing a treatment for adults with ADHD, we focused on difficulties largely in the cognitive/attentive and executive function domains. Executive function refers to the self-regulation of behavior across time so as to anticipate and prepare for future events and to effectively pursue one's goals [21]. Time-management, organization, and planning are typically included under this rubric. We chose to target executive functions because difficulties in this domain are virtually universal among adults with ADHD, whereas problems with impulse control, mood regulation, and interpersonal interaction, though significant and important, are limited to subsets of patients. Recent research has supported this approach in documenting that problems in the domains of inattention [22] and executive function [21] are more highly associated with impairment for adults with ADHD than those which emerge from the hyperactive–impulsive domain. Furthermore, our clinical experience indicated that addressing problems emerging from the impulse control domain of symptoms requires a separate, equally intensive program of treatment employing different methods. By focusing on executive dysfunction we hoped to generate greater and more long-lasting improvement than can be achieved by attempting to address multiple domains of symptoms and dysfunction.

The Mount Sinai program was therefore designed to address many of the most common problems and complaints that are documented as areas of deficit for adults with ADHD and freely voiced by patients as sources of distress and frustration: inefficiency, failure to complete tasks, difficulty initiating and terminating tasks and activities in a timely manner, disorganization, difficulty prioritizing, poor planning, tardiness, forgetfulness, indecisiveness, and perfectionism.

A cognitive-behavioral approach

Our manualized treatment [23] is grounded in cognitive-behavioral principles and methods. Some components aim to change behavior by imparting new skills and new habits. Other components focus on changing cognitions while also imparting skills. Some of these new cognitions may be considered adaptive internal speech or self-instruction to guide behavior. The unique utility of the cognitive-behavioral approach is that these interventions are synergistic. The cognitive changes generate adaptive behavioral changes; when these behavioral changes are reinforced they serve in turn to generate more positive cognitions and self-attributions.

An important goal of our treatment design was to foster generalization and maintenance such that the adaptive behaviors and cognitions would be assimilated into all the activities of daily life in a way that they would become habitual and automatic. The development of new skills and strategies is fostered via intensive practice during the session and during the home exercise which follows each session, as well as by group support and positive reinforcement from the therapist and group members. The Home Exercise is central to the program in that it is the opportunity for the participant to actually apply and practice the strategy in the "real-world" environment of work, school, or home.

Behavioral strategies

Examples of explicit skills imparted in the program are the use of the planner for scheduling and prioritizing, and setting up a filing system. New habits related to these skills are checking the planner regularly during the day, and restoring possessions to their places in order to maintain organizational systems. Behavioral strategies also include the practice of contingent self-reinforcement upon completion of difficult or aversive tasks, and breaking down complex tasks into manageable parts. These practices are intended to intensify the participant's experience of reinforcement, thereby counteracting an apparently reduced centrally mediated experience of reinforcement in individuals with ADHD [24, 25].

Visualization of long-term rewards of present behavior is another example of a strategy that is neuropsychologically informed. This strategy is intended to counteract the steeper temporal discounting of reinforcement in individuals with ADHD. The delay of reinforcement gradient describes the fall-off in the reinforcing values of distant rewards as a function of time into the future. Thus, the more distantly a reward will occur, the less power it has to motivate behavior in the present. Although applicable to everyone, this delay gradient appears to be steeper for individuals with ADHD. This has been demonstrated in findings that children with ADHD are more likely than typical children to choose an immediate reward in

preference to a larger, but delayed reward [26]. Adults with ADHD appear to be similarly more inclined to prefer activities which promise to deliver immediate gratification over those which entail protracted effort over long periods of time before they reach fruition. Since the latter include many of the important rewards of life – for example, higher academic degrees, job advancement, saving money for the purchase of a home – it seems clear that this scenario, repeated many thousands of times during the course of development to and through adulthood, may help to account for the lower academic and occupational attainment of adults with ADHD.

In our treatment program, the problem of delay discounting is addressed by a strategy to make distant rewards more salient such that they can serve to motivate effortful behavior in the present. The participant is guided to generate a well-elaborated rewards scenario for a long-term goal, imagining as vividly as possible the material and non-material rewards which will be available upon achievement of the goal. Each participant is encouraged to review this rewards scenario at junctures when choosing between an immediate reinforcer (e.g., watching television) and an effortful task that is one step of a project which will yield reinforcement only in the long term (e.g., setting to work on a new business proposal).

Other behavioral strategies include modifications of the physical environment to decrease distraction and increase efficiency.

Cognitive strategies

Among the cognitive interventions, the program aims to impart "rules" for daily scheduling, prioritizing, and organization. An example of such a rule is the advice to enter all appointments and tasks into a planner. Participants are also helped to develop adaptive cognitions to facilitate task initiation, completion, and planning. For example, the aphorism "Getting started is the hardest part" confers the expectation that anything that aids in starting a task will have significant payoff, and assures the participant that, once started, the process will become easier. Some of these adaptive cognitions are encompassed in the form of "mantras" which are maxims to self-cue the application of the strategy in daily life. These mantras are repeated strategically throughout the program so that they will become internalized and thereby facilitate the maintenance of treatment benefits. One example is "If it's not in the planner, it doesn't exist," meaning that unless appointments and tasks are entered into the planner they are highly unlikely to be accomplished. Another mantra is "If I'm having trouble getting started, then the first step is too big," which is the cue to break down a difficult or aversive task into more manageable parts.

In addition to employing these methods developed specifically to treat ADHD, the program also incorporates traditional CBT as it has been used to address anxiety, depression, and demoralization [27], which, as described, are common among individuals with ADHD. In this context, participants are taught to recognize and challenge irrational automatic thoughts such as "all-or-none thinking" (perfectionism), over-generalization, selective attention, and catastrophizing. During the sessions following their introduction into the program, these irrational cognitions are flagged as appropriate for individual participants.

Treatment parameters

The treatment is rendered in a group modality, consisting of six to eight adults meeting for 12 weekly sessions of 2 hours each. Although easily adapted for individual treatment, the group-based intervention offers unique advantages of mutual support and encouragement, modeling and vicarious reinforcement of successful strategies. The structured set of skills to be learned also lends itself to presentation in a group format.

Each session has four parts: the review of the previous week's Home Exercise, presentation of new material, the In-Session exercise, and discussion of the next week's Home Exercise. Given the importance of the Home Exercise for generalization and maintenance of treatment gains, fully the first hour of the session is devoted to a roundtable review of each participant's experience with the Home Exercise, including successes, failures, and partial successes, which are analyzed to ascertain what additional or alternate strategies might be utilized in the next iteration. Positive efforts as well as positive outcomes are reinforced and it is emphasized to the participants that long-term improvement occurs only through "successive approximations" of the desired behaviors. Following the review of the Home Exercise, the new material for the session is presented using the Socratic Method, which encourages active participation by group members. The session proceeds with an In-Session exercise to illustrate application of the strategies discussed during the session. Material for the exercise is taken from the participants' own experiences, difficulties, and goals. One particularly important tool is the Project Flow Sheet that is introduced in the first session on Planning. This flow sheet is an aid in planning out a multistep, multicomponent project that involves coordination over time. It is intended to help adults with ADHD counteract their tendency to overlook the multiple steps in the planning process and to "telescope" time, with results that are typically inadequate, incomplete, or late.

The session concludes with a presentation and anticipatory trouble-shooting of the next Home Exercise. Weekly handouts include not only the next Home Exercise, but also a pithy summary of the content of the session, intended to serve as an aid to learning (particularly for those whose attention may have wandered during the session), and which can be emailed to any who missed the session.

Randomized trials with controls for non-specific effects of treatment

Group treatment

Despite yielding evidence of apparent benefits of CBT, our preliminary investigation [28] did not control for expectancy of change or for spontaneous diminution of symptoms over time, nor did it take into account the non-specific effects of therapy (e.g., mutual support and information sharing). Therefore, with the support of NIMH[1], we undertook a randomized controlled trial [8], hypothesizing that more robust therapeutic change would occur for individuals receiving CBT compared to a supportive psychotherapy (SP) group that controlled for non-specific therapeutic elements, such as the attention and support of the therapist and the other group members. In addition, despite the absence of effects of medication in our small open trial, it was hypothesized that medication would interact with the treatment group such that CBT participants taking ADHD medications would better assimilate the treatment techniques and more successfully apply the interventions between sessions, thereby achieving better outcomes.

In the pivotal efficacy study [8], 88 adults rigorously diagnosed as having ADHD (combined or predominantly inattentive subtype) were stratified by

[1] The study was supported by NIMH Grant 1R34MH071721 to the author.

medication use and otherwise randomly assigned to receive either the group CBT intervention or a parallel support group designed to control for non-specific effects of therapy. Outcomes were measured via independent evaluator ratings on a structured interview (the Adult ADHD Investigator Symptom Rating Scale or AISRS) [29], as well as self-report and collateral report on the Conners' Adult ADHD Rating Scale (CAARS-IN) [30]. General linear models comparing change from baseline between treatments revealed statistically superior effects for the CBT group on all measures. The response rate, defined as 30% reduction in inattentive symptoms on the AISRS, was 42.2% for CBT, compared to 12% in the support group, yielding an odds ratio of 5.41 in favor of CBT. Response rate as defined by a decrease of at least one standard deviation on the Inattention/Memory subscale of the CAARS (CAARS-IN) was 53% compared to 28% in the support group. Only one statistically significant interaction was observed between baseline score and response to treatment: the larger (more severe) the CAARS-IN score at baseline, the greater the differential improvement with CBT; change in the support group, by contrast, was stable across the entire range of initial CAARS-IN scores.

Additional analyses revealed no significant differences between groups vis-à-vis expectancy ratings obtained pretreatment or after the first two treatment sessions. Moreover, age, gender, ethnicity, education, household income, marital status, employment status, IQ, ADHD subtype, concurrent medication for ADHD, and presence of a comorbid mood and/or anxiety disorder did not interact with the effects of treatment and in each analysis, the effect of CBT vs. support remained significant while controlling for each of the above variables. However, within the CBT group, completion of the Home Exercise was positively related to change in AISRS-IN score, highlighting the importance of this treatment component.

Several factors may have accounted for the fact that medication did not interact with treatment group to moderate treatment response. First, the fact that participants were required to meet entry criteria for minimum levels of symptom severity may have resulted in oversampling for non-responders or suboptimal responders to medication. This may have been especially likely given that medicated and non-medicated participants did not differ with respect to baseline levels of ADHD severity. Although analyses were repeated using a subset of participants considered to be adequately medicated, with the same result, it is conceivable that specific medication(s) and dosage(s) may not have been optimally titrated by individual practitioners in the community. A final possibility, and one that is consistent with findings from our initial investigation of primarily medicated participants [28], is that the CBT intervention is sufficiently structured that participants benefit irrespective of medication status.

Individual treatment

Shortly after initial publication of our study, Safren and colleagues published the results of a randomized controlled trial examining the effectiveness of individual CBT for medicated adults with ADHD who continued to display clinically significant symptoms [9]. The CBT was the same as that in the earlier study with wait-list controls by this team [7]. Eighty-eight adults were randomized to receive either CBT or a comparison treatment consisting of relaxation training with psychoeducation. Results indicated that a significantly greater proportion of individuals assigned to CBT (vs. comparison) were classified as treatment responders on the basis of blind clinician ratings on the Clinical Global Index and the ADHD Rating Scale consisting of all 18 DSM-IV symptoms of ADHD: CGI: 53% vs. 23%; ADHD-RS: 67% vs. 33%. Analogous findings were observed using self-report ratings. Post-treatment assessments indicated that gains were maintained at 6 and 12 months for those who received CBT.

A comparison of these two randomized controlled trials revealed robust effect sizes of 0.73 for DSM-IV Inattentive symptoms for the group intervention [8] and 0.60 for total DSM-IV symptoms in the study of individual treatment [9]. It is interesting to note that in both these studies the participants benefited about half as much from the supportive intervention as they did from the active treatment. This may have occurred because the support of the group or the therapist mobilized the participants to discover new compensatory strategies on their own and/or to more regularly practice strategies of which they were already aware.

Conclusions and future directions

As demonstrated by the above studies, CBT, delivered in individual or group modalities, in the presence or absence of psychopharmacological intervention, can help to mitigate the core features of ADHD and associated impairments in executive skills (e.g., time management, organization, and planning skills). Although effective compared with control interventions, there is room for improvement in response rate to psychosocial treatments, which, where reported, ranged from 30% to 67%. Efficacy may be further enhanced by increasing the length of the program to allow more time for rehearsal and consolidation of the new adaptive cognitive and behavioral habits. In the interest of enhancing outcomes, it would also be useful to ascertain the relative contributions of the treatment components (e.g., contingent self-reinforcement, visualization of long-term rewards) to overall outcome. Further studies are also needed of the duration of improvement beyond the end point of treatment and the utility of "booster" sessions to maintain benefits. In addition, there is a need to develop more specialized treatment programs that intensively address problems resulting from poor impulse control, and difficulties in interpersonal interactions.

Studies thus far provide no evidence that concurrent medication impacts response to psychosocial treatment [6, 8, 18, 28]. In addition, more recent studies have shown that methylphenidate alone did not improve executive function in adults with ADHD [31], and that dextroamphetamine did not add to the benefit of treatment with CBT in a secondary analysis [32]. The separate and combined effects of stimulant medication and psychosocial treatment, however, can best be studied in a 2×2 design in which patients are randomly assigned to receive medication (individually titrated within the study proper), psychosocial treatment, the combination of both treatments, or neither treatment. Of particular interest would be examination of possible differential mediation of the therapeutic effects of medication and of CBT. Larger-scale studies of this type may also allow for identification of individual clinical variables that predict differential response to medication and psychosocial treatment.

Several of the studies reviewed in this chapter indicated that the psychosocial treatment yielded secondary beneficial effects for anxiety and depression in open trials [7, 12, 16, 18, 20]. However, this was not demonstrated in either of the fully controlled studies [8, 9], suggesting that this result may be a non-specific effect of intervention. Differences between studies in the components of treatment that directly address internalizing symptoms (e.g., challenging irrational beliefs) as well as differences in the range of severity of internalizing symptoms represented in the samples may also account for these disparities, which should be explored in further research. Studies thus far are consistent, however, in finding that *pretreatment* levels of depression did *not* moderate the effects of treatment on ADHD symptoms [6, 8, 18]. On the one hand, this result suggests that patients' improvement in ADHD-related symptomatology after psychosocial treatment cannot be attributed merely to their generally "feeling better." On the other hand, one might have predicted that patients who are less depressed at the outset might have been able to more fully and effortfully participate in the treatment and thus achieve greater improvement in their ADHD. This and other potential demographic and clinical moderators and mediators of treatment response can best be explored fully in large-scale studies that include more comprehensive assessment of potential cognitive mediators of change.

Finally, neuroimaging may have utility in documenting changes in patterns of activation (functional MRI) as a function of treatment and may also identify neurophysiological predictors of response.

Although there is increasing support from *efficacy* studies that psychosocial treatments, particularly CBT, are beneficial in the treatment of adult ADHD, *effectiveness* studies in "real-world" clinical settings are needed before these interventions can be widely adopted in the community. Furthermore, there is a need to develop cost-effective and efficient methods of training practitioners.

All in all, evidence-based psychosocial treatments have the potential to significantly improve the functioning of adults with ADHD, and we look forward to continued developments in this field.

References

1. Kessler RC, Adler LA, Barkley RA, et al. The prevalence and correlates of adult ADHD in the United States: results from the national comorbidity survey replication. *Am J Psychiatry*. 2006;**163**: 716–23.

2. Barkley RA, Fischer M, Smallish L, Fletcher K. Young adult outcome of hyperactive children: adaptive functioning in major life areas. *J Am Acad Child Adolesc Psychiatry*. 2006;**45**:192–202.

3. Wilens TE, Spencer TJ, Biederman J. A review of the pharmacotherapy of adults with attention-deficit/ hyperactivity disorder. *J Atten Disord*. 2002;**5**: 189–202.

4. Weiss M, Safren SA, Solanto MV, *et al.* Research forum on psychological treatment of adults with ADHD. *J Atten Disord.* 2008;**11**:642–51.

5. Knouse LE, Safren SA. Current status of cognitive behavioral therapy for adult attention-deficit hyperactivity disorder. *Psychiatr Clin North Am.* 2010;**33**:497–509.

6. Stevenson CS, Whitmont S, Bornholt L, Livesey D, Stevenson RJ. A cognitive remediation programme for adults with attention deficit hyperactivity disorder. *Aust N Z J Psychiatry.* 2002;**36**:610–16.

7. Safren SA, Otto MW, Sprich S, *et al.* Cognitive-behavioral therapy for ADHD in medication-treated adults with continued symptoms. *Behav Res Ther.* 2005;**43**:831–42.

8. Solanto MV, Marks DJ, Wasserstein J, *et al.* Efficacy of meta-cognitive therapy (MCT) for adult ADHD. *Am J Psychiatry.* 2010;**167**:958–68.

9. Safren SA, Sprich S, Mimiaga MJ, *et al.* Cognitive behavioral therapy vs. relaxation with educational support for medication-treated adults with ADHD and persistent symptoms: a randomized controlled trial. *JAMA.* 2010;**304**:875–80.

10. Goodwin RE, Corgiat MD. Cognitive rehabilitation of adult attention deficit disorder: a case study. *J Cogn Rehabil.* 1992;**10**:28–35.

11. Weinstein C. Cognitive remediation strategies. An adjunct to the psychotherapy of adults with attention deficit hyperactivity disorder. *J Psychother Pract Res.* 1994;**3**:44–57.

12. Hesslinger B, Tebartz van Elst L, Nyberg E, *et al.* Psychotherapy of attention deficit hyperactivity disorder in adults – a pilot study using a structured skills training program. *Eur Arch Psychiatry Clin Neurosci.* 2002;**252**:177–84.

13. Wiggins D, Singh K, Getz H, Hutchins D. Effects of a brief group intervention for adults with attention-deficit/hyperactivity disorder. *J Ment Health Couns.* 1999;**21**:82–92.

14. Wilens TE, McDermott S, Biederman J, *et al.* Cognitive therapy in the treatment of adults with ADHD: a systematic chart review of 26 cases. *J Cogn Psychother.* 1999;**13**:215–26.

15. McDermott SP, Wilens TE. Cognitive therapy for adults with ADHD. In: Brown T, ed. *Attention Deficit Disorders and Comorbidities in Children, Adolescents, and Adults.* Washington, DC: American Psychiatric Press. 2000; 569–606.

16. Rostain AL, Ramsay JR. A combined treatment approach for adults with ADHD – results of an open study of 43 patients. *J Atten Disord.* 2006;**10**:150–9.

17. Ramsay JR, Rostain AL. *Cognitive-Behavioral Therapy for Adult ADHD: An Integrative Psychosocial and Medical Approach.* New York, NY: Routledge; 2008.

18. Philipsen A, Richter H, Peters J, *et al.* Structured group psychotherapy in adults with attention deficit hyperactivity disorder: results of an open multicentre study. *J Nerv Ment Dis.* 2007;**195**:1013–19.

19. Virta M, Vedenpaa A, Gronroos N, *et al.* Adults with ADHD benefit from cognitive-behaviorally oriented group rehabilitation: a study of 29 participants. *J Atten Disord.* 2008;**12**:218–26.

20. Zylowska L, Ackerman DL, Yang MH, *et al.* Mindfulness meditation training in adults and adolescents with ADHD: a feasibility study. *J Atten Disord.* 2008;**11**:737–46.

21. Barkley RA, Fischer M. Predicting impairment in major life activities in hyperactive children as adults: self-reported executive function (EF) deficits vs. EF tests. *Dev Neuropsychol.* 2010;**36**:137–61.

22. Safren SA, Sprich SE, Cooper-Vince C, Knouse LE, Lerner JA. Life impairments in adults with medication-treated ADHD. *J Atten Disord.* 2010;**13**:524–31.

23. Solanto MV. *Cognitive-Behavioral Therapy for Adult ADHD: Targeting Executive Dysfunction.* New York, NY: Guilford Press; 2010.

24. Luman M, Oosterlaan J, Sergeant JA. The impact of reinforcement contingencies on AD/HD: a review and theoretical appraisal. *Clin Psychol Rev.* 2004;**25**:183–213. Erratum in *Clin Psychol Rev.* 2005;**25**:533.

25. Volkow ND, Wang GJ, Kollins SH, *et al.* Evaluating dopamine reward pathway in ADHD: clinical implications. *JAMA.* 2009;**302**:1084–91.

26. Aase H, Sagvolden T. Infrequent, but not frequent, reinforcers produce more variable responding and deficient sustained attention in young children with attention-deficit/hyperactivity disorder (ADHD). *J Child Psychol Psychiatry.* 2006;**47**:457–71.

27. Beck JS. *Cognitive Therapy: Basics and Beyond.* New York, NY: Guilford Press; 1995.

28. Solanto MV, Marks DJ, Mitchell K, Wasserstein J, Kofman MD. Development of a new psychosocial treatment for adults with AD/HD. *J Atten Disord.* 2008;**11**:728–36.

29. Spencer RJ, Adler LA, Qiao M, *et al.* Validation of the Adult ADHD Investigator Symptom Rating Scale (AISRS). *J Atten Disord.* 2010;**14**:57–68.

30. Conners CK, Erhardt D, Epstein JN, *et al.* Self-ratings of ADHD symptoms in adults I: Factor structure and normative data. *J Atten Disord.* 1999;**3**:141–51.

31. Biederman J, Mick E, Fried R, *et al.* Are stimulants effective in the treatment of executive function deficits? Results from a randomized double-blind study of OROS-methylphenidate in adults with ADHD. *Eur Neuropsychopharmacol.* 2011;**21**:508–15.

32. Weiss M, Murray C, Wasdall M, *et al.* A randomized controlled trial of CBT therapy for adults with ADHD with and without medication. *BMC Psychiatry.* 2012;**12**:12–30.

Complementary and alternative treatments for pediatric and adult ADHD

Nicholas Lofthouse, Elizabeth Hurt, and L. Eugene Arnold

Introduction

Despite most patients with attention-deficit hyper-activity disorder (ADHD) benefiting from evidence-based treatments such as medication and behavioral/cognitive-behavioral therapy, some youth and adults with ADHD find these treatments ineffective, intolerable because of side effects, or unpalatable. To help these patients, several complementary (i.e., used together with established treatment) and alternative (i.e., used in place of established treatment) interventions have been proposed. Complementary and alternative medicine (CAM) is technically a misnomer for these treatments as a complementary or alternative treatment should only be designated as such if incremental effects when added or similar effects when compared to established treatment, respectively, are empirically demonstrated. Therefore, the current interventions are for the most part more accurately considered experimental treatments with the potential to become CAMs. Nevertheless, the popular term CAMs is generally applied to these "CAM wannabes." As these treatments can be either ingestible (i.e., orally administered) or noningestible (i.e., externally administered), instead of CAMs we refer to them as complementary and alternative treatments (CATs).

Some limited scientific evidence of efficacy exists for some CATs but key safety and efficacy questions remain for the majority [1]. Because many of them are in popular use, practitioners and researchers need to know about their current status. To assist with this, we will present information about ingestible and non-ingestible CATs for pediatric and adult ADHD by describing each intervention's specific approach and rationale; associated research in terms of the number and design of studies, total number of subjects (n), overall results (including effect size [ES] d where

available), study limitations, and future directions; and our evaluation of whether it is *recommended, acceptable,* or *not recommended.* Our evaluation is based on current evidence and a guideline suggesting that treatments that are safe, easy, cheap, and sensible (SECS) do not require as much evidence to justify an individual patient trial as do treatments that are risky, unrealistic, difficult, or expensive (RUDE). As none of these CATs currently have enough empirical support to be considered a stand-alone treatment for ADHD, a major risk for any CAT is the delay of other, more established treatments should it not improve ADHD symptoms.

All the studies in this chapter are based on recent (2012) PsychInfo and Medline searches and references from prior publications. For brevity, most of the treatment studies are cited succinctly but covered in more detail in our recent comprehensive reviews of ingestible and noningestible CAT treatments for ADHD [2–4]. Ingestible CATs not included here but previously reviewed [2] include thyroid treatment and deleading, which are only recommended for a small percentage of ADHD patients with thyroid abnormality or clinical blood lead levels. Similarly, several other noningestible CATs currently used in the community despite a lack of evidence are not included although previously reviewed [3].

Ingestible CATs for pediatric ADHD

Elimination (few-foods, defined, or oligoantigenic) diets are based on the hypothesis that many children are sensitive to dietary salicylates and artificially added colors, flavors, and preservatives, or certain foods, so eliminating these substances may ameliorate learning and behavioral problems, such as ADHD [5]. Nine controlled studies (three randomized controlled trials [RCTs] and six placebo challenges [PBOC], total

Attention-Deficit Hyperactivity Disorder in Adults and Children, ed. Lenard A. Adler, Thomas J. Spencer and Timothy E. Wilens.
Published by Cambridge University Press. © Cambridge University Press 2015.

n = 704) have reported ESs of 0.5–2.0 or significant (p = 0.05–001) improvements in ADHD symptoms. However, two large studies reported a small deleterious behavioral effect of artificial food dyes for all children, not just those with ADHD. Thus, dietary management, at least restriction of food dyes, may not be a specific treatment for ADHD, but a general behavioral health issue for all children. As few of the studies used subjects with actual ADHD diagnoses, future research needs to include these in their samples.

Restriction of artificial food dyes and other dietary components known to affect a given individual child appears sensible and relatively safe, but potential risks of an oligoantigenic ("few-foods") diet include family stress of implementation and nutritional imbalance. Given these concerns; the research findings; and the time, effort, and expense in maintaining this type of diet, we suggest such diets in addition to, rather than as replacements for, conventional treatments and only *recommend* them for youth with a documented history of reactions to certain food substances. It may be more *acceptable* for youth with ADHD without a prior history of reaction to these substances to have a 2-week trial if they are not in need of immediate symptom relief. If there is no benefit, the diet should be abandoned; if benefit, foods should be added back one at a time to find the problem foods. Due to the high level of organization needed for elimination diets, families may require consultations from dietitians to ensure nutritional adequacy and clinicians to develop behavioral plans to assist with adherence to the diet.

An associated dietary approach, **elimination of sugar** alone, despite widespread public belief, has not received convincing scientific support from 12 double-blind (DB) PBOC studies (n = 296), a meta-analysis of 23 DB-PBOC studies (n = 531), or even a DB well-controlled 3-week trial (n = 48) of a sugar-restricted diet. However, a recent study reported the natural increase of inattentiveness during the course of a morning in the classroom was significantly (p < 0.0025) worsened by a glucose-drink breakfast but lessened by a same-calorie whole-grain cereal breakfast with milk (n = 29, children were not selected for ADHD) [6]. In view of the potential parent–child conflict associated with restricting sugar and time to monitor a youth's eating habits, elimination of sugar by itself is *not recommended* for treating pediatric ADHD, unless the youth has pre-diabetic symptoms. Nevertheless, reasonable reduction of sugar has

general health benefits (i.e., is sensible), is safe and cheap, and so is *acceptable* even if not easy.

In a sense, **nutritional supplementation** is the opposite of elimination diets; it is based on the assumption that something is lacking in the diet and should be added. Seven types of nutritional supplements have been considered, including essential fatty acids (EFAs), carnitine, amino acids, dimethylaminoethanol (DMAE), vitamins, minerals, glyconutritional and melatonin hormone.

EFA deficiency in ADHD has been documented in some [7], but not all [8], comparisons to non-affected children. EFA supplementation is one of the better studied CATs for ADHD with 16 DB PBO RCTs (n = 1069) and documented benefit in ADHD symptoms (ES ~ 0.4, p = 0.1–0.01). The most promising EFA combination appears to be eicosapentaenoic acid (EPA), docosahexaenoic acid (DHA), and gamma-linolenic acid (GLA), but EPA is probably the most critical component, and it showed a meta-analytic dose–response curve [9]. Unfortunately, many studies were limited by non-diagnosed samples and dropouts, possibly because of the long 3- to 6-month wait for EFAs to take effect. As few studies used subjects with actual ADHD diagnoses, future research needs to include these in their samples. Due to cardiovascular health and brain development benefits, EFAs appear sensible, and are easy, inexpensive, and safe as long as mercury-free oils are used (indicated on the label or by USP seal). Even though EFAs do not decrease ADHD symptoms to the same extent as US Food and Drug Administration (FDA)-approved medications, a trial of EFA supplementation is *recommended* for youth who do not eat oily wild ocean fish at least 3 times a week and it is *acceptable* for all youth. A recent meta-analysis concluded that their use is "reasonable" [9].

Carnitine is essential for fatty acid metabolism, transporting lipids across the microsomal inner membrane [10], and supporting EFA elongation [11]. In three DB PBO RCTs of youth with ADHD (n = 168), L-carnitine supplementation failed to show significant benefit on intent-to-treat analysis but in secondary analyses in two of them it either significantly (p = 0.02) improved attention in children with inattentive type but not combined type or improved attention on a timed arithmetic test (p = 0.02, d = 0.67). Future research requires a RCT specifically on ADHD-Inattentive type. With documented general cardiovascular benefits, L-carnitine appears sensible, safe, easy, and inexpensive. Thus, L-carnitine may be an *acceptable* option for youth with inattentive type ADHD who have not responded well to more conventional treatments although it is not recommended for combined type.

Amino acid supplementation has been tried in response to reports of low levels of amino acids in children with ADHD, including the precursors of catecholamines and serotonin [12–14]. Although four open and PBO trials (n = 43) reported promising results (p = 0.01), no studies have documented long-term benefit as tolerance typically developed after 2 to 3 months. This is not promising for future research for pediatric ADHD. Because of some metabolic risk, it is *not recommended* for pediatric ADHD.

Dimethylaminoethanol (DMAE) – also called deanol and dimethylethanolamine – is a precursor of choline involved in acetylcholine synthesis, which is an important neurotransmitter. Initially marketed as a drug (Deaner®) for ADHD, this was modified to dietary supplement following a 1980 FDA decision necessitating evidence of efficacy as well as safety. Four PBO-controlled studies reported promising results (ESs 0.1–0.6, 0.1 > p > 0.05). However, most have methodological flaws and other studies showed no effect, or even PBO superiority, so further controlled studies are required. As a few studies showed encouraging results, this CAT can be seen as sensible. Although safe, cheap, and easy, DMAE will probably not yield the effect seen with medication so it may be only an *acceptable* option for youth with mild symptoms.

Three strategies for **vitamin supplementation** include recommended daily allowance/recommended intake (RDA/RDI) multivitamins, megavitamin multiple combinations, and megadoses of specific vitamins. RDA/RDI multivitamins have not been systematically examined in ADHD; but, in two DB PBO RCTs (n = 137) of typically developing children, subjects improved, relative to a PBO, in non-verbal intelligence (p < 0.001 and p < 0.001), concentration (p < 0.05), sustained attention (ES = 1.3, p < 0.05) and excess motor behavior (p < 0.05). However, another RCT (n = 86) found no significant advantage over PBO on tests of reasoning. This approach appears sensible, inexpensive, easy, and, unless the patient has a rare genetic disorder, safe. Therefore, even if it does not specifically improve ADHD symptoms, RDA/RDI is recommended for all youth, especially for picky eaters or with stimulant-suppressed appetites at risk for vitamin deficiency. In contrast, megadoses

of single or multiple vitamins are *not recommended* because the former has not been adequately explored despite some encouraging early reports, the latter has not been found effective in three (n = 92) DB PBO 2-week and 6-month RCTs, and there are some concerns about toxicity.

Regarding **iron, zinc, and magnesium supplements**, it is currently unclear whether a lack of these nutrients is related to ADHD as some studies have found an inverse relation between their level and ADHD severity [15] whereas other studies do not support this relation [16]. For iron, two treatment studies exist, with the first an open trial with 17 nonanemic ADHD boys that reported an improvement in parents' ADHD ratings (ES = 1.0), but not in teachers' ratings. A DB PBO-controlled RCT of 23 nonanemic children with ADHD and borderline deficient iron status found significant decreases (ESs = 0.20–0.68) in parent-reported ADHD symptoms compared to placebo. Four DB PBO RCTs exist on zinc (n = 507), with three conducted in the Middle East reporting significant decreases (ESs = 0.35–1.62) in ADHD symptoms compared to placebo; however, a fourth from the USA found no significant benefit. The difference may be associated with the different zinc formulations used (sulfate in the Middle East, glycinate in the USA) and/or samples with different endemic diets. For magnesium, four open trials (n = 173) found significant (p < 0.05) decreases in inattention and hyperactivity. Research on iron and magnesium need large DB PBO RTC's with follow-up (FU) while zinc needs further controlled studies to explore different types of zinc and different sample locations and diets. Although easy to administer, an excess can cause hemochromatosis (iron), aplasia and interference with iron/copper absorption (zinc), and aggression or diarrhea (magnesium). Therefore, as controlled research has not supported their use for youth with ADHD, iron, zinc, and magnesium supplements are only *recommended* for youth with ADHD who have documented deficiency or borderline levels or are living in areas of endemic mineral deficiency.

Glyconutritional supplementation involves eight specific sugars integral to the body's cell-to-cell communication of which only two are abundant in a typical diet. Two open trials (n = 35) reported significant (p < 0.05–0.002) decreases in parent ratings of inattention, hyperactivity/impulsivity, and oppositionality. However, further DB PBO RCTs with FU are needed. Although easy and cheap, safety and efficacy (i.e., sensible) have not been demonstrated so glyconutritional supplementation is *not recommended* for pediatric ADHD.

Melatonin supplementation has been suggested because melatonin is a natural hormone involved in the regulation of circadian rhythm and sleep problems are associated with ADHD. Three studies of melatonin (n = 159, open, crossover and DB PBO RCT) did not report any significant decreases of ADHD symptoms but did find significant improvements of sleep (ES = 0.59–1.02). Although additional larger DB PBO RCTs with FU are needed, as melatonin is relatively safe, cheap, sensible, and easy, it is *recommended* for sleep problems in children with ADHD.

The **combination of dietary supplements** has been examined by three trials. The first, an open trial (n = 20), gave parents the choice of a combined dietary supplement or stimulant medication and reported both groups of children improved on computerized tests of inattention and impulsivity; with no differences between groups. The second, an open trial of EMPower+ (36 vitamins/minerals, n = 11), in a group of children with mood and behavioral problems, found significant (p < 0.01) decreases in parent-rated inattention and disruptive behaviors. Finally, a DB PBO RCT of a combination of supplements (i.e., EFAs, phospholipids, amino acids, B-vitamins, minerals, and other micronutrients needed for normal brain growth and development) significantly improved visual attention (ES = 0.56–1.13). Future DB PBO RCTs with FU are warranted. Combination supplements can be expensive and a nuisance because of the quantity of capsules, and their safety is unknown. Therefore, any particular combination supplement is *not recommended* for ADHD at this time.

Herbal interventions, using plant extracts, have been examined for the treatment of ADHD because many plants synthesize substances that are potentially useful. Despite lack of systematic testing and most of the existing literature being anecdotal, based on case study, or in other disorders with overlapping symptoms, many consumers are willing to spend large amounts on "natural" substances for these herbal remedies [17]. **Ningdong granules** (a traditional Chinese medicine preparation of plants, animal substances and human placenta) were examined in a methylphenidate (MPH)-controlled DB RCT (n = 72), and produced significant (p < 0.01) decreases in teacher- and a downward trend in parent-reported ADHD symptoms, both comparable to the MPH group. Pycnogenol (French maritime pine bark extract) led to significant improvements in hyperactivity, inattention, and visual-motor coordination in a DB PBO RTC (n = 61); similar findings were not found in the placebo group and children in the Pycnogenol group had a return of symptoms a month after discontinuation of treatment. A DB RCT (n = 50) of ginkgo biloba (ginkgo tree leaves) found significantly (p < 0.001) more improvement on parent and teacher ADHD symptoms for MPH (ES = 1.36–1.62 vs. 0.02–0.55). Results from an open-label trial (n = 36) combining ginkgo biloba with ginseng were promising, with 74% of participants rated as improved on ADHD parent ratings. A single DB PBO RCT of St. John's wort (n = 50) did not demonstrate benefit relative to PBO for children with ADHD. Future research on herbal approaches requires more DB PBO RCTs with FU. Despite being easy to use and relatively inexpensive, some herbs can cause side effects such as strokes and bleeding (ginkgo biloba) and convulsions in children with epilepsy and other neurological problems, and lead contamination has been reported for some Indian and Chinese herbs. Therefore, given minimal but promising empirical support and involved risks, Pycnogenol is *acceptable* if other, safer treatments have failed. As patients may assume that herbal remedies are safer than prescription medication because they are "natural," practitioners need to educate patients that herbs are essentially "crude drugs" not regulated by the FDA, their overall quality/safety may vary across manufacturers, they may have significant side effects, they may be contaminated with heavy metals, and they may interact with prescription drugs. The following herbs are commonly used with patients with ADHD, without evidence, but with associated risks: valerian, kava, and chamomile.

Homeopathic remedies are based on Hahnemann's Law of Similars, which posits that if a substance leads to sickness in a healthy person then a lower concentration of that substance (remedy) may cure that sickness [18]. Unlike herbal medicine, homeopathy uses ultradiluted plant, mineral, or other natural substances [18]. Of five studies (one open-label, one crossover, three DB PBO RCT, n = 283), three found significant (p < 0.05) improvement in ADHD symptoms while no significant differences were found in a PBO RCT and a RCT comparison with MPH. This area needs better-controlled studies, use of standard treatment outcome measures, and the examination of specific patient factors affecting response. Although homeopathy appears safe and relatively easy, it can be expensive due to lengthy (average response time 3.5 months) and repeated doctor visits. However, short trials may be *acceptable* for patients unresponsive to or unwilling to try conventional treatment.

Noningestible CATs for pediatric ADHD

Biofeedback and its specialized subcategory of neurofeedback work via operant conditioning to train the body/brain to modify its physiological activity to improve health and performance by giving it real-time video/audio information about its electrical activity. Electromyographic **biofeedback** (BF) and **relaxation** approaches typically have been combined in treatment studies of ADHD. Most studies regulated muscle tension in the forehead via visual feedback from an electromyograph (EMG), whereas relaxation typically involved audio-taped instructions for progressive muscle relaxation. Based on the theory that muscle tension and an inability to relax contribute to and increase hyperactivity [19], both EMG-BF and relaxation training attempt to induce overall muscle relaxation. Six RCTs (n = 247) of EMG-BF/relaxation-training reported significant decreases, compared with controls, for overall (ES = 1.31), inattentive (ES = 0.91), and impulsive (ES = 0.93) symptoms [20]. Unfortunately, none of the studies were DB and only one used a sham control. As 83% of the studies combined EMG-BF with relaxation, it is not known which treatment component or combination caused the reported results. More recently, a RCT of heart-rate variability (HRV) BF significantly (p < 0.05) improved cognitive functioning and participant- and teacher-rated overall behaviors compared with an active control. Both EMG-BF and HRV-BF appear safe, relatively easy, and sensible although not cheap as they require expensive equipment and a technician. Because some studies reported response with only four treatments, both forms of BF are *acceptable* for pediatric ADHD. However, the progressive muscle relaxation with which it was often paired seems safe, easy, cheap, and sensible and produced similar results across a few sessions; it is *recommended*.

Neurofeedback (NF, EEG biofeedback) typically attempts to modify certain electroencephalogram (EEG) rhythms (brainwaves) thought to be associated with ADHD, including increasing the power of beta rhythms (12–21 hertz [Hz]) and suppressing theta rhythms (4–8 Hz). Twelve randomized studies of NF have been conducted showing significant

improvements compared with control conditions for overall ADHD (ES = 0.62), inattention (ES = 0.72), hyperactivity/impulsivity (ES = 0.70) and neurophysiological changes [21]. However, except for one study that also had limitations, these results have not been replicated in the few existing small DB studies, although those studies also had some limitations.

NF appears sensible and safe (although this has not been empirically examined), but because of the 20–40 twice/thrice-weekly sessions incorporating expensive equipment/trained technicians, it is neither easy nor cheap. Although the evidence for NF is increasing in quantity and quality, because of some questions about methodology and laborious intensity and cost, it is *not recommended* for pediatric ADHD for most families at this time, although for families with surplus resources of time and money, it would be acceptable.

Executive function (EF) training, also called cognitive control, involves systematic computerized exercises to improve the core components of EF: inhibition, working memory, and cognitive flexibility. These skills are deficient in children with ADHD [22]. One RCT and two open-label trials of EF have been conducted. The RCT, a pilot study of 40 school-age children, demonstrated significantly greater improvement on parent ratings of EF and ADHD than a wait-list condition (but non-significant teacher ratings), with effects maintained at follow-up 9 weeks later. The two open-label trials of EF involved group training of preschoolers, diagnosed with ADHD, games to improve EF skills, and teaching parents, in a separate group, on how to apply these skills at home. Both studies reported significant improvements in parent-rated ADHD symptoms and one study found 3-month maintenance of gains on parent-rated measures of ADHD. However, results for teacher ratings of ADHD and psychometric measures of EF were mixed.

In addition to EF training, there are also more specific attention and working memory programs designed to remediate impairments in working memory and selective and sustained attention related to ADHD. For **attention training** there exist two open-label studies, two non-randomized, but controlled trials in children with ADHD. These studies document consistent improvement on psychometric measures of visual and auditory attention and one study found 9-month post-treatment maintenance of parent-reported improvements of ADHD. However, improvements on other outcomes, such as parent- and teacher-rated ADHD symptoms and academic functioning, were mixed.

For **working memory training**, five RCTs exist on school-aged children diagnosed with ADHD and comparing computerized training with a sham or alternative treatment. These studies reported significant improvements on neuropsychological verbal and visual-spatial working memory tasks; one study found improvements in EEG-evoked response potentials; another demonstrated improvement in observed behavior on a simulated academic task; and one study reported gains were maintained at 3-month post-treatment. However, results for parent- and teacher-rated ADHD, parent-rated EF, and academic performance were inconsistent.

Future investigations on EF, attention, and working memory training require RCTs, DB treatment outcome measures, sham/alternative control groups, and more follow-up assessments. Despite promising results and appearing sensible and safe, these types of training are not cheap or easy in terms of time/effort because of the need for specialized equipment/technicians. Therefore, if it is not too burdensome for a given family's resources, such training may be *acceptable,* but if not, it is *not recommended* for pediatric ADHD. New web-based applications may drive the cost down to an acceptable level.

Yoga involves changing the body's physiology by practicing physical and mental exercises such as postures and breathing techniques. It is thought to work via disengaging the sympathetic nervous system while engaging the parasympathetic system, leading to a sense of calm, emotional balance, and increased concentration [23]. Three studies (n = 69), including two open trials and one RCT, reported several significant decreases in overall ADHD (ES = 0.6), inattention (ES = 0.48), and hyperactivity/impulsivity (ES = 0.10). Although promising, future research needs blinded sham-controlled RCTs with FU and larger samples. Yoga appears safe, cheap, and sensible; whether it is easy for children with ADHD to learn and use is not clear, therefore a short trial as utilized by the three studies, for an average of 45 minutes per session, twice weekly for 10 weeks, may be *acceptable.*

Meditation/mindfulness involves the practicing of certain techniques (e.g., listening to the breath, repeating a mantra, being mindful of the present) to train the brain to eliminate unnecessary thoughts and increase alertness, awareness and attention in the present moment [24]. It is hypothesized to work by relaxing the sympathetic nervous system, activating parasympathetic-limbic pathways, and reducing theta while increasing beta EEG frequencies [24]. Results from four open studies and two RCTs include significant ($p < 0.05{-} \le 0.001$) improvements on overall ADHD ($d = 0.35$), inattention ($d = 0.50$), "on task" behavior ($d = 2.15$), anxiety ($d = 0.70$), depression ($d = 0.35$), and executive functioning ($d = 0.40$). A 2010 Cochrane review concluded, "As a result of the limited number of included studies, the small sample sizes and the high risk of bias, we are unable to draw any conclusions regarding the effectiveness of meditation therapy for ADHD" [25, p. 4]. Future studies require sham/alternative treatment groups with blinded RCTs, FU, and larger samples. Given these results, as meditation is also beneficial for cardiovascular health, it seems sensible, and is safe, reasonably cheap, and easy. Therefore, a short trial, as utilized by the four studies, for an average of 18 minutes/session, four times/week for 7 weeks with regular practice at home, is *recommended* for pediatric ADHD.

Vestibular stimulation uses indirect physical arousal of the sensory system associated with movement and balance in the inner ear via stimulation of either the otoliths or semicircular canals. It has been examined as a CAT for pediatric ADHD because past research reported associated vestibular processing impairments [26]. Two single-blind sham-controlled crossover studies of rotational vestibular stimulation, which stimulates the semicircular canals, reported significant/marginally significant ($p < 0.05$, ES = 0.5) decreases in ADHD symptoms compared to the control condition. A RCT utilizing vestibular stimulation across all vectors via complex motion, stimulating semicircular canals mildly and otoliths more intensely, did not find significant differences between treatment and PBO conditions. Future research involving larger, blinded PBO RCTs with FU on rotational vestibular stimulation is needed. Despite appearing relatively safe and sensible, structured vestibular stimulation in clinical settings is not cheap and therefore *not recommended*. However, home activities utilizing appropriate, available play activities/equipments (e.g., "Sit'N'Spin" toy, swivel chairs, single-suspension swings, carousels, spinning games) to stimulate the semicircular canals are *acceptable*.

Massage therapy involves the physical manipulation of superficial layers of muscle and connective tissue to enhance function, relaxation, and well-being. It is thought to improve ADHD symptoms, increase relaxation, and increase alertness by altering brain waves, increasing vagal tone, improving parasympathetic activity, and increasing vagal control of the heart by enhancing a deficient physiological inhibitory system [27]. Two RCTs (n = 58) reported significantly (p < 0.05–0.01) less hyperactivity, daydreaming/inattention, overall ADHD symptoms, and anxiety, and more on-task time and happiness. Future research needs standardized clinical assessments to validate ADHD and control of confounds in ongoing treatments. Being sensible, seemingly safe, easy, and cheap if parents can be taught to administer it, massage might provide an *acceptable* addition to bedtime ritual, improving sleep onset and parent–child relationship even if it does not improve ADHD symptoms.

Exercise may improve EF in children and has therefore been suggested as a CAT for children with ADHD [28]. Three small non-randomized, control group studies examining exercise for pediatric ADHD have been published. Although the earliest study found no significant improvement on parent-rated ADHD symptoms, the two more recent studies appeared more effective. One found significant improvements on parent-rated ADHD symptoms (p = 0.01) and on 2/5 measures of EF. The other reported improvements in teacher-rated ADHD symptoms ($d = 0.70$), motor skills ($d = 0.96$), and psychometric measures of EF (average $d = 0.22$). Future research on exercise for ADHD requires RCTs, DB designs, alternative treatment control groups, and follow-up assessments. As exercise appears sensible, safe, cheap, and easy a brief trial, as used in the aforementioned studies (e.g., 30 min/day, 5× per week, 5 weeks), is recommended.

Electro-acupuncture involves the use of a small needle with a pulsating electrical current to stimulate certain acupoints on the body. An intervention from Traditional Chinese Medicine, this approach is based on the hypothesis that ADHD is caused by "effulgent gallbladder fire, Yin-Yang disharmony and noninteraction of heart and kidney" [29, p. 176]. One large (n = 213) RCT of 4- to 6-year-olds with DSM-IV ADHD (and typical ADHD-related comorbidities) compared electro-acupuncture plus behavior therapy with sham electro-acupuncture and behavior therapy [29]. Based on blinded 4-point ratings of ADHD symptom improvement from two pediatric psychologists, this study reported electro-acupuncture had significantly (p < 0.05) more improvement than the control group immediately post-treatment, and at 6-month follow-up (p < 0.05). Although few adverse effects were

reported there was a high dropout rate (9% treatment noncompliant and 20% dropped out at 6-months).

Although promising preliminary data, future studies of electro-acupuncture require testing the validity of the blind, testing the valid inertness of the sham, standard treatment outcome measures with reported validity or reliability. Therefore, as this approach appears safe, seems sensible (from a traditional Chinese medicine perspective), and easy, if it is not too expensive, a 12-week trial combined with behavior therapy, as used in this study, may be acceptable for some children with ADHD. A recent Cochrane review concluded there was "no evidence base of randomized or quasi-randomized controlled trials to support" the use of other types of acupuncture for ADHD [30, p. 4].

Ingestible CATs for adult ADHD

Four studies (n = 41, two open, two DB PBO crossover) have been conducted on **amino acid supplementation** with some promising results, but no study has documented long-term benefit as tolerance typically developed after 2 to 3 months. An open trial of a **combined micronutrient supplement** (EMPower+) for 14 adults, selected for ADHD and severe mood dysregulation found large improvements in ADHD symptoms (ESs = 0.7–1.58, p = 0.01–0.001) and mood (ESs = 1.29–1.45, p = 0.001), greater than ordinarily expected from PBO. Thus, it appears that DB PBO RCTs for adult ADHD are warranted. This combination supplement can be expensive and a nuisance to swallow. Therefore, given the uncontrolled nature of the data, it is *not recommended* for ADHD at this time. Finally, as a single DB PBO crossover study on the **herbal supplement** of Pycnogenol (n = 24) found similar treatment effects to a PBO [31], it is *not recommended* for adult ADHD.

It is possible that some of the more effective, safe, easy, cheap, and sensible ingestible CATs for pediatric ADHD previously discussed could help some adults with ADHD. However, as they have not been empirically examined in adults, they should only be considered after standard treatments for adult ADHD have been tried.

Noningestible CATs for adult ADHD

For **neurofeedback** (NF) in the treatment of adult ADHD, only a chart review [32] and an open-label pilot study [33] have been published. The chart review included 13 adults, along with 111 children, and reported results for each group separately; all patients received NF with metacognitive training. For the adult patients, significant (p < 0.03–0.0001) improvements were reported on computerized measures of attention span, reaction time, and variability; a standardized math test; and overall IQ; and marginally significant (p = 0.08) improvements in EEG theta/beta ratio. The open-label pilot study included 14 adults and 7 children who received quantitative EEG-informed NF; results were presented for the entire sample because the adult/child by time interactions were non-significant. Significant improvements (all p < 0.01) were reported on rating scales of ADHD symptoms and depression; for a subsample with pre- to post-treatment data available (n = 6), sensorimotor rhythm power was decreased from pre to post treatment. Unlike the evidence for pediatric ADHD, research on NF for adult ADHD lacks even open RCTs, let alone DB, sham-controls, FU, large samples, and standardized diagnostic procedures. Despite making sense and appearing safe, NF is time-consuming and expensive and, given existing data, is therefore *not recommended* for adult ADHD.

Mindfulness meditation training (MMT) involves a calm, non-judgmental, and accepting awareness of one's "in-the-moment" experiences. It has been suggested as a treatment because it trains self-regulation of attention and emotion. Two open trials [34, 35] and one waitlist-controlled study [36] have been published, two of which included MMT as part of a larger psychotherapy program [34, 36], and the third examined it alone in a mixed adult/adolescent sample [35]. Significant (p < 0.001–0.05) improvements were reported on self-rated ADHD, anxiety, depressive, and overall symptoms; personal health; and computerized tests of attention and impulsivity. In addition to MMT being sensible, it appears safe, easy, and relatively inexpensive (8–13 sessions). Therefore, a short (2.5 hours/week for 8 weeks with daily at-home practice) trial is *acceptable* for adult ADHD.

Light therapy, traditionally used to treat seasonal affective disorder, involves the use of a light box radiating specific light wavelengths, equivalent to natural outdoor light, thought to release brain chemicals associated with mood. It has been suggested because of studies reporting a delayed sleep/activity rhythm and/or seasonal mood symptoms in some adults with ADHD [37]. In the single existing open-label study of adult ADHD (n = 29) morning bright light therapy, given daily for 3 weeks from November to December, was found to significantly (p = 0.001– < 0.05, ESs = 0.21–0.85) improve several subjective and objective measures of ADHD, primarily inattention, improve self-rated mood symptoms, and change circadian phase preference from being an "evening" to a "morning person" [38]. Seemingly safe (unless comorbid mania is present), easy, and relatively inexpensive, light therapy is sensible and *recommended* for adults with ADHD reporting a delayed sleep/activity rhythm and/or seasonal mood symptoms.

Although the published research evaluating **cognitive training** (including attention training, working memory training, and executive functioning training) for pediatric ADHD has increased significantly in the last decade, only one study of computerized training of EF for adult ADHD has been published. Adults with ADHD were randomized into four conditions: individual cognitive-behavioral therapy (CBT), hypnotherapy (comparisons not discussed in the article), computerized cognitive training, and a no-treatment control condition [39]. Relative to placebo, there were no significant effects of cognitive training on self-reported ADHD symptoms or blinded evaluator global ratings; CBT was found to be superior to computerized cognitive training on self-reported ratings of attention (p = 0.09) and blinded evaluator global ratings (p < 0.05). Thus, computerized cognitive training is not currently recommended as a treatment for adult ADHD.

It is possible that some of the more effective, safe, easy, cheap and sensible noningestible treatments for pediatric ADHD previously discussed could help some adults with ADHD. However, as none of these approaches have been empirically examined they should only be considered after standard treatments for adult ADHD have been tried.

Conclusion

In general, research on CATs for pediatric and adult ADHD is increasing in quantity and quality with several promising treatment approaches. However, due to a lack of comparative research with established treatments, none of these currently meet criteria for complementary or alternative treatments for pediatric or adult ADHD. Future research needs to include more DB, PBO/sham-controlled RCTs with FU and reliably diagnosed samples with ADHD; definitive trials and replications of promising interventions that may have some advantage (benefit–risk ratio) over standard treatments if proven effective; controlled clinical trials of promising interventions for which a controlled trial is easy and cheap; and open pilot trials of well-considered hypotheses for which there are no pilot data and for which a controlled trial would be expensive or difficult. Finally, before being designated as a complementary or alternative treatment, well-controlled research studies are required to demonstrate, with replication, incremental or similar effects when added or compared to established treatments.

Clinically, although research evidence is currently limited, individual treatment needs cannot always wait for the science to improve. Thus, for those who do not respond completely to established treatments, practitioners are often expected to advise patients about alternatives or adjuncts. If patients sense practitioners are reluctant or unknowledgeable about such interventions they may experiment with them by themselves. Therefore, it is imperative that practitioners have the knowledge to discuss and guide individual patient trials of currently available CATs. To assist practitioners we offer the following clinical recommendations:

1. As several CATs target specific causes, they should be *considered* (not necessarily used) early during the diagnostic evaluation. Therefore, a good history, physical exam, and, as indicated, a blood count, electrolyte/mineral screen, vitamin D assay, and, in areas with high rates of subclinical lead poisoning, serum lead assessment are needed. Once causes associated with specific treatments are ruled out, standard conventional treatments (medication and behavioral treatment) may be more confidently utilized.

2. Clinicians and patients need to request data/evidence associated with specific CATs as many claim scientific proof, but merely provide anecdote, case history, or testimonial data.

3. Comparisons to established treatments are not convincing unless subject assignment to treatment conditions is random.

4. Failure to find a significant difference from established treatment does not make the treatment equal or effective because a small sample can easily fail to find a significant difference when one really exists.

5. Investing family resources (money, time, effort) to an intervention that does not work is a risk to be

considered for the patient and other family members.

6. For some individuals, a CAT may work better than established treatment even though it is not proven by group averages.

7. Whether a particular CAT is worth a short monitored trial for an individual patient depends partly on the SECS criterion and on the accessibility and response to established treatments.

8. When trying any treatment, change only one thing at a time and monitor the results (and potential adverse affects) carefully with specific ADHD rating scales [40–42]. If clinically significant benefit is not noted in the expected time, move on to another treatment.

9. Patients and their families should discuss with their prescribing physician all ingestible CATs they are considering, even "natural" herbs, so as to identify any possible interactions with currently prescribed medications.

10. All patients and their families should be provided with biopsychosocial information or psychoeducation about ADHD and its treatment. Psychoeducational resources may be accessed from Children and Adults with Attention Deficit/Hyperactivity Disorder (*CHADD*, www.chadd.org).

References

1. National Center for Complementary and Alternative Medicine Publication No. D347 (2007). What is CAT? http://nccam.nih.gov/health/whatiscam (accessed May 25, 2014).

2. Arnold LE, Hurt E, Mayes T, Lofthouse N. Ingestible alternative and complementary treatments for attention-deficit/hyperactivity disorder. In: Evans E., Hoza B, eds. *Treating Attention Deficit Disorder*. New Jersey: Civic Research Institute. 2011; 14–1 to 14–40.

3. Hurt E, Lofthouse N, Arnold LE. Noningestible alternative and complementary treatments for attention-deficit/hyperactivity disorder. In: Evans E., Hoza B, eds. *Treating Attention Deficit Disorder*. New Jersey: Civic Research Institute; 2011; 15–1 to 15–26.

4. Lofthouse N, Hurt E. Complementary and alternative treatments for pre-school children with attention-deficit/hyperactivity disorder. In Guhman H., Guhman J, eds. *ADHD in Preschool Children: Assessment and Treatment:* Oxford: Oxford University Press. 2014; 180–209.

5. Feingold BF. *Why Your Child is Hyperactive*. New York, NY: Random House; 1975.

6. Wesnes KA, Pincock C, Richardson D, Helm G, Hails S. Breakfast reduces declines in attention and memory over the morning in schoolchildren. *Appetite*. 2003; **41**:329–31.

7 Stevens LJ, Zentall SS, Deck JL, et al. Essential fatty acid metabolism in boys with attention-deficit hyperactivity disorder. *Am J Clin Nutr*. 1995;**62**:761–8.

8. Spahis S, Vanasse M, Belanger SA, et al. Lipid profile, fatty acid composition and pro- and anti-oxidant status in pediatric patients with attention-deficit/hyperactivity disorder. *Prostaglandins Leukot Essent Fatty Acids*. 2008;**79**:47–53.

9. Bloch MH, Qawasmi A. Omega-3 fatty acid supplementation for the treatment of children with attention-deficit/hyperactivity disorder: Systematic review and meta-analysis. *J Am Acad Child Adolesc Psychiatry*. 2011;**50**:991–1000.

10. Arduini A, Denisova N, Virmani A, et al. Evidence for the involvement of carnitine-dependent long-chain acyltransferases in neuronal triglyceride and phospholipid fatty acid turnover. *J Neurochem*. 1994;**62**:1530–8.

11. Ricciolini R, Scalibastri M, Kelleher JK, et al. Role of acetyl-l-carnitine in rat brain lipogenesis: implications for polyunsaturated fatty acid synthesis. *J Neurochem*. 1998;**71**:2510–17.

12. Bornstein RA, Baker GB, Carroll A, et al. Plasma amino acids in attention deficit disorder. *Psychiatry Res*. 1990;**33**:301–6.

13. Baker GB, Bornstein RA, Rouget AC, et al. Phenylethylaminergic mechanisms in attention-deficit disorder. *Biol Psychiatry*. 1991;**29**:15–22.

14. Stein TP, Sammaritano AM. Nitrogen metabolism in normal and hyperkinetic boys. *Am J Clin Nutr*. 1984;**39**:520–4.

15. Cortese S, Konofal E, Bernadina BD, et al. Sleep disturbance and serum ferritin levels in attention-deficit hyperactivity disorder. *Eur Child Adolesc Psychiatry*. 2009;**18**:393–9.

16. McGee R, Williams S, Anderson J, et al. Hyperactivity and serum hair zinc in 11-year-old children from the general population. *Biol Psychiatry*. 1990;**28**:165–8.

17. Vickers A, Zollman C, Lee R. Herbal medicine. *West J Med*. 2001;**175**:125–98.

18. National Center for Homeopathy. What is homeopathy? http://www.homeopathycenter.org/learn-about-homeopathy (accessed May 25, 2014).

19. Braud LW, Lupin MN, Braud WG. The use of electromyographic biofeedback in the control of hyperactivity. *J Learn Disabil*. 1975;**8**:21–6.

20. Lofthouse N, McBurnett K, Hurt E, Arnold LE. Biofeedback and neurofeedback treatments for ADHD. *Psychiatr Ann*. 2011;**41**:42–8.

21. Lofthouse N, Arnold LE, Hurt E. Current status of neurofeedback for attention-deficit hyperactivity disorder. *Curr Psychiatry Rep*. 2012;**14**(5):536–42.

22. Barkley RA. Behavioral inhibition, sustained attention, and executive functions: constructing a unifying theory of ADHD. *Psychol Bull*. 1997;**121**:65–94.

23. Peck HL, Kehle TS, Bray MA, Theodore LA. Yoga as an intervention for children with attention problems. *School Psych Rev*. 2005;**34**:415–24.

24. Harrison LJ, Manocha R, Rubin K. Sahaja yoga meditation as a family treatment programme for children with attention deficit-hyperactivity disorder. *Clin Child Psychol Psychiatry*. 2004;**9**:479–97.

25. Krisanaprakornkit T, Ngamjarus C, Witoonchart C, Piyavhatkul N. Meditation therapies for attention-deficit/hyperactivity disorder (ADHD). *Cochrane Database Syst Rev*. 2010;(6):CD006507.

26. Mulligan S. An analysis of score patterns of children with attention disorders on the sensory integration and praxis tests. *Am J Occup Ther*. 1996;**50**:647–54.

27. Khilnani S, Field T, Hernandez-Reif M, Schanberg S. Massage therapy improves mood and behavior of students with attention-deficit/hyperactivity disorder. *Adolescence*. 2003;**38**:623–38.

28. Berwid OG, Halperin JM. Emerging support for a role of exercise in attention-deficit/hyperactivity disorder intervention planning. *Curr Psychiatry Rep*. 2012; **14**:543–51.

29. Li S, Yu B, Lin Z, et al. Randomized-controlled study of treating attention deficit hyperactivity disorder of preschool children with combined electro-acupuncture and behavior therapy. *Complement Ther Med*. 2010;**18**:175–83.

30. Li S, Yu B, Zhou D, et al. Acupuncture for attention deficit hyperactivity disorder (ADHD) in children and adolescents. *Cochrane Database Syst Rev*. 2011;(4): CD007839.

31. Tenenbaum S, Paull JC, Sparrow EP, et al. An experimental comparison of Pycnogenol and methylphenidate in adults with attention-deficit/hyperactivity disorder. *J Atten Disord*. 2002;**6**:49–60.

32. Thompson L, Thompson M. Neurofeedback combined with training in metacognitive strategies: effectiveness in students with ADD. *Appl Psychophysiol Biofeedback*. 1998;**23**:243–63.

33. Arns M, Drinkenburg W, Kenemans JL. The effects of QEEG-informed neurofeedback in ADHD: an open-label pilot study. *Appl Psychophysiol Biofeedback*. 2012;**37**:171–80.

34. Philipsen A, Richter H, Peters J, *et al.* Structured group psychotherapy in adults with attention deficit hyperactivity disorder: results of an open multicentre study. *J Nerv Ment Dis.* 2007;**195**:1013–19.

35. Zylowska L, Ackerman DL, Yang MH, *et al.* Mindfulness meditation training in adult and adolescent with ADHD: a feasibility study. *J Atten Dis.* 2008;**11**:737–46.

36. Hesslinger B, Tebartz van Elst L, Nyberg E, *et al.* Psychotherapy of attention deficit hyperactivity disorder in adults – a pilot study using a structured skills training program. *Eur Arch Psychiatry Clin Neurosci.* 2002;**252**:177–84.

37. Rybak YE, McNeely HE, Mackenzie BE, *et al.* Seasonality and circadian preference in adult attention-deficit/hyperactivity disorder: clinical and neuropsychological correlates. *Compr Psychiatry.* 2007;**48**:562–71.

38. Rybak YE, McNeely HE, Mackenzie BE, *et al.* An open trial of light therapy in adult attention-deficit/hyperactivity disorder. *J Clin Psychiatry.* 2006;**67**:1527–35.

39. Virta M, Saslakari A, Antila M, *et al.* Short cognitive behavioral therapy and cognitive training for adults with ADHD – a randomized controlled pilot study. *Neuropsychiatr Dis Treat.* 2010;**6**:443–53.

40. Swanson, Nolan and Pelham IV Rating Scales (SNAP-IV). http://www.adhd.net/snap-iv-form.pdf (accessed November 23, 2010).

41. Vanderbilt scales. http://www.psychiatrictimes.com/clinical-scales/adhd/vadrs/ (accessed November 29, 2010).

42. Adult Self-Report Scale (ASRS). http://webdoc.nyumc.org/nyumc/files/psych/attachments/psych_adhd_checklist.pdf (accessed October 6, 2010).

Chapter 25

Preschool ADHD treatment

Brigette S. Vaughan, Joan M. Daughton, and Christopher J. Kratochvil

Introduction

Preschool psychopharmacology is nearly entirely off-label [1], and the use of psychopharmacological interventions essentially exposes a young child to agents whose potential risks and benefits may not be entirely known. In addition to potentially unintended central nervous system (CNS) and other adverse effects, children display more rapid hepatic and renal metabolisms which may change the dosing and administration strategy for psychopharmacological intervention in this age group. Few studies examine the effects of psychiatric medications on preschool-aged children, and even fewer offer data on long-term outcomes. The limited support of pharmacotherapy as a safe and efficacious treatment for young children with attention-deficit hyperactivity disorder (ADHD) no doubt provides the rationale for recommending behavioral therapy as the initial intervention for these patients, or at a minimum, as a key part of a comprehensive treatment plan. The lack of US Food and Drug Administration (FDA) approval for many of the ADHD pharmacotherapies for use in the preschool age group, however, does not suggest that available approved medications cannot be used. It does, however, emphasize the importance of a careful and thorough assessment of the young child, and cautious determination of the degree of impairment and the need for treatment. This risk–benefit analysis is a crucial aspect of treatment planning. If pharmacotherapy is ultimately determined to be warranted, the prescribing clinician is obligated to provide a detailed and collaborative informed consent process.

Epidemiology

One epidemiological study found that 12% of preschool-aged children met criteria for an impairing

Diagnostic and Statistical Manual of Mental Disorders (DSM)-IV disorder [2], with 9% meeting criteria for a behavioral disorder. Carter *et al.* also found that 21.6% of children entering formal schooling (kindergarten or first grade) met criteria for an impairing DSM-IV disorder [3]. In school-age children, ADHD has a 5.7% worldwide prevalence [4–6], while epidemiological surveys of community samples have reported 2–6% of preschoolers meet full criteria for ADHD [7–9]. Symptoms of the disorder are very common in the preschool population. Two studies have reported that 59–86% of 2- to 6-year-olds referred to psychiatric clinics have at least some symptoms of the disorder [9, 10]. A careful assessment by a skilled clinician is necessary to differentiate "true" ADHD from other disorders with overlapping symptoms, or even from "normal" development.

Preschool children with ADHD are at higher risk for functional impairment in home, academic, and social settings [11–13], and their presentation and comorbidity is comparable to that seen in school-aged children with disruptive behavior disorders [13]. Early onset of ADHD appears to correlate with increased risk for accidents and/or injuries [14, 15]. Preschool-aged boys with ADHD and comorbid oppositional defiant disorder (ODD) have significantly higher rates of unintentional injury than their unaffected counterparts [16]. With data supporting high rates of impairing disorders in preschool children, the question is raised regarding how to intervene and when, and what the safest and most effective interventions are.

Disruptive behavior disorders, including ADHD, appear to have higher stability over time than other disorders [17–20]. In studies of preschoolers with ADHD, 75–80% continued to meet criteria 3–5 years later [18, 21]. Preschoolers with a disruptive behavior disorder appear to be at higher risk over time to

Attention-Deficit Hyperactivity Disorder in Adults and Children, ed. Lenard A. Adler, Thomas J. Spencer and Timothy E. Wilens. Published by Cambridge University Press. © Cambridge University Press 2015.

develop a second disorder, with 70% meeting criteria for an additional disorder within 3 years [20, 22]. Children with comorbid disorders have been found to be more likely to have impairment, and their diagnoses were also more likely to persist [3]. The presence of an impairing diagnosis was associated with more significant family burden and poorer social competence on the part of the affected child.

Diagnosis/assessment

Efforts have been made to improve the specificity of diagnostic tools for young children. The Preschool Age Psychiatric Assessment (PAPA) [2], a semi-structured diagnostic interview conducted with the parent, for example, is a research instrument not generally used in clinical practice but sets the stage for a more developmentally appropriate assessment and application of diagnostic criteria. Using the PAPA, 5.1% of a sample of 1073 preschoolers from a pediatric clinic met diagnostic criteria for ADHD, with 2.9% of the sample identified as having the hyperactive/impulsive subtype, 2.1% the combined type, and only 0.1% meeting criteria for the primarily inattentive subtype [2].

Screening for ADHD in clinical practice is often done with the assistance of rating scales. Not all instruments, however, are normed for use in the preschool population. The long and short versions of the Conners' Rating Scales (CRS) are normed for preschoolers and are available in French, Spanish, and English. Parent and teacher versions have been standardized for boys and girls ages 3 to 17 years using a normative database compiled from over 200 data collection sites throughout North America, on ethnically diverse samples [23]. The long forms allow for screening across a broad range of symptom domains beyond ADHD, while the short versions of the CRS are useful for repeated administration when monitoring treatment response [24]. Clinicians must note that preschoolers who are referred for treatment of behavioral problems do not necessarily present with the same symptoms on ADHD checklists as school-aged children [25]. Young children frequently present with predominantly hyperactive symptoms [25], while older children, teens, and adults are more likely to demonstrate inattention. The lack of age and developmentally specific symptom criteria places the burden on the clinician to decide if the activity level and inattention in a particular child are excessive and inappropriate, rather than relying solely on symptom checklists, which, if used exclusively in this population, may result in over-identification of ADHD [26]. The presenting complaint at the time of evaluation may indicate a reaction to a challenge in the midst of "typical" development, a delay in a developmental process, or a pathological symptom warranting psychiatric intervention. A thorough assessment, including prenatal and birth history, developmental history, family and social history, and an assessment of the parent–child relationship, is required in order to limit the possibility that another psychiatric disorder, general medical condition, or developmental disorder is misdiagnosed as ADHD.

Preschool ADHD Treatment Study (PATS)

Despite limited safety and efficacy data, prescription of psychotropic medications to preschoolers has increased significantly in the last 20 years [27]. In a 2007 study, Zito et al. found that 2.3% of 2- to 4-year-old Medicaid recipients were receiving at least one psychotropic prescription [28]. Between 1997 and 2002, 0.3% of preschoolers in one Medicaid database were being prescribed a psychostimulant [29]. The efficacy of methylphenidate for treating ADHD in school-aged children has been well documented [1]; unfortunately, controlled data on its safety and efficacy in preschoolers have been much more limited. Prior to the Preschool ADHD Treatment Study (PATS), there were 11 small controlled trials of methylphenidate in preschoolers with ADHD [30], all of which varied in diagnostic standards, methods, length, and outcomes. Greater variability in response [31], as well as differences in side effects compared with those seen in school-aged children [32], was observed in these earlier trials.

The PATS is the only multisite, randomized controlled study of a psychotropic medication in preschool children with a psychiatric disorder (Table 25.1). Greenhill et al. examined the efficacy and tolerability of immediate-release methylphenidate in 3- to 5.5-year-olds with either hyperactive–impulsive or combined type ADHD [33]. Symptoms had to be of at least moderate severity as evidenced by scores 1.5 standard deviations (SD) above age and gender norms for hyperactivity on both the Conners' Parent Rating Scale (CPRS) and Conners' Teacher Rating Scale (CTRS). Children also had to demonstrate at least 9 months of significant impairment as evidenced by a Children's Global Assessment Scale (CGAS)

Table 25.1. Key findings from the Preschool ADHD Treatment Study (PATS)

Population:
- 303 3- to 5.5-year-olds
- 261 completed 10 weeks of parent training
  - 37 showed either "significant" or "satisfactory" improvement
- 165 randomized (74% male, 63% White, 75% ADHD, combined subtype) to acute pharmacotherapy phase

Efficacy, safety and tolerability of immediate-release methylphenidate (MPH):
- TID dosing: placebo, 1.25 mg, 2.5 mg, 5 mg, 7.5 mg
  - Received each treatment condition for 1 week
- Linear dose response (p < 0.0001) for all active conditions except 1.25 mg TID
- Mean optimal total daily dose 14.22 ± 8.1 mg/day (0.7 ± 0.4 mg/kg/day)
- Most common adverse events: appetite loss, trouble sleeping, stomachaches, social withdrawal and lethargy
  - appetite loss, trouble sleeping, and feeling worried/anxious persisted over time
  - appetite loss appeared to increase with dose increase
- Changes in blood pressure and heart rate were mild and not clinically significant
- 21 discontinuations due to adverse events (AEs)
  - emotional lability was significantly related to study withdrawal (p < 0.0002)

Growth rates in PATS over first 12 months:
- Subjects were larger at baseline for height and weight compared to age-based norms
- Achieved 1.38 cm less in expected height per year, and 1.32 kg less in expected weight per year
- Higher weight at baseline was predictive of greater weight change

Pharmacogenetics and MPH response:
- 81 samples collected
- No significant association between MPH dose–response and genotype
- Associations found between certain genotypes and specific AEs (irritability, motor tics, buccal-lingual movements, and picking/biting)

Functional outcomes [63]:
- Significant medication effects noted on clinician ratings of ADHD severity (p < 0.0001), and teacher social competence ratings (p < 0.03)
- Parent ratings of child depression (p < 0.02) and dysthymia (p < 0.001) worsened with MPH

Source: Lubberstedt *et al.* [62].

of 55 or less. The presence of adjustment disorder, pervasive developmental disorders, psychosis, or other psychiatric disorder requiring treatment with medication was exclusionary.

Subjects were thoroughly screened and the diagnosis was confirmed by a consensus panel prior to participation in the treatment portion of the study. The parents of eligible subjects were first required to participate in ten 2-hour weekly sessions of parent training. Subjects who did not demonstrate at least a 30% decrease in their CPRS and CTRS hyperactivity scores or improvement on the Clinical Global Impression Severity (CGI-S) scale as rated by two of three raters (parent, teacher, clinician) after completion of parent training were eligible for the pharmacotherapy phase of the study. Only 7.2% of the 261 PATS subjects who completed the 10-week parent training intervention demonstrated significant improvement; however, the relatively high ADHD symptom severity in these preschoolers may have been less responsive to the initial stand-alone psychosocial intervention.

The crossover titration phase of the study enrolled 165 subjects (74% male, 63% White, mean age 4.74 years). During this phase, subjects were randomly assigned to 1 week of treatment with either placebo, 1.25 mg TID, 2.5 mg TID, 5 mg TID, or 7.5 mg TID immediate-release methylphenidate. At the conclusion of the 5-week crossover period, a linear dose response was observed (p < 0.0001) with the majority of subjects responding best to 7.5 mg TID (22%). The mean optimal dose was 14.22 ± 8.1 mg/day divided TID (0.7 ± 0.4 mg/kg/day).

Short-acting methylphenidate was generally well tolerated in PATS, although moderate or severe adverse events were reported by 16–20% of subjects on 1.25 mg TID, 19–24% on 2.5 mg TID, 25–30% on 5 mg TID, and 25–30% of those on 7.5 mg TID. Six moderate or severe adverse events, appetite loss, trouble sleeping, stomachache, tired/dull/listless, social withdrawal, and buccal-lingual movements, occurred significantly more often in subjects on methylphenidate compared to those on placebo. Eleven percent of subjects (n = 21) discontinued from the PATS due to adverse events: emotionality/irritability, tics, tactile hallucinations, possible seizure, rash, and insomnia. Only emotional lability was significantly related to discontinuation from the study (p < 0.0002). In the 10-month open-label maintenance treatment phase, appetite loss, trouble sleeping, and feeling worried or anxious persisted. Reports of crabbiness/irritability, prone to crying, tearful/sad/depression and listless/tired, however, decreased over time. Increases in blood pressure and/or pulse were not clinically significant. Growth rates in the PATS showed decreases in expected height (1.38 cm/year less than expected) and weight (1.32 kg/year less than expected) with methylphenidate treatment over the first 12 months. It is important to note that this was only 12-month data and longer observational data are needed to

Table 25.2. Gleason *et al.*'s Treatment Algorithm for Preschoolers with ADHD

Stage 0: Evaluation, diagnosis and psychotherapeutic intervention

Stage 1: Trial of methylphenidate

Stage 2: Trial of amphetamine

Stage 3: Trial of α-adrenergic agents or atomoxetine

General principles
- Assessment and diagnosis should be comprehensive, developmentally appropriate, and ongoing
- Psychosocial intervention should precede pharmacotherapy, and should continue even if medication is used
- Pharmacotherapy should be considered in the context of the clinical diagnosis and degree of functional impairment
- Referral of the parent for treatment, if appropriate, may optimize family mental health
- Medication discontinuation trials are recommended after 6 months of treatment
- The use of additional medication to manage side effects of medication is discouraged

Source: Gleason et al. [56].

fully assess the impact of stimulant treatment over time.

A 6-year follow-up study of 207 of the original PATS subjects evaluated longitudinal changes in severity of ADHD symptoms and diagnostic status [34]. At the 6-year point, 89% of participants still met criteria for ADHD based on symptom ratings from parents and teachers, and clinician diagnostic assessment. Those with comorbid oppositional defiant disorder or conduct disorder were 30% more likely to meet criteria for ADHD at year 6. Medication status between years 3 and 6 was not predictive of symptom severity change during that time. This study supports the notion that ADHD diagnosed in preschool is not only symptomatically severe and impairing for the child and family, but also chronic in nature. Predictors of impairment and comorbidity, and issues related to why, when, and how medications are used need to be determined.

Treatment guidelines (AAP, AACAP, Gleason)

Education of the parents and other caregivers is a key element in the treatment plan for a preschooler with ADHD (Table 25.2). Materials such as websites, handouts, and other literature developed by experts for the lay population are readily available, easily accessible, and offer translation of clinical expertise into "real life." The National Initiative for Children's

Healthcare Quality (NICHQ) specifically recommends that children with ADHD and their families receive individualized treatment with ongoing support and education [35, 36]. Additionally, NICHQ recommends that parent training, behavioral modification and social skills training, and school-based interventions be included in an effective ADHD management plan. For preschool children specifically, the American Academy of Child and Adolescent Psychiatry (AACAP) [37] and American Academy of Pediatrics (AAP) [38] recommend behavioral intervention prior to pharmacotherapy. Studies have shown that while behavioral therapies offer some benefit, they may have limited effectiveness as a monotherapy for treating moderate to severe ADHD. Ultimately, for the majority of cases, behavioral interventions are only one component of a more extensive treatment plan.

Behavioral intervention

Behavioral parent training has strong empirical support for a positive outcome when applied to younger school-age children [39], and parent management training [40, 41], is supported by randomized controlled trials. Sonuga-Barke and colleagues conducted one of the few controlled investigations of parent training in the treatment of preschool ADHD [42], randomizing children in a community sample to either a home-based parent-training intervention (n = 30), parent-counseling and support therapy (n = 29), or a wait-list control group (n = 20). ADHD symptoms were significantly reduced by the home-based parent training compared to the other two groups, with 53% of children in the parent-training group demonstrating clinically significant improvement. The maternal sense of well-being was also significantly improved with the home-based parent-training intervention. In a related study of 96 2- to 5-year-olds, parent–child interaction training also reduced ADHD and internalizing symptoms [43].

Behavioral outcomes of preschool children with ADHD are impacted by parenting variables [11, 44], poor maternal coping correlating with higher reported levels of hyperactivity. Negative, inconsistent parental behavior and high levels of family adversity are associated with early-onset and persistent behavioral problems. Parents of preschoolers with ADHD displayed twice as many controlling/negative behavior management strategies as positive preventive strategies

[45]. The presence of ADHD in preschool-aged boys has been associated with inconsistent parental discipline strategies, limited parental coping, decreased father–child communication, and strained mother–child interactions [46]. Interventions aimed at improving parenting skills, then, may positively affect child behavior, as well as parent–child interactions.

Parental psychopathology can further affect the efficacy of parent training, with the presence and severity of maternal ADHD being shown to limit the effectiveness of parent-training interventions for preschoolers with ADHD [47]. Maternal depression also interferes with successful implementation of parent-training interventions [45]. Treating parental psychopathology is required in order to maximize the potential benefit from parent-training programs [47].

Parent training has been shown to augment the efficacy of other psychological therapies for young children [48]. In a study of 55 families of 4- to 8-year-olds, a combination of group parent training and child group training was superior to the child intervention alone in improving child behavior and parental behavioral management ability. Both groups experienced significant improvement in child externalizing behaviors, social skills, child self-concept, parental stress, and parental efficacy. Pisterman et al. found that parent training improved parental outcomes, even though there was little change in child symptomatology [49]. Behavioral family intervention has been shown to lower levels of dysfunctional parenting and improved parental competence for parents of preschoolers [50]. Barkley et al., however, compared a school-year-long parent-training program and classroom interventions in a group of 158 kindergarten children with inattention and disruptive behavior [51]. While the classroom intervention yielded improvements on direct observation of classroom behavior, as well as teacher ratings of in-class attention, aggression, self-control, and social skills, neither intervention reduced problem behaviors at home.

Preschool parent-training interventions have been studied outside the United States and across cultures. A study of 23 Taiwanese families found that a 10-week parent-training intervention significantly improved ADHD and ODD symptoms in preschoolers [52]. In an Australian sample of 87 preschoolers with ADHD, a behavioral family intervention program was associated with significant reductions in parent-reported child behavior problems and directly observed child

negative behavior [50]. Gains were maintained at 1-year follow-up, with 80% continuing to demonstrate clinical improvement. In contrast, Shelton and colleagues reported that the 2-year post-treatment follow-up evidenced no enduring benefits [53].

Pharmacotherapy

Reduction in core ADHD symptoms is the most obvious benefit of pharmacotherapy, and by reducing inattention, hyperactivity, and impulsivity, patients with ADHD are better able to perform academically and socially. The evidence for the efficacy of psychosocial interventions for school-age children with ADHD, however, has been weaker than that for psychopharmacological treatments [54], and the National Institute of Mental Health (NIMH)-sponsored Multimodal Treatment Study of Children with ADHD (MTA) showed that an intensive psychosocial intervention was less effective than a medication management strategy in school-aged children. When combined with medication treatment, behavioral intervention provided only negligible benefit on the core symptoms of ADHD in school-age children with ADHD [55]. The PATS study differed in that failure of a parent-training program was required before pharmacotherapy was started; however, with less than 10% of subjects who completed parent training demonstrating sufficient improvement in ADHD, it appears that in these severe cases, parent training alone was insufficient.

The PATS study gives us the most extensive data on the safety and efficacy of pharmacotherapy for preschool ADHD, and supports use of immediate-release methylphenidate as the first-line medication for this age group. Unfortunately, a comparison of the PATS data with the MTA data demonstrates that preschoolers appeared to benefit less and have more adverse effects with methylphenidate treatment. Effect sizes were smaller (PATS 0.35 parent, 0.43 teacher; MTA 0.52 parent, 0.75 teacher) at "best" doses. It should be noted, however, that doses above 7.5 mg TID were not examined in PATS, so an optimal dose may not necessarily have been attained in all cases.

Despite a lack of randomized controlled trials examining any amphetamine preparation in preschool ADHD, the FDA approved d-amphetamine for children ages 3 years and up [41]. This was several decades ago, when approval criteria were much less rigorous.

Table 25.3. Pediatric friendly formulations of ADHD pharmacotherapies

Beaded capsules (can be sprinkled)
- Adderall XR
- Ritalin LA
- Metadate CD
- Focalin XR
- Dexedrine Spansules

Liquid concentrate
- Methylin
- Clonidine
- Quillivant XR

Chewable tablets
- Methylin

Transdermal
- Daytrana
- Clonidine patch[*]

Only amphetamine is FDA approved for children < 6 years of age.
[*] Not FDA-approved for ADHD.

Given data in older children which suggest comparable effectiveness between classes of psychostimulants, mixed amphetamine salts have been recommended as a second-line pharmacotherapy for preschool ADHD [56].

Long-acting stimulant formulations have not been extensively studied in preschool-aged children, due at least in part to administration challenges of formulations historically available. Fortunately recent development of beaded preparations which can be sprinkled, liquid formulations, and transdermal preparations have helped to address this concern (Table 25.3). Ritalin LA, a beaded capsule which can be opened and sprinkled, was used in a small open-label study in eleven 4- and 5-year-olds with ADHD [57] and was shown to reduce ADHD symptoms. The beaded methylphenidate preparation was well-tolerated, with decreased appetite reported as the most common side effect.

Data on non-stimulant pharmacotherapies are even more limited. Two open-label trials of atomoxetine [41, 58] in young children demonstrated reductions in ADHD symptoms, with generally good tolerability. In a 10-week study of 12 preschoolers [41], a mean decrease of 42% in parent-rated ADHD symptoms and 10% improvement in teacher ratings were seen at an average dose of 1.6 mg/kg/day. Five of the twelve subjects developed irritability, aggression and/or defiance, and one child withdrew due to chest ache. In Kratochvil et al.'s 2007 8-week study of atomoxetine in twenty-two 5- and 6-year-olds with ADHD,

significant decreases in parent ADHD-IV Rating Scale total score and hyperactive–impulsive and inattentive subscale scores ($p < 0.001$) were observed. The mean final dose of atomoxetine was 1.25 mg/kg/day. Over half of the subjects reported mood lability ($n = 12$), and 11 subjects reported decreased appetite. Vital sign changes were mild and not clinically significant. No subjects discontinued due to adverse events [58].

One double-blind placebo-controlled trial has been recently completed on the use of atomoxetine in 101 5- and 6-year-olds. The parents received education on ADHD and behavioral interventions at each study visit. Improvements were noted on parent and teacher ADHD-IV ratings for children who received atomoxetine compared to those who received placebo ($p < 0.05$). Three subjects withdrew from the study due to adverse events (atomoxetine = 0, placebo = 3). The mean final daily dose of atomoxetine was 1.38 mg/kg/day. Despite statistically significant improvements in ADHD symptoms, the children continued to have ADHD-IV (parent) scores above the 86th percentile for age and gender at study completion [59].

A meta-analysis of data from clinical trials of atomoxetine in 272 6- and 7-year-old children was done by Kratochvil et al. [60]. Ninety-seven of these children completed 2 years of treatment. Adverse events in the 6- and 7-year-olds in these studies were similar to those reported in short- and long-term studies of atomoxetine in adolescents. Observed heights and weights at 2 years were lower than predicted based on baseline measurements, and it was unclear if this was due to appetite having been decreased, or a direct metabolic effect. The decrement in growth rates appeared reversible, with normalization of growth after 18 months. A regression toward the mean was also observed, with younger children who were larger at baseline experiencing a greater decrement in growth than children who were smaller.

Limited data are also available on the use of the alpha (α)-adrenergic agents, guanfacine and clonidine. No controlled data are available on the use of either agent in preschoolers with ADHD, but there is a small double-blind, placebo-controlled crossover study of clonidine in children as young as age 5 with autistic disorder which showed it to be helpful for aggression and hyperactivity in some subjects [61]. Both clonidine and guanfacine have recently received FDA approval for ADHD in long-acting formulations for children ages 6 years and older.

Conclusion

ADHD symptoms account for the majority of referrals of preschool-aged children for psychiatric care. While not all of these children meet full criteria for the disorder, the symptoms can cause significant impairment in academic, social, and family functioning. The knowledge base about preschool ADHD and the tools available to diagnose and manage the disorder are increasing. Behavioral intervention, including parent management training and, potentially, school intervention, is a key component of treatment for young children with ADHD, or those with subthreshold symptoms. When behavioral intervention is inadequate, pharmacotherapy may be indicated.

The PATS offers data on the safety and efficacy of immediate-release methylphenidate for treating moderate to severe ADHD in preschool children; however, many treatment decisions are made based on the more extensive data on pharmacotherapies used in school-aged children with the disorder. Clinicians must take extra care to consider the special needs of the young child when extrapolating data to guide use of medications such as long-acting stimulant formulations, amphetamine-based stimulants, atomoxetine, and α-adrenergic agents.

Practice parameters and treatment algorithms offer reasonable clinical strategies for managing ADHD in preschoolers, however, the recommendations remain general, and a case-by-case assessment is warranted when developing a treatment plan. Parents and clinicians should have open and ongoing discussions of the available data on ADHD treatments, especially in regards to pharmacotherapy. While challenges exist, such as ease of administration, duration of effect, assessment of benefit, and management of side effects, medication should not be omitted from a treatment plan due to the presence or absence of FDA guidelines. In severe cases, it may not be in the child's or family's best interest to delay pharmacotherapy until a behavioral intervention has failed; however, behavioral therapy should be included and remain a key component throughout preschool ADHD treatment.

References

1. Greenhill LL. The use of psychotropic medication in preschoolers: indications, safety, and efficacy. *Can J Psychiatry*. 1998;**43**(6):576–81.

2. Egger HL, Angold A. The preschool age psychiatric assessment (PAPA): A structured parent interview for diagnosing psychiatric disorders in preschool children. In: Del Carmen-Wiggins R, Carter A, eds. *Handbook of Infant, Toddler, and Preschool Mental Assessment.* New York, NY: Oxford University Press. 2004; 223–43.

3. Carter AS, Wagmiller RJ, Gray SA, *et al.* Prevalence of DSM-IV disorder in a representative, healthy birth cohort at school entry: sociodemographic risks and social adaptation. *J Am Acad Child Adolesc Psychiatry*. 2010;**49**(7):686–98.

4. Barbaresi W, Katusic S, Colligan R, *et al.* How common is attention-deficit/hyperactivity disorder? Towards resolution of the controversy: results from a population-based study. *Acta Paediatr Suppl.* 2004; **93**(445):55–9.

5. Costello EJ, Angold A, Burns BJ, *et al.* The Great Smoky Mountains Study of Youth. Goals, design, methods, and the prevalence of DSM-III-R disorders. *Arch Gen Psychiatry*. 1996;**53**(12):1129–36.

6. Polanczyk G, de Lima MS, Horta BL, Biederman J, Rohde LA. The worldwide prevalence of ADHD: a systematic review and metaregression analysis. *Am J Psychiatry*. 2007;**164**(6):942–8.

7. Lavigne JV, Gibbons RD, Christoffel KK, *et al.* Prevalence rates and correlates of psychiatric disorders among preschool children. *J Am Acad Child Adolesc Psychiatry*. 1996;**35**(2):204–14.

8. Angold A, Erkanli A, Egger HL, Costello EJ. Stimulant treatment for children: a community perspective. *J Am Acad Child Adolesc Psychiatry*. 2000;**39**(8):975–84; discussion 984–94.

9. Keenan K, Wakschlag LS. More than the terrible twos: the nature and severity of behavior problems in clinic-referred preschool children. *J Abnorm Child Psychol*. 2000;**28**(1):33–46.

10. Wilens TE, Biederman J, Brown S, *et al.* Patterns of psychopathology and dysfunction in clinically referred preschoolers. *J Dev Behav Pediatr*. 2002;**23**(1 Suppl): S31–6.

11. DuPaul GJ, McGoey KE, Eckert TL, VanBrakle J. Preschool children with attention-deficit/hyperactivity disorder: impairments in behavioral, social, and school functioning. *J Am Acad Child Adolesc Psychiatry*. 2001;**40**(5):508–15.

12. Lahey BB, Applegate B. Validity of DSM-IV ADHD. *J Am Acad Child Adolesc Psychiatry*. 2001;**40**(5):502–4.

13. Wilens TE, Biederman J, Brown S, *et al.* Psychiatric comorbidity and functioning in clinically referred preschool children and school-age youths with ADHD. *J Am Acad Child Adolesc Psychiatry*. 2002;**41**(3):262–8.

14. Rappley MD, Mullan PB, Alvarez FJ, *et al.* Diagnosis of attention-deficit/hyperactivity disorder and use of psychotropic medication in very young children. *Arch Pediatr Adolesc Med*. 1999;**153**(10):1039–45.

15. Lahey BB, Pelham WE, Stein MA, *et al.* Validity of DSM-IV attention-deficit/hyperactivity disorder for younger children. *J Am Acad Child Adolesc Psychiatry.* 1998;**37**(7):695–702.

16. Schwebel DC, Speltz ML, Jones K, Bardina P. Unintentional injury in preschool boys with and without early onset of disruptive behavior. *J Pediatr Psychol.* 2002;**27**(8):727–37.

17. Briggs-Gowan MJ, Carter AS, Bosson-Heenan J, Guyer AE, Horwitz SM. Are infant-toddler social-emotional and behavioral problems transient? *J Am Acad Child Adolesc Psychiatry.* 2006;**45**(7):849–58.

18. Lahey BB, Pelham WE, Loney J, *et al.* Three-year predictive validity of DSM-IV attention deficit hyperactivity disorder in children diagnosed at 4–6 years of age. *Am J Psychiatry.* 2004;**161**(11):2014–20.

19. Leblanc N, Boivin M, Dionne G, *et al.* The development of hyperactive-impulsive behaviors during the preschool years: the predictive validity of parental assessments. *J Abnorm Child Psychol.* 2008;**36**(7):977–87.

20. Lavigne JV, Arend R, Rosenbaum D, *et al.* Psychiatric disorders with onset in the preschool years: I. Stability of diagnoses. *J Am Acad Child Adolesc Psychiatry.* 1998;**37**(12):1246–54.

21. Harvey EA, Youngwirth SD, Thakar DA, Errazuriz PA. Predicting attention-deficit/hyperactivity disorder and oppositional defiant disorder from preschool diagnostic assessments. *J Consult Clin Psychol.* 2009;**77**(2):349–54.

22. Cesena M, Gonzalez-Heydrich J, Szigethy E, Kohlenberg TM, DeMaso DR. A case series of eight aggressive young children treated with risperidone. *J Child Adolesc Psychopharmacol.* 2002;**12**(4):337–45.

23. Conners CK. *Conners' Rating Scales-Revised, Technical Manual.* Toronto: Multi-Health Systems Inc.; 1997.

24. Madaan V, Daughton J, Lubberstedt B, *et al.* Assessing the efficacy of treatments for ADHD: overview of methodological issues. *CNS Drugs.* 2008;**22**(4):275–90.

25. Hardy KK, Kollins SH, Murray DW, *et al.* Factor structure of parent- and teacher-rated ADHD symptoms in preschoolers in the preschoolers with ADHD treatment study (PATS). *J Child Adolesc Psychopharmacol.* 2007;**17**(5):621–34.

26. Gimpel GA, Kuhn BR. Maternal report of attention deficit hyperactivity disorder symptoms in preschool children. *Child Care Health Dev.* 2000;**26**(3):163–76; discussion 176–9.

27. Zito JM, Safer DJ, dosReis S, *et al.* Trends in the prescribing of psychotropic medications to preschoolers. *JAMA.* 2000;**283**(8):1025–30.

28. Zito JM, Safer DJ, Valluri S, *et al.* Psychotherapeutic medication prevalence in Medicaid-insured preschoolers. *J Child Adolesc Psychopharmacol.* 2007;**17**(2):195–203.

29. Zuvekas SH, Vitiello B, Norquist GS. Recent trends in stimulant medication use among U.S. children. *Am J Psychiatry.* 2006;**163**(4):579–85.

30. Greenhill LL, Posner K, Vaughan BS, Kratochvil CJ. Attention deficit hyperactivity disorder in preschool children. *Child Adolesc Psychiatr Clin N Am.* 2008;**17**(2):347–66, ix.

31. Connor DF. Preschool attention deficit hyperactivity disorder: a review of prevalence, diagnosis, neurobiology, and stimulant treatment. *J Dev Behav Pediatr.* 2002;**23**(1 Suppl):S1–9.

32. Firestone P, Musten LM, Pisterman S, Mercer J, Bennett S. Short-term side effects of stimulant medication are increased in preschool children with attention-deficit/hyperactivity disorder: a double-blind placebo-controlled study. *J Child Adolesc Psychopharmacol.* 1998;**8**(1):13–25.

33. Greenhill L, Kollins S, Abikoff H, *et al.* Efficacy and safety of immediate-release methylphenidate treatment for preschoolers with ADHD. *J Am Acad Child Adolesc Psychiatry.* 2006;**45**(11):1284–93.

34. Riddle MA, Yershova K, Lazzaretto D, *et al.* The Preschool Attention-Deficit/Hyperactivity Disorder Treatment Study (PATS) 6-year follow-up. *J Am Acad Child Adolesc Psychiatry.* 2013;**52**(3):264–78.e2.

35. Bodenheimer T, Wagner EH, Grumbach K. Improving primary care for patients with chronic illness: the chronic care model, Part 2. *JAMA.* 2002;**288**(15):1909–14.

36. Bodenheimer T, Wagner EH, Grumbach K. Improving primary care for patients with chronic illness. *JAMA.* 2002;**288**(14):1775–9.

37. Pliszka S. Practice parameter for the assessment and treatment of children and adolescents with attention-deficit/hyperactivity disorder. *J Am Acad Child Adolesc Psychiatry.* 2007;**46**(7):894–921.

38. American Academy of Pediatrics. Subcommittee on Attention-Deficit/Hyperactivity Disorder and Committee on Quality Improvement. Clinical practice guideline: treatment of the school-aged child with attention-deficit/hyperactivity disorder. *Pediatrics.* 2001;**108**(4):1033–44.

39. Pelham WE, Jr., Wheeler T, Chronis A. Empirically supported psychosocial treatments for attention deficit hyperactivity disorder. *J Clin Child Psychol.* 1998;**27**(2):190–205.

40. Eyberg SM, Nelson MM, Boggs SR. Evidence-based psychosocial treatments for children and adolescents

with disruptive behavior. *J Clin Child Adolesc Psychol.* 2008;**37**(1):215–37.

41. Ghuman JK, Arnold LE, Anthony BJ. Psychopharmacological and other treatments in preschool children with attention-deficit/hyperactivity disorder: current evidence and practice. *J Child Adolesc Psychopharmacol.* 2008;**18**(5):413–47.

42. Sonuga-Barke EJ, Daley D, Thompson M, Laver-Bradbury C, Weeks A. Parent-based therapies for preschool attention-deficit/hyperactivity disorder: a randomized, controlled trial with a community sample. *J Am Acad Child Adolesc Psychiatry.* 2001;**40**(4):402–8.

43. Strayhorn JM, Weidman C. Reduction of attention deficit and internalizing symptoms in preschoolers through parent-child interaction training. *J Am Acad Child Adolesc Psychiatry.* 1989;**28**(6):888–96.

44. Campbell SB. Behavior problems in preschool children: a review of recent research. *J Child Psychol Psychiatry.* 1995;**36**(1):113–49.

45. Cunningham CE, Boyle MH. Preschoolers at risk for attention-deficit hyperactivity disorder and oppositional defiant disorder: family, parenting, and behavioral correlates. *J Abnorm Child Psychol.* 2002;**30**(6):555–69.

46. Keown LJ, Woodward LJ. Early parent-child relations and family functioning of preschool boys with pervasive hyperactivity. *J Abnorm Child Psychol.* 2002;**30**(6):541–53.

47. Sonuga-Barke EJ, Daley D, Thompson M. Does maternal ADHD reduce the effectiveness of parent training for preschool children's ADHD? *J Am Acad Child Adolesc Psychiatry.* 2002;**41**(6):696–702.

48. Corrin EG. Child group training versus parent and child group training for young children with ADHD. In: *Dissertation Abstracts International: Section B: The Sciences & Engineering*; 2004.

49. Pisterman S, Firestone P, McGrath P, *et al.* The role of parent training in treatment of preschoolers with ADDH. *Am J Orthopsychiatry.* 1992;**62**(3):397–408.

50. Bor W, Sanders MR, Markie-Dadds C. The effects of the triple p-positive parenting program on preschool children with co-occurring disruptive behavior and attentional/hyperactive difficulties. *J Abnorm Child Psychol.* 2002;**30**(6):571–87.

51. Barkley RA, Shelton TL, Crosswait C, *et al.* Multi-method psycho-educational intervention for preschool children with disruptive behavior: preliminary results at post-treatment. *J Child Psychol Psychiatry.* 2000;**41**(3):319–32.

52. Huang HL, Chao CC, Tu CC, Yang PC. Behavioral parent training for Taiwanese parents of children with

attention-deficit/hyperactivity disorder. *Psychiatry Clin Neurosci.* 2003;**57**(3):275–81.

53. Shelton TL, Barkley RA, Crosswait C, *et al.* Multimethod psychoeducational intervention for preschool children with disruptive behavior: two-year post-treatment follow-up. *J Abnorm Child Psychol.* 2000;**28**(3):253–66.

54. Diagnosis and treatment of attention deficit hyperactivity disorder (ADHD). *NIH Consens Statement.* 1998;**16**(2):1–37.

55. MTA Cooperative Group. A 14-month randomized clinical trial of treatment strategies for attention-deficit/hyperactivity disorder. The MTA Cooperative Group. Multimodal Treatment Study of Children with ADHD. *Arch Gen Psychiatry.* 1999;**56**(12):1073–86.

56. Gleason MM, Egger HL, Emslie GJ, *et al.* Psychopharmacological treatment for very young children: contexts and guidelines. *J Am Acad Child Adolesc Psychiatry.* 2007;**46**(12):1532–72.

57. Maayan L, Paykina N, Fried J, *et al.* The open-label treatment of attention-deficit/hyperactivity disorder in 4- and 5-year-old children with beaded methylphenidate. *J Child Adolesc Psychopharmacol.* 2009;**19**(2):147–53.

58. Kratochvil CJ, Vaughan BS, Mayfield-Jorgensen ML, *et al.* A pilot study of atomoxetine in young children with attention-deficit/hyperactivity disorder. *J Child Adolesc Psychopharmacol.* 2007;**17**(2):175–85.

59. Kratochvil CJ, Vaughan BS, Daughton JM, *et al.* Atomoxetine vs placebo for the treatment of ADHD in 5- and 6-year-old children. 55th Annual Meeting of the American Academy of Child and Adolescent Psychiatry; 2008 October 27–31; Chicago, IL; 2008.

60. Kratochvil CJ, Wilens TE, Greenhill LL, *et al.* Effects of long-term atomoxetine treatment for young children with attention-deficit/hyperactivity disorder. *J Am Acad Child Adolesc Psychiatry.* 2006;**45**(8):919–27.

61. Jaselskis CA, Cook EH, Jr., Fletcher KE, Leventhal BL. Clonidine treatment of hyperactive and impulsive children with autistic disorder. *J Clin Psychopharmacol.* 1992;**12**(5):322–7.

62. Lubberstedt B, Vaughan B, Kratochvil C. Treatment of preschool ADHD: overview of the Preschool ADHD Treatment Study (PATS). *Child Adolesc Psychopharmacol News.* 2007;**12**(3):1–6.

63. Abikoff H, Vitiello B, Riddle M, *et al.* Methylphenidate effects on functional outcomes in the Preschoolers with Attention-Deficit/Hyperactivity Disorder Treatment Study (PATS). *J Child Adolesc Psychopharmacol.* 2007;**17**(5):581–92.

Chapter 26

ADHD and smoking

Scott Haden Kollins and Francis Joseph McClernon

Introduction

Cigarette smoking is the leading preventable cause of death and disability in the United States. Annually, smoking leads to more than 400 000 premature deaths in the USA and nearly 5 million deaths worldwide [1]. In the USA alone, $150 billion in annual costs are attributable to smoking-related illnesses and lost worker productivity [2].

Several large-scale, epidemiological studies have reported that individuals who have psychiatric disorders are significantly more likely to smoke than individuals from the general population [3, 4]. The prevalence of smoking among individuals with a current psychiatric condition is nearly double that of individuals without current mental illness [4, 5]. While individuals who reported a psychiatric diagnosis in the past month make up approximately 30% of the US population, they consume an estimated 44.3% of all cigarettes [4]. The number of co-occurring psychiatric disorders in an individual is also associated with higher levels of nicotine dependence and greater withdrawal severity [4, 6].

Most population- and clinic-based studies of smoking/psychiatric illness comorbidity have excluded attention-deficit hyperactivity disorder (ADHD). This may be because ADHD is often considered a disorder of childhood and is thus not included as a psychiatric condition category when studying samples of adults. However, in the few studies in which the disorder has been examined, ADHD shows comparable rates of comorbidity with cigarette smoking as other psychiatric disorders (approximately 40%) [7]. Moreover, recent evidence suggests that ADHD symptoms, even at levels below the threshold required to make a clinical diagnosis, are significantly associated with risk for smoking [8]. As such, a more thorough understanding of the relationship between ADHD and smoking has the potential to inform researchers and clinicians concerning mechanisms that underlie smoking risk in both ADHD diagnosed and non-ADHD individuals. Despite the well-established associations between ADHD and smoking, comparatively little experimental research has focused on this comorbidity.

In this chapter, we will first provide a brief overview of the clinical characteristics of both ADHD and cigarette smoking. We will describe current knowledge about the prevalence of comorbid ADHD and smoking (ADHD–smoking). We will concentrate on how ADHD and related problems influence different stages of smoking (e.g., initiation, maintenance, and relapse). The common potential molecular genetic substrates of ADHD and smoking will then be reviewed, with an emphasis on genes that regulate monoaminergic neurotransmission. Following directly from this review of the potential genetic substrates of this comorbidity, we will describe what is known about the behavioral and neuropharmacological bases of comorbid ADHD–smoking, focusing on nicotinic-acetylcholine receptor (nAChR) and dopamine (DA) systems that influence cognitive functions. Finally, we will discuss the clinical implications of the smoking–ADHD comorbidity and discuss the need to develop novel prevention and treatment efforts.

Attention-deficit hyperactivity disorder (ADHD)

ADHD is a genetically heritable, biologically driven disorder that involves developmentally inappropriate levels of inattention, hyperactivity, and impulsivity [9]. Details regarding the diagnosis and epidemiology of

Attention-Deficit Hyperactivity Disorder in Adults and Children, ed. Lenard A. Adler, Thomas J. Spencer and Timothy E. Wilens. Published by Cambridge University Press. © Cambridge University Press 2015.

ADHD are found elsewhere in this volume. It is important to consider, however, one aspect of the ADHD phenotype as pertains to risk for smoking. As is the case with many, if not most, psychiatric disorders, the prevalence of ADHD symptoms is distributed continuously in the population [10]. In other words, individuals may present with symptoms without meeting full criteria for the disorder. Data from several population-based studies have found that ADHD *symptoms* can be associated with smoking behavior, whether or not ADHD *diagnoses* are present [8, 11]. These and other studies will be explored further in subsequent sections of this review.

Cigarette smoking and nicotine dependence

Nicotine dependence is characterized by chronic and repetitive use of nicotine-containing products, withdrawal symptoms following cessation of use (e.g., depressed mood, irritability, restlessness), and inability to successfully quit despite knowledge that using such products is harmful to one's health [9]. Though a small number of individuals are able to maintain smoking behavior at low rates (i.e., <5 cigarettes/day), the majority of individuals who smoke do so at high rates [12]. However, not all smokers develop nicotine dependence: nearly 40% of individuals who smoke ≥10 cigarettes/day do not meet criteria for nicotine dependence [13].

Despite decreases in prevalence over the last three decades, approximately 20% of the adult US population smokes daily or nearly daily [14]. These rates are higher among individuals with lower education levels and who work in blue collar settings (both of which are more common among adults with ADHD) [15]. Experimentation with smoking typically begins during adolescent years. Regular, daily smoking typically starts soon thereafter [16, 17]. Quitting attempts among adult US smokers are frequent, but long-term unassisted quit rates are less than 5% at 6 months [2, 18, 19]. This is in spite of the fact that the majority of current smokers (nearly 69%) express interest in quitting [14]. Moreover, pharmacologically and behaviorally supported smoking cessation treatments typically result in overall low success rates. For instance, nicotine replacement therapies result in long-term abstinence rates (6–12 months) of less than 20% [20, 21]. Newer prescription medications including the nicotinic partial agonist varenicline have been shown to improve success rates [22].

Overall prevalence of ADHD/smoking

Clinical samples of individuals with ADHD smoke at rates significantly higher than the general population and/or non-diagnosed controls among both adults (41–42% vs. 26% for ADHD and non-ADHD, respectively) and adolescents (19.0–46% vs. 10–24% for ADHD and non-ADHD, respectively) [7, 23–25]. A number of studies have reported that the co-occurrence of ADHD and substance use disorders in general can be accounted for almost completely by the presence of comorbid conduct disorder (CD) [26–28]. However, ADHD has been shown to be a specific, independent risk factor for tobacco use in clinical and high-risk samples after controlling for comorbid CD [25, 29]. Moreover, there is evidence that specific problems with ADHD symptoms and related deficits in executive functioning significantly predict smoking, again even after controlling for conduct problems [25, 30, 31].

In addition to research with clinical samples, several studies have found significant associations between ADHD symptoms and smoking behavior in community samples of adolescents [11, 32]. In a population-based sample of over 15 000 young adults, a linear relation was identified between the number of retrospectively, self-reported ADHD symptoms and lifetime risk of regular smoking [8]. This study also found an inverse association between the number of ADHD symptoms and age of onset of smoking. Among current smokers, it identified a positive association between ADHD symptoms and number of cigarettes smoked per day. These findings are important because they raise the possibility that it is abnormalities in the underlying attentional processes that engender smoking risk, as opposed to categorical diagnoses of ADHD per se.

Influence of ADHD/ADHD symptoms on stages of smoking

Both ADHD and smoking are complex and heterogeneous phenotypes. As a result, there are myriad and complex ways in which ADHD-related phenotypes might facilitate transition to and through different smoking stages (i.e., initiation, progression, relapse). Independent evaluation of these associations can provide a more refined understanding of the mechanisms underlying the ADHD–smoking comorbidity, and lead to more targeted prevention and treatment strategies.

Initiation of smoking

There is evidence that ADHD individuals start smoking at an earlier age [24]. In a longitudinal study of 140 children with ADHD and 120 non-psychiatric controls, one study found that at 4-year follow-up (mean age = 15.0 ± 3.6 years), the children with ADHD smoked at rates nearly twice as high as the control children (19% vs. 10%, respectively). Moreover, the mean age of onset of smoking for the ADHD group was 15.5 ± 2.0 years versus 17.4 ± 2.3 years for the controls. In addition, 75% of the ADHD smokers began smoking prior to age 16 versus only 27% of the non-ADHD smokers [24]. These findings are comparable to another retrospective study that found earlier ages of both first cigarette use and regular use for smokers with ADHD compared to those without [33]. In a non-clinical, population-based study of young adults, age of onset of regular smoking was found to be significantly associated with the number of retrospectively reported ADHD symptoms. Individuals reporting the highest levels of symptoms started smoking approximately 1.25 years earlier than individuals reporting the lowest levels of symptoms (16.67–16.73 years versus 15.44–15.48 years) [8].

Progression to regular smoking

ADHD symptoms have also been shown to influence the trajectory of smoking behavior from initial use to regular use/dependence. One study found that a lifetime diagnosis of ADHD was a significant predictor of progression from initiation of smoking to daily use [34]. Another more recent study evaluated the relative contributions of inattentive versus hyperactive–impulsive ADHD symptoms on the progression of smoking behavior in a population-based study of young adults [35]. When compared to individuals reporting low levels of ADHD symptoms, those reporting high levels of hyperactive–impulsive ADHD symptoms were 1.9 times as likely to progress from no smoking at Wave 1 (mean age = 15.7 years) to regular smoking at Wave 3 (22.96 years). They were 3.25 times as likely to progress from experimentation at Wave 1 to regular smoking at Wave 3. This study also found that high levels of

Inattentive ADHD symptoms did not predict smoking progression [35].

Severity of regular smoking

Two studies in population-based samples have shown that levels of ADHD symptoms predict levels of nicotine use/dependence. Among current regular smokers, self-reported numbers of both hyperactive–impulsive and inattentive ADHD symptoms significantly predicted the number of cigarettes smoked/day [8]. A second study conducted using the same sample found that both ADHD symptom domains were associated with levels of nicotine dependence, as measured by the Fagerström Test of Nicotine Dependence, among current smokers [35]. These studies stand in contrast to two studies that have found no differences in numbers of cigarettes smoked or levels of nicotine dependence in adult smokers with ADHD compared with non-ADHD control groups [33, 36]. The differences across these studies may well relate to the sampling strategies used. The latter two studies were conducted with samples selected for both ADHD diagnosis and smoking status. The former studies were population-based samples; subjects were included in ways that did not depend on either of these factors. These differences highlight the importance of distinguishing between ADHD diagnoses and continuously measured ADHD symptoms.

Smoking cessation and relapse

There is evidence that ADHD and non-ADHD individuals may differ in their rates of quitting smoking and their ability to maintain smoking abstinence. The percentage of ever-smokers who became ex-smokers is lower among adults with ADHD (29%) compared to the general population (48.5%). Individuals with ADHD may thus have greater difficulty quitting [7]. Histories of childhood ADHD can predict worse smoking cessation outcomes, even after controlling for demographic, baseline smoking variables, and depression symptoms [37].

One possible explanation for these differences in quit rates and cessation outcomes is that smokers with ADHD can differ from non-ADHD smokers in the severity of withdrawal symptoms. Individuals with non-ADHD psychiatric comorbidities exhibit greater smoking withdrawal severity. Conceivably, this observation might help to explain why psychiatrically ill patients smoke at such high rates [4, 38].

Several studies have directly compared ADHD and non-ADHD smokers' withdrawal symptoms severities. In one study, retrospective smoking withdrawal symptoms were evaluated in adult smokers with current ADHD, adult smokers with a history of childhood but not current ADHD, and adult smokers who report neither childhood nor current ADHD. Individuals in the ADHD groups reported experiencing greater irritability and difficulty concentrating during quit attempts compared to smokers without a history of or current ADHD [33].

In another study, ADHD symptoms were measured prospectively in ADHD and non-ADHD smokers in a laboratory setting [36]. No significant differences in self-reported withdrawal symptom severity were observed between the two groups following 12-hour abstinence. However, following abstinence, ADHD smokers exhibited greater worsening of performance on a continuous performance test, with greater numbers of errors of commissions and greater reaction time variability than did non-ADHD smokers.

Another study examined adult smokers with and without ADHD during a longer-term abstinence period (2 weeks) [39]. In this study, smokers were paid to stop smoking for up to 2 weeks and withdrawal symptoms were measured each day. In general, smokers with ADHD exhibited greater withdrawal severity, particularly during the first 5 days of abstinence. Interestingly, this effect was largely driven by female smokers with ADHD, who endorsed higher levels of craving, somatic symptoms, and negative affect compared to smokers without ADHD and compared to male smokers with ADHD. Importantly, this study also showed that increases in withdrawal symptoms occurred independently of changes in ADHD symptoms [39].

Collectively, these findings suggest that ADHD smokers may be differentially sensitive to the effects of smoking abstinence, and that these withdrawal effects are likely related to both sex and the perceived duration of abstinence. This differential sensitivity might encompass effects on both withdrawal symptomatology and changes in cognitive function. These changes may also lead to increased risk for relapse in individuals with ADHD or high levels of ADHD symptoms that accompany quit attempts.

Section summary

ADHD phenotypes, defined either as *Diagnostic and Statistical Manual of Mental Disorders* (DSM)-based clinical diagnoses or as continuously distributed symptom counts, have each been shown to be significantly associated with all stages of smoking, including smoking initiation, progression to regular use, level of smoking/nicotine dependence, and withdrawal/relapse. While these studies demonstrate important links between ADHD and various aspects of smoking behavior as it develops over time, they have largely been retrospective in nature, thus limiting our ability to draw conclusions about underlying mechanisms or causality. Studies that are both prospective and longitudinal in nature and studies that track the trajectory of ADHD symptoms/diagnosis and smoking outcomes are needed to further understanding of the mechanisms for this ADHD–smoking comorbidity.

Common genetic substrates of ADHD and tobacco smoking

Both ADHD and smoking are highly heritable; genetic factors account for 60–80% and 56% of the two phenotypes, respectively [40, 41]. Candidate gene studies have identified a number of similar genetic markers associated with both ADHD and smoking phenotypes, suggesting that several common neurobiological mechanisms may give rise to ADHD–smoking comorbidity [42–45].

Molecular genetics of ADHD and treatment response

A recent meta-analytic review identified variants in seven genes that have been shown to have statistically significant evidence of association with ADHD on the basis of pooled odds ratios across at least three studies [40]. Four of these genes are involved in DA neurotransmission and metabolism: the DA D_4 and D_5 receptor genes (*DRD4*, *DRD5*), the DA transporter gene (*DAT1*), and the dopamine beta-hydroxylase gene (*DBH*). Two additional genes are involved in serotonin neurotransmission: the serotonin receptor 1B gene (*HTR1B*) and the serotonin transporter gene (*5HTT*). Finally, the synaptosomal-association protein 25 gene (*SNAP-25*), variants of which result in significant hyperactivity in mouse models and are related to exocytotic neurotransmitter release, has been shown to have significant evidence of association with ADHD.

There is also evidence that the efficacy of stimulant drugs such as methylphenidate in the treatment of ADHD is moderated, in part, by genetic factors [46]. For example, variations of both the *DRD4* and *DAT1* genes have been shown to influence efficacy of methylphenidate in trials with pediatric populations [47–49]. In addition, there is some evidence that genetic variants are also associated with the potential for side effects associated with stimulant treatment in children diagnosed with ADHD [50].

Several genome-wide linkage-based studies of ADHD have been published [51]. Considered separately, three of the studies have reported logarithm of the odds (LOD) scores indicating definite or suggestive linkage on three different chromosomes (16p13, 15q, and 11q22) [52–54]. The only chromosomal region that has been shown to have a LOD score >1 in more than one of the separate studies was located at 5p13 [53–55]. Interestingly, this region is also close to the location for the candidate gene *DAT1*; variation in the *DAT1* gene might conceivably contribute to the linkage findings at the 5p13 locus. A number of large-scale efforts are currently underway throughout the world that will greatly increase power to detect meaningful linkage in larger samples [56].

Smoking

Candidate gene studies of smoking behavior have focused on many of the same monoamine regulating genes as have ADHD studies. Variants of the *DRD4*, *DAT*, and *DBH* genes, as well as the *HTR1B* and *5HTT* genes have been shown to be associated with higher levels of smoking behavior in a range of populations [57–65]. In addition, a haplotype of the *DRD5* gene has been shown to be protective against smoking phenotypes [66]. In a meta-analytic review of candidate genes associated with multiple smoking phenotypes, modest yet significant associations were observed between *DRD2* and both smoking initiation and consumption; and the long promoter region of the *5HTT* gene (*5HTTLPR*) and smoking cessation outcomes [44]. The 7-repeat (or longer) allele of the *DRD4* VNTR has also been associated with behavioral and brain responses to smoking-related cues, suggesting the D$_4$ receptor system potentially plays a critical role in cue-provoked smoking and relapse [58, 67].

More recently, greater attention has been paid to candidate genes involved in nicotinic receptor system activity [68, 69]. Single nucleotide polymorphisms (SNPs) of the nicotinic receptor alpha4 subunit gene (*CHRNA4*) have been associated with a range of

smoking phenotypes [69, 70]. SNPs of the beta2 subunit gene (*CRHNB2*) have been shown to be associated with initial response to smoking but not with nicotine dependence [70, 71].

As with ADHD, a growing number of genome-wide linkage studies have been conducted in a search for the genetic bases for smoking phenotypes. To date, regions on chromosomes 9, 10, 11, and 17 have been most reliably replicated [72]. Genes within these regions regulate a wide range of functions, some with obvious connections to neurotransmitter function (e.g., GABA receptor 2 on chromosome 9).

Recent data also suggest genetic factors account for approximately half of the variability in relapse following a quit attempt [38]. Pharmacogenetic trials have provided preliminary evidence that many of the same genes associated with nicotine dependence are modestly related to smoking cessation outcomes [73]. For instance, the *Taq*1 A2/A2 allele at the *DRD2/ANKK1* gene locus was associated with better nicotine replacement therapy outcomes, but only among female smokers [74]. Similarly, the *Taq*1A allele of the *DRD2/ANKK1* locus was associated with less responsiveness to bupropion [75].

Overlap in genetic substrates of ADHD and smoking

Clearly, there is considerable overlap in the genetic substrates of ADHD and smoking behavior, with a number of candidate genes exhibiting associations with both phenotypes, most notably *DRD4* and *DAT1* [40, 44]. In addition, several studies have examined the relationship among genes, smoking, and ADHD. A study that examined interactions between gene and ADHD symptoms found effects for both *DRD2* and, among females, *MAO-A* [76]. In that study, carriers of the *DRD2/ANKK1 Taq*1 A2/A2 allele with six or more hyperactivity/impulsivity symptoms were almost twice as likely to have a history of smoking as individuals carrying the A1 allele. Another study observed significant interactive effects of in utero exposure to smoking and either *DAT1* or *DRD4* polymorphisms in predicting combined type ADHD [77]. This same group observed a similar interaction between in utero smoke exposure and an exon 5 polymorphism of the *CHRNA4* gene in predicting combined type ADHD [78].

Genes regulating nicotinic receptor functioning are another group of potential targets that might allow us to identify genetic overlaps between ADHD and smoking. As noted above, a number of studies have found that variation in these genes can relate to smoking behavior. In addition, at least five studies have examined relations between the *CHRNA4* gene and ADHD. However, findings have been mixed. One study found significant association between variation in this gene and a quantitative phenotype of ADHD while another study failed to identify any significant association between the gene and ADHD [79, 80]. Three additional studies have reported nominally significant association between the *CHRNA4* gene and ADHD phenotypes [81–83]. No association was observed between ADHD and *CHRNA7* microsatellite markers [84]. Although the interactive effects of nicotinic receptor genes and psychiatric symptomatology has been studied in the context of schizophrenia, no similar studies have been conducted for ADHD. This provides an obvious area for additional research [85].

Section summary

The literature presented here suggests a great deal of commonality in the genetic substrates underlying both ADHD and smoking. Most of this overlap involves genes that regulate monoaminergic transmission, with a particular focus on DA system genes, especially *DRD4* and *DAT1*. Evidence also suggests that nicotinic receptor genes may also be associated with both smoking and ADHD. The few studies that have examined relations among genes, smoking, and ADHD have shown that (1) ADHD symptoms interact with genes to increase smoking risk; and (2) in utero smoke exposure may interact with genes to increase the odds of ADHD. These studies highlight the need for additional work to more precisely characterize the pathways from genetic variation to both smoking and ADHD-related phenotypes. Additionally, while genome-wide linkage studies are available for both ADHD and smoking phenotypes, these studies have not shown common areas of linkage. Future genome-wide association analyses of samples that include both ADHD and smoking status as phenotypes may be required to determine whether specific chromosomal regions confer risk for both conditions. Pharmacogenetic studies have identified genetic markers for ADHD and smoking cessation treatment response separately. Future research might seek to identify whether smoking status interacts with genotype to predict ADHD treatment outcomes; or conversely whether ADHD status interacts with genotype to predict smoking cessation outcomes.

Neuropharmacological and behavioral factors in ADHD–smoking

Despite the relative lack of direct work concerning the mechanisms responsible for increased risks of smoking in individuals with ADHD, several lines of research provide convergent evidence that neurobiological and behavioral factors may both contribute to the high rates of smoking in these individuals.

Neurobiological/neuropharmacological factors

From a neuropharmacological perspective, ADHD is hypothesized to be the result of an aberrant striatal dopaminergic system that results in disrupted dopaminergic transmission in corticostriatal circuits. These disruptions in turn give rise to the characteristic deficits in executive functioning observed in ADHD patients [86, 87]. This altered DA hypothesis is supported by studies showing differences in DA transporter (DAT) density in relevant striatal areas in ADHD patients compared to controls [88–97]. Although these studies have reported discrepant findings with respect to the direction of DAT density change (i.e., some report higher levels, some report lower levels in ADHD), collectively they suggest associations of DAT density and its consequent effects on DA neurotransmission with the clinical condition of ADHD.

Drawing on both preclinical and clinical studies, one possible implication of altered DA functioning is that ADHD patients exhibit lower DA tone due to lower than normal activation of presynaptic DA autoreceptors, resulting in exaggerated phasic DA responses to salient stimuli [86]. Nicotine has been shown to stimulate DA release in the striatum of both animals and human smokers [98, 99]. We therefore propose that nicotine-stimulated phasic DA release may be more rewarding in ADHD compared to non-ADHD individuals. This enhanced reward salience would lead to higher levels of nicotine reinforcement after first use, thus facilitating the transition to continued use in this population. In other words, ADHD patients might experience higher initial rewarding effects of nicotine than those without ADHD due to fundamental differences in DA function.

Behavioral mechanisms: attention, behavior inhibition, and ADHD symptoms

At a behavioral level of analysis, several different processes could account for the higher rates of smoking among individuals with ADHD or with high levels of ADHD symptoms. It has been proposed that nicotine use may be negatively reinforced in some individuals by reducing the characteristic symptoms of ADHD, even if those symptoms do not reach clinical thresholds [32]. This so-called "self-medication" explanation has garnered considerable speculation, though empirical evidence for the validity of such a mechanism is lacking [100]. Specific processes that might contribute to the high rates of smoking in individuals with ADHD include increased withdrawal severity (*reviewed above*) and the direct effects of nicotine on attention, behavioral inhibition, and ADHD symptoms.

Attention

Nicotine has been shown to improve performance on a range of attentional tasks in both human and non-humans [101–103]. In human studies, nicotine administration has been shown to improve performance on attentional tasks in regular smokers and in non-smokers [104, 105]. For example, one study found that smoking improved abstinence-related cognitive disruptions in smokers with schizophrenia [106]. Nicotine administration has also been shown to enhance attentional performance in smoking and non-smoking adults diagnosed with ADHD. Specifically, transdermal nicotine (7 mg or 21 mg administered to non-smokers and smokers, respectively) decreased both reaction time and reaction time variability on a continuous performance task (CPT) [107].

Behavioral inhibition

Behavioral inhibition is a broad construct relating to an individual's ability to withhold an inappropriate or maladaptive response. Deficits in behavioral inhibition are theorized to be central distinguishing features of individuals with ADHD versus non-diagnosed individuals [108]. The effects of nicotine on behavioral inhibition may be more subtle than those observed for attention. Studies of non-smokers suggest that nicotine only marginally improves behavioral inhibition as measured by errors of commission on a CPT [104, 109]. Among non-smoking adolescents and young individuals with ADHD, nicotine enhanced one measure of response inhibition, Stop Signal reaction time, but had no effect on a CPT measure of response inhibition in adult non-smokers [110–112].

ADHD symptoms

Nicotine has also demonstrated clinical efficacy for individuals with ADHD. One study in ADHD patients showed that transdermal nicotine (7 mg/day) improved clinical global impressions of ADHD symptomatology while it increased self-ratings of positive affect [107]. Two other studies have shown that novel nicotinic agonists display efficacy in reducing both inattentive and hyperactive–impulsive symptoms in adults with ADHD [113, 114]. Efficacy in these latter studies were not altered by current or lifetime smoking status.

The above evidence indicates that nicotine and nicotinic agonists improve symptoms of ADHD, lending support to "self-medication" hypotheses of smoking among individuals with ADHD. Several caveats to this conceptualization are worth mentioning, however. First, studies demonstrating beneficial effects of nicotine on cognition in smokers cannot distinguish between absolute effects of nicotine versus their benefits in alleviating withdrawal. Further, most of the small number of human studies that show beneficial effects of nicotine on attention, impulsivity, and ADHD symptoms in non-smokers had small sample sizes and produced effects of relatively small magnitude. Thus, while a small but growing body of evidence points to negatively reinforced reduction in ADHD symptoms by smoking, additional research is needed to accurately evaluate both the magnitude and scope of this phenomenon.

Clinical implications of the smoking–ADHD comorbidity

One of the front-line treatments for children and adults with ADHD is stimulant medication, including both methylphenidate-based and amphetamine-based products. Hundreds of studies have documented the efficacy and safety of these products for treating the core symptoms of ADHD, including inattention, impulsivity, and hyperactivity in both adults and children [115, 116]. However, the role that stimulant medication may play both as a precursor or risk factor for subsequent cigarette smoking, and as a precipitant for *increased* smoking in already regular smokers has been a controversial topic for a number of years.

Regarding the former issue, an early study raised the possibility that early stimulant treatment increased the risk for regular cigarette smoking in adults in a longitudinal cohort of hyperactive and control children ([23] but see Mick *et al.* [117]). A number of other longitudinal studies, however, have failed to replicate these findings, and report that early stimulant treatment either has no effect on subsequent risk of cigarette smoking, or actually reduces the risk [118–120]. Similarly, a naturalistic study of medicated and unmedicated youth with ADHD reported that the unmedicated children were more likely to smoke and had higher mean salivary cotinine levels (a biomarker for tobacco use) across the early years of high school compared to their medicated peers [121].

Both clinical and laboratory studies have addressed the question of how stimulant medications affect cigarette smoking among individuals who are already regular smokers with somewhat discrepant findings. Several laboratory-based studies have shown that both amphetamine and methylphenidate increase cigarette smoking in psychiatrically healthy regular smokers. Two studies demonstrated that d-amphetamine significantly increased the relative reinforcing effects of smoking versus money measured using a progressive ratio task or a choice procedure in regular adult smokers [122, 123]. Similarly, methylphenidate has been reported to dose-dependently increase both ad libitum smoking and choices of cigarette puffs over money in psychiatrically healthy regular adult smokers [124, 125].

As noted, all of these laboratory studies of stimulant drug effects on cigarette smoking were conducted with psychiatrically healthy individuals. More recently, Vansickel and colleagues reported a similar finding in regular adult smokers diagnosed with ADHD. In this study, nine regular smokers (10–20 cigarettes/day) who met criteria for adult ADHD were exposed to placebo and three different doses of immediate-release methylphenidate (10 mg, 20 mg, 40 mg) in separate experimental sessions under double-blind conditions. Outcome measures included total number of cigarette puffs per 4-hour session, exhaled carbon monoxide (CO), and total cigarettes smoked per session. Results showed that under the 10 mg and 40 mg conditions, adult smokers with ADHD smoked significantly more cigarettes than under the placebo conditions. Similar findings were reported for the number of cigarette puffs and exhaled CO [126].

In contrast to these laboratory findings, several clinical/naturalistic studies have shown that stimulant medication either has no effect on or reduces cigarette smoking in patients with ADHD. For example, smokers with ADHD who took their regularly prescribed stimulant medication (either methylphenidate or amphetamine based) during a naturalistic study had lower salivary cotinine levels than when they took placebo, suggesting that they smoked less while taking stimulants [127]. Similarly, in a large (n = 255) randomized, double-blind, placebo-controlled trial of osmotic-release methylphenidate in adult smokers with ADHD, stimulant-treated smokers showed a small but significant reduction in cigarettes smoked per day compared to those treated with placebo [128].

An integrated model of ADHD–smoking comorbidity

Despite the considerable amount of descriptive work that has characterized associations between ADHD and smoking, relatively little research has been conducted to elucidate the mechanisms underlying this common comorbidity. In an effort to consolidate what is known and to also generate hypotheses to be tested in future research we have developed a multifactor model of nicotine use and dependence in ADHD. Relevant aspects of this model are reviewed below.

Individuals with ADHD exhibit psychological and biological vulnerabilities that influence both the likelihood that they might experiment with nicotine and the reinforcing effects of initial use. With respect to risk for experimentation, individuals with ADHD are more impulsive, score higher on measures of novelty seeking, and have more problematic peer interactions than non-diagnosed individuals. Each of these factors is considered an independent risk factor for smoking [129–136]. This overlap in psychological/social risk is likely to be driven, in part, by common genetic and neurobiological factors.

From a neuropharmacological perspective, ADHD is hypothesized to result from aberrant striatal dopaminergic systems that result in disrupted dopaminergic transmission in corticostriatal circuits. These disruptions in turn can give rise to the characteristic deficits in executive functioning observed in ADHD patients. They have important implications for several aspects of smoking behavior as reviewed above. First, individuals with ADHD are hypothesized to have lower tonic DA which may amplify the phasic DA response stimulated by nicotine which in turn may enhance the reward salience of smoking in this population. Second, deficits in attentional and inhibitory control functions are reduced by nicotine, which negatively reinforces continued use. Third, upon quitting smoking, individuals with ADHD experience greater withdrawal symptom severity and greater disruption of inhibitory control, increasing the likelihood of relapse. Finally, higher baseline levels of impulsivity and greater sensitivity to salient reward-related cues may confound efforts to maintain smoking abstinence.

There are a number of family/social variables represented in this model that have not been thoroughly evaluated in this review, but that represent important moderators/mediators of the association between ADHD and smoking. For example, it is well established that deviant peer relations and parenting styles are associated with both ADHD and smoking [137–141]. Delineating more precisely the manner in which these and related constructs interact should help us to better understand the developmental trajectory of smoking behavior in individuals with ADHD and/or with high levels of ADHD symptoms.

Prevention and treatment implications

The above model highlights a number of compelling research questions that could help us to elucidate mechanisms underlying the prevalent comorbidity of ADHD and smoking. A critical aspect of any model of maladaptive behavior, however, is the extent to which it can inform clinical and community-based interventions.

The foregoing review and proposed framework suggest several applications for preventing and reducing smoking/nicotine dependence in individuals who are vulnerable as a result of ADHD and related risk factors. As reviewed above, a number of studies have shown that both a diagnosis of ADHD and ADHD symptomatology (independent of clinical diagnosis) are associated with lifetime risk of regular smoking, higher levels of smoking, and earlier initiation of smoking. These findings suggest that young people with ADHD and/or those who manifest a number of ADHD symptoms might be preferentially targeted for prevention efforts. A sizable literature exists

on community- and school-based smoking prevention programs [142, 143]. It is not known, however, whether individuals at risk for smoking as a result of ADHD-related problems would benefit from existing prevention programs, or if they would require novel alternative approaches. Several of the more successful current prevention programs focus on peer and family influences [142, 143]. It is well established, however, that individuals with ADHD have significant deficits in peer relationships [144]. Further, coping skills and parent–child communication have been shown to mediate the association between ADHD and smoking outcomes [145]. As such, individuals with ADHD or related symptomatology may benefit from prevention programs that specifically target these important mediating processes.

As noted previously, the question of whether early pharmacotherapy for ADHD influences risk for subsequent cigarette smoking is controversial. The data to date, however, suggest that, at worst, treatment of children with ADHD using medication has no effect on subsequent risk of smoking. One small randomized prevention study even demonstrated a positive protective effect of stimulant drug use [146]. Given the demonstrated beneficial effects of pharmacotherapy on a number of other factors known to mediate risk for smoking, and the lack of consistent evidence of a deleterious effect, increasing risk for cigarette smoking should not be an important consideration when deciding on pharmacotherapy for youth with ADHD.

Our review and proposed model also form the basis for several innovative approaches to treating individuals with ADHD and related problems who have initiated regular smoking. It has been shown that individuals with ADHD have a harder time quitting smoking and show more significant signs and symptoms of smoking withdrawal [7, 33, 36]. Based on these findings and much of the other literature reviewed, an argument could be made that individuals with ADHD and related problems smoke, in part, to reduce the requisite symptoms of inattention, hyperactivity, and impulsivity. Based on this conceptualization, treatment strategies that improve these deficits prior to and during a quit attempt may be successful in facilitating smoking cessation among individuals with ADHD. Although a recent study evaluated the effects of osmotic-release methylphenidate on smoking cessation in adults with ADHD and found no difference in abstinence rates compared with placebo

[128], additional work is needed to determine whether there may be subgroups of ADHD smokers who differentially benefit from stimulant treatment. For example in a secondary analysis of the Winhusen study [128], a recent report indicated that among heavily dependent smokers, osmotic-release oral system (OROS) methylphenidate worked particularly well to maintain abstinence compared with placebo among combined type patients, but the opposite was true for Inattentive type patients [147].

Considering the literature, it would seem that at least among adult smokers with ADHD who are interested in quitting, treatment with stimulant medication has little effect on smoking behavior and can be effective in reducing ADHD symptoms and impairment [128]. However, there is evidence, albeit limited, that among adult smokers with ADHD who are not interested in quitting, that immediate-release stimulants may increase rates of smoking behavior [126]. Collectively, these data suggest that clinicians working with adults with ADHD should be mindful both of the smoking status of their patients and their motivation level for quitting when considering treatment options. For those patients who are smokers, clinicians should address cessation options as part of treatment and monitor rates of smoking if pharmacotherapy is initiated.

Novel pharmacological interventions that target either cholinergic or dopaminergic systems have shown some promise in treating both smoking and ADHD. For example, bupropion has shown efficacy in treating adults with ADHD and is also a US Food and Drug Administration (FDA)-approved aid to smoking cessation [146, 148, 149]. Novel cholinergic agents have also shown promise in treating adults with ADHD [113, 114]. Whether these agents would work for treating comorbid ADHD–smoking is largely unknown, although one open-label pilot study with adolescents reported positive results [150].

Based on the conceptualization reported here for how ADHD and smoking behavior might be related, it stands to reason that non-pharmacological approaches to treating ADHD might also be useful in facilitating smoking cessation. Emerging work shows promise for the use of cognitive-behavioral treatment of adults with ADHD. It would be important to evaluate whether these treatment approaches would serve as useful adjuncts to smoking cessation in those with ADHD [151].

Conclusions

Tobacco use among individuals diagnosed with ADHD or among individuals with elevated ADHD symptoms represents a significant public health problem. Significant progress has been made in the last 5–10 years to understand the prevalence and developmental trajectory of ADHD and smoking. More recent work has begun to focus on the genetic and neural underpinnings of these comorbid problems. Significantly more work is necessary before a full picture of the mechanisms underlying this association is available. As these underlying mechanisms are elucidated more fully, progress can be made in developing novel prevention and treatment strategies for reducing the harm associated with tobacco smoking in this population.

References

1. Ezzati M, Lopez AD. Estimates of global mortality attributable to smoking in 2000. *Lancet*. 2003;**362**: 847–52.

2. Centers for Disease Control and Prevention (CDC). Cigarette smoking among adults – United States, 2006. *MMWR Morb Mortal Wkly Rep*. 2007;**56**:1157–61.

3. Grant BF, Hasin DS, Chou SP, Stinson FS, Dawson DA. Nicotine dependence and psychiatric disorders in the United States: results from the national epidemiologic survey on alcohol and related conditions. *Arch Gen Psychiatry*. 2004;**61**:1107–15.

4. Lasser K, Boyd JW, Woolhandler S, *et al*. Smoking and mental illness: a population-based prevalence study. *JAMA*. 2000;**284**:2606–10.

5. Breslau N. Psychiatric comorbidity of smoking and nicotine dependence. *Behav Genet*. 1995;**25**:95–101.

6. John U, Meyer C, Rumpf HJ, Hapke U. Smoking, nicotine dependence and psychiatric comorbidity–a population-based study including smoking cessation after three years. *Drug Alcohol Depend*. 2004;**76**: 287–95.

7. Pomerleau OF, Downey KK, Stelson FW, Pomerleau CS. Cigarette smoking in adult patients diagnosed with attention deficit hyperactivity disorder. *J Subst Abuse*. 1995;**7**:373–8.

8. Kollins SH, McClernon FJ, Fuemmeler BF. Association between smoking and attention-deficit/hyperactivity disorder symptoms in a population-based sample of young adults. *Arch Gen Psychiatry*. 2005;**62**:1142–7.

9. American Psychiatric Association. *Diagnostic and Statistical Manual of Mental Disorders*, 4th edn., text rev. (DSM-IV-TR). Washington, DC: American Psychiatric Association; 2000.

10. Rasmussen ER, Todd RD, Neuman RJ, *et al.* Comparison of male adolescent-report of attention-deficit/hyperactivity disorder (ADHD) symptoms across two cultures using latent class and principal components analysis. *J Child Psychol Psychiatry.* 2002;**43**:797–805.

11. Tercyak KP, Lerman C, Audrain J. Association of attention-deficit/hyperactivity disorder symptoms with levels of cigarette smoking in a community sample of adolescents. *J Am Acad Child Adolesc Psychiatry.* 2002;**41**:799–805.

12. Shiffman S. Tobacco "chippers"–individual differences in tobacco dependence. *Psychopharmacology (Berl).* 1989;**97**:539–47.

13. Donny EC, Dierker LC. The absence of DSM-IV nicotine dependence in moderate-to-heavy daily smokers. *Drug Alcohol Depend.* 2007;**89**:93–6.

14. CDC. Quitting smoking among adults–United States, 2001–2010. *MMWR Morb Mortal Wkly Rep.* 2011;**60**:1513–19.

15. CDC. Current cigarette smoking prevalence among working adults–United States, 2004–2010. *MMWR Morb Mortal Wkly Rep.* 2011;**60**:1305–9.

16. Gilpin EA, Choi WS, Berry C, Pierce JP. How many adolescents start smoking each day in the United States? *J Adolesc Health.* 1999;**25**:248–55.

17. Tucker JS, Ellickson PL, Klein DJ. Predictors of the transition to regular smoking during adolescence and young adulthood. *J Adolesc Health.* 2003;**32**:314–24.

18. Gritz ER, Carr CR, Marcus AC. The tobacco withdrawal syndrome in unaided quitters. *Br J Addict.* 1991;**86**:57–69.

19. Hughes JR, Gulliver SB, Fenwick JW *et al.* Smoking cessation among self-quitters. *Health Psychol.* 1992;**11**:331–4.

20. Croghan GA, Sloan JA, Croghan IT, *et al.* Comparison of nicotine patch alone versus nicotine nasal spray alone versus a combination for treating smokers: a minimal intervention, randomized multicenter trial in a nonspecialized setting. *Nicotine Tob Res.* 2003;**5**:181–7.

21. Lerman C, Kaufmann V, Rukstalis M, *et al.* Individualizing nicotine replacement therapy for the treatment of tobacco dependence: a randomized trial. *Ann Intern Med.* 2004;**140**:426–33.

22. Nides M, Oncken C, Gonzales D, *et al.* Smoking cessation with varenicline, a selective alpha4beta2 nicotinic receptor partial agonist: results from a 7-week, randomized, placebo- and bupropion-controlled trial with 1-year follow-up. *Arch Intern Med.* 2006,**166**.1561–8.

23. Lambert NM, Hartsough CS. Prospective study of tobacco smoking and substance dependencies among

samples of ADHD and non-ADHD participants. *J Learn Disabil.* 1998;**31**:533–44.

24. Milberger S, Biederman J, Faraone SV, Chen L, Jones J. ADHD is associated with early initiation of cigarette smoking in children and adolescents. *J Am Acad Child Adolesc Psychiatry.* 1997;**36**:37–44.

25. Molina BS, Pelham WE, Jr. Childhood predictors of adolescent substance use in a longitudinal study of children with ADHD. *J Abnorm Psychol.* 2003;**112**:497–507.

26. Barkley RA, Fischer M, Edelbrock CS, Smallish L. The adolescent outcome of hyperactive children diagnosed by research criteria: I. An 8-year prospective follow-up study. *J Am Acad Child Adolesc Psychiatry.* 1990;**29**:546–57.

27. Biederman J, Wilens T, Mick E, *et al.* Is ADHD a risk factor for psychoactive substance use disorders? Findings from a four-year prospective follow-up study. *J Am Acad Child Adolesc Psychiatry.* 1997;**36**:21–9.

28. Boyle MH, Offord DR. Psychiatric disorder and substance use in adolescence. *Can J Psychiatry.* 1991;**36**:699–705.

29. Milberger S, Biederman J, Faraone SV, Wilens T, Chu MP. Associations between ADHD and psychoactive substance use disorders. Findings from a longitudinal study of high-risk siblings of ADHD children. *Am J Addict.* 1997;**6**:318–29.

30. Aytaclar S, Tarter RE, Kirisci L, Lu S. Association between hyperactivity and executive cognitive functioning in childhood and substance use in early adolescence. *J Am Acad Child Adolesc Psychiatry.* 1999;**38**:172–8.

31. Burke JD, Loeber R, Lahey BB. Which aspects of ADHD are associated with tobacco use in early adolescence? *J Child Psychol Psychiatry.* 2001;**42**:493–502.

32. Whalen CK, Jamner LD, Henker B, Delfino RJ, Lozano JM. The ADHD spectrum and everyday life: experience sampling of adolescent moods, activities, smoking, and drinking. *Child Dev.* 2002;**73**:209–27.

33. Pomerleau CS, Downey KK, Snedecor SM, *et al.* Smoking patterns and abstinence effects in smokers with no ADHD, childhood ADHD, and adult ADHD symptomatology. *Addict Behav.* 2003;**28**:1149–57.

34. Rohde P, Kahler CW, Lewinsohn PM, Brown RA. Psychiatric disorders, familial factors, and cigarette smoking: II. Associations with progression to daily smoking. *Nicotine Tob Res.* 2004;**6**:119–32.

35. Fuemmeler BF, Kollins SH, McClernon FJ. Attention deficit hyperactivity disorder symptoms predict nicotine dependence and progression to regular

smoking from adolescence to young adulthood. *J Pediatr Psychol.* 2007;**32**:1203–13.

36. McClernon FJ, Kollins SH, Lutz AM, *et al.* Effects of smoking abstinence on adult smokers with and without attention deficit hyperactivity disorder: results of a preliminary study. *Psychopharmacology (Berl).* 2008;**197**:95–105.

37. Humfleet GL, Prochaska JJ, Mengis M, *et al.* Preliminary evidence of the association between the history of childhood attention-deficit/hyperactivity disorder and smoking treatment failure. *Nicotine Tob Res.* 2005;**7**:453–60.

38. Xian H, Scherrer JF, Madden PA, *et al.* The heritability of failed smoking cessation and nicotine withdrawal in twins who smoked and attempted to quit. *Nicotine Tob Res.* 2003;**5**:245–54.

39. McClernon FJ, Van Voorhees EE, English J, *et al.* Smoking withdrawal symptoms are more severe among smokers with ADHD and independent of ADHD symptom change: results from a 12-day contingency-managed abstinence trial. *Nicotine Tob Res.* 2011;**13**:784–92.

40. Faraone SV, Perlis RH, Doyle AE, *et al.* Molecular genetics of attention-deficit/hyperactivity disorder. *Biol Psychiatry.* 2005;**57**:1313–23.

41. Li MD, Cheng R, Ma JZ, Swan GE. A meta-analysis of estimated genetic and environmental effects on smoking behavior in male and female adult twins. *Addiction.* 2003;**98**:23–31.

42. Li MD, Ma JZ, Beuten J. Progress in searching for susceptibility loci and genes for smoking-related behaviour. *Clin Genet.* 2004;**66**:382–92.

43. Maher BS, Marazita ML, Ferrell RE, Vanyukov MM. Dopamine system genes and attention deficit hyperactivity disorder: a meta-analysis. *Psychiatr Genet.* 2002;**12**:207–15.

44. Munafo M, Clark T, Johnstone E, Murphy M, Walton R. The genetic basis for smoking behavior: a systematic review and meta-analysis. *Nicotine Tob Res.* 2004;**6**:583–97.

45. Todd RD, Huang H, Smalley SL, *et al.* Collaborative analysis of DRD4 and DAT genotypes in population-defined ADHD subtypes. *J Child Psychol Psychiatry.* 2005;**46**:1067–73.

46. McGough JJ. Attention-deficit/hyperactivity disorder pharmacogenomics. *Biol Psychiatry.* 2005;**57**: 1367–73.

47. Hamarman S, Fossella J, Ulger C, Brimacombe M, Dermody J. Dopamine receptor 4 (DRD4) 7-repeat allele predicts methylphenidate dose response in children with attention deficit hyperactivity disorder: a pharmacogenetic study. *J Child Adolesc Psychopharmacol.* 2004;**14**:564–74.

48. Joober R, Grizenko N, Sengupta S, *et al.* Dopamine transporter 3′-UTR VNTR genotype and ADHD: a pharmaco-behavioural genetic study with methylphenidate. *Neuropsychopharmacology.* 2007;**32**:1370–6.

49. Stein MA, Waldman ID, Sarampote CS, *et al.* Dopamine transporter genotype and methylphenidate dose response in children with ADHD. *Neuropsychopharmacology.* 2005;**30**:1374–82.

50. McGough J, McCracken J, Swanson J, *et al.* Pharmacogenetics of methylphenidate response in preschoolers with ADHD. *J Am Acad Child Adolesc Psychiatry.* 2006;**45**:1314–22.

51. Albayrak O, Friedel S, Schimmelmann BG, Hinney A, Hebebrand J. Genetic aspects in attention-deficit/ hyperactivity disorder. *J Neural Transm.* 2008;**115**: 305–15.

52. Arcos-Burgos M, Castellanos FX, Pineda D, *et al.* Attention-deficit/hyperactivity disorder in a population isolate: linkage to loci at 4q13.2, 5q33.3, 11q22, and 17p11. *Am J Hum Genet.* 2004;**75**: 998–1014.

53. Bakker SC, van der Meulen EM, Buitelaar JK, *et al.* A whole-genome scan in 164 Dutch sib pairs with attention-deficit/hyperactivity disorder: suggestive evidence for linkage on chromosomes 7p and 15q. *Am J Hum Genet.* 2003;**72**:1251–60.

54. Ogdie MN, Bakker SC, Fisher SE, *et al.* Pooled genome-wide linkage data on 424 ADHD ASPs suggests genetic heterogeneity and a common risk locus at 5p13. *Mol Psychiatry.* 2006;**11**:5–8.

55. Hebebrand J, Dempfle A, Saar K, *et al.* A genome-wide scan for attention-deficit/hyperactivity disorder in 155 German sib-pairs. *Mol Psychiatry.* 2006;**11**: 196–205.

56. Manolio TA, Rodriguez LL, Brooks L, *et al.* New models of collaboration in genome-wide association studies: the Genetic Association Information Network. *Nat Genet.* 2007;**39**:1045–51.

57. Gerra G, Garofano L, Zaimovic A, *et al.* Association of the serotonin transporter promoter polymorphism with smoking behavior among adolescents. *Am J Med Genet B Neuropsychiatr Genet.* 2005;**135**:73–8.

58. Hutchison KE, LaChance H, Niaura R, Bryan A, Smolen A. The DRD4 VNTR polymorphism influences reactivity to smoking cues. *J Abnorm Psychol.* 2002;**111**:134–43.

59. Ishikawa H, Ohtsuki T, Ishiguro H, *et al.* Association between serotonin transporter gene polymorphism and smoking among Japanese males. *Cancer Epidemiol Biomarkers Prev.* 1999;**8**:831–3.

60. Lerer E, Kanyas K, Karni O, Ebstein RP, Lerer B. Why do young women smoke? II. Role of traumatic life

experience, psychological characteristics and serotonergic genes. *Mol Psychiatry*. 2006;**11**: 771–81.

61. Lerman C, Caporaso N, Main D, *et al*. Depression and self-medication with nicotine: the modifying influence of the dopamine D4 receptor gene. *Health Psychology*. 1998;**17**:56–62.

62. Luciano M, Zhu G, Kirk KM, *et al*. Effects of dopamine receptor D4 variation on alcohol and tobacco use and on novelty seeking: multivariate linkage and association analysis. *Am J Med Genet B Neuropsychiatr Genet*. 2004;**124**:113–23.

63. Skowronek MH, Laucht M, Hohm E, Becker K, Schmidt MH. Interaction between the dopamine D4 receptor and the serotonin transporter promoter polymorphisms in alcohol and tobacco use among 15-year-olds. *Neurogenetics*. 2006;**7**:239–46.

64. Tapper AR, McKinney SL, Nashmi R, *et al*. Nicotine activation of alpha4* receptors: sufficient for reward, tolerance, and sensitization. *Science*. 2004;**306**: 1029–32.

65. Timberlake DS, Haberstick BC, Lessem JM, *et al*. An association between the DAT1 polymorphism and smoking behavior in young adults from the National Longitudinal Study of Adolescent Health. *Health Psychol*. 2006;**25**:190–7.

66. Sullivan PF, Neale MC, Silverman MA, *et al*. An association study of DRD5 with smoking initiation and progression to nicotine dependence. *Am J Med Genet*. 2001;**105**:259–65.

67. McClernon FJ, Hutchison KE, Rose JE, Kozink RV. DRD4 VNTR polymorphism is associated with transient fMRI-BOLD responses to smoking cues. *Psychopharmacology (Berl)*. 2007;**194**:433–41.

68. Greenbaum L, Kanyas K, Karni O, *et al*. Why do young women smoke? I. Direct and interactive effects of environment, psychological characteristics and nicotinic cholinergic receptor genes. *Mol Psychiatry*. 2006;**11**:312–22, 223.

69. Hutchison KE, Allen DL, Filbey FM, *et al*. CHRNA4 and tobacco dependence: from gene regulation to treatment outcome. *Arch Gen Psychiatry*. 2007; **64**:1078–86.

70. Li MD, Beuten J, Ma JZ, *et al*. Ethnic- and gender-specific association of the nicotinic acetylcholine receptor alpha4 subunit gene (CHRNA4) with nicotine dependence. *Hum Mol Genet*. 2005; **14**:1211–19.

71. Ehringer MA, Clegg HV, Collins AC, *et al*. Association of the neuronal nicotinic receptor beta2 subunit gene (CHRNB2) with subjective responses to alcohol and nicotine. *Am J Med Genet B Neuropsychiatr Genet*. 2007;**144B**:596–604.

72. Li MD. Identifying susceptibility loci for nicotine dependence: 2008 update based on recent genome-wide linkage analyses. *Hum Genet*. 2008;**123**:119–31.

73. Lerman CE, Schnoll RA, Munafo MR. Genetics and smoking cessation improving outcomes in smokers at risk. *Am J Prev Med*. 2007;**33**: S398–405.

74. Yudkin P, Munafo M, Hey K, *et al*. Effectiveness of nicotine patches in relation to genotype in women versus men: randomised controlled trial. *BMJ*. 2004;**328**:989–90.

75. David SP, Brown RA, Papandonatos GD, *et al*. Pharmacogenetic clinical trial of sustained-release bupropion for smoking cessation. *Nicotine Tob Res*. 2007;**9**:821–33.

76. McClernon FJ, Fuemmeler BF, Kollins SH, Kail ME, Ashley-Koch AE. Interactions between genotype and retrospective ADHD symptoms predict lifetime smoking risk in a sample of young adults. *Nicotine Tob Res*. 2008;**10**:117–27.

77. Neuman RJ, Lobos E, Reich W, *et al*. Prenatal smoking exposure and dopaminergic genotypes interact to cause a severe ADHD subtype. *Biol Psychiatry*. 2007;**61**:1320–8.

78. Todd RD, Neuman RJ. Gene-environment interactions in the development of combined type ADHD: evidence for a synapse-based model. *Am J Med Genet B Neuropsychiatr Genet*. 2007;**144**: 971–5.

79. Kent L, Middle F, Hawi Z, *et al*. Nicotinic acetylcholine receptor alpha4 subunit gene polymorphism and attention deficit hyperactivity disorder. *Psychiatr Genet*. 2001;**11**:37–40.

80. Todd RD, Lobos EA, Sun LW, Neuman RJ. Mutational analysis of the nicotinic acetylcholine receptor alpha 4 subunit gene in attention deficit/hyperactivity disorder: evidence for association of an intronic polymorphism with attention problems. *Mol Psychiatry*. 2003;**8**:103–8.

81. Brookes K, Xu X, Chen W, *et al*. The analysis of 51 genes in DSM-IV combined type attention deficit hyperactivity disorder: association signals in DRD4, DAT1 and 16 other genes. *Mol Psychiatry*. 2006; **11**:934–53.

82. Guan L, Wang B, Chen Y, *et al*. A high-density single-nucleotide polymorphism screen of 23 candidate genes in attention deficit hyperactivity disorder: suggesting multiple susceptibility genes among Chinese Han population. *Mol Psychiatry*. 2009;**14**:546–54.

83. Lee J, Laurin N, Crosbie J, *et al*. Association study of the nicotinic acetylcholine receptor alpha4 subunit

gene, CHRNA4, in attention-deficit hyperactivity disorder. *Genes Brain Behav.* 2008;7:53–60.

84. Kent L, Green E, Holmes J, *et al.* No association between CHRNA7 microsatellite markers and attention-deficit hyperactivity disorder. *Am J Med Genet.* 2001;**105**:686–9.

85. Voineskos S, De Luca V, Mensah A, *et al.* Association of alpha4beta2 nicotinic receptor and heavy smoking in schizophrenia. *J Psychiatry Neurosci.* 2007;**32**:412–16.

86. Grace AA. Psychostimulant actions on dopamine and limbic system function: relevance to the pathophysiology and treatment of ADHD. In: Solanto M, Arnsten A, Castellanos F, eds. *Stimulant Drugs and ADHD: Basic and Clinical Neuroscience.* London: Oxford University Press. 2001; 134–57.

87. Solanto MV. Neuropsychopharmacological mechanisms of stimulant drug action in attention-deficit hyperactivity disorder: a review and integration. *Behav Brain Res.* 1998;**94**:127–52.

88. Cheon KA, Ryu YH, Kim YK, *et al.* Dopamine transporter density in the basal ganglia assessed with [123I]IPT SPET in children with attention deficit hyperactivity disorder. *Eur J Nucl Med Mol Imaging.* 2003;**30**:306–11.

89. Dougherty DD, Bonab AA, Spencer TJ, *et al.* Dopamine transporter density in patients with attention deficit hyperactivity disorder. *Lancet.* 1999;**354**:2132–3.

90. Dresel S, Krause J, Krause KH, *et al.* Attention deficit hyperactivity disorder: binding of [99mTc]TRODAT-1 to the dopamine transporter before and after methylphenidate treatment. *Eur J Nucl Med.* 2000;**27**:1518–24.

91. Krause KH, Dresel SH, Krause J, Kung HF, Tatsch K. Increased striatal dopamine transporter in adult patients with attention deficit hyperactivity disorder: effects of methylphenidate as measured by single photon emission computed tomography. *Neurosci Lett.* 2000;**285**:107–10.

92. Krause KH, Dresel SH, Krause J, *et al.* Stimulant-like action of nicotine on striatal dopamine transporter in the brain of adults with attention deficit hyperactivity disorder. *Int J Neuropsychopharmacol.* 2002;**5**:111–13.

93. Krause KH, Dresel SH, Krause J, la Fougere C, Ackenheil M. The dopamine transporter and neuroimaging in attention deficit hyperactivity disorder. *Neurosci Biobehav Rev.* 2003;**27**:605–13.

94. Larisch R, Sitte W, Antke C, *et al.* Striatal dopamine transporter density in drug naive patients with attention-deficit/hyperactivity disorder. *Nucl Med Commun.* 2006;**27**:267–70.

95. Spencer TJ, Biederman J, Madras BK, *et al.* In vivo neuroreceptor imaging in attention-deficit/hyperactivity disorder: a focus on the dopamine transporter. *Biol Psychiatry.* 2005;**57**:1293–300.

96. Volkow ND, Wang GJ, Newcorn J, *et al.* Brain dopamine transporter levels in treatment and drug naive adults with ADHD. *Neuroimage.* 2007;**34**:1182–90.

97. Volkow ND, Wang GJ, Kollins SH, *et al.* Evaluating dopamine reward pathway in ADHD: clinical implications. *JAMA.* 2009;**302**:1084–91.

98. Brody AL, Olmstead RE, London ED, *et al.* Smoking-induced ventral striatum dopamine release. *Am J Psychiatry.* 2004;**161**:1211–18.

99. Corrigall WA, Coen KM, Adamson KL. Self-administered nicotine activates the mesolimbic dopamine system through the ventral tegmental area. *Brain Res.* 1994;**653**:278–84.

100. Glass K, Flory K. Why does ADHD confer risk for cigarette smoking? A review of psychosocial mechanisms. *Clin Child Fam Psychol Rev.* 2010;**13**:291–313.

101. Hahn B, Stolerman IP. Nicotine-induced attentional enhancement in rats: effects of chronic exposure to nicotine. *Neuropsychopharmacology.* 2002;**27**:712–22.

102. Koelega HS. Stimulant drugs and vigilance performance: a review. *Psychopharmacology (Berl).* 1993;**111**:1–16.

103. Rezvani AH, Levin ED. Cognitive effects of nicotine. *Biol Psychiatry.* 2001;**49**:258–67.

104. Levin ED, Conners CK, Silva D, *et al.* Transdermal nicotine effects on attention. *Psychopharmacology (Berl).* 1998;**140**:135–41.

105. Warburton DM, Mancuso G. Evaluation of the information processing and mood effects of a transdermal nicotine patch. *Psychopharmacology (Berl).* 1998;**135**:305–10.

106. Sacco KA, Termine A, Seyal A, *et al.* Effects of cigarette smoking on spatial working memory and attentional deficits in schizophrenia: involvement of nicotinic receptor mechanisms. *Arch Gen Psychiatry.* 2005;**62**:649–69.

107. Levin ED, Conners CK, Sparrow E, *et al.* Nicotine effects on adults with attention-deficit/hyperactivity disorder. *Psychopharmacology (Berl).* 1996;**123**:55–63.

108. Barkley RA. Behavioral inhibition, sustained attention, and executive functions: constructing a unifying theory of ADHD. *Psychol Bull.* 1997;**121**:65–94.

109. McClernon FJ, Hiott FB, Westman EC, Rose JE, Levin ED. Transdermal nicotine attenuates depression symptoms in nonsmokers: a double-blind,

placebo-controlled trial. *Psychopharmacology (Berl)*. 2006;**189**:125–33.

110. Levin ED, Conners CK, Silva D, Canu W, March J. Effects of chronic nicotine and methylphenidate in adults with attention deficit/hyperactivity disorder. *Exp Clin Psychopharmacol*. 2001;**9**: 83–90.

111. Potter AS, Newhouse PA. Effects of acute nicotine administration on behavioral inhibition in adolescents with attention-deficit/hyperactivity disorder. *Psychopharmacology (Berl)*. 2004;**176**: 182–94.

112. Potter AS, Newhouse PA. Acute nicotine improves cognitive deficits in young adults with attention-deficit/hyperactivity disorder. *Pharmacol Biochem Behav*. 2008;**88**:407–17.

113. Wilens TE, Biederman J, Spencer TJ, *et al*. A pilot controlled clinical trial of ABT-418, a cholinergic agonist, in the treatment of adults with attention deficit hyperactivity disorder. *Am J Psychiatry*. 1999;**156**:1931–7.

114. Wilens TE, Verlinden MH, Adler LA, Wozniak PJ, West SA. ABT-089, a neuronal nicotinic receptor partial agonist, for the treatment of attention-deficit/hyperactivity disorder in adults: results of a pilot study. *Biol Psychiatry*. 2006;**59**:1065–70.

115. Faraone SV, Buitelaar J. Comparing the efficacy of stimulants for ADHD in children and adolescents using meta-analysis. *Eur Child Adolesc Psychiatry*. 2010;**19**:353–64.

116. Faraone SV, Glatt SJ. A comparison of the efficacy of medications for adult attention-deficit/hyperactivity disorder using meta-analysis of effect sizes. *J Clin Psychiatry*. 2010;**71**:754–63.

117. Mick E, Biederman J, Faraone SV. Comment on Lambert and Hartsough (1998). *J Learn Disabil*. 2000;**33**:314.

118. Barkley RA, Fischer M, Smallish L, Fletcher K. Does the treatment of attention-deficit/hyperactivity disorder with stimulants contribute to drug use/abuse? A 13-year prospective study. *Pediatrics*. 2003;**111**: 97–109.

119. Faraone SV, Biederman J, Wilens TE, Adamson J. A naturalistic study of the effects of pharmacotherapy on substance use disorders among ADHD adults. *Psychol Med*. 2007;**37**:1743–52.

120. Wilens TE, Vitulano M, Upadhyaya H, *et al*. Concordance between cigarette smoking and the modified Fagerstrom Tolerance Questionnaire in controlled studies of ADHD. *Am J Addict*. 2008; **17**:491–6.

121. Whalen CK, Jamner LD, Henker B, Gehricke JG, King PS. Is there a link between adolescent cigarette smoking and pharmacotherapy for ADHD? *Psychol Addict Behav*. 2003;**17**:332–5.

122. Sigmon SC, Tidey JW, Badger GJ, Higgins ST. Acute effects of D-amphetamine on progressive-ratio performance maintained by cigarette smoking and money. *Psychopharmacology (Berl)*. 2003;**167**: 393–402.

123. Tidey JW, O'Neill SC, Higgins ST. d-amphetamine increases choice of cigarette smoking over monetary reinforcement. *Psychopharmacology (Berl)*. 2000; **153**:85–92.

124. Rush CR, Higgins ST, Vansickel AR, Stoops WW, Lile JA, Glaser PE. *et al*. Methylphenidate increases cigarette smoking. *Psychopharmacology (Berl)*. 2005;**181**:781–9.

125. Stoops WW, Poole MM, Vansickel AR, *et al*. Methylphenidate increases choice of cigarettes over money. *Nicotine Tob Res*. 2011;**13**:29–33.

126. Vansickel AR, Stoops WW, Glaser PE, Poole MM, Rush CR. Methylphenidate increases cigarette smoking in participants with ADHD. *Psychopharmacology (Berl)*. 2011;**218**:381–90.

127. Gehricke JG, Hong N, Wigal TL, Chan V, Doan A. ADHD medication reduces cotinine levels and withdrawal in smokers with ADHD. *Pharmacol Biochem Behav*. 2011;**98**:485–91.

128. Winhusen TM, Somoza EC, Brigham GS, *et al*. Impact of attention-deficit/hyperactivity disorder (ADHD) treatment on smoking cessation intervention in ADHD smokers: a randomized, double-blind, placebo-controlled trial. *J Clin Psychiatry*. 2010; **71**:1680–8.

129. Bagwell CL, Molina BS, Pelham WE, Jr., Hoza B. Attention-deficit hyperactivity disorder and problems in peer relations: predictions from childhood to adolescence. *J Am Acad Child Adolesc Psychiatry*. 2001;**40**:1285–92.

130. Doran N, Spring B, McChargue D, Pergadia M, Richmond M. Impulsivity and smoking relapse. *Nicotine Tob Res*. 2004;**6**:641–7.

131. Downey KK, Pomerleau CS, Pomerleau OF. Personality differences related to smoking and adult attention deficit hyperactivity disorder. *J Subst Abuse*. 1996;**8**:129–35.

132. DuBois DL, Silverthorn N. Do deviant peer associations mediate the contributions of self-esteem to problem behavior during early adolescence? A 2-year longitudinal study. *J Clin Child Adolesc Psychol*. 2004;**33**:382–8.

133. Lejuez CW, Aklin WM, Jones HA, *et al*. The Balloon Analogue Risk Task (BART) differentiates smokers and nonsmokers. *Exp Clin Psychopharmacol*. 2003; **11**:26–33.

134. Mitchell SH. Measures of impulsivity in cigarette smokers and non-smokers. *Psychopharmacology (Berl)*. 1999;**146**:455–64.

135. Pomerleau CS. Co-factors for smoking and evolutionary psychobiology. *Addiction*. 1997;**92**: 397–408.

136. Reynolds B, Richards JB, Horn K, Karraker K. Delay discounting and probability discounting as related to cigarette smoking status in adults. *Behav Processes*. 2004;**65**:35–42.

137. Finzi-Dottan R, Manor I, Tyano S. ADHD, temperament, and parental style as predictors of the child's attachment patterns. *Child Psychiatry Hum Dev*. 2006;**37**:103–14.

138. Harakeh Z, Scholte RH, Vermulst AA, de Vries H, Engels RC. Parental factors and adolescents' smoking behavior: an extension of the theory of planned behavior. *Prev Med*. 2004;**39**: 951–61.

139. Laucht M, Hohm E, Esser G, Schmidt MH, Becker K. Association between ADHD and smoking in adolescence: shared genetic, environmental and psychopathological factors. *J Neural Transm*. 2007; **114**:1097–104.

140. Marshal MP, Molina BS. Antisocial behaviors moderate the deviant peer pathway to substance use in children with ADHD. *J Clin Child Adolesc Psychol*. 2006;**35**:216–26.

141. Simons-Morton B, Haynie DL, Crump AD, Eitel SP, Saylor KE. Peer and parent influences on smoking and drinking among early adolescents. *Health Educ Behav*. 2001;**28**:95–107.

142. Dobbins M, Decorby K, Manske S, Goldblatt E. Effective practices for school-based tobacco use prevention. *Prev Med*. 2008;**46**:289–97.

143. Thomas R, Perera R. School-based programmes for preventing smoking. *Cochrane Database Syst Rev*. 2006;**3**:CD001293.

144. Hoza B. Peer functioning in children with ADHD. *J Pediatr Psychol*. 2007;**32**:655–63.

145. Molina BS, Marshal MP, Pelham WE, Jr., Wirth RJ. Coping skills and parent support mediate the association between childhood attention-deficit/ hyperactivity disorder and adolescent cigarette use. *J Pediatr Psychol*. 2005;**30**:345–57.

146. Monuteaux MC, Spencer TJ, Faraone SV, Wilson AM, Biederman J. A randomized, placebo-controlled clinical trial of bupropion for the prevention of smoking in children and adolescents with attention-deficit/hyperactivity disorder. *J Clin Psychiatry*. 2007;**68**:1094–101.

147. Covey LS, Hu MC, Weissman J, *et al*. Divergence by ADHD subtype in smoking cessation response to OROS-methylphenidate. *Nicotine Tob Res*. 2011; **13**:1003–8.

148. Dwoskin LP, Rauhut AS, King-Pospisil KA, Bardo MT. Review of the pharmacology and clinical profile of bupropion, an antidepressant and tobacco use cessation agent. *CNS Drug Rev*. 2006;**12**:178–207.

149. Wilens TE, Haight BR, Horrigan JP, *et al*. Bupropion XL in adults with attention-deficit/hyperactivity disorder: a randomized, placebo-controlled study. *Biol Psychiatry*. 2005;**57**:793–801.

150. Upadhyaya HP, Brady KT, Wang W. Bupropion SR in adolescents with comorbid ADHD and nicotine dependence: a pilot study. *J Am Acad Child Adolesc Psychiatry*. 2004;**43**:199–205.

151. Safren SA. Cognitive-behavioral approaches to ADHD treatment in adulthood. *J Clin Psychiatry*. 2006;**67**(Suppl 8):46–50.

ADHD and tic disorders

Rahil Jummani and Barbara J. Coffey

Bidirectional overlap between attention-deficit hyperactivity disorder (ADHD) and tic disorders has long been described. Twenty percent of individuals with ADHD may meet diagnostic criteria for a tic disorder, and the prevalence of ADHD in individuals with Tourette Syndrome (TS), also known as Tourette's Disorder is reported to be as high as 55% [1]. ADHD, obsessive–compulsive disorder (OCD), and mood and anxiety disorders often co-occur in clinically referred youth and adults with TS. A recent epidemiological TS study from the National Survey of Children's Health (2007) reported that over 60% of children ages 6–17 in the community had also been diagnosed with ADHD [2]. While comorbid presentation of ADHD and tic disorders is firmly established, underlying genetic and pathophysiological mechanisms remain elusive. However, the etiology and pathophysiology of tics is being demystified by current neurobiological studies.

Most studies indicate that ADHD places a greater burden on patients than do tics. Optimal patient outcomes may depend on management of both ADHD symptoms and tics when they co-occur. Research in the past decade has shown that these conditions can be safely treated simultaneously. Most recently, non-pharmacological treatments have been developed as first-line interventions for tics that are as successful as pharmacotherapy.

This chapter provides an updated review with a special focus on ADHD and chronic tic disorders.

Definitions and diagnostic criteria

Definitions

Tics are stereotyped, rapid, recurring motor movements or vocalizations that are non-rhythmic, involuntary or semi-voluntary, and sudden in onset. They result from the movement of one muscle or a group of muscles and are characterized by their anatomical location, number, frequency, duration, and complexity. They are classified as either *simple or complex*. Simple tics involve one muscle group or sound. Complex tics are slower and more purposeful, involving multiple muscle groups or multiple sounds.

Simple motor tics are the most common presentation of tic disorders. They are categorized as clonic, dystonic, or tonic. *Clonic tics* involve brief jerking movements such as eye blinking, shoulder shrugging, or head turning. Eye blinking is the most common initial tic in TS. *Dystonic tics* are briefly sustained abnormal postures. Examples include sustained eye closure (blepharospasm), mouth opening, neck twisting, and shoulder rotation. *Tonic tics* are isometric contractions and include tensing of abdominal or limb muscles. *Complex motor tics* may include touching objects, jumping, and imitating others' gestures (echopraxia). Less frequently occurring complex motor tics are the involuntary production of obscene gestures (copropraxia).

Simple vocal tics include throat clearing, coughing, and sniffing; *complex vocal tics* include repeating syllables, words, or phrases (palilalia) or repeating others' words or phrases (echolalia). Less common vocal tics include involuntary vocalization of obscenities (coprolalia).

Complex motor tics may be difficult to distinguish from compulsions, which are repetitive behaviors enacted to reduce anxiety or prevent a feared outcome. As OCD frequently co-occurs with tics, the difference between some complex tics and compulsive behaviors is subtle. The distinction may be made by establishing whether the behavior is pursued to

Attention-Deficit Hyperactivity Disorder in Adults and Children, ed. Lenard A. Adler, Thomas J. Spencer and Timothy E. Wilens.
Published by Cambridge University Press. © Cambridge University Press 2015.

prevent or reduce anxiety, or simply to satisfy an inner urge or sensation.

Premonitory sensations are uncomfortable physical or mental feelings or urges that may precede tics. Most individuals with TS describe this phenomenon. Premonitory sensations distinguish tic disorders from other movement disorders. An example is a burning sensation in the eye before an eye blink. In addition, many individuals with tics report "just right" phenomena; to relieve an uncomfortable urge, the individual feels that he or she must repeat a particular movement or vocalization until "it feels just right." The urge is experienced as aversive, and the tic relieves the negative experience; and thus, the tic is reinforced [3].

Tics fluctuate and often occur in bouts over variable periods. They change in frequency, location, number, complexity, and severity over minutes, hours, days, and much longer time periods [4]. Tics may persist during sleep [5]. They are experienced as irresistible, but may be suppressed for varying periods of time. Some individuals experience a decrease in frequency and severity of tics during concentration on mental or physical tasks such as reading. Stress, excitement, boredom, fatigue, and temperature extremes may increase tics [6].

Diagnostic criteria

Diagnostic criteria are found in the *Diagnostic and Statistical Manual of Mental Disorders*, fifth edition (DSM-5) [7] and the *International Statistical Classification of Diseases and Related Health Problems*, 10th revision (ICD-10) [8]. According to DSM-5 and ICD-10, tic disorders include provisional tic disorder (transient tic disorder in previous editions of the DSM and in ICD-10), persistent motor tic disorder, chronic vocal tic disorder, TS (combined vocal and multiple motor tics disorder [de la Tourette] in ICD-10), and unspecified tic disorder (tic disorder not otherwise specified in previous editions of the DSM and in ICD-10).

According to DSM-5, provisional tic disorder (transient tic disorder in ICD-10) is defined by the presence of motor and/or vocal tics for less than a year. Persistent motor or vocal tic disorder is the occurrence of either motor or vocal tics, but not both, for more than a year. Diagnostic criteria for TS are the presence of multiple motor and one or more vocal tics for a period greater than 1 year. According to DSM-5, unspecified tic disorder is diagnosed when a tic

disorder does not meet criteria for any of the other tic disorders.

In addition to tic disorder diagnostic criteria shared by DSM-5 and ICD-10, DSM-5 specifies a few common criteria that must be met to diagnose tic disorders: onset of tics before age 18 years and absence of a causal link to a general medical condition or substance.

Epidemiology and clinical phenomenology

Transient or provisional tic disorder is the most common tic disorder; prevalence estimates suggest occurrence in up to 20% of school-age children [9]. By contrast, a recent study of more than 800 children ages 4 to 16 years in Spain reported a prevalence of approximately 6.5% for all tic disorders. The vast majority of tics were mild in severity and of short duration [10]. The prevalence of persistent tic disorders is estimated to be between 2% and 4% [11].

Prevalence estimates for TS also vary. Current lifetime rate estimates vary from 1 to 30 per 1000 children in European and Asian populations; a common prevalence figure for TS is 1% [12]. A study conducted by the United States Centers for Disease Control in 2007 reported a TS prevalence rate between 0.3 and 1% of children ages 6–17 [2]. Studies in both adults and children demonstrate that males are at least three to four times more likely than females to have TS [13].

In most cases, TS symptoms are present before age 11 years, typically beginning between ages 3 and 8. Average age of onset is about 6 years. The course of TS is characterized by onset of simple motor tics in the eyes, face, head, and/or neck at around age 6 or 7, followed by head-to-toe progression of shoulder, trunk, and extremity tics over several years. Phonic tics typically start at age 8 to 9 years and initially may not be concurrent with motor tics. More complex tics often begin later, around age 11 to 12 [14]. Tics range from mild to severe and tend to stabilize over time. Most children, including those evaluated in specialty clinics, have mild to moderate tics. Recent studies indicate that tic severity usually improves significantly by mid adolescence. Some children experience lengthy periods of time during which most or all symptoms diminish or remit. Twenty percent or fewer of those with TS continue to experience notable functional impairment by age 20 years [14]. Rarely, patients experience tic onset or an exacerbation in adulthood. Adult TS largely represents re-emergence or exacerbation of childhood-onset TS [15].

Comorbidity of tics with psychiatric disorders such as ADHD and OCD is very common in clinical settings. The most common comorbid diagnosis in children with TS is ADHD, reported in more than 60% of children ages 6–17 [2]. As many as half of clinically referred TS patients show signs of ADHD prior to onset of tics, usually preceding the onset of tics by 2 to 3 years. Some researchers have reported that 50% to 75% of TS patients also meet criteria for ADHD, whereas 20–30% of ADHD patients meet criteria for a tic disorder [1, 16]. One population-based study of school-age children found comorbid psychiatric disorders in 92% of the children with TS. ADHD was the most frequent co-occurring condition [17].

Full criteria for OCD are met in 20–60% of TS patients [18]. OCD symptoms typically emerge at about age 11 to 12 years after simple tics have been present for some time. Some studies have reported that as tics improve in early adolescence, OCD symptoms may increase. In addition to ADHD and OCD, oppositional defiant disorder, mood disorders, and other non-OCD anxiety disorders have been reported in individuals with TS [18].

Co-occurring psychiatric disorders confer a more difficult clinical course and outcome [19]. Coffey and colleagues reported in one study that comorbid mood disorders were the strongest predictors of psychiatric hospitalization and illness severity in a cohort of TS patients [20]. Tic severity was only minimally significant as a predictor of psychiatric hospitalization. ADHD and OCD often interfere more with overall functioning than do tics. Co-occurring TS and ADHD often manifest with academic difficulties, peer rejection, family conflict, and disruptive behaviors. It has been clearly demonstrated that comorbid ADHD and/or OCD leads to greater disability than tic disorders alone [21–25].

A Tourette Syndrome International Database Consortium study of 6805 cases reported that TS plus ADHD was associated with an earlier TS diagnosis and a much higher rate of anger control problems and oppositional defiant disorder, sleep difficulties, learning disability, mood disorders, social skills deficits, sexually inappropriate behavior, and self-injurious behavior than TS alone [1]. In another study, parent ratings of aggression and delinquent behavior and teacher ratings of conduct problems were elevated in those with ADHD alone and those with ADHD and TS [23]. Carter and co-investigators found that children with TS plus ADHD experienced more emotional and behavioral problems and more difficulty with social adaption than control subjects and those with TS alone [26]. Finally, learning and academic problems are common in children with TS. In a database of 5450 patients with TS, 1235 (22.7%) had learning disabilities. Learning disorders should always be considered in the evaluation of TS patients [27]. Other research examining the impact of tics on the course and prognosis of ADHD [28, 29] demonstrates that co-occurrence of these disorders leads to a more complicated course and outcome.

Gorman and colleagues examined psychosocial functioning in late adolescents with TS compared to age-matched peers. Compared with controls, those with TS had higher rates of ADHD, depression, learning, and conduct disorders. TS subjects had poorer psychosocial outcomes which were associated with greater ADHD, OCD, and tic severity [30]. When controlled for ADHD, TS youth still had higher overall rates of comorbidity and major depression compared with healthy controls. These findings are supported by numerous studies [31].

Adults with TS and comorbid conditions are also reported to experience a more severe course. In one study, adults with TS plus ADHD demonstrated significantly more depression, anxiety, obsessive–compulsive symptoms, and maladaptive behaviors than adults with TS only [32]. However, Spencer and colleagues reported that although adults with ADHD have higher lifetime rates of tic disorders than controls, the tics did not impact the course of ADHD [33].

Nevertheless, tics may have significant impact in some individuals. Persistent tic symptoms can cause distress and may directly interfere with daily activities, depending on tic severity [34]. Figure 27.1 shows a suggested evidence-based ADHD/tics/TS treatment algorithm.

Etiology and pathophysiology

The etiology and pathophysiology of tic disorders remain unknown. Research suggests a diffuse process in the brain involving cortico-striato-thalamic-cortical (CSTC) pathways in the basal ganglia, striatum, and frontal lobes with dysregulation involving dopamine, serotonin, glutamate, and endogenous opioids.

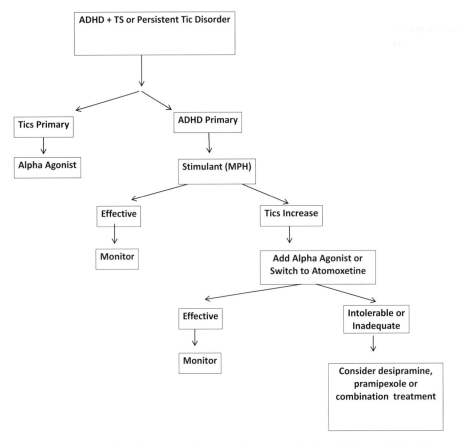

Figure 27.1. Evidence-based ADHD/tics/TS suggested treatment algorithm. MPH = methylphenidate.

Neurobiological studies support conceptualization of TS as an inherited neurodevelopmental condition. Twin studies have demonstrated 87–94% concordance [35], but environmental factors are also implicated. Gestational and perinatal insults, including hypoxia, androgen exposure, heat, and infections may contribute to pathophysiology; prenatal ischemia may alter dopamine signaling, leading to the development of tics [36].

Environmental factors possibly common to the pathophysiology of both TS and ADHD have been assessed. One study found that children with both ADHD and TS had greater odds of low birth weight status, prematurity, breathing problems, and maternal smoking compared to children with TS only [37]. Motlagh and coworkers retrospectively evaluated presence of heavy maternal smoking and severe psychosocial stress during pregnancy in youth with TS alone, ADHD alone, TS plus ADHD, or neither. All clinical groups demonstrated higher rates of heavy maternal smoking and severe psychosocial stress during preg-

nancy than controls, but the difference was statistically significant only for the ADHD alone group [38].

Stress hormones may play a role in the strong association of tics and anxiety. TS patients have been found to have higher levels of cerebrospinal fluid corticotrophin-releasing factor than normal controls [39]. A stress diathesis model modulated by the hypothalamic–pituitary–adrenal axis, associated stress-related neurotransmitters, and hormones and their targets may be the final common pathway accounting for variable tic expression.

That abnormal dopamine neurotransmission contributes to the pathophysiology of TS is supported by increased levels of dopaminergic innervation of the striatum of TS subjects in single photon emission computed tomography (SPECT) studies [40]. Neuroimaging findings explain the efficacy of neuroleptic drugs that block dopamine receptors in the treatment of tics. TS patients have been shown to release more dopamine in response to amphetamine at dopaminergic synapses than healthy controls.

Dopamine-releasing drugs, such as stimulants, may precipitate or exacerbate tics in some individuals.

Midbrain dopaminergic neurons play a central role in motor control and attentional processes through direct connections to the striatum and cortex, respectively. The role of dopaminergic pathways is compelling when considering the high comorbidity of tic disorders with ADHD, which is also considered a neurodevelopmental disorder associated with dysregulated dopaminergic neurotransmission.

Peterson and colleagues demonstrated increased overall hippocampus and amygdala volumes in TS patients, with a decline in volume with age in the group with TS but not in healthy controls. In children and adults with TS, volumes were correlated inversely with tic, OCD, and ADHD severity. An explanation for these findings is that the subregion plays a compensatory and neuromodulatory role with tic, OCD, and ADHD symptoms [41]. In addition, cerebral hyperintensities, bright patches in brain tissue on T2-weighted magnetic resonance imaging indicative of neuroinflammatory or neurodegenerative processes, have been detected at increased rates in youth with TS, OCD, or ADHD in subcortical regions (primarily the basal ganglia and thalamus). This finding supports a role of subcortical injury in the pathophysiology of these conditions [42].

Tic disorders cluster in families. Twin studies show 50–90% concordance for tic disorders among monozygotic pairs, in contrast to about 20% concordance among dizygotic twins [43]. Other studies have confirmed a higher percentage of tic disorders in first-degree relatives of TS patients than of normal controls. The largest TS genetic linkage study, by the Tourette Syndrome Association International Consortium for Genetics (TSAIGC) and consisting of over 2000 participants, found strong evidence of linkage for a region on chromosome 2p. Current understanding of TS points to multiple susceptibility genes; however, the recently published TSAICG genome-wide association study (GWAS) reported that no genes reached threshold significance [44].

Evaluation and treatment of tic disorders and ADHD

As the onset of ADHD occurs before age 12, and in most cases before age 7, ADHD symptoms usually precede onset of tics. Especially if motoric hyperactivity and restlessness are present, tics may

be overlooked, or assumed to be part of the ADHD picture. Diagnosis is based on a detailed history of tics and, to a lesser extent, on the observation of tics in the office. It is not uncommon for tics to be suppressed during clinical evaluation. Generally, neurological, laboratory, and neuroimaging assessments are normal. Baseline laboratory tests, including a comprehensive metabolic panel, complete blood count (CBC), thyroid panel, lipid panel, and urine toxicology screen should be obtained to rule out possible underlying medical conditions or substance abuse.

Careful history, physical examination, and review of records are necessary. If there are no findings, further evaluation with neuroimaging or electroencephalogram (EEG) is likely to be low yield. A meticulous tic history should be taken, including onset, course, severity, premonitory sensations, and prior treatments. Use of standardized rating scales such as the Yale Global Tic Severity Scale is helpful.

Psychiatric assessment of patients with ADHD and tics should include systematic review of comorbid disorders, including OCD, anxiety, and mood disorders. The Child Behavior Checklist (CBCL), Swanson, Nolan, and Pelham IV Questionnaire (SNAP-IV), Yale–Brown Obsessive Compulsive Scale (YBOCS), and Children's Yale–Brown Obsessive Compulsive Scale (CYBOCS) are considered gold standard quantitative assessments.

Treatment is based on a consideration of the impact of tics, in the context of ADHD, on social, emotional, family, and academic/occupational functioning. If tics are not causing significant distress or impairment, treatment may not be necessary. Mild to moderate tics may only require support and monitoring. Treatment is indicated when tics cause distress or impairment. In general, ADHD is more likely to be associated with both short-term and, left untreated, longer-term problems for patients.

The first step of treatment is psychoeducation. Clarification that the tics are involuntary is critical. Advocacy for an optimal school/occupational environment is often necessary. Support groups, such as the Tourette Syndrome Association (http://www.tsa-usa.org), are a valuable resource.

Pharmacotherapy

Pharmacotherapy must be tailored to the specific needs of the patient. Prior to medication initiation, workup should include physical, neurological, and psychiatric examination, basic laboratory screening, and electrocardiogram (EKG).

The next step is evaluation of the impact of both ADHD and tics on the patient's overall functioning and quality of life. ADHD symptoms are usually more impairing than tics, and treatment should target the most impairing symptoms first. When tics are treated, the goal of intervention is not elimination, but relief of tic-related impairment and/or distress, and achievement of a degree of control over tics that allows the patient to function as normally as possible.

Medication should generally be initiated at the lowest dose with gradual titration. When possible, a single medication should be used initially. Targeted combined pharmacotherapy is indicated when monotherapy has not been efficacious or has resulted in limiting adverse effects.

Bloch and colleagues examined pharmacotherapy treatment for youth with ADHD and tic disorders in a meta-analysis. Methylphenidate, alpha-2 (α_2) agonists, desipramine, and atomoxetine were effective for ADHD symptoms with comorbid tics. Supratherapeutic doses of dextroamphetamine reportedly worsened tics, but therapeutic doses did not. There was no evidence that methylphenidate exacerbated tics in the short term [45].

Alpha-adrenergic agonists

The α-adrenergic agonists clonidine and guanfacine are first-line pharmacotherapy for mild to moderate tics in the context of ADHD and are also effective for ADHD symptoms. Low-dose clonidine produces presynaptic noradrenergic effects that decrease tics and reduce impulsivity, hyperactivity, and inattention. Clonidine was examined in a retrospective chart review over a 4-year period in children with ADHD with and without tic disorders and resulted in improvement of both ADHD and tic symptoms in a significant majority of patients [46]. Guanfacine activates postsynaptic prefrontal α-adrenergic cortical receptors and is also efficacious for hyperactivity, impulsivity, and tics [47–49].

Both medications are available in short- and long-acting formulations. There is established evidence for the efficacy of the short-acting α-adrenergic agonists for tic disorders and for the efficacy of long-acting agents for ADHD, but there is not yet evidence for the efficacy of long-acting agents for tics. Clonidine is also available in a transdermal patch form that may be applied for up to a 1-week period. Adverse effects

include sedation, hypotension, headache, dry mouth, mid-sleep awakening, and irritability. Sedation often dissipates over a few weeks. Hypotension is unlikely at the low doses used, but blood pressure, heart rate, and EKG should be monitored at baseline and follow-up visits. Rebound hypertension, anxiety, and tics are risks if medication is abruptly discontinued.

Stimulants

Controversy has surrounded the use of stimulants for ADHD symptoms in tic disorder patients. Since the publication of case reports in 1963, and particularly due to an influential case series in the early 1980s [50]. US Food and Drug Administration (FDA) recommendations still caution against the use of stimulants in individuals with tics due to potential exacerbation. There have been accumulating data over the last two decades, however, showing that stimulants may be used safely and effectively for ADHD symptoms in patients with tics [51, 52].

The only placebo-controlled crossover study to compare methylphenidate with dextroamphetamine in youth with ADHD and TS demonstrated that relatively high doses of methylphenidate and dextroamphetamine exacerbated tics in a minority of subjects, which later diminished on methylphenidate but persisted in dextroamphetamine. The majority experienced improvement of ADHD symptoms with acceptable tic effects [53].

The contemporary understanding is that no significant risk of tics is present when stimulants are used in patients with ADHD and tics. However, some patients may experience at least a transient increase in tics. Stimulants may be used judiciously in the treatment of ADHD in the context of tic disorders, monitoring for tic exacerbation. If tics worsen, the stimulant dose may be adjusted, or the patient switched to another agent.

Atomoxetine (Strattera)

Atomoxetine, a selective norepinephrine reuptake inhibitor, has been studied in youth with ADHD and chronic tics. Studies have reported that atomoxetine improved both ADHD symptoms and tics in youth with ADHD and tics. Adverse effects included tachycardia, nausea, and decreased appetite and weight [54, 55].

Tricyclic antidepressants

Studies of desipramine have documented efficacy for treatment of tics in patients with ADHD. One retrospective chart review of children with chronic tics and ADHD showed significant improvement of both tics and ADHD symptoms in a majority of patients without major adverse effects over an average follow-up period of 16 months [56]. A placebo controlled study by Spencer and colleagues reported desipramine as superior to placebo in the management of tics and ADHD symptoms [57]. A controlled trial comparing clonidine and desipramine in children with ADHD and TS demonstrated superior efficacy of desipramine over clonidine for ADHD symptoms. Neither exacerbated nor significantly improved tics [58]. Though desipramine has proven efficacy, it is not considered a first-line agent due to associated electrocardiographic changes [59]. Careful cardiac monitoring is necessary.

Neuroleptics

Though first-generation neuroleptics haloperidol and pimozide are the only FDA-approved tic suppressing medications, these agents are generally only used for the treatment of moderate to severe tics that have not responded to behavioral interventions or α-adrenergic agonists. The mechanism of action is blockade of D_2 (dopamine) receptors in the basal ganglia, leading to tic reduction through decreased dopaminergic input from the substantia nigra and ventral tegmentum. Neuroleptics are generally not recommended for treatment of comorbid ADHD symptoms. Controlled trials have demonstrated efficacy for haloperidol and pimozide in tic treatment. However, adverse effects are considerable; most problematic are the extrapyramidal effects. As a result, these are recommended only for severe tics.

The second-generation agents block both D_2 receptors and 5-HT_2 (serotonin) receptors. Multiple trials have demonstrated efficacy of risperidone for tics comparable to pimozide [60] and clonidine. These agents tend to cause fewer extrapyramidal adverse effects than conventional neuroleptics. Common adverse effects include appetite increase, weight gain, lipid and glucose metabolism abnormalities, and sedation. Ziprasidone was shown in one placebo-controlled trial to be as efficacious as risperidone for treatment of tics [61]. Weight gain is less likely. Because QTC prolongation may occur, EKG monitoring is recommended. Aripiprazole is a novel atypical neuroleptic with partial agonist–antagonist effects on dopamine and serotonin systems. Several open-label trials and one controlled trial have been published on its use and tolerability in TS [62–65].

Metabolic and extrapyramidal effects are common to all neuroleptic agents. Fasting glucose and lipid panel are recommended before treatment initiation, upon reaching the maintenance dose, and at regular follow-up intervals. Weight, waist circumference, and body mass index (BMI) should be monitored. Education, exercise, and nutritional consultation are recommended.

Alternatives

When established treatments are unsuccessful, alternatives may be considered. Omega 3 fatty acids and pramipexole show some promise [66, 67]. Botulinum toxin may be useful for isolated dystonias or laryngeal tics [68]. Surgical intervention, including deep brain stimulation, is another option, but is reserved for severe, intractable, and highly debilitating tics, and data are limited [69].

Behavior therapy for tics

Comprehensive behavioral intervention for tics (CBIT), including habit reversal training or therapy (HRT), is a specific behavioral treatment for tics that is as successful as pharmacotherapy. Research has demonstrated the superiority of CBIT/HRT over supportive therapy and psychoeducation alone in the management of tics in both youth and adults [70, 71]. CBIT/HRT is now considered first-line treatment for mild to moderate tics when intervention is warranted. Treatment components include awareness training, competing response training, relaxation training, contingency management, social support, and relapse prevention. Teaching patients a competing response to target tics to prevent emergence is a central feature.

In summary, optimal patient outcomes depend on management of both ADHD symptoms and tics when they co-occur. Recent research has demonstrated safe treatment of both conditions simultaneously.

References

1. Freeman RD. Tourette Syndrome International Database Consortium. Tic disorders and ADHD: answers from a world-wide clinical dataset on Tourette syndrome. *Eur Child Adolesc Psychiatry*. 2007;**16**(Suppl 1):15–23. Erratum in: *Eur Child Adolesc Psychiatry*. 2007;**16**(8):536.

2. Centers for Disease Control and Prevention (CDC). Prevalence of diagnosed Tourette syndrome in persons aged 6–17 years – United States, 2007. *MMWR Morb Mortal Wkly Rep.* 2009;**58**(21):581–5.

3. Steinberg T., Shmuel Baruch S, Harush A, *et al.* Tic disorders and the premonitory urge. *J Neural Transm.* 2010;**117**(2):277–84.

4. Peterson BS, Leckman JF. The temporal dynamics of tics in Gilles de la Tourette syndrome. *Biol Psychiatry.* 1998;**44**:1337–48.

5. Cohrs S, Rasch T, Altmeyer S, *et al.* Decreased sleep quality and increased sleep related movements in patients with Tourette's syndrome. *J Neurol Neurosurg Psychiatry.* 2001;**70**:192–7.

6. Findley DB, Leckman JF, Katsovich L, *et al.* Development of the Yale Children's Global Stress Index (YCGSI) and its application in children and adolescents with Tourette's syndrome and obsessive-compulsive disorder. *J Am Acad Child Adolesc Psychiatry.* 2003;**42**:450–7.

7. American Psychiatric Association. *Diagnostic and Statistical Manual of Mental Disorders*, 5th edn (DSM-5). Arlington, VA: American Psychiatric Publishing; 2013.

8. World Health Organization. *The International Statistical Classification of Diseases and Related Health Problems*, 10th Revision (ICD-10). Geneva: World Health Organization; 1993.

9. Khalifa N, Von Knorring AL. Prevalence of tic disorders and Tourette syndrome in a Swedish school population. *Dev Med Child Neurol.* 2003;**45**:315–19.

10. Linazasoro G, Van Blercom N, de Zárate CO. Prevalence of tic disorder in two schools in the Basque country: results and methodological caveats. *Mov Disord.* 2006; **21**(12):106–9.

11. Mason A, Banerjee S, Eapen V, *et al.* The prevalence of Tourette syndrome in a mainstream school population. *Dev Med Child Neurol.* 1998;**40**:292–6.

12. Robertson MM, Eapen V, Cavanna AE. The international prevalence, epidemiology, and clinical phenomenology of Tourette syndrome: a cross-cultural perspective. *J Psychosom Res.* 2009;**67**:475–83.

13. Kurlan R, McDermott MP, Deeley C, *et al.* Prevalence of tics in school children and association with placement in special education. *Neurology.* 2001; **57**:1383–8.

14. Bloch MH, Peterson BS, Scahill L, *et al.* Adulthood outcome of tic and obsessive-compulsive symptom severity in children with Tourette syndrome. *Arch Pediatr Adolesc Med.* 2006;**160**:65–9.

15. Jankovic J, Gelineau-Kattner R, Davidson A. Tourette's syndrome in adults. *Mov Disord.* 2010;**25**(13):2171–5.

16. Spencer T, Biederman J, Wilens T. Attention-deficit/hyperactivity disorder and comorbidity. *Pediatr Clin North Am.* 1999;**46**(5):915–27.

17. Khalifa N, Von Knorring AL. Psychopathology in a Swedish population of school children with tic disorders. *J Am Acad Child Adolesc Psychiatry.* 2006;**45**(11):1346–53.

18. Kurlan R, Como PG, Miller B, *et al.* The behavioral spectrum of tic disorders: a community-based study. *Neurology.* 2002;**59**(3):414–20.

19. Debes NM, Hjalgrim H, Skov L. The presence of comorbidity in Tourette syndrome increases the need for pharmacological treatment. *J Child Neurol.* 2009;**24**(12):1504–12.

20. Coffey B, Biederman J, Geller D, *et al.* Distinguishing illness severity from tic severity in children and adolescents with Tourette's disorder. *J Am Acad Child Adolesc Psychiatry.* 2000;**39**(5):556–61.

21. Storch EA, Merlo LJ, Lack C, *et al.* Quality of life in youth with Tourette's syndrome and chronic tic disorder. *J Clin Child Adolesc Psychol.* 2007; **36**(2):217–27.

22. Rizzo R, Gulisano M, Cali PV, *et al.* Long term clinical course of Tourette syndrome. *Brain Dev.* 2012; **34**(8):667–73.

23. Sukhodolsky DG, Landeros-Weisenberger A, Scahill L, Leckman JF, Schultz RT. Neuropsychological functioning in children with Tourette syndrome with and without attention-deficit/hyperactivity disorder. *J Am Acad Child Adolesc Psychiatry.* 2010;**49**(11): 1155–64.

24. Lebowitz R, Motlagh MG, Katsovich L, *et al.* Tourette syndrome in youth with and without obsessive compulsive disorder and attention deficit hyperactivity disorder. *Eur Child Adolesc Psychiatry.* 2012;**21**(8): 451–7.

25. Budman CL, Bruun RD, Park KS, Lesser M, Olson M. Explosive outbursts in children with Tourette's disorder. *J Am Acad Child Adolesc Psychiatry.* 2000;**39**(10):1270–6.

26. Carter AS, O'Donnell DA, Schultz RT, *et al.* Social and emotional adjustment in children affected with Gilles de la Tourette's syndrome: associations with ADHD and family functioning. *J Child Psychol Psychiatry.* 2000;**41**(2):215–23.

27. Burd L, Freeman RD, Klug MG, Kerbeshian J. Tourette syndrome and learning disabilities. *BMC Pediatr.* 2005;**5**:34.

28. Spencer T, Biederman J, Harding M, *et al.* Disentangling the overlap between Tourette's disorder and ADHD. *J Child Psychol Psychiatry.* 1998;**39**(7): 1037–44.

29. Pierre BC, Nolan E, Gadow K, *et al.* Comparison of internalizing and externalizing symptoms in children with attention-deficit hyperactivity disorder with and without comorbid tic disorder. *J Dev Behav Pediatr.* 1999;**20**(3):170–6.

30. Gorman DA, Thompson N, Plessen KJ, *et al.* Psychosocial outcome and psychiatric comorbidity in older adolescents with Tourette syndrome: controlled study. *Br J Psychiatry.* 2010;**197**(1):36–44.

31. Robertson MM, Orth M. Behavioral and affective disorders in Tourette syndrome. *Adv Neurol.* 2006;**99**:39–60.

32. Haddad AD, Umoh G, Bhatia V, Robertson MM. Adults with Tourette's syndrome with and without attention deficit hyperactivity disorder. *Acta Psychiatr Scand.* 2009;**120**(4):299–307.

33. Spencer TJ, Biederman J, Faraone S, *et al.* Impact of tic disorders on ADHD outcome across the life cycle: findings from a large group of adults with and without ADHD. *Am J Psychiatry.* 2001;**158**:611–17.

34. Zhu Y, Leung KM, Liu PZ, *et al.* Comorbid behavioral problems in Tourette's syndrome are positively correlated with the severity of tic symptoms. *Aust N Z J Psychiatry.* 2006;**40**(1):67–73.

35. Hyde TM, Aaronson BA, Randolph C, *et al.* Relationship of birth weight to the phenotypic expression of Gilles de la Tourette's syndrome in monozygotic twins. *Neurology.* 1992;**42**:652–8.

36. Mathews CA, Bimson B, Lowe TL, *et al.* Association between maternal smoking and increased symptom severity in Tourette's syndrome. *Am J Psychiatry.* 2006;**163**(6):1066–73.

37. Pringsheim T, Lang A, Kurlan R, Pearce M, Sandor P. Understanding disability in Tourette syndrome. *Dev Med Child Neurol.* 2009;**51**(6):468–72.

38. Motlagh MG, Katsovich L, Thompson N, *et al.* Severe psychosocial stress and heavy cigarette smoking during pregnancy: an examination of the pre- and perinatal risk factors associated with ADHD and Tourette syndrome. *Eur Child Adolesc Psychiatry.* 2010;**19**(10):755–64.

39. Swain JE, Scahill L, Lombroso PJ, *et al.* Tourette syndrome and tic disorders: a decade of progress. *J Am Acad Child Adolesc Psychiatry.* 2007;**46**(8):947–68.

40. Wolf SS, Jones DW, Knable MB, *et al.* Tourette syndrome: prediction of phenotypic variation in monozygotic twins by caudate nucleus D2 receptor binding. *Science.* 1996;**273**:1225–7.

41. Peterson BS, Choi HA, Hao X, *et al.* Morphologic features of the amygdala and hippocampus in children and adults with Tourette syndrome. *Arch Gen Psychiatry.* 2007;**64**(11):1281–91.

42. Amat JA, Bronen RA, Saluja S, *et al.* Increased number of subcortical hyperintensities on MRI in children and adolescents with Tourette's syndrome, obsessive-compulsive disorder, and attention deficit hyperactivity disorder. *Am J Psychiatry.* 2006;**163**(6):1106–8.

43. Price RA, Kidd KK, Cohen DJ, *et al.* A twin study of Tourette syndrome. *Arch Gen Psychiatry.* 1985;**42**:815–20.

44. Scharf JM, Yu D, Mathews CA, *et al.* Genome-wide association study of Tourette's syndrome. *Mol Psychiatry.* 2013;**18**:721–8.

45. Bloch MH, Panza KE, Landeros-Weisenberger A, Leckman JF. Meta-analysis: treatment of attention-deficit/hyperactivity disorder in children with comorbid tic disorders. *J Am Acad Child Adolesc Psychiatry.* 2009;**48**(9):884–93.

46. Steingard R, Biederman J, Spencer T, Wilens T, Gonzalez A. Comparison of clonidine response in the treatment of attention-deficit hyperactivity disorder with and without comorbid tic disorders. *J Am Acad Child Adolesc Psychiatry.* 1993;**32**(2):350–3.

47. Scahill L, Erenberg G, Berlin CM, Jr., *et al.*; Tourette Syndrome Association Medical Advisory Board: Practice Committee. Contemporary assessment and pharmacotherapy of Tourette syndrome. *NeuroRx.* 2006;**3**(2):192–206. Review.

48. Boon-yasidhi V, Kim YS, Scahill L. An open-label, prospective study of guanfacine in children with ADHD and tic disorders. *J Med Assoc Thai.* 2005;**88**(8):S156–62.

49. Chappell PB, Riddle MA, Scahill L, *et al.* Guanfacine treatment of comorbid attention-deficit hyperactivity disorder and Tourette's syndrome: preliminary clinical experiences. *J Am Acad Child Adolesc Psychiatry.* 1995;**34**:1140–6.

50. Lowe TL, Cohen DJ, Detlor J, Kremenitzer MW, Shaywitz BA. Stimulant medications precipitate Tourette's syndrome. *JAMA.* 1982;**247**(12):1729–31.

51. Gadow KD, Sverd J, Sprafkin J, Nolan EE, Enzor SN. Efficacy of methylphenidate for attention-deficit hyperactivity disorder in children with tic disorder. *Arch Gen Psychiatry.* 1995;**52**(6):444–55.

52. Tourette's Syndrome Study Group. Treatment of ADHD in children with tics: a randomized controlled trial. *Neurology.* 2002;**58**(4):527–36.

53. Castellanos X, Giedd J, Elia J, *et al.* Controlled stimulant treatment of ADHD and comorbid Tourette's syndrome: effects of stimulant and dose. *J Am Acad Child Adolesc Psychiatry.* 1997;**36**:589–96.

54. Allen AJ, Kurlan RM, Gilbert DL, *et al.* Atomoxetine treatment in children and adolescents with ADHD and comorbid tic disorders. *Neurology.* 2005;**65**(12): 1941–9.

55. Spencer TJ, Sallee FR, Gilbert DL, *et al.* Atomoxetine treatment of ADHD in children with comorbid Tourette syndrome. *J Atten Disord.* 2008;**11**(4):470–81.

56. Spencer T, Biederman J, Kerman K, Steingard R, Wilens T. Desipramine treatment of children with attention-deficit hyperactivity disorder and tic disorder or Tourette's syndrome. *J Am Acad Child Adolesc Psychiatry.* 1993;**32**(2):354–60.

57. Spencer T, Biederman J, Coffey B, *et al.* A double-blind comparison of desipramine and placebo in children and adolescents with chronic tic disorder and comorbid attention-deficit/hyperactivity disorder. *Arch Gen Psychiatry.* 2002;**59**:649–56.

58. Singer HS, Brown J, Quaskey S, *et al.* The treatment of attention-deficit hyperactivity disorder in Tourette's syndrome: a double-blind placebo-controlled study with clonidine and desipramine. *Pediatrics.* 1995; **95**(1):74–81.

59. Biederman J, Baldessarini RJ, Wright V, Knee D, Harmat JS. A double-blind placebo controlled study of desipramine in the treatment of ADD: I. Efficacy. *J Am Acad Child Adolesc Psychiatry.* 1989;**28**(5): 777–84.

60. Bruggeman R, Van der Linden C, Buitelaar JK, *et al.* Risperidone versus pimozide in Tourette's disorder: a comparative double-blind parallel-group study. *J Clin Psychiatry.* 2001;**62**(1):50–6.

61. Sallee FR, Kurlan R, Goetz CG, *et al.* Ziprasidone treatment of children and adolescents with Tourette's disorder: a pilot study. *J Am Acad Child Adolesc Psychiatry.* 2000;**39**:292–9.

62. Budman C, Coffey BJ, Shechter R, *et al.* Aripiprazole in children and adolescents with Tourette disorder with and without explosive outbursts. *J Child Adolesc Psychopharmacol.* 2008;**18**(5):509–15.

63. Lyon GJ, Samar S, Jummani R, *et al.* Aripiprazole in children and adolescents with Tourette's disorder: an open-label safety and tolerability study. *J Child Adolesc Psychopharmacol.* 2009;**19**(6):623–33.

64. Murphy TK, Mutch PJ, Reid JM, *et al.* Open label aripiprazole in the treatment of youth with tic disorders. *J Child Adolesc Psychopharmacol.* 2009;**19**(4):441–7.

65. Yoo H, Joung YS, Lee JS, *et al.* A multicenter, randomized, double-blind, placebo-controlled study of aripiprazole in children and adolescents with Tourette's disorder. *J Clin Psychiatry.* 2013;**78**(8):e722–80.

66. Gabbay V, Babb JS, Klein RG, *et al.* A double-blind, placebo-controlled trial of ω-3 fatty acids in Tourette's disorder. *Pediatrics.* 2012;**129**(6):e1493–500.

67. Kurlan R, Crespi G, Coffey B, *et al.*; Pramipexole for TS Trial Investigators. A multicenter randomized placebo-controlled clinical trial of pramipexole for Tourette's syndrome. *Mov Disord.* 2012;**27**(6):775–8.

68. Scott BL, Jankovic J, Donovan DT. Botulinum toxin injection into vocal cord in the treatment of malignant coprolalia associated with Tourette's syndrome. *Mov Disord.* 1996;**11**(4):431–3.

69. Neuner I, Podoll K, Janouschek H, *et al.* From psychosurgery to neuromodulation: deep brain stimulation for intractable Tourette syndrome. *World J Biol Psychiatry.* 2009;**10**(4 Pt 2):366–76.

70. Azrin NH, Nunn RG. Habit-reversal: a method of eliminating nervous habits and tics. *Behav Res Ther.* 1973;**11**(4):619–28.

71. Piacentini J, Woods DW, Scahill L, *et al.* Behavior therapy for children with Tourette disorder: a randomized controlled trial. *JAMA.* 2010; **303**(19):1929–37.

Chapter 28

Sustainable change
Treatment adherence in ADHD

Michael J. Manos

Introduction

"The good that I would do, that I do not; that which I hate, that do I." St. Paul

"We know the good and recognize it, but we cannot do it." Euripides *Hippolytus*

Attention-deficit hyperactivity disorder (ADHD) affects an estimated 11% of the school-aged population in the United States [1]. It is a chronic condition that can have adverse effects extending beyond childhood into adolescence and adulthood [2]. Children, teens, and adults with ADHD struggle to manage domains of functioning that range across the lifespan from experiencing success in school to achieving fulfillment in work, from making friends in childhood to building social networks in adulthood, and from sustaining family trust and intimacy to contributing to community life [3, 4]. Though many people with ADHD "muddle through" in managing the affairs of life, evidence indicates that people diagnosed with ADHD are at higher risk for mental health problems and life adversity [5–8] and families of children with ADHD experience considerable emotional and financial stressors [9, 10]. These adverse outcomes make a strong case that ADHD is a public health concern requiring careful attention to appropriate independent and multimodal treatment approaches. The pervasiveness of symptoms in domains of daily functioning supports the need for ongoing treatment across settings, through the day, and over years. Research and clinical expertise have provided practical treatments for children and adults with ADHD, but despite successes, sustained application of interventions remains problematic. This chapter reviews pharmacotherapy treatment adherence for

ADHD across the lifespan, overviews psychosocial intervention adherence, and provides suggestions to clinicians to improve treatment adherence over time.

ADHD is a treatable neurocognitive condition

Medical interventions

> To see a single daily dose of benzedrine produce a greater improvement in school performance than the combined efforts of a capable staff working in a most favorable setting would have been all but demoralizing to the teachers had not the improvement been so gratifying from a practical viewpoint. Charles Bradley, MD 1937 [11].

Since Bradley's comments on the effects of medical treatment in children with "morbid defect of volition" [12], ADHD treatments are available through increasingly sophisticated modes of delivery. Successful intervention has been demonstrated in preschoolers, children, adolescents, and adults.

Preschoolers

This neurodevelopmental disorder is usually diagnosed in school-age children though symptoms are diagnosable as young as 3 years of age. Initial results from the Preschoolers with ADHD Treatment Study (PATS) indicate that pharmacotherapy with preschoolers can be safe and effective though it should be applied cautiously [13]. In addition, long-term follow-up of young children treated with medication and psychosocial intervention is likely to impact outcomes favorably [14, 15].

Attention-Deficit Hyperactivity Disorder in Adults and Children, ed. Lenard A. Adler, Thomas J. Spencer and Timothy E. Wilens. Published by Cambridge University Press. © Cambridge University Press 2015.

School-age children

Children of school age (6–12 years) are the most studied group of children with ADHD. Pharmacotherapy and psychosocial interventions have been demonstrated to be effective with this age group and symptom reduction has been related to improvements in quality of life and family functioning.

Adolescents

The belief that ADHD symptoms do not extend beyond the teen years is no longer substantive. Only a minority of children diagnosed with ADHD in childhood exhibit normalized behavior in adolescence and even when symptoms improve in the teen years, notable impairment in social, emotional, and behavioral domains may continue [16]. Though with increasing age, symptoms of hyperactivity tend to diminish, difficulties associated with inattention, disorganization, distractibility, low task persistence, and emotional dysregulation become more obvious and problematic [17]. Adolescents have been shown to respond to treatment [18] though the extent to which behavior normalizes or remits is an open question [19].

Adults

ADHD in adults has received increasing attention in the last decade since the dissemination of the World Health Organization (WHO) Adult ADHD Self-Report Scale (ASRS) [20]. ADHD symptoms were initially framed for childhood expression and these have been redefined to better reflect expression in adulthood. Treatment of adults has been demonstrated to be effective over the last several decades [21, 22], and multimodal options combining pharmacotherapy and psychosocial treatment can improve behavioral functioning in the affairs of daily life [23].

Psychosocial interventions

Psychosocial interventions for individuals with ADHD across the lifespan have a demonstrated effectiveness in some studies but an equivocal contribution in others. Cognitive-behavioral psychotherapy for adults [24], parent and teacher skills training for work with children, and behavioral coaching for adolescents [25] are effective in themselves and can give added benefit to pharmacological treatment. Multicenter trials, the most noteworthy of which is the NIMH Collaborative Multisite Multimodal Treatment Study of Children with Attention-Deficit/Hyperactivity

Disorder (MTA) [26, 27], and the Treatment for Adolescents with Depression Study (TADS) [28] report specific advantages of multimodal treatment separate from and in conjunction with psychopharmacology. However, in other studies, no effect of psychosocial intervention was noted when stimulant medication was optimally titrated [29]. Psychosocial interventions may be hard to access and implement [28] so families often find it difficult to start them, much less sustain them. The benefit of psychosocial treatment must be weighed against the ability of a family to carry out the recommended program because some interventions may place undue strain on family functioning through costs in time and money.

Adherence to pharmacotherapy for ADHD is uncommon despite effective treatments

Treatment adherence is the extent to which a prescribed treatment has been completed [30, p. 590]. Its corollary, non-adherence, is defined as the "decreased exposure to a given medical treatment which can subsequently influence multiple medical and psychological outcomes" [31]. Even though logic and evidence support the position that effective treatments, when adhered to, produce beneficial effects over time [32–34], 13.2–64% of children and adults do not adhere to stimulant treatment [35]. When proximal adherence to treatment declines, distal outcomes are drastically affected – healthcare costs increase, family functioning deteriorates, demand placed on medical institutions rises, and ongoing healthcare use persists.

In studies of adherence to ADHD pharmacotherapy, adherent behavior is confirmed prospectively by measures such as saliva assays and pill counts, and retrospectively through prescription refills. New methods using technology allow more refined measurements. The Medication Event Monitoring System (MEMS®) records whether pills (1) were taken, (2) taken as many times as prescribed, and (3) taken on time [36]. Though no measure is likely to be unerringly accurate as patients tend to find ways to circumvent extant recording systems, MEMS® is the most sophisticated system to date and is also relatively easily managed.

In the MTA study [26], treatment adherence in children was studied using rigorous measures (i.e., saliva assay) and high physician contact (rather than by parent report alone). One-fourth (24.5%) of the saliva samples indicated that there was non-adherence and one-quarter (24.8%) of participants did not adhere to treatment at least half of the time. In the sophisticated dosing and monitoring of treatment that characterized the MTA study, just slightly over half (53.5%) of participants followed pharmacotherapy treatment regimens at every time point [37].

Unlike the MTA study, treatment adherence research is typically assessed by parent report and by claims analyses of prescription refills (i.e., monitoring the number of prescriptions filled over time). Findings indicate that medication use abruptly decreases in early to mid adolescence and the trend continues into early adulthood [32]. In addition, clinicians such as physicians and behavior therapists who are in a position to intervene to support adherence tend not to have consistent contact with patients to actively influence the course of treatment. Thus, despite strong evidence that pharmacological treatment works for ADHD, treatment adherent behavior *declines* by age and over time.

Rates of adherence show significant individual variation. In the case of chronic conditions such as ADHD, when prescriptive measures require exposure to treatment over months and years, poor and non-adherence become common; clinicians only get re-engaged in the absence of treatment to manage emerging adverse consequences [38, 39]. The problem of treatment adherence is not confined to mental health conditions either. Estimates indicate that up to 20% of children in the USA have a chronic health condition such as asthma or diabetes and only 50% of these maintain consistent engagement with prescribed treatments [31]. It is as if opposing forces delimit treatment engagement and these forces are more compelling than relief from symptoms.

Explaining treatment adherence in ADHD

Why would treatment adherence in ADHD be so low when the evidence for its benefit is so high? Successful management of personal behavior, referred to as self-control, is at the heart of treatment adherence for individuals with symptoms of ADHD. We will explore this phenomenon in human beings and apply it to the problem of treatment adherence with ADHD.

Though myriad descriptions of self-control are offered from different theoretical perspectives, we adopt B. F. Skinner's operant analysis [40] and

its evolution into Relational Frame Theory [41]. In Skinner's original description of self-control, he observed:

> …[We] must consider the possibility that the individual may control his own behavior…He is often able to do something about the variables affecting him. Some degree of 'self-determination' of conduct is usually recognized in the creative behavior of the artist and scientist, in the self-exploratory behavior of the writer, and in the self-discipline of the ascetic. Humbler versions of self-determination are more familiar. The individual 'chooses' between alternative courses of action, 'thinks through' a problem while isolated from the relevant environment, and guards his health or his position in society through the exercise of 'self-control.' [40, p. 228]

From this perspective, the emphasis is on the *behaving* of the individual, not on the behaver, not on a self that is the source of behaving. This conception differs significantly from common notions of "willpower" that describe behavioral control as volitional. Self-control is less a function of an autonomous self "deciding" what to do and more on arranging the circumstances in which behavior occurs. One who does not have the "self-discipline" to exercise regularly, simply has not arranged the conditions that allow exercise to occur (e.g., joining an exercise class; arranging to meet a friend daily at a specified time and place to run). Thus the person is not controlling a "self" but controlling the circumstances that yield an outcome in which the "self" participates.

Adherence is a behavior, and as such it is subject to the contingencies that control behavior. If a person repeatedly engages a prescribed treatment, it is the behavior of engaging the treatment that produces an outcome. If a person avoids or terminates a treatment, that too performs a function – it results in escape from an aversive condition such as eliminating the daily "chore" of taking medicine at a given time, terminating medicine side effects, or reducing the disapproval of a social network (e.g., in-laws blame parents for being "lazy" for using drugs instead of being "good parents").

Complex behavior such as self-control is also assisted by a function that occurs inside the individual – the function of language. Dr. Russell Barkley described the relation of language and behavior as "a matchless capacity for delaying a motor response to a signal [that] formed the central feature in the evolution of human language from a system of social communication to one of personal reflection and self-regulation" [42, p. 320]. This ability to use language to mediate behavior allows a person to inhibit a prepotent response that yields an immediate consequence (e.g., pleasure of eating an extra dessert) in favor of a new response that yields a delayed but more productive outcome in a distal future (e.g., maintaining a diet to lose weight). From Barkley's perspective, the executive functions that predispose a person to engage behavior consistent with a long-term outcome are suboptimal in individuals with ADHD; current behavior is not controlled to favor *long-term* consequences but rather functions to access *immediate* consequences. The "matchless capacity" of language, however, can improve a person's disposition and tendency to favor distal outcomes.

Relational Frame Theory [41] evolved from an operant approach to behavior analysis to include a broader understanding of the functions and true power of language. Language creates a context for behavior. It can free behavior from the control of immediate contingencies – which produce unwanted future outcomes – to produce behavior that results in desirable outcomes in the distal future.

Two distinctions from the Relational Frame Theory give insight to sustaining treatment adherence in individuals with ADHD. *Values* are new verbal constructions that make it possible to engage behaviors that produce life outcomes not as yet realized. *Rules* (or rule-governed behavior) are *previously* generated verbal constructions that establish relations among events; because they are derived from a person's history, however, they function in the person's present life to reproduce, not a new future, but event relations that have *already* occurred. Behavior changes when *values,* representing a future that was unlikely to occur, replace *rules* that repeat what has already occurred. These two principles – values and rule-governed behavior – can be applied in real life by change agents such as parents, teachers, spouses, and friends.

Values and rule-governed behavior may be described in an example of a clinical case of a 9-year-old boy diagnosed with ADHD predominantly inattentive type. Danny's maternal grandfather, "Papa," did not believe that ADHD was a legitimate diagnosis (the rule) and would not allow discussion of pharmacotherapy as a treatment. Papa stated his rule-governed position: "All it requires is discipline.

His attention span will increase with discipline," and noted that this was what his own father told him when he was growing up. This placed the focus on Danny and created the context that inattention is under volitional control and can be corrected with willpower. Danny himself adopted his Papa's perspective, saying, "I want to do it myself; all it requires is discipline. I'm like Papa, I'm not sure about drugs." This subjective, verbally reinforced rule was derived from an important person in Danny's life and generated actions consistent with the rule that "I can do it myself." The rule subsequently allowed no possibility for pharmacotherapy, an acknowledged effective treatment. Papa worked on school work with Danny every day. In the 6-month follow-up visit, school records indicated that Danny had made virtually no progress in school. The clinician again raised the discussion of pharmacotherapy, and the family initiated medical intervention within a reframed perspective: "Do you think it can work? Let's find out if it does." Papa continued his work with Danny such that in 3 months, with the combined approach of pharmacotherapy and Papa's daily tutoring, Danny made 9 months progress. The perpetuation of rule-governed behavior ("just needs discipline") gave way to a revised perspective that produced valued outcomes.

To bring about effective change in the real world, people work with people. A triadic model of intervention [43] best describes the relationships – the *clinician* is the consultant who both prescribes treatment and supports its implementation; the mediator is a *change agent*, such as a parent, teacher, or other caregiver; and the target is the *client* – the child, adolescent, or adult. Clinicians are experts who have knowledge of available treatments and how to implement them. Change agents directly control the conditions that replace rule-governed behavior with valued behavior. They reduce the occurrence of reactive rule-governed behavior and increase the occasion for behavior consistent with future outcomes. Change agents change across the lifespan. In younger children, valued behaviors such as placing homework in assigned folders or using medicine to improve task orientation are mediated by parents and teachers; in older children – adolescents and in some cases even young adults – change agency is shared among parents, teachers, counsellors, and others such as friends and classmates. Change agents and teens negotiate what is valued and make agreements as to when medicine is to be taken, when structured treatment interruptions (i.e., "drug holidays") are scheduled, and under what conditions homework will be monitored and by whom – decision-making is collaborative. In adults, the change agent is the client him/herself, though spouses or colleagues may also be recruited.

Treatment adherence: lessons learned from other chronic conditions

Moderators of treatment adherence are conditions that are present prior to initiation of a treatment protocol and influence whether or not a person sustains treatment. Mediators are factors that influence the course of treatment as they arise after treatment is initiated. Given the paucity of evidence for the moderators and mediators of treatment adherence in ADHD, we examine the conditions that promote adherence in other disorders in order to apply them to ADHD.

World Health Organization short course

In a review of direct observation therapy (DOT) (i.e., supervised swallowing of drugs to improve adherence) in the WHO's short course in treating tuberculosis worldwide, Volmink and colleagues described five factors that increased treatment adherence: (1) political commitment, (2) improved lab analysis, (3) direct observation of the patient swallowing a pill, (4) a drug supply that provides free drug therapy or reduced cost access, and (5) efficient reporting systems to track prescription use [44]. These factors were derived from managing a disease on a macro-scale, but they can be applied to managing dysfunction on a micro-scale within a contemporary behavioral perspective of treatment adherence in ADHD.

Political commitment created incentives (e.g., returned wages when treatments were completed) and punishers (e.g., involuntary hospital admissions for non-adherers). Applied to ADHD, clinicians encourage change agents who in turn incentivize and reinforce treatment adherence in the home using behavior modification. Improved lab analysis in DOT demonstrated the effectiveness of a medication in the absence of intrusive side effects and provided hard evidence that a treatment worked. In ADHD, the interchange between clinicians and change agents can demonstrate gains in real-life conditions, and via titration strategies, in varying degrees of complexity

[45]; in other words, the clinician assists the family to systematically observe benefits of treatment. Direct observation of the patient swallowing the dose needs no elaboration in its application to ADHD. Available drug access is essential, thus change agents should have access to a medication supply at manageable costs, available at most pharmacies, and with competitive pricing across drugs and drug delivery systems. Finally, a reliable reporting system is widely missing for clinicians who treat ADHD. The monitoring used in the MTA study, for example, is seldom reproduced; thus clinicians cannot intervene in a timely way to insure that treatment works and benefit outweighs side effects.

The other factors that impact treatment adherence that were reported in the WHO's short course but are not quantifiable include the enthusiasm of change agents, the physician's confidence in treatment, reminder letters to patients, assistance by lay people not directly related to treatment (e.g., teachers or family members), unpredictable incentives such as the simple act of observed positive changes by others, increased social supervision of people in treatment, patient-centered contacts with medical professionals, and accounting for the needs and preferences of patients.

Physician behavior

In a review of the association of health outcomes and treatment adherence for chronic disorders such as diabetes and asthma, Drotar described the importance of how clients perceived the level of interest of their physician "in me as opposed to my condition" [46, p. 247]. The less clients perceived the physician understood their need for support, the less consistent was adherence; the more personally engaged the physician was, the more adherent clients were. This principle was especially salient with adolescents.

One pediatric endocrinologist with high rates of adherence in children with diabetes depicted his unswerving interest in his patients' well-being:

> I only care about whether my patients live full lives, and they can only do that if they take care of themselves. If parents don't set standards for kids and tell them they have to do this – I do that for them. I threaten, cajole, praise, tell the parents to take the car away and give it back when the child is adherent. I've even taken a young girl's cell phone and told her she

could have it back when her blood sugars were down. The one thing I never do, however, is cast a moral judgment or use my authority as a doctor when blood sugars go up – I mean, I never get mad at them if blood sugars are down. They won't come back if I do that. (Chair, Pediatric Endocrinology, Cleveland Clinic, personal communication, August, 2010)

Authoritarian models of medical care severely limit treatment adherence [47]. The physician who relies solely on his or her authority as a physician limits the time spent with clients, restricts client understanding of why treatment works, and precludes collaborative decision-making. Collaborative decision-making and shared goal-setting, however, are positively related to treatment adherence. Treatment adherence increases with children and adolescents when physicians: (1) increase knowledge of the chronic illness, (2) describe its biological basis; (3) explain how treatment would impact the illness; (4) authentically give a realistic perspective of treatment; (5) set achievable expectations (valued outcomes), (6) review short-term treatment goals; (7) engage change agents as collaborators; (8) shed the coercive role of authority, and (9) pay special attention to collaboration of change agents and clients [46].

Ongoing monitoring of treatment

Adherence is not routinely and consistently assessed in standard treatment of many disorders [46]. Clinicians are often unaware of when to change interventions that are unsuccessful. In some conditions, treatment can be interrupted for long periods because symptoms go unnoticed until caregivers and clients return for assistance because intruding symptoms have emerged.

Multicomponent adherence interventions

Interventions tend to be adhered to when they combine multiple strategies to sustain treatment engagement rather than relying on single measures that coerce and rely on fear of consequences of nontreatment. In diabetes, when behavior therapy and psychological consultation was implemented in the presence of interventions to address emotional, social, and family processes, more robust effects of improvement in metabolic control were reported [48]. In general, psychological consultation has a positive impact on specific health outcomes [49].

Treatment adherence: lessons learned from ADHD

Functional conditions for adherence to medical treatments for ADHD are highly varied across individuals. Thiruchelvam and colleagues found moderators of high adherence were the absence of teacher-rated oppositional defiant disorder, greater initial severity of symptoms on teacher-rated ADHD scales, and younger age at baseline. Interestingly, the primary predictor associated with ongoing use of pharmacotherapy was a distal effect – success at symptom management in school after 1 year [39]. Nevertheless, only half the sample (52%) adhered to stimulant treatment after 3 years. Other factors associated with adherence to treatment in ADHD are low patient cognitive ability and ongoing treatment at a medical center [50].

Moderators of low adherence were (1) lower severity of ADHD, (2) presence of oppositional defiant/conduct disorder, (3) learning difficulties, (4) anxiety, (5) older age, (6) family dysfunction, and (7) socioeconomic adversity at baseline. Other factors associated with low adherence to pharmacotherapy are low and possibly ineffective starting doses and minority ethnic status [38].

Poor treatment adherence can be *logistical* in nature – families are unable to afford prescribed treatments, doses are forgotten, medicine runs out and prescriptions are not filled. Such barriers to continuous treatment are more common in patients with ADHD than is indicated in patients with diabetes or asthma [51]. A descriptive profile of pharmacological treatment patterns derived from a claims database analysis [52], for example, showed that stimulants were more frequently used over time than non-stimulants, longer-acting medications were preferred over immediate-release formulations [53], and augmentation of treatment was lower with long-acting medications. In children, timing of dosing with immediate-release medicines can especially interfere with continuity of treatment as medicines have differing durations of action. Adherence tends to accrue if clinicians check response to treatment with more frequency [54]; individualize length of time between follow-up appointments to prevent initial suboptimal outcomes [55]; monitor adverse events, however mild, especially in the initial course of treatment [56]; choose the easiest and most appropriate delivery system (e.g., long-acting treatments preferred over immediate-release formulations) [57]; simplify dose administration [58, 59]; monitor treatment in a variety of ways with scheduled office visits, phone calls, email, or through pharmacy database monitoring [60–62]; and, incorporate self-responsibility for medication management as children and adolescents with greater self-responsibility are more likely to report medication dosing error [51]. All of these factors may also be described as psychological side effects such as *perceived* ineffectiveness of treatment [63].

Another logistical reality is that as one grows and matures, fundamental lifestyle changes impact long-term treatment. Inadequate change agent supervision contributes to low ADHD adherence rates and results in missed doses. (Recall that many children with ADHD have parents who themselves are disorganized and distractible.) Change agents' influence significantly wanes over time as students leave the supervision of their parents to attend college. In some instances, change agents have less time and availability to monitor ongoing treatment when circumstances, such as job responsibilities or the birth of a child, change. In other families where adherence was maintained through threat of punishment for non-use, treatments tend to be abandoned when children gain independence and the threat of punishment is withdrawn.

Adherence rates are also *rule-governed* – members of a family may hold the perspective that medicine is a "cure" used only by bad parents or they may believe that individuals taking controlled substances have "something wrong with them that needs to be fixed." Rule-governed behavior is especially pernicious in this latter context because taking medicine becomes a daily reminder of a fault in the individual – medication confirms disease [64]. Stopping treatment – an action consistent with the rule – alleviates this social derision but prevents the emergence of positive effects that take weeks or months to change (i.e., grades or changes in friendships). Other debilitating perceptions are associated with resistance to taking pills; the requirement for long-term treatment that may, dauntingly, extend across the lifespan; reluctance to take medicine due to disinformation about it (e.g., "If I give medicine to my child when she's younger, she'll use drugs when she's older."); uninformed and misinformed social pressures; and a poor understanding of treatment goals and target outcomes.

Strategies from evidence and theory to promote adherence in ADHD

The methods of control used to maintain treatment adherence ultimately belong to the community [40, p. 240]. With focus on the client's social network, treatment adherence is not an effort of one individual acting upon him- or herself alone. Children, teenagers, and adults with ADHD who have difficulty valuing longer-term consequences may be assisted via their network of relationships – parents, teachers, spouses, colleagues, relatives, and friends. Within a community, valued behavior replaces impulsive or non-functional rule-governed action. Ultimately, a person adopts the perspective of the community to sustain health promotion through self-generated verbal facility. In ADHD, the process begins with the interaction of clinician and change agent to influence the client. The clinician ties treatment to valued outcomes and does so with conscious intent. Clients and change agents can then observe that treatment gives greater control over current circumstances that produce valued outcomes, rather than that treatment violates social rules or misinformed perspectives. Treatment ultimately gives control over the factors that control behavior – it gives control back to the volition of client and change agent rather than assuming control is there from the beginning, existing only in the individual.

How does a Relational Frame perspective translate to clinical practices that support treatment adherence in ADHD? It starts in the initial conversation the client has with the clinician. The discerning clinician discloses the "rule" about pharmacotherapy that controls a change agent's actions and begins a fresh conversation about what is possible regarding treatment and what valued outcome may derive from a recommended treatment. The role of authority assumed by many clinicians gives way to a role of collaborator in sustainable change.

Potential approaches to enhance ADHD treatment adherence fall into two broad categories – *easing logistics* and *transforming rules*. Logistics are the simple, organized delivery of services. These fall largely under the purview of the clinician (usually the primary care physician) and the pharmaceutical industry to insure monitored access to treatment. Rules are personal, however, and they live in the client's community of relationships; they are modified in relationships and are accessed only in the verbal community surrounding the patient. Rules are transformed in change agents by those who speak to change agents. The role of the clinician is critical as he or she can strengthen valued behavior and point out the pitfalls of impulsive adherence to rule-governed behavior. The clinician makes the distal future more salient while clarifying the pitfalls of impulsive outcomes. The following are guidelines for easing logistics and transforming rules.

Easing logistics

- Deliberately include strategies of treatment adherence in the treatment protocol.
- Systematically and sufficiently monitor ongoing treatment response. Treatment adherence should not be assumed but rather should be confirmed by frequent contact with the clinician and by reliable evidence of change over time.
- Individualize continuity of care. Insure that the frequency and duration of follow-up sessions are workable for each family and client. Sessions should follow a standard protocol querying symptom reduction, quality of relationship, and review of side effects. Schedule feedback sessions with change agents. It is best to use direct contact (i.e., phone or office visit) or email.
- Create a structure (i.e., regular programmed procedures) for office staff to communicate with change agents. Communication opportunities should be frequent at the beginning of treatment and gradually built into the schedule of monthly, quarterly, and annual visits to the clinician. (See Baumgaertel and Wolraich, for practical office management of this process [65].)
- Create incentives for treatment adherence. Though social reinforcers are ubiquitously used in raising children, they may also be applied to the behavior of change agents. Clinicians can point out treatment gains and encourage change agents to sustain treatment. Primary care physicians can adjust treatment to remove or control side effects or manage difficulties with treatment administration. Above all, clinicians and change agents should avoid nagging, begging, or cajoling as this is usually counterproductive.
- Recommend that parents are present and engaged with teens. When teens begin to assume responsibility for managing symptoms, encourage parents to monitor (i.e., observe) but not to coerce the adolescent's self-administration of medication in order to provide reliable feedback to clinicians.
- Track individuals who have terminated treatment. Feedback on medication use can be monitored through databases or by using an office manager to check on treatment progress.
- Provide client and family education, behavior therapy, and behavioral coaching that emphasize active participation in treatment. These help to select coping skills to effectively implement medical and psychosocial interventions. In adults, they may identify potential self-managed work accommodations.
- Inquire about conditions in the family. In order to offer treatment options that accommodate family needs and optimize patient convenience, knowledge of family stressors such as hectic routines, problematic family members, and job stress can be useful.
- Provide change agents with readily available and affordable medications within guidelines provided by regulating agencies.
- Use extended-duration formulations to provide maximum coverage over the course of the day's activities. When possible, avoid dosing regimens that require multiple daily dosing.
- Encourage change agents to integrate pharmacotherapy into the routine of the day as a habitual practice.
- In general, continue to supervise treatment over time to resolve logistical factors that lead clients to disengage treatment.

Transforming rules

- Expect treatment adherence to fade. This dictates the need to incorporate systematic logistical strategies to handle adherence as part of the treatment protocol.
- Prior to pharmacotherapy, enroll the patient and change agents by accurately informing and correcting change agents' and client's disinformation about medicine and speaking to the person's commitment to improve (i.e., valued outcomes).
- Develop a strong therapeutic alliance to form a clinician–change agent partnership in problem

solving. The doctor is a collaborator. This requires following up regularly with clients to adjust dose, address side effects, and to discuss problems obtaining medication. Adherence tends to improve with feedback to the clinician; in turn, empowering the clinician to act as an effective change agent to change agents.

- In the teenage years, turn over control to the teen as a privilege rather than using coercive control through shame, guilt, or anger.
- Provide education to change agents regarding ADHD as a biological condition. Transform the perception about ADHD behavior itself away from the idea that it is a result of people not engaging their disruptive behavior out of willfulness.
- Re-frame the relationship of medicine to the condition. The client uses medicine to manage attention in difficult conditions such as effortful attention tasks. Medicine is not daily evidence of the presence of a disease, it is the occasion for people to exercise greater control over their own attention.
- When improvement is noted during initial treatment, generate a discussion (i.e., create the verbal context) to re-frame improvement. The client is the source of success, medicine did not "do it to him/her." Medicine assists attention but it is still the person who *directs* attention toward useful activity. Pharmacotherapy assists the treatment protocol that includes skill acquisition and modifying school or work conditions; it does not change the person.
- Use language that conveys respect for change agents' disinformation and convey that their point of view matters. Pharmacotherapy may not be a treatment option for the rest of the child's life but may certainly be needed to manage conditions in the present.
- Speak to the change agents' commitment to improve. In conversations about the treatment process, create a distal outcome that presents as salient.
- Encourage active participation in treatment by clients and change agents. Include multiple members of the client's social network or family in discussions about pharmacotherapy so that side conversations about "bad parenting" are illuminated for what they are (i.e., disinformation).

- When possible, combine behavioral skill acquisition with medical intervention to strengthen perceptions that the client is the source of change due to his/her engagement rather than that treatment is being "done to" him/her. Design a treatment protocol that gives greater participation of the client and change agents and is more likely to tie personal effort to treatment. Psychosocial treatments for adults in pharmacotherapy are more consistently adhered to when they target interpersonal relationships and include skills for managing distress associated with relationships [66, 67].
- Recommend or provide skills training in decision-making for teens and adults. Decision-making competence in adolescence and adulthood may be a mediator in adherence. It is defined as "the ability or capacity to form flexible and effective plans for managing different situations in the midst of pursuing one's goals" [68, p. 178].
- Underscore that the change agent is primary in the treatment process.
- Focus potential school and work accommodations for adolescents and adults on those that can be self- or social network-managed rather than on those that require the conciliations from authority in the school or workplace.
- Build in structured treatment interruptions (i.e., drug holidays) for those with managed side effects and for those whose rule-governed behavior can only be postponed rather than transformed. Treatment interruptions are typically of longer duration (several weeks or months rather than weekends) and occur at periods of low demand that have a reduced requirement for directed attention.
- In general, continue to supervise treatment over time to resolve intruding percepts that lead clients to disengage treatment and abandon focus on distal outcomes.

From patients to participant-collaborators in lifestyles that work

Based on current evidence, avoidance is more the rule than the exception in ADHD treatment. For clinicians using multiple facets of engagement, the consistent treatment of people with ADHD across the lifespan requires a recurrent cycle of other-to-self assistance. Physicians, psychologists, and other professionals assist the actions of change agents to change the behavior of clients. The efforts of clinicians and change agents, however, are hampered by logistics and rule-governed behavior. It can become the role of the clinician to assist in managing the logistics and transforming rules.

The very nature of ADHD precludes consistent adherence to treatment, and actually predisposes a person to escape from the demand imposed by treatment. It inclines a person toward impulsive acts that yield a short-term effect and repels them from valued acts that yield valued distal effects. Reversing this ultimately occurs by increasing the salience or "realness" of the delayed outcome. This is accomplished within the individual but seldom by the individual acting alone. It is accomplished in the verbal community around the individual, by the engagement of others in the person's life.

Feedback to the clinician is a critical factor in assisting treatment adherence. That no readily available biomarkers exist in ADHD creates a compelling need to design methods that measure adherence. Treatment adherence impact (TAI), the outcome measure of the effects of adherence to pharmacotherapy or behavioral treatment, is largely missing in most chronic conditions [31] and is especially missing from ADHD treatment. TAI quantifies the ongoing effects of sustained treatment using a variety of methods – "An ideal operational definition of TAI would be a clinical cutoff on an adherence measure for which scores above (or below depending on the directionality of the measure) indicate a level of non-adherence that results in change in medical or psychological outcomes (improvement or decline)" [31, p. 384]. By systematically examining TAI in adherence studies across the lifespan of individuals with ADHD, we may advance our understanding of strategies that promote adherence to the treatment of a condition that militates against treatment.

Conclusion

Sustainable change in ADHD is possible by removing the physical barriers to treatment such as costs and access and by modifying the way we commonly talk and think about ADHD. Strategies to modify logistics

and rules are little understood, thus research, awareness of, and training in recognizing the barriers to adherence, especially rule-governed behavior, is essential. A fruitful first step may be to simply observe clinicians with strong adherence rates to determine what they do that works.

References

1. Visser S, Danielson M, Bitsko R, et al. Trends in the Parent-Report of Health Care Provider-Diagnosed and Medicated Attention-Deficit/Hyperactivity Disorder: United States 2003–2011. *J Am Acad Child Adolesc Psychiatry*. 2013;**53**(1):34–46 e32.

2. Biederman J, Faraone SV. Attention-deficit hyperactivity disorder. *Lancet*. 2005;**366**(9481): 237–48.

3. Minde K, Lewin D, Weiss G, et al. The hyperactive child in elementary school: a 5 year, controlled, followup. *Except Child*. 1971;**38**(3):215–21.

4. Adesman AR. The diagnosis and management of attention-deficit/hyperactivity disorder in pediatric patients. *Prim Care Companion J Clin Psychiatry*. 2001;**3**(2):66–77.

5. Spencer TJ. Issues in the management of patients with complex attention-deficit hyperactivity disorder symptoms. *CNS Drugs*. 2009;**23**(Suppl 1):9–20.

6. Biederman J, Petty CR, Fried R, et al. Educational and occupational underattainment in adults with attention-deficit/hyperactivity disorder: a controlled study. *J Clin Psychiatry*. 2008;**69**(8):1217–22.

7. Biederman J, Faraone S, Milberger S, et al. A prospective 4-year follow-up study of attention-deficit hyperactivity and related disorders. *Arch Gen Psychiatry*. 1996;**53**(5):437–46.

8. Biederman J, Milberger S, Faraone SV, et al. Impact of adversity on functioning and comorbidity in children with attention-deficit hyperactivity disorder. *J Am Acad Child Adolesc Psychiatry*. 1995;**34**(11):1495–503.

9. Johnston C, Mash EJ. Families of children with attention-deficit/hyperactivity disorder: review and recommendations for future research. *Clin Child Fam Psychol Rev*. 2001;**4**(3):183–207.

10. Swensen AR, Birnbaum HG, Secnik K, et al. Attention-deficit/hyperactivity disorder: increased costs for patients and their families. *J Am Acad Child Adolesc Psychiatry*. 2003;**42**(12):1415–23.

11. Bradley C. The behavior of children receiving benzedrine. *Am J Psychiatry*. 1937;**94**:577–85.

12. Still GF. Some abnormal psychical conditions in children: excerpts from three lectures. *J Atten Disord*. 2006;**10**(2):126–36.

13. Greenhill L, Kollins S, Abikoff H, *et al*. Efficacy and safety of immediate-release methylphenidate treatment for preschoolers with ADHD. *J Am Acad Child Adolesc Psychiatry*. 2006;**45**(11): 1284–93.

14. Greenhill LL, Posner K, Vaughan BS, Kratochvil CJ. Attention deficit hyperactivity disorder in preschool children. *Child Adolesc Psychiatr Clin N Am*. 2008; **17**(2):347–66, ix.

15. Murray DW. Treatment of preschoolers with attention-deficit/hyperactivity disorder. *Curr Psychiatry Rep*. 2010;**12**(5):374–81.

16. Lee SS, Lahey BB, Owens EB, Hinshaw SP. Few preschool boys and girls with ADHD are well-adjusted during adolescence. *J Abnorm Child Psychol*. 2008; **36**(3):373–83.

17. Krause J, Krause KH, Dresel SH, la Fougere C, Ackenheil M. ADHD in adolescence and adulthood, with a special focus on the dopamine transporter and nicotine. *Dialogues Clin Neurosci*. 2006;**8**(1): 29–36.

18. Newcorn JH, Stein MA, Cooper KM. Dose-response characteristics in adolescents with attention-deficit/hyperactivity disorder treated with OROS methylphenidate in a 4-week, open-label, dose-titration study. *J Child Adolesc Psychopharmacol*. 2010;**20**(3):187–96.

19. Ramos-Quiroga JA, Casas M. Achieving remission as a routine goal of pharmacotherapy in attention-deficit hyperactivity disorder. *CNS Drugs*. 2011;**25**(1):17–36.

20. Kessler RC, Adler L, Ames M, *et al*. The World Health Organization Adult ADHD Self-Report Scale (ASRS): a short screening scale for use in the general population. *Psychol Med*. 2005;**35**(2):245–56.

21. Wender PH, Reimherr FW, Wood DR. Attention deficit disorder ('minimal brain dysfunction') in adults. A replication study of diagnosis and drug treatment. *Arch Gen Psychiatry*. 1981;**38**(4):449–56.

22. Spencer T, Biederman J, Wilens T, *et al*. Pharmacotherapy of attention-deficit hyperactivity disorder across the life cycle. *J Am Acad Child Adolesc Psychiatry*. 1996;**35**(4):409–32.

23. Faraone SV, Antshel KM. Diagnosing and treating attention-deficit/hyperactivity disorder in adults. *World Psychiatry*. 2008;**7**(3):131–6.

24. Ramsay JR. Current status of cognitive-behavioral therapy as a psychosocial treatment for adult attention-deficit/hyperactivity disorder. *Curr Psychiatry Rep*. 2007;**9**(5):427–33.

25. Pelham WE, Jr., Fabiano GA. Evidence-based psychosocial treatments for attention-deficit/ hyperactivity disorder. *J Clin Child Adolesc Psychol*. 2008;**37**(1):184–214.

26. A 14-month randomized clinical trial of treatment strategies for attention-deficit/hyperactivity disorder. The MTA Cooperative Group. Multimodal Treatment Study of Children with ADHD. *Arch Gen Psychiatry*. 1999;**56**(12):1073–86.

27. Richters JE, Arnold LE, Jensen PS, *et al*. NIMH collaborative multisite multimodal treatment study of children with ADHD: I. Background and rationale. *J Am Acad Child Adolesc Psychiatry*. 1995;**34**(8): 987–1000.

28. Reeves G, Anthony B. Multimodal treatments versus pharmacotherapy alone in children with psychiatric disorders: implications of access, effectiveness, and contextual treatment. *Paediatr Drugs*. 2009;**11**(3): 165–9.

29. van der Oord S, Prins PJ, Oosterlaan J, Emmelkamp PM. Does brief, clinically based, intensive multimodal behavior therapy enhance the effects of methylphenidate in children with ADHD? *Eur Child Adolesc Psychiatry*. 2007;**16**(1):48–57.

30. Kahana S, Drotar D, Frazier T. Meta-analysis of psychological interventions to promote adherence to treatment in pediatric chronic health conditions. *J Pediatr Psychol*. 2008;**33**(6):590–611.

31. Pai AL, Drotar D. Treatment adherence impact: the systematic assessment and quantification of the impact of treatment adherence on pediatric medical and psychological outcomes. *J Pediatr Psychol*. 2010; **35**(4):383–93.

32. Charach A, Ickowicz A, Schachar R. Stimulant treatment over five years: adherence, effectiveness, and adverse effects. *J Am Acad Child Adolesc Psychiatry*. 2004;**43**(5):559–67.

33. Torgersen T, Gjervan B, Rasmussen K. Treatment of adult ADHD: is current knowledge useful to clinicians? *Neuropsychiatr Dis Treat*. 2008;**4**(1): 177–86.

34. Swanson J, Arnold LE, Kraemer H, *et al*. Evidence, interpretation, and qualification from multiple reports of long-term outcomes in the Multimodal Treatment Study of children with ADHD (MTA): Part II: supporting details. *J Atten Disord*. 2008;**12**(1):15–43.

35. Adler LD, Nierenberg AA. Review of medication adherence in children and adults with ADHD. *Postgrad Med*. 2010;**122**(1):184–91.

36. Adler LA, Lynch LR, Shaw DM, *et al*. Medication adherence and symptom reduction in adults treated with mixed amphetamine salts in a randomized crossover study. *Postgrad Med*. 2011;**123**(5):71–9.

37. Pappadopulos E, Jensen PS, Chait AR, *et al*. Medication adherence in the MTA: saliva methylphenidate samples versus parent report and mediating effect of concomitant behavioral treatment.

J Am Acad Child Adolesc Psychiatry. 2009;**48**(5): 501–10.

38. Faraone SV, Biederman J, Zimmerman B. An analysis of patient adherence to treatment during a 1-year, open-label study of OROS methylphenidate in children with ADHD. *J Atten Disord*. 2007;**11**(2): 157–66.

39. Thiruchelvam D, Charach A, Schachar RJ. Moderators and mediators of long-term adherence to stimulant treatment in children with ADHD. *J Am Acad Child Adolesc Psychiatry*. 2001;**40**(8):922–8.

40. Skinner BF. *Science and Human Behavior*. New York, NY: Macmillan; 1953.

41. Barnes-Holmes Y, Hayes SC, Barnes-Holmes D, Roche B. Relational frame theory: a post-Skinnerian account of human language and cognition. *Adv Child Dev Behav*. 2001;**28**:101–38.

42. Barkley R. Linkages between attention and executive functions. In: Lyon GR, Krasnegor NA, eds. *Attention, Memory and Executive Function*. Baltimore, MD: Brookes. 1996; 307–25.

43. Tharp RG, Wetzel RJ. *Behavior Modification in the Natural Environment*. New York, NY: Academic Press; 1969.

44. Volmink J, Matchaba P, Garner P. Directly observed therapy and treatment adherence. *Lancet*. 2000; **355**(9212):1345–50.

45. Manos MJ, Tom-Revzon C, Bukstein OG, Crismon ML. Changes and challenges: managing ADHD in a fast-paced world. *J Manag Care Pharm*. 2007;**13** (9 Suppl B):S2–13; quiz S14–16.

46. Drotar D. Physician behavior in the care of pediatric chronic illness: association with health outcomes and treatment adherence. *J Dev Behav Pediatr*. 2009;**30**(3): 246–54.

47. Drotar D, Crawford P, Bonner M. Collaborative decision-making and promoting treatment adherence in pediatric chronic illness. *Patient Intelligence*. 2010;**2**:1–7.

48. Hood KK, Rohan JM, Peterson CM, Drotar D. Interventions with adherence-promoting components in pediatric type 1 diabetes: meta-analysis of their impact on glycemic control. *Diabetes Care*. 2010; **33**(7):1658–64.

49. Gelfand K, Geffken G, Lewin A, *et al*. An initial evaluation of the design of pediatric psychology consultation service with children with diabetes. *J Child Health Care*. 2004;**8**(2):113–23.

50. Gau SS, Chen SJ, Chou WJ, *et al*. National survey of adherence, efficacy, and side effects of methylphenidate in children with attention-deficit/

51. Clay D, Farris K, McCarthy AM, Kelly MW, Howarth R. Family perceptions of medication administration at school: errors, risk factors, and consequences. *J Sch Nurs*. 2008;**24**(2):95–102.

52. Christensen L, Sasane R, Hodgkins P, Harley C, Tetali S. Pharmacological treatment patterns among patients with attention-deficit/hyperactivity disorder: retrospective claims-based analysis of a managed care population. *Curr Med Res Opin*. 2010;**26**(4):977–89.

53. Lachaine J, Beauchemin C, Sasane R, Hodgkins PS. Treatment patterns, adherence, and persistence in ADHD: a Canadian perspective. *Postgrad Med*. 2012;**124**(3):139–48.

54. Pliszka SR. Pharmacologic treatment of attention-deficit/hyperactivity disorder: efficacy, safety and mechanisms of action. *Neuropsychol Rev*. 2007; **17**(1):61–72.

55. Pliszka S. Practice parameter for the assessment and treatment of children and adolescents with attention-deficit/hyperactivity disorder. *J Am Acad Child Adolesc Psychiatry*. 2007;**46**(7):894–921.

56. Pliszka SR. Texas Children's Medication Algorithm for ADHD: clarification. *J Am Acad Child Adolesc Psychiatry*. 2001;**40**(9):991.

57. Swanson J. Compliance with stimulants for attention-deficit/hyperactivity disorder: issues and approaches for improvement. *CNS Drugs*. 2003;**17** (2):117–31.

58. Kripalani S, Yao X, Haynes RB. Interventions to enhance medication adherence in chronic medical conditions: a systematic review. *Arch Intern Med*. 2007;**167**(6):540–50.

59. Sanchez RJ, Crismon ML, Barner JC, Bettinger T, Wilson JP. Assessment of adherence measures with different stimulants among children and adolescents. *Pharmacotherapy*. 2005;**25**(7):909–17.

60. Dopheide JA. The role of pharmacotherapy and managed care pharmacy interventions in the treatment of ADHD. *Am J Manag Care*. 2009; **15**(5 Suppl):S141–50.

61. Ramos-Quiroga JA, Bosch R, Castells X, *et al*. Effect of switching drug formulations from immediate-release to extended-release OROS methylphenidate : a chart review of Spanish adults with attention-deficit hyperactivity disorder. *CNS Drugs*. 2008;**22**(7): 603–11.

62. Chou WJ, Chou MC, Tzang RF, *et al*. Better efficacy for the osmotic release oral system methylphenidate among poor adherents to immediate-release

methylphenidate in the three ADHD subtypes. *Psychiatry Clin Neurosci.* 2009;**63**(2):167–75.

63. Toomey SL, Sox CM, Rusinak D, Finkelstein JA. Why do children with ADHD discontinue their medication? *Clin Pediatr.* 2012;**51**(8):763–9.

64. Manos M. Nuances of assessment and treatment of ADHD in adults: a guide for psychologists. *Prof Psychol Res Pract.* 2010;**41**(6):511–17.

65. Baumgaertel A, Wolraich M. Practice guideline for the diagnosis and management of attention deficit hyperactivity disorder. *Ambulatory Child Health.* 1998;**4**:45–58.

66. Meijer WM, Faber A, van den Ban E, Tobi H. Current issues around the pharmacotherapy of ADHD in children and adults. *Pharm World Sci.* 2009;**31**(5): 509–16.

67. Safren SA, Sprich SE, Cooper-Vince C, Knouse LE, Lerner JA. Life impairments in adults with medication-treated ADHD. *J Atten Disord.* 2010; **13**(5):524–31.

68. Miller VA, Drotar D. Decision-making competence and adherence to treatment in adolescents with diabetes. *J Pediatr Psychol.* 2007;**32** (2):178–88.

Chapter 29

College students with ADHD

J. Russell Ramsay and Anthony L. Rostain

Introduction

Young adults with attention-deficit hyperactivity disorder (ADHD) are at risk for experiencing numerous life difficulties as a consequence of impairments in the cognitive skills that undergird self-control, also known as the executive functions [1, 2]. Moreover, coming as they do during this period of life during which there are long-term effects of decisions made (e.g., education, career, relationships), the manner in which these life difficulties are managed may have lingering effects on one's sense of self and one's future.

The aim of this chapter is to review how ADHD affects the experiences of young adults, roughly defined as 18- to 30-year-olds, who are enrolled in post-secondary educational programs. In particular, the current review will start with a discussion of the typical difficulties encountered by these students that might lead them to seek help. The components of a competent assessment of ADHD in young adults, as well as some areas of concern in their evaluation will be outlined. The chapter will conclude with an overview of the different treatments available to college and university students with ADHD, including discussions of the available outcome research on these approaches.

Symptoms and functional impairments

As a group, individuals with ADHD are less likely to attend college and are more likely to drop out of college than individuals without ADHD [3, 4]. Surveys have found that between 2% and 9% of college students fulfill diagnostic criteria for ADHD [5–7], although only about 1% of students formally identify themselves with ADHD [4]. Nevertheless, increasing numbers of students are arriving at college with learning disabilities associated with ADHD. Although the prevalence of college students with any sort of disability has

consistently fallen around 9%, the number of students with learning disabilities (including ADHD) comprises a growing portion of this percentage of students with disabilities despite the likely under-identification of ADHD.

In terms of dealing with the demands of college, students with ADHD are likely to experience numerous adjustment issues, including using ineffective coping skills to manage the academic and social demands of college, reporting higher levels of internal restlessness, experiencing more distracting thoughts, reporting more depressive symptoms, having lower grades, and being more likely to be placed on academic probation when compared with non-ADHD students [7–13]. Higher education students with ADHD do not seem to be at greater risk for psychiatric diagnoses than their non-ADHD peers [9], although students with ADHD often report clinical complaints related to mild mood or anxiety symptoms, substance use, and self-esteem issues [12, 14–16]. They also perform about as well on intelligence tests as their non-ADHD peers [7]. Thus, it is reasonable to conclude that higher education students with ADHD, particularly if they are not diagnosed until young adulthood, may represent a distinct population with lower levels of impairment than individuals whose ADHD was first identified in childhood [3].

Regarding specific academic strategies used by college students with ADHD, these students scored lower than both students with learning disabilities and control group students on measures of time management, concentration, selecting main ideas, and test strategies [17]. ADHD and learning disabled students both scored lower than control group students on measures of motivation, anxiety, information processing, and self-testing, with measures of motivation and time management being the strongest predictors of college

Attention-Deficit Hyperactivity Disorder in Adults and Children, ed. Lenard A. Adler, Thomas J. Spencer and Timothy E. Wilens. Published by Cambridge University Press. © Cambridge University Press 2015.

grade [18]; both of these factors are common problems for students with ADHD.

It is clear that college presents ADHD students with many challenges that may be difficult for them to manage effectively. However, the aforementioned research is based on students already diagnosed with ADHD. Many individuals arrive at college who have exhibited features of ADHD but have never been diagnosed because they heretofore have not encountered significant coping difficulties until facing the myriad demands of college or university life. The next section will review the key components of a comprehensive assessment for ADHD in young adults.

Assessment

The majority of college students without ADHD report multiple domains of learning-related challenges, with the main areas classified as information processing (e.g., concentration, memory), reading and writing (e.g., slow reading, poor comprehension, difficulty organizing thoughts while writing), motivation (e.g., getting started on academic tasks), mathematics, and test taking [19]. Consequently, some college students encountering academic difficulties for the first time may mistakenly attribute these problems to ADHD. A small minority of college students may exaggerate or fabricate symptoms of ADHD in an attempt to seek academic accommodations or prescription medication for purposes of cognitive enhancement or other types of misuse [20–23]. Thus, it is important that assessments for ADHD in college students incorporate corroborative information regarding symptoms (e.g., parent reports) and impairments (e.g., academic underperformance, poor class attendance) in addition to the standard assessment of symptoms (including use of ADHD screening instruments) in order to establish a definitive diagnosis. To be sure, it is often difficult to disentangle the various factors contributing to academic underperformance and/or poor adjustment to college; hence, sufficient time should be set aside to explore all facets of the student's functioning (see Table 29.1) [24].

A comprehensive assessment for ADHD in college or university students begins with a clinical interview in which the reason for referral, presenting problems, and the history of these problems are reviewed. The degree of impairment associated with these difficulties should be assessed to determine the impact of

Table 29.1. Summary of recommended considerations when assessing and treating college students with Attention-Deficit Hyperactivity Disorder

Comprehensive diagnostic assessment
Childhood and current symptom checklists
Norm-based adult ADHD inventories
Norm-based executive function inventories
Gather corroborative information (observer ratings, old reports, report cards)
Structured diagnostic interview to assess for differential or comorbid conditions
Consider possible malingering or secondary gain with a diagnosis of ADHD

Treatment options
Academic accommodations
    Formal accommodations (require evidence of a learning disability to qualify)
    Informal accommodations (coping strategies)
ADHD coaching
Medication treatment
    Stimulant medications for ADHD
    Non-stimulant medications for ADHD
    Other medication options
        Off-label treatments for ADHD
        Treatment options for comorbid conditions
    Monitor for misuse of medications
Psychosocial treatment
Cognitive-behavioral therapy for adult ADHD
Cognitive-behavioral therapy for comorbid conditions

Abbreviation: ADHD = attention-deficit hyperactivity disorder.

coping difficulties on a student's adaptation to school. Academic difficulties are the primary reasons these students seek help for ADHD, often at the behest of concerned family, faculty, or other college/university personnel. The clinical interview should explore the potential role of disorganization, poor time management, and procrastination on academic performance, as well as collateral problems in other areas of life, such as keeping up with non-academic tasks, handling social relationships, etc.

Even if the student did not experience significant impairment until reaching college, there must be ample evidence of the emergence of ADHD symptoms by early adolescence in order for the diagnosis to be established. Hence, the clinical interview should include a thorough developmental history. Family input regarding a student's childhood is often essential in the review of various developmental factors, hence it is important to include parents at some point in the evaluation. The family medical, psychiatric, and learning histories should be reviewed, with particular attention paid to whether there is history of ADHD and/or learning problems in the family. It is useful to have parental input regarding the student's educational history and experiences at different levels of school. Parents can provide corroborative evidence in the form of past report cards, evaluations, and/or recollections of past behaviors and teachers' comments. College personnel who refer students for evaluation, such as college counselors or advisors, may also be able to provide useful insights about the student's functioning at college.

Screening for comorbid diagnoses should occur throughout the interview. It is useful to follow up on suspected coexisting symptoms using structured clinical interview and to listen to concerns expressed by significant others about the student's mental functioning. The evidence regarding comorbidity among college students with ADHD is mixed, inasmuch as these students are generally high functioning but may report issues related to low self-esteem, poor use of coping skills, and increased sensitivity to the potentially disruptive effects of "typical college life," such as poor sleep habits, the behavior of roommates, lack of structured routine, etc.

ADHD symptoms should be assessed throughout the evaluation, but it is essential to quantify these by using symptom checklists and other normative self-report inventories and by reviewing *Diagnostic and Statistical Manual of Mental Disorders* (DSM) criteria. There are easy-to-use symptom checklists that are based on DSM-IV criteria that include separate forms for childhood and adult functioning as well as both self- and observer-reports [3, 25]. Other available symptom checklists may generally assess similar items (ADHD Rating Scale-IV; [26]), with some recent inventories having been developed specifically for adults (World Health Organization Adult ADHD Self-Report Scale; [27]).

A drawback of current DSM criteria for ADHD is that they were developed for children and some symptoms may not be relevant for young adults. Consequently, inventories have been developed for and normative data gathered on adults in order to reflect developmentally relevant features of adult ADHD. The Brown Attention Deficit Disorders Scale – Adult Version (BADDS; [28]) is a very useful scale that yields useful subscale scores that are clinically useful in identifying common areas of difficulty and includes space for observer ratings of symptoms, though there are no norms for observer ratings. The Conners' Adult ADHD Rating Scales (CAARS; [29]) offers several self-report versions as well as observer reports. The Long Version includes subscales associated with DSM-IV subtypes but also offers other subscales related to

common features of ADHD, including issues related to self-concept.

An organizing conceptualization of ADHD is the view that it is a developmental disorder of impaired executive functions, or those self-directed actions that comprise self-regulation [30]. Students often experience functional difficulties managing the academic and social demands of their education without exhibiting impaired performance on neuropsychological tests. Self-report measures of the executive functions, such as the Barkley Deficits in Executive Functioning Scale (BDEFS; [30]) have emerged as a specific, reliable diagnostic indicator of adult ADHD although the executive functions – time management, organization/problem solving, self-motivation, impulse control, and emotional management – are not well represented in the extant diagnostic criteria [31].

The DSM-5 is introducing several modifications to the diagnosis of ADHD. The age of onset has been increased from 7 to 12 years of age, specifiers have been introduced to characterize the current manifestation of ADHD at the time of assessment, key symptoms have been elaborated to increase their developmental sensitivity and salience for adolescent and adult patients, and new impulsivity items have been added. Proposals to lower the symptom threshold for adult patients from six to four items were not incorporated into the latest version of DSM-5 [32].

The diagnosis of ADHD must be based on the presence of specific symptoms that emerged in childhood and that cause clinically significant impairments in domains of life functioning. Neuropsychological and/or psychoeducational testing has not demonstrated adequate reliability as a diagnostic indicator of ADHD, although it can be useful for identifying norm-based evidence of learning impairment that interferes with academic functioning. Thus, comprehensive testing is often required if a student seeks official academic accommodations for a learning disability, as protected by the Americans with Disabilities Act.

The end goal of any evaluation should be to confirm (or rule out) the diagnosis of ADHD and to determine the primary sources of a student's coping difficulties so as to develop a feasible treatment plan. For a sizable minority, there will not be sufficient evidence to make a diagnosis of ADHD. In these instances there will be better explanations for a student's coping difficulty, ranging from issues related to adjustment to college, inefficient study habits, poor sleep hygiene, excessive socializing, or problems secondary to anxiety and/or mood disorders. In cases in which ADHD plays a prominent role in the student's coping difficulties, there are multimodal treatment options that can be personalized to the needs of the patient. The next section provides a review of the various treatment options available to college and university students with ADHD.

Treatment options

The following sections provide summaries of different treatment approaches available for college students with ADHD who are seeking help to improve their functioning. Not every student will require all interventions; rather, these sections provide a menu of options and an appropriate multimodal treatment plan can be assembled from these based on the individual's needs.

Academic accommodations

Academic accommodations are commonly recommended for students with ADHD who demonstrate learning impairments. These accommodations include "formal" modifications of the standard teaching and testing approaches and informal environmental adjustments, the use of assistive technology, and specialized educational support; there also are many "informal" accommodations of coping strategies that can be instituted by students, including study groups, tutoring sessions, and coaching sessions (see next section).

Students with documented learning disabilities who otherwise fulfill requirements for attending college (i.e., meeting admission requirements and enrolling in the school) are protected under federal disability laws (see Latham and Latham [33] for extended discussions of these laws as they pertain to students with ADHD). That is, students with a learning disability (or other documented disabilities affecting physical, emotional, or sensory functioning) have the legally protected right to be provided with equal access to classrooms and educational materials, including the right to be granted reasonable modifications to courses and testing and access to auxiliary learning aids (e.g., assistive technology). The purpose of each accommodation is to compensate for some aspect of a disability that puts an affected student at a disadvantage in traditional academic settings inasmuch as the disability interferes with the demonstration of one's knowledge. There also are accommodations that may

be granted for high stakes standardized testing, such as the Scholastic Aptitude Test and various tests for admissions to graduate and professional programs that are beyond the purview of this chapter (see Gregg [34] and Mapou [35]).

The effectiveness of academic accommodations and use of assistive technologies for college students with ADHD has not been well studied, despite the logic underlying their use and anecdotal reports of their usefulness [7]. However, there are some accommodations that are commonly used to address difficulties faced by many college and university students with ADHD. Extended time on tests to help compensate for distractibility and slow processing speed is probably the most common accommodation granted to college students with ADHD. The common extension increments are 50% and 100% added to the scheduled length of a test. The format and/or location of testing can also be adapted to address issues of distractibility, including small group or individual formats or separate testing locations (i.e., distraction-reduced settings).

There is a variety of accommodations to address the negative impact of a learning disability on an otherwise qualified student's ability to manage the demands of an academic environment. Common difficulties for which accommodations are sought include the ability to demonstrate one's knowledge (e.g., laptop computer testing), to manage day-to-day classroom and studying environments (e.g., preferential seating), to process information presented in the classroom (e.g., note-taking service), and to deal with bureaucratic details (e.g., priority registration, reduced course load, individual housing). Reduced course load usually results in an extension of the time needed to fulfill graduation requirements beyond the traditional 4-year program. These extra semesters translate into increased costs for tuition and housing expenses, not to mention the possibility that status as a full-time student might be a requirement to obtain financial aid or to be covered under a parent's health insurance plan, although recent federal healthcare reforms are designed to address the latter concern. In some cases, ADHD with accompanying learning disabilities might be a justification for exemption from or course substitution for required classes, most often a foreign language or math courses [33, 35]. Of course, it is incumbent on students with ADHD to follow through on and make use of the accommodations in order to derive their benefits. This can become a major clinical challenge as many students with ADHD are reluctant to pursue these options.

In addition to official accommodations, there are many proactive steps students with ADHD can take to manage the effects of their symptoms on their academic functioning. For example, they need to become aware of their propensity for distraction while studying. They may have to seek out or set up reduced-distraction locations conducive to studying, such as remote sections of a library or empty classrooms. This is particularly true for students who have difficulties studying in their dorm room or apartment. If possible, it is helpful for students to set up designated "study areas" of their residence that are designed to promote their productivity.

Regardless of the studying environment, students with ADHD often struggle with developing an adaptive relationship with their computers and other technologies (e.g., cell phones, gaming systems). There are many assistive devices and computer features that can be extremely beneficial [34, 35]; however, students with ADHD are particularly prone to fall into patterns of problematic computer use inasmuch as excessive recreational use distracts them from focusing on their work [36]. Issues related to unhealthy computer use are often prominent in psychosocial and academic coaching interventions. Moreover, issues of stimulus control regarding distracting technologies are important to implement (e.g., remove gaming system from study area, limit access to social media sites during study periods).

There are many other elements of college life about which students with ADHD must be mindful. For instance, increasing numbers of students with ADHD attend local community colleges for both academic and financial reasons. Community college may offer an intermediate step toward independence, allowing a student to adjust to increased academic demands while living at home before enrolling in and moving away to a traditional college. Moreover, students with ADHD who enroll in college after high school but who experience significant academic problems, perhaps necessitating a leave of absence, often take classes at a community college before re-enrolling in college. Many choose to postpone a return to college until after they earn a 2-year degree.

Academic support: ADHD coaching

Most colleges and universities have a learning center that is staffed by learning specialists who provide academic support services to the student body at large, such as sessions on effective study strategies, time management, and organization skills. Learning specialists are also usually available to provide individual support to students struggling with various school-related tasks, such as setting up a study schedule or developing an outline for a paper. Either by design or by necessity, learning specialists are becoming more familiar with the needs of students with ADHD and are starting to provide specialized academic support to help moderate the effects of executive dysfunction on academic performance.

Similar to the role of learning specialists serving as "executive function" coaches for students with ADHD, ADHD coaching has emerged as an increasingly visible and popular treatment option for adults with ADHD that is easily adapted to be relevant for college students. The field of ADHD coaching developed from a metaphor in a popular book on ADHD that suggested that adults with ADHD could benefit from having persons in their lives who functioned as "coaches," providing reminders, encouragement, and assistance for follow through on various tasks [37]. ADHD coaching subsequently arose as a profession designed to help adults with ADHD develop and implement the necessary organization, time management, and other skills to handle the challenges of daily life [38]. More specifically, ADHD coaches help individuals identify and develop action-oriented approaches for completing personally valued tasks and goals [39]. Said differently, coaching may focus on "how" and "when" an individual can obtain a goal rather than review "why" he or she may be having difficulties doing so [38]. Consequently, "academic coaching" would seem to be a particularly good fit for college students with ADHD because (1) many do not experience comorbid psychiatric problems or wide-ranging coping problems that would require comprehensive psychosocial treatment and (2) coping with the academic and social demands of college requires efficient executive functioning skills.

There have been preliminary studies of the efficacy of what could be considered "academic coaching" programs that have revealed positive outcomes, including a single-case study of a college student with ADHD [40], a controlled study of a peer-based coaching program for college students with ADHD and/or learning disabilities [41], a multi-institution study of course-specific learning strategy instruction for college students with ADHD and/or learning disability, about half of whom were on academic probation or suspension [42], and a study of coaches' ratings of the follow through of college students with ADHD on between sessions assignments [43]. Most recently, there has been a randomized controlled study of an ADHD coaching approach designed specifically for college students [44]. All participants in the studies were college students experiencing academic impairments. Most students were identified with ADHD and/or a learning disability and several sought help after having been placed on academic probation. Interventions focused on helping students improve their academic performance by the implementation of various learning strategies and studying skills, time management and reducing procrastination in order to implement and maintain consistent study schedules, and organization of deadlines for projects, exam dates, and working backwards from these dates to set up work plans. Not surprisingly, students who consistently attended coaching sessions and implemented the coping strategies reported improve outcome on coaching goals, improved academic performance, and improved executive functioning skills [42–44].

Academic coaching would seem to be a promising intervention option for many college students with ADHD. It could serve as an adjunctive psychosocial approach in combination with pharmacotherapy for students who do not require comprehensive psychosocial treatment, such as cognitive-behavioral therapy (CBT). It could also be employed concurrently with psychosocial treatment for students who require specialized learning support.

Most students with ADHD report substantial benefits from environmental restructuring, accommodations (either formal or informal), and academic coaching that serve to enhance their school performance and psychosocial functioning. Nevertheless, even with these interventions in place, many students with ADHD experience pervasive difficulties in post-secondary educational settings and struggle with the effects of mounting emotional symptoms and (dis)stress that necessitate other interventions, such as medications and psychosocial treatment.

Medications

The efficacy of medication for the treatment of ADHD in adults has been well documented in dozens of clinical trials over the past two decades. While the literature is not as extensive as published research on

children and adolescents, it is now generally accepted that pharmacotherapy is both safe and effective for adults. Since there are few studies conducted exclusively on college students with ADHD, clinicians are obliged to extrapolate from published studies that include subjects between 18 and 50 years of age (see Rostain [45] and Wilens and Spencer [46] for reviews of the published literature). DuPaul et al. conducted the first randomized, placebo-controlled trial of medication treatment for college students using lisdexamfetamine and found significant improvements in both ADHD symptoms and executive functioning across the various dosages administered (30, 50, and 70 mg) as compared with placebo [47]. The medication proved safe and effective, although impact on academic and social functioning was not studied.

Other recent studies of stimulant treatment for ADHD in adults have documented that osmotic-release oral system (OROS) methylphenidate is safe and effective [48–50]; that once-daily dextromethylphenidate extended release from 20 to 40 mg is safe and effective [51]; that mixed amphetamine salts, both immediate release and extended release, are safe and effective, with the latter leading to better adherence using objective measures [52]; and that extended-release methylphenidate is well tolerated and associated with ADHD symptom improvement [53] as well as with a reduction in emotional symptoms associated with ADHD [54]. Reimherr et al. reported that atomoxetine was also effective in reducing emotional lability that often accompanies ADHD in adults [55]. Finally, given the relevance of executive functioning to academic success for college and university students, it is important to note that stimulant treatment of adult ADHD has not been shown to improve measures of executive function [56, 57].

Relatively little is known about the effectiveness of medications for college and university students with ADHD, and about the impact that taking medication has on academic success. Rabiner et al. reported there was no correlation between treatment status and college adjustment, including academic concerns, depressive symptoms, social satisfaction, and alcohol/drug use [11]. In a follow-up study with a larger sample, Blasé et al. also found that adjustment to college was unrelated to treatment status [8]. Advokat et al. reported no medication treatment-related differences in the grade of college students with ADHD [58]. Baker et al. found that students with ADHD who were taking medication were more likely than those who were not taking medication to engage in problematic drinking behaviors [59]. Taken together, these papers suggest that it is not clear what impact ADHD medication treatment has on college performance and adjustment. Factors that might account for this include sample selection bias, variable treatment adherence, inadequate dosing of medication, and the unique characteristics of college and university life (including longer hours for studying and less supervision and structure than when living at home). It is also important to consider the role that alcohol and substance use may play in moderating the impact of medication treatment, especially given the higher rates of these behaviors that are seen in medication-treated college students.

In view of these facts, along with previously mentioned concerns regarding stimulant misuse, abuse, and diversion, a rational approach to the medication treatment of college and university students with ADHD should employ sound clinical principles, including specifying target symptoms and behavioral objectives, educating the patient about the effects of medication, integrating medications into other coping strategies, promoting adherence, minimizing health risks, establishing good communication, and monitoring the patient closely.

For most young adult patients with ADHD, stimulant medication is usually the first line of treatment. The advantages of stimulants include rapidity of onset, immediate efficacy, tolerability, ability to titrate dose to different demands, and the scientific evidence that has led to US Food and Drug Administration (FDA) approval of these agents. At the present time, four of the five medications approved for adults with ADHD are stimulants (Focalin XR®, Vyvanse®, Adderall XR®, Concerta®), which lends further weight to the selection process.

Disadvantages of stimulant treatment include time limitation of medication effects (i.e., no effects in early morning and late evening), variability of effects throughout the day, subjective reports of altered mentation that are undesirable (e.g., "personality blunting," "rote thinking"); and the emergence of side effects, most notably anorexia, sleep disturbance, jitteriness, and cardiovascular toxicity. The misuse and abuse potential of stimulants also needs to be carefully considered. College and university students are often tempted to misuse these medications in order to stay up late and complete assignments or study for exams [60–62]. They are also used by some to lose weight or to minimize the soporific effects of alcohol. There is a growing literature on the misuse and abuse of stimulants on college campuses that should lead clinicians to be careful when prescribing these medications and to advise their patients about the risks of misuse and abuse [63, 64]. Clinicians are generally advised to choose long-acting stimulants over immediate-release preparations in order to reduce the chances for misuse/abuse (see Chapter 10).

Prior to the clinician writing a stimulant prescription, patients and family members need to be informed of the risks involved in taking these medications to college. The high demand for stimulants as "study aids" and cognitive enhancers makes it critical for students to take steps to insure that their medications are not diverted or stolen. For instance, it is strongly recommended that ADHD medications be stored in a locked box or safe in the student's room, and that others are not told about the prescription. It is also vital for students to understand the legal implications of sharing their medications with others; namely, to do so is illegal because it is considered to be distribution and/or trafficking of narcotics. Most universities have a disciplinary code that specifically sanctions the sharing or selling of prescription medications, and being caught doing so can lead to the student's suspension or expulsion from school. Last but not least, there are ethical concerns involved in providing stimulants to others. Direct physical harm can result from the use of these compounds, and dependence and addiction can also result (for a useful guide to instruct college students about their medications, see Quinn [65]; also, www.chadd.org).

Once the educational process is completed, careful protocols should be followed by prescribing clinicians. Practice parameters by the American Academy of Child and Adolescent Psychiatry (AACAP) include using recommended starting dose of each stimulant, deciding on both a minimum and maximum dose, using a consistent titration schedule, deciding on a method of assessing drug response, managing treatment-related side effects, providing a schedule for initial titration and monitoring, and providing a schedule for monitoring the drug maintenance phase [66].

In addition to these parameters, it is important to educate patient and family about their responsibility for avoiding misuse of medication, to use consent forms to document discussions, to record conversations between clinician and patient/family in the medical record, to monitor carefully the number of pills and refills prescribed, to order urine toxicology if substance abuse is suspected, and to watch for any signs ("red flags") that indicate the presence of misuse, diversion, and/or abuse. These include patient demands for immediate-release stimulants instead of extended-release or non-stimulant medications, repeatedly discordant pill counts, running short of medication, frequently lost/misplaced prescriptions, requests to increase dosage, or repeated claims that the medication has been stolen. Signs and symptoms of stimulant misuse/abuse may include worsening academic performance, anxiety, excited speech, anorexia, confusion, depression, tachycardia and hypertension, increased wakefulness, irritability, memory loss, paranoia, aggression, mania, psychosis, tremors, seizures, and even coma [67, 68].

Atomoxetine is the only non-stimulant medication that is FDA approved for ADHD in adults [69, 70]. It has a long duration of action (>12 hours) and has a longer onset period, so that positive effects emerge after 4 to 6 weeks. It is most helpful with patients who do not tolerate stimulants, who are highly anxious, and/or who express a preference for a medication that works "around the clock." It has also shown to be effective in ADHD patients with comorbid social anxiety disorder [71]. Atomoxetine does not have any reported abuse potential nor can it be used for weight loss or for staying up late. The most common side effects from atomoxetine are nausea, gastrointestinal upset, headache, sedation, fatigue, reduced sexual drive, and difficulty with urination. Mild increases in heart rate and blood pressure have been reported, but these are rarely significant enough to require discontinuation.

There is some evidence that the alpha-2 agonists can improve symptoms in adults with ADHD. A double-blind placebo-controlled study comparing guanfacine with dextroamphetamine in adults with ADHD found that they were comparable in their clinical effects as well as their impact on neuropsychological measures [72]. Recently, an extended-release preparation of guanfacine has been given FDA approval for ADHD in children and adolescents, although the compound was never tested in the adult population.

Bupropion is a medication with proven efficacy for treatment of depression, smoking cessation, and adult ADHD [73, 74]. It is a potent dopamine reuptake inhibitor with less potent inhibition of norepinephrine

reuptake. Like other non-stimulants, it has little abuse potential, although it can cause interference with sleep onset. The most significant side effect of bupropion is an increased incidence of seizures, reported in 0.4% of patients taking the immediate-release preparation. Seizures remit with discontinuation of the medication. Other adverse effects include dry mouth, constipation, nausea, vomiting, anorexia, weight loss, headache, dizziness, fainting spells, insomnia, tremor, restlessness, excitability, mood swings, and irritability.

There are no existing professional practice parameters stipulating which clinicians should be prescribing ADHD medications for college students, and how patient monitoring should be carried out. Clinical wisdom suggests that medication treatment should be individualized, and that regular follow-up should be arranged in advance of the student's departure for school. For patients who are well known to their prescribers, quarterly follow-up during academic break is adequate. More frequent visits are indicated in cases where the diagnosis of ADHD is recently made, or where there are comorbid conditions (e.g., depression, anxiety, learning disabilities) that might interfere with successful adaptation to the college setting. In cases where the student needs close monitoring, transfer of care to college mental health services and/or to practitioners near the student's campus is indicated. In all cases, it is imperative for prescribers to establish professional contact with college/university service providers that can directly monitor the student's adjustment to college and can provide additional resources where these are needed.

Psychosocial treatments

Of the non-medication treatments for adult ADHD, the psychosocial approaches have the strongest research support and have consistently produced positive results in clinical research (see Knouse *et al.* [75]; Knouse and Safren [76]; Ramsay [77, 78] for reviews). Although the majority of early clinical outcome studies of psychosocial treatments comprised open or uncontrolled studies, there have been recent studies employing randomized controlled designs that have yielded similarly positive results. The aforementioned studies did not specifically target college or university students, although most studies included participants in this age range and the intervention approaches are relevant for post-secondary students with ADHD.

There is variety among the different psychosocial treatments for adult ADHD, though there are many more similarities than differences among these therapies. CBT approaches, in particular, have demonstrated efficacy in numerous preliminary clinical outcome studies (see Ramsay [78]) as well as recent randomized controlled studies [79–81]. CBT for ADHD emphasizes the implementation of various coping skills to counteract executive dysfunction. In particular, CBT's focus on planning, time management, organization, and dealing with procrastination is particularly relevant for college students with ADHD. Cognitive interventions are also vital to enhance patient follow through and maintenance of these coping skills, and to address the rationalizations that could undo effective coping patterns. Issues related to motivation for treatment and follow through also are addressed through cognitive interventions to promote behavioral implementation.

There are several CBT-oriented group treatments designed particularly to target the executive functioning problems common to ADHD and to provide mutual support (see Solanto [81]). Structured group treatments have the benefit of being time-limited, utilizing manualized content, and being implementable over the course of a semester. However, clinical experience suggests that it can be difficult to recruit a group of college and university students with ADHD in sufficient number to commit to a standing meeting time and to have adequate attendance in order to sustain a cohesive group experience over a semester. Issues of ambivalence about treatment may further interfere with group composition and attendance.

Individual CBT approaches have also been developed and studied and are conducive for use with post-secondary students with ADHD and cover the same coping strategies as the group treatments but allow for greater individualization. There are manualized individual approaches that can be adapted for use over the course of an academic semester. Treatment for comorbid difficulties may also be integrated into individual CBT for adult ADHD.

Based on available clinical outcome data, CBT-oriented approaches are the adjunctive treatment of choice for the treatment of adult ADHD. These approaches will also be useful for college and university students with ADHD, particularly if accommodations and medications alone are insufficient. Not all students with ADHD, however, will require comprehensive psychosocial treatment. Many students may

Table 29.2. Suggested college ADHD resources

ADD Warehouse www.addwarehouse.com

American College Health Association www.acha.org

American Professional Association of ADHD and Related Disorders (APSARD) www.apsard.org

Children and Adults with Attention-Deficit/Hyperactivity Disorder (CHADD) www.chadd.org

Edge Foundation www.edgefoundation.org

Learning Disabilities Association of America National Resources Center on ADHD www.ldanatl.org

National Attention Deficit Disorder Association (ADDA) www.add.org

National Resource Center on ADHD www.help4adhd.org

WebMD www.webmd.com

only need focused support on managing their academic coping difficulties.

Conclusion

The transition to higher education can be a challenging one for many students, but is particularly difficult for students with ADHD. Otherwise qualified college and university students may find themselves struggling with the increased amount, pace, and difficulty of school work at the post-secondary level based on difficulties related to disorganization, poor time management, distractibility, and other features of ADHD that interfere with learning. Thus, most students with ADHD will require some sort of specialized support or treatment during college in order to effectively manage these demands. The various difficulties commonly reported by these students as well as the key components of a thorough, competent assessment for ADHD were described.

Encouragingly, there are several options for support and treatment available to college students diagnosed with ADHD that also have been reviewed in this chapter (Table 29.2). Academic accommodations, ADHD coaching, medications, and psychosocial treatment represent the most promising and relevant adjunctive treatments for college and university students with ADHD insofar as they are designed to target the specific areas of functional impairments experienced by these students. Consequently, although ADHD is associated with various coping problems that can interfere with academic performance, there are many treatment and coping options that are available to assist students with ADHD to make the most of their post-secondary education.

References

1. Barkley RA. *ADHD and the Nature of Self-Control.* New York, NY: Guilford Press; 1997.

2. Brown TE. *Attention Deficit Disorder: The Unfocused Mind in Children and Adults.* New Haven, CT: Yale University Press; 2005.

3. Barkley RA, Murphy KR, Fischer M. *ADHD in Adults: What the Science Says.* New York, NY: Guilford Press; 2008.

4. DuPaul GJ, Weyandt LL, O'Dell SM, Varejao M. College students with ADHD: current status and future directions. *J Atten Disord.* 2009;**13**:234–50.

5. DuPaul GJ, Schaughency EA, Weyandt LL, *et al.* Self-report of ADHD symptoms in university students: Cross-gender and cross-national prevalence. *J Learn Disabil.* 2001;**34**:370–9.

6. McKee TE. Comparison of a norm-based versus criterion-based approach to measuring ADHD symptomatology in college students. *J Atten Disord.* 2008;**11**:677–88.

7. Weyandt LL, DuPaul G. ADHD in college students. *J Atten Disord.* 2006;**10**:9–19.

8. Blase SL, Gilbert AN, Anastopoulos AD, *et al.* Self-reported ADHD and adjustment to college: cross-sectional and longitudinal findings. *J Atten Disord.* 2009;**13**:297–309.

9. Heiligenstein E, Guenther G, Levy A, Savino F, Fulwiler J. Psychological and academic functioning in college students with attention deficit hyperactivity disorder. *J Am Coll Health.* 1999;**47**:181–5.

10. Norwalk K, Norvilitis JM, MacLean MG. ADHD symptomatology and its relationship to factors associated with college adjustment. *J Atten Disord.* 2009;**13**:251–8.

11. Rabiner DL, Anastopoulos AD, Costello J, Hoyle RH, Swartzwelder HS. Adjustment to college in students with ADHD. *J Atten Disord.* 2008;**11**:689–99.

12. Shaw-Zirt B, Popali-Lehane L, Chaplin W, Bergman A. Adjustment, social skills, and self-esteem in college students with symptoms of ADHD. *J Atten Disord.* 2005;**8**:109–20.

13. Weyandt LL, Iwaszuk W, Fulton K, *et al.* The internal restlessness scale: performance of college students with and without ADHD. *J Learn Disabil.* 2003;**36**:382–9.

14. Dooling-Litfin JK, Rosén LA. Self-esteem in college students with a childhood history of attention deficit hyperactivity disorder. *J Coll Stud Psychother.* 1997;**11**:69–82.

15. Heiligenstein E, Keeling RP. Presentation of unrecognized attention deficit hyperactivity disorder in college students. *J Am Coll Health.* 1995;**43**:226–8.

16. Richards TL, Rosen LA, Ramirez CA. Psychological functioning differences among college students with confirmed ADHD, ADHD by self-report only, and without ADHD. *J Coll Stud Dev.* 1999;**40**:299–304.

17. Reaser A, Prevatt F, Petscher Y, Proctor B. The learning and study strategies of college students with ADHD. *Psychol Sch.* 2007;**44**:627–38.

18. Rugsaken KT, Robertson JA, Jones JA. Using the learning and study strategies inventory scores as additional predictors of student academic performance. *NACADA Journal.* 1998;**18**:20–6.

19. Rachal KC, Daigle S, Rachal WS. Learning problems reported by college students: are they using learning strategies? *J Instruct Psychol.* 2007;**34**:191–9.

20. Harrison AG. An investigation of reported symptoms of ADHD in a university population. *ADHD Rep.* 2004;**12**(6):8–11.

21. Harrison AG. Adults faking ADHD: you must be kidding! *ADHD Rep.* 2006;**14**(4):1–7.

22. Booksh RL, Pella RD, Singh AN, Gouvier WD. Ability of college students to simulate ADHD on objective measures of attention. *J Atten Disord.* 2010;**13**(4):325–38.

23. Sollman MJ, Ranseen JD, Berry DT. Detection of feigned ADHD in college students. *Psychol Assess.* 2010;**22**:325–35.

24. Rostain AL, Ramsay JR. College Students with Attention-Deficit Hyperactivity Disorder: New Directions in Assessment and Treatment. *Monograph American College Health Association.* Millstone Township, NJ: Princeton Media Associates. 2006; 7–16.

25. Barkley RA, Murphy KR. *Attention-Deficit Hyperactivity Disorder: A Clinical Workbook*, 3rd edn. New York, NY: Guilford Press; 2006.

26. DuPaul G, Power T, Anastopoulos A, Reid R. *ADHD Rating Scale – IV: Checklist, Norms, and Clinical Interpretation.* New York, NY: Guilford Press; 1998.

27. Adler L, Kessler R, Spencer T. *Adult Self Report Scale, ASRS-v1.1 Screener.* New York, NY: World Health Organization; 2003.

28. Brown TE. *Brown Attention Deficit Disorder Scales.* San Antonio, TX: The Psychological Corporation; 1996.

29. Conners CK, Erhardt D, Sparrow E. *Conners' Adult ADHD Rating Scales.* North Tonawanda, NY: Multi-Health Systems, Inc.; 1999.

30. Barkley RA. *Barkley Deficits in Executive Functioning Scale.* New York, NY: Guilford Press; 2011.

31. Kessler RC, Green JG, Adler LA, *et al.* Structure and diagnosis of adult attention-deficit/hyperactivity disorder: analysis of expanded diagnostic criteria from the adult ADHD clinical diagnostic scale. *Arch Gen Psychiatry.* 2010;**67**:1168–78.

32. Tannock R. Rethinking ADHD and LD in DSM-5: proposed changes in diagnostic criteria. *J Learn Disabil.* 2012;**46**:5–25.

33. Latham PS, Latham PH. *Learning Disabilities, ADHD and the Law in Higher Education and Employment.* Washington, DC: JKL Communications; 2007.

34. Gregg N. *Adolescents and Adults with Learning Disabilities and ADHD: Assessment and Accommodations.* New York, NY: Guilford Press; 2009.

35. Mapou RL. *Adult Learning Disabilities and ADHD: Research Informed Assessment.* New York, NY: Oxford University Press; 2009.

36. Ko CH, Yen JY, Chen CS, Chen CC, Yen CF. Psychiatric comorbidity of internet addiction in college students: an interview study. *CNS Spectr.* 2008;**13**:147–53.

37. Hallowell EM, Ratey JJ. *Driven to Distraction.* New York, NY: Touchstone; 1994.

38. National Resource Center on AD/HD. *What we Know: Coaching for Adults with AD/HD.* Landover, MD: Children and Adults with Attention Deficit Hyperactivity Disorder; 2003.

39. Kubik JA. Efficacy of ADHD coaching for adults with attention deficit disorder. *J Atten Disord.* 2010; **13**:442–3.

40. Swartz SL, Prevatt F, Proctor BE. A coaching intervention for college students with attention deficit/hyperactivity disorder. *Psychol Sch.* 2005;**46**:647–56.

41. Zwart LM, Kallemeyn LM. Peer-based coaching for college students with ADHD and learning disabilities. *J Postsec Educ Disabil.* 2001;**15**:5–20.

42. Allsopp DH, Minskoff EH, Bolt L. Individualized course-specific strategy instruction for college students with learning disabilities and ADHD: lessons learned from a model demonstration program. *Learn Disabil Res Pract.* 2005;**20**:103–18.

43. Prevatt F, Lampropoulos GK, Bowles V, Garrett L. The use of between session assignments in ADHD coaching with college students. *J Atten Disord.* 2011;**15**:18–27. doi: 10.1177/1087054709356181.

44. Parker DR, Hoffman SF, Sawilowsky S, Rolands L. An examination of the effects of ADHD coaching on university students' executive functioning. *J Postsec Educ Disabil.* 2011;**24**:115–32.

45. Rostain AL. Attention-deficit/hyperactivity disorder in adults: evidence-based recomendations for management. *Postgrad Med.* 2008;**120**:27–37.

46. Wilens T, Spencer T. Understanding attention-deficit/hyperactivity disorder from childhood to adulthood. *Postgrad Med.* 2010; **122**:97–109.

47. DuPaul GJ, Weyandt LL, Rossi JS, *et al.* Double-blind, placebo-controlled, crossover study of the efficacy and safety of lisdexamfetamine dimesylate in college students with ADHD. *J Atten Disord.* 2012;**16**:202–20. doi: 10.1177/1087054711427299.

48. Adler LA, Zimmerman B, Starr HL, *et al.* Efficacy and safety of OROS methylphenidate in adults with attention-deficit/hyperactivity disorder: a randomized, placebo-controlled, double-blind, parallel group, dose-escalation study. *J Clin Psychopharmacol.* 2009;**29**:239–47.

49. Adler LA, Orman C, Starr HL, *et al.* Long-term safety of OROS methylphenidate in adults with attention-deficit/hyperactivity disorder: an open-label, dose-titration, 1-year study. *J Clin Psychopharmacol.* 2011;**31**:108–14.

50. Buitelaar JK, Casas M, Philipsen A, *et al.* Functional improvement and correlations with symptomatic improvement in adults with attention deficit hyperactivity disorder receiving long-acting methylphenidate. *Psychol Med.* 2012;**42**:195–204.

51. Adler LA, Spencer T, McGough JJ, Jiang H, Muniz R. Long-term effectiveness and safety of dexmethylphenidate extended-release capsules in adult ADHD. *J Atten Disord.* 2009;**12**:449–59.

52. Adler LA, Lynch LR, Shaw DM, *et al.* Medication adherence and symptom reduction in adults treated with mixed amphetamine salts in a randomized crossover study. *Postgrad Med.* 2011;**123**:71–9.

53. Retz W, Rösler M, Ose C, *et al.*; Study Group. Multiscale assessment of treatment efficacy in adults with ADHD: a randomized placebo-controlled, multi-centre study with extended-release methylphenidate. *World J Biol Psychiatry.* 2010; **13**:48–59.

54. Rösler M, Retz W, Fischer R, *et al.* Twenty-four-week treatment with extended release methylphenidate improves emotional symptoms in adult ADHD. *World J Biol Psychiatry.* 2010;**11**:709–18.

55. Reimherr FW, Marchant BK, Strong RE, *et al.* Emotional dysregulation in adult ADHD and response to atomoxetine. *Biol Psychiatry.* 2005;**58**(2): 125–31.

56. Biederman J, Seidman LJ, Petty CR, *et al.* Effects of stimulant medication on neuropsychological functioning in young adults with attention-deficit/hyperactivity disorder. *J Clin Psychiatry.* 2008; **69**:1150–6.

57. Biederman J, Mick E, Fried R, *et al.* Are stimulants effective in the treatment of executive function deficits? Results from a randomized double blind study of OROS-methylphenidate in adults with ADHD. *Eur Neuropsychopharmacol.* 2011;**21**:508–15.

58. Advokat C, Lane SM, Luo C. College students with and without ADHD: comparison of self-report of medication usage, study habits, and academic achievement. *J Atten Disord*. 2011;**15**:656–66. doi: 10.1177/1087054710371168.

59. Baker L, Prevatt F, Proctor B. Drug and alcohol use in college students with and without ADHD. *J Atten Disord*. 2012;**16**:255–63. doi: 10.1177/1087054711416314.

60. McCabe SE, Boyd CJ, Teter CJ. Subtypes of nonmedical prescription drug misuse. *Drugs Alcohol Depend*. 2009;**102**:63–70.

61. Rabiner DL, Anastopoulos AD, Costello EJ, *et al.* The misuse and diversion of prescribed ADHD medications by college students. *J Atten Disord*. 2009;**13**:144–53.

62. Garnier LM, Arria AM, Caldeira KM, *et al.* Sharing and selling of prescription medications in a college student sample *J Clin Psychiatry*. 2010;**71**: 262–9.

63. Rostain AL. Addressing the misuse and abuse of stimulant medications on college campuses. *Curr Psychiatry Rep*. 2006;**8**:335–6.

64. Wilens TE, Adler L, Adams K, *et al.* Misuse and diversion of stimulants prescribed for ADHD: A systematic review of the literature. *J Am Acad Child Adolesc Psychiatry*. 2008;**47**:21–31.

65. Quinn PO. *AD/HD and the College Student*. Washington, DC: Magination Press; 2012.

66. American Academy of Child and Adolescent Psychiatry. Summary of the practice parameter for the use of stimulant medications in the treatment of children, adolescents and adults. *J Am Acad Child Adolesc Psychiatry*. 2001;**40**:1352–5.

67. Staufer WB, Greydanus DE. Attention-deficit/hyperactivity disorder psychopharmacology for college students. *Pediatr Clin North Am*. 2005;**52**: 71–84.

68. Greydanus DE. Stimulant Misues: Strategies to Manage a Growing Problem. *Monograph American College Health Association*, Millstone Township, NJ: Princeton Media Associates. 2006; 17–26.

69. Michelson D, Adler L, Spencer T, *et al.* Adults with ADHD: two randomized, placebo-controlled trials. *Biol Psychiatry*. 2003;**53**(2):112–20.

70. Simpson D, Plosker GL. Atomoxetine: a review of its use in adults with attention deficit hyperactivity disorder. *Drug*. 2004;**64**:205–22.

71. Adler LA, Liebowitz M, Kronenberger W, *et al.* Atomoxetine treatment in adults with attention-deficit/hyperactivity disorder and comorbid social anxiety disorder. *Depress Anxiety*. 2009; **26**:212–21.

72. Taylor FB, Russo J. Comparing guanfacine and dextroamphetamine for the treatment of adult attention-deficit/hyperactivity disorder. *J Clin Psychopharmacol*. 2001;**21**:223–8.

73. Wilens TE, Spencer TJ, Biederman J, *et al.* A controlled clinical trial of bupropion for attention deficit hyperactivity disorder in adults. *Am J Psychiatry*. 2001;**158**(2):282–8.

74. Wilens TE, Haight BR, Horrigan JP, *et al.* Bupropion XL in adults with attention-deficit/hyperactivity disorder: a randomized, placebo-controlled study. *Biol Psychiatry*. 2005;**57**:793–801.

75. Knouse LE, Cooper-Vince C, Sprich S, Safren SA. Recent developments in the psychosocial treatment of adult ADHD. *Expert Rev Neurother*. 2008;**8**:1537–48.

76. Knouse LE, Safren SA. Current status of cognitive behavioral therapy for adult attention-deficit hyperactivity disorder. *Psychiatr Clin North Am*. 2010;**33**:497–509. doi: 10.1016/j.psc.2010.04.001.

77. Ramsay JR. Evidence-based psychosocial treatments for adult ADHD: a review. *Curr Atten Disord Rep*. 2009;**1**:85–91.

78. Ramsay JR. *Nonmedication Treatments for Adult ADHD: Evaluating Impact on Daily Functioning and Well-Being*. Washington, DC: American Psychological Association; 2010.

79. Safren SA, Sprich S, Mimiaga MJ, *et al.* Cognitive behavioral therapy vs relaxation with educational support for medication-treated adults with ADHD and persistent symptoms: a randomized controlled trial. *JAMA*. 2010;**304**:875–80.

80. Solanto MV, Marks DJ, Wasserstein J, *et al.* Efficacy of meta-cognitive therapy for adult ADHD. *Am J Psychiatry*. 2010;**167**(8):958–68.

81. Solanto MV. *Cognitive Behavior Therapy for Adult ADHD: Targeting Executive Dysfunction*. New York, NY: Guilford Press; 2011.

Index

psychiatric disorders
comorbidity with ADHD in
children, 18
comorbidity with adult ADHD,
31–2
psychiatric disorders in ADHD
protective potential of stimulant
treatment, 253–4
psychopharmacology of ADHD
discovery of effects of stimulant
drugs, 5–6
early history, 5–7
psychosis
associated with stimulant
medications, 251
psychosocial treatment of adult ADHD
features of adult ADHD, 298
future directions, 303–4
limitations of stimulant medications
in adults, 298
Mount Sinai CBT program for adult
ADHD, 300–4
treatment literature before 2010,
298–300
psychosocial treatments
for college students with ADHD,
373–4
for comorbid depression and
ADHD, 91–2
psychostimulants
effects on prefrontal cortical
function, 163–5
Pycnogenol, 310, 313

quality of life
and ADHD, 49
assessment scales, 229–30
concept, 42
quetiapine, 147

Rafalovich, A., 1, 4–5
Rapaport, Judith, 10
rating scales for ADHD
assessment issues in adolescents,
238–9
assessment issues in preschool
children, 239–40
choice of, 236
description and use, 234–5
for functional impairment, 236–7
function, 233–4
history, 233–4
recommendations for clinical use,
240
to aid diagnosis of ADHD in
children, 19
to assess treatment response in
adults, 276
to track adverse events, 237–8

to track side effects, 237–8
See also diagnostic scales; symptom
rating scales
reading disorder
differential diagnosis case study,
219–20
DSM-IV criteria, 125
reading disorder and ADHD, 127
case study, 127–30
neurobiology of reading disorders,
124
recurrent brief depression (RBD) and
ADHD, 85
region-of-interest quantification
neuroimaging of ADHD, 199
Relational Frame Theory, 355, 356
approach to ADHD treatment,
359–60
relaxation therapies, 311
resistance to thyroid hormone
and ADHD, 157
restless legs syndrome (RLS), 154, 155
Rey–Osterreith Complex Figure
(ROCF) test, 217
rheumatoid arthritis, 158
risperidone, 76, 147, 349
Ritalin LA, 323
Rutter, M., 9

Safer, D. J., 10
Schedule for Affective Disorders and
Schizophrenia (SADS), 218
Schedule for Affective Disorders and
Schizophrenia for School Age
Children (K-SADS), 183, 238
schizophrenia, 152
seasonal affective disorder (SAD) and
ADHD in adults, 85
seizure disorders
differential diagnosis of ADHD,
152–4
seizure disorders and ADHD
stimulant medications for pediatric
use, 253
selective serotonin reuptake inhibitors
(SSRIs), 90–1, 147, 165
selegiline, 90, 267, 288
self-control
and treatment adherence, 355–7
sensorimotor skills
neuropsychological assessment,
214–15
sensory deficits
differential diagnosis for ADHD, 152
sensory functions
neuropsychological tests, 217
separation anxiety disorder in
children, 99
serotonergic genes

ADHD association studies, 180–2
serotonin receptor (*HTR1B*)
ADHD association studies, 180–1
serotonin receptor (*HTR2A, 5HT2A*)
ADHD association studies, 181
serotonin receptor (*HTR2C*)
ADHD association studies, 181
serotonin transporter (*HTT, SLC6A4*)
ADHD association studies, 181
severe mood dysregulation (SMD)
phenotype, 66
SF-36 measure, 42
Side Effect Rating Scale (SERS), 237
side effects
rating scales to track, 237–8
Skinner, B. F., 355
sleep apnea, 155
sleep disorders
differential diagnosis of ADHD,
154–5
sleep problems, 49
sluggish cognitive tempo (SCT), 59, 60,
123
smoking
morbidity and mortality caused by,
327
rates among individuals with
psychiatric disorders, 327
smoking and ADHD
ADHD as risk factor for smoking,
112–13, 327–8
behavioral mechanisms, 333
clinical implications, 333–4
common genetic substrates, 330–1
consequences of smoking during
pregnancy, 143
effects of ADHD treatment, 112
effects of maternal smoking, 346
effects of nicotine on ADHD
symptoms, 333
effects of nicotine on attentional
performance, 333
effects of nicotine on behavioral
inhibition, 333
effects of stimulant medications,
333–4
evidence for association, 327
genetic substrates of smoking and
ADHD, 330–1
influence of ADHD on the stages of
smoking, 328–30
integrated model of ADHD–
smoking comorbidity, 334–5
neurobiological/
neuropharmacological factors,
332
nicotine dependence among
smokers, 328
prevalence, 328

tricyclic antidepressants (TCAs), 90,
147
drug–drug interactions, 248,
283
use in ADHD treatment, 267
use in adult ADHD, 288
use in tic disorders and ADHD,
348–9
use in Tourette syndrome and
ADHD, 348–9
tryptophan hydroxylase (*TPH* and
TPH2)
ADHD association studies, 181–2
tuberous sclerosis, 155
Turner syndrome, 152
Twain, Mark, 3

valerian, 310
valproate semisodium, 147
Vanderbilt ADHD Diagnostic Parent/
Teacher Rating Scales, 234, 236
vasopressor drugs, 248
velo-cardio-facial syndrome (VCFS),
152
venlafaxine, 90–1, 261, 266
Verbal Comprehension Index (in
WISC-IV), 126
vestibular stimulation, 312
Vineland Scales of Adaptive Behavior,
237
visual functions
neuropsychological tests, 216–17
visual-spatial skills
neuropsychological assessment,
213–14
vitamin supplementation, 309

von Economo's encephalitis, 5–6
voxel-based morphometry studies in
ADHD, 199–200
Vyvanse®, 89, 93, 372

Wechsler Adult Intelligence Scale –
Fourth Edition (WAIS-IV), 126
Wechsler Individual Achievement
Test – Third Edition (WIAT-III),
126, 218
Wechsler Intelligence Scale for
Children – Fourth Edition
(WISC-IV), 126, 216
Wechsler Intelligence tests, 215
language tests, 216
tests of visual and spatial abilities,
216
Wechsler Memory Scale – Fourth
Edition (WMS-IV), 217
weight
effects of stimulant medications, 250
Weiss Functional Impairment Rating
Scale, 42, 45, 237
Weiss Functional Impairment Rating
Scale Self-Report (WFIRS-S), 230
Wellbutrin, 93
Wender–Reimherr Adult ADHD
Rating Scale, 276
Wender, P., 8, 10
Wender–Reimherr Adult Attention
Deficit Disorder Scale
(WRAADDS), 229
WHO Disability Assessment Schedule,
32
WHO Disability Assessment Schedule
2 (WHODAS 2), 42

WHO short course in tuberculosis
treatment, 357
Wide Range Assessment of Memory of
Learning – Second Edition
(WRAML2), 217
Williams syndrome, 152
Wisconsin Card Sorting Test (WCST),
216
Woodcock–Johnson Tests of Academic
Achievement, Third Edition
(WJ-III), 126, 218
work environment
and functional impairment in
ADHD, 46–7
work performance
adults with ADHD, 20
Working Memory Index (in
WISC-IV), 126
working memory training, 311–12,
314
workplace screening programs for
ADHD, 34
written expression disorder
and ADHD, 127
DSM-IV criteria, 126

Yale–Brown Obsessive Compulsive
Scale (YBOCS), 347
Yale Global Tic Severity Scale,
347
yoga, 312

Zeitgeist explanation for scientific
progress, 2–5
zinc supplements, 309
ziprasidone, 147, 349

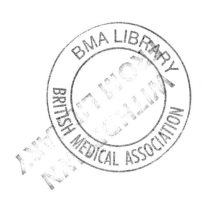